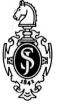

P. Lanzer   J. Rösch (Eds.)

Vascular Diagnostics

Noninvasive and Invasive Techniques
Periinterventional Evaluations

Foreword by W. W. Parmley and G. Schettler

With Contributions by
C. J. G. Bakker, R. E. Barton, G. Biamino, P. Bösinger, E. G. Cape, J. Carreira,
L. E. Crooks, P. de Jaegere, C. M. Gross, E. Gussenhoven, K. Haag, M. J. Hartkamp,
J. Haase, D. Hausmann, M. Hennerici, J. Hennig, J. B. Hermiller, R. T. Higaschida,
N. Hylton, D. Keane, F. S. Keller, M. Kouwenhoven, W. Krause, P. C. Lakin,
P. Lanzer, W. Li, W. März, W. P. Th. M. Mali, M. R. Malinow, M. Maynar, K. Mizuno,
G. L. Moneta, M. Nauck, J. Niepel, J. Noordzij, C. M. Orr, T. Peters, H. Pieterman,
C. A. Pinkerton, L. J. Polman, J. M. Porter, J. M. Pulido-Duque, W. Rautenberg,
H. Refsum, N. Reifart, R. Reyes, J. Rösch, P. J. Rubio, R. R. Saxon, M. Scheidegger,
P. W. Serruys, W. Steinke, B. H. Strauss, G. P. Teitelbaum, S. H. K. The, P. M. Ueland,
V. A. W. M. Umans, A. van der Lugt, F. C. van Egmond, M. S. van Leeuwen,
J. van Tassel, H. van Urk, B. Velthuis, I. Wendelhag, K. U. Wentz, H. Wieland,
J. Wikstrand, P. G. Yock, A. P. Yoganathan, E. Zeitler

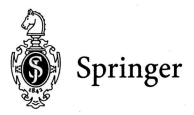

Springer

Dr. Peter Lanzer

Kardiologische Gemeinschaftspraxis
Saalbaustraße 27

D-64283 Darmstadt, FRG

Prof. Dr. Josef Rösch

Oregon Health Sciences University
Charles Dotter Institute of Interventional Therapy
3181 S.W. Sam Jackson Park Road
Portland, Oregon 97201-3098
USA

ISBN 3-540-57939-7 Springer-Verlag Berlin Heidelberg New York
ISBN 0-387-57939-7 Springer-Verlag New York Berlin Heidelberg

Library of Congress Cataloging-in-Publication Data. Vascular diagnostics : noninvasive and invasive techniques : periinterventional evaluations / P. Lanzer, J. Rösch (eds.). p. cm. Includes bibliographical references and index.
ISBN 3-540-57939-7 (alk. paper)
ISBN 0-387-57939-7 (alk. paper)
1. Blood-vessels-Diseases-Diagnosis. I. Lanzer, P. (Peter), 1950– . II. Rösch, J. (Josef), 1925– . [DNLM: 1. Vascular Diseases-diagnosis. 2. Diagnostic Imaging. WG 500 V33125 1994] RC691.5.V37 1994 616.1'30754-dc20 DNLM/DLC

© Springer-Verlag Berlin Heidelberg 1994
Printed in Germany

Production and Supervision: W. Bischoff, Heidelberg
Cover Design: E. Kirchner, Heidelberg
Reproduction of Figures and Typesetting: Mitterweger Werksatz GmbH, Plankstadt

23/3130 – 5 4 3 2 1 0 – Printed on acid-free paper

Foreword

Vascular disease is the number one cause of mobidity and mortality in developed countries. Although diagnostic techniques have been available for decades to assess the severity of vascular disease, there has been a recent development of new techniques and new applications of old techniques which have greatly enhanced our ability to characterize the anatomic location and severity of vascular involvement. This textbook on vascular diagnostics performs a great service for the clinician dealing with vascular disease by bringing together in one volume excellent multiauthor reviews of the most important techniques available for vascular evaluation. There is particular emphasis on newer techniques and the additional information which they can provide. Those who deal with the coronary circulation, the cerebral circulation, and the rest of the peripheral circulation will find this an important collection of critical reviews of the field. In expressing enthusiasm for newer diagnostic techniques, however, the authors have not neglected the basic fundamentals of the physical examination, basic laboratory examinations, and evaluation of lipoprotein metabolism. I believe that the reader will be rewarded for the time spent in reviewing specific chapters of interest or, more importantly, gaining an overview of a field which is under continuing, rapid development. A glance at the international authorship of this book reveals some of the most well – known researchers in their respective areas. Thus this book is authoritative and relatively comprehensive for its size in providing the reader with a current snapshot of the ever-changing arena of vascular diagnostics. It is a much needed and welcome addition to the library of cardiologists, neurologists, radiologists, vascular surgeons, and others.

William W. Parmley

Foreword

The textbook provides a long awaited interdisciplinary perspective of the state-of-the-art vascular diagnostics. The editors have succeeded in presenting the reader with a comprehensive and authoritative review of the noninvasive and invasive diagnostic methods utilized to assess cerebrovascular, coronary and peripheral vascular disease. The individual chapters are written by competent, internationally recognized vascular specialists. The style is clear, definitive and critical. The sections on metabolic and periinterventional evaluations employed in preventive and interventional vascular medicine are appropriately emphasized and to the specializing as well as the general reader of particular interest. The sections on new upcomming vascular diagnostic methodologies are informative and complete.

I wish to compliment the editors, the authors and the publishers for providing the readers with an outstanding textbook and with the much needed information on modern means and ways to evaluate vascular patients. I hope that "Vascular Diagnostics" will be widely read and consulted not only in the english but also in german speaking medical communities.

Gerhard Schettler

Preface

Modern vascular diagnostics is a complex, interdisciplinary enterprise. Recognizing the nosologic unity of the vascular organs as well as the systemic character of vascular pathogenesis, this area spans a wide range of metabolic, functional, and morphologic diagnostic measure.

The textbook *Vascular Diagnostics* has been designed to provide an interdisciplinary perspective of the clinically applicable noninvasive and invasive diagnostic evaluations of the cerebral, coronary, visceral, and peripheral vasculature, and where appropriate, of the corresponding vascular-related end-organ functions. Due to the growing importance of prevention and intervention in vascular medicine, the metabolic and periinterventional techniques have been strongly emphasized. To avoid repetition, standard examination techniques have not been systematically reviewed in this context. We have chosen to preview the most promising vascular imaging technologies, whereas we felt that inclusion of upcoming hemostaseologic, immunologic, and molecular biologic vascular diagnostic techniques in this volume would have been premature.

The textbook is divided into three parts and nine sections based on the noninvasive or invasive nature of the individual diagnostic technique and on the specific vascular territory in question. Each diagnostic method is discussed under individualized headings, allowing the reader both a systematic and a random review of the topics presented. The text advances from noninstrumentel to instrumental nonimaging, noninvasive imaging, and invasive imaging diagnostic strategies. Parts I and II are devoted to current clinical methods, and in Part III upcoming imaging technology is discussed.

Quite obviously, a properly conducted physical examination still retains its importance in selecting the most efficient vascular diagnostic cascade. Among the nonivasive techniques, vascular ultrasound has become the primary method in the initial and follow-up assessment of vascular disease in nearly all major vascular territories. Clinical ultrasonographic applications pertinent to the individual vascular territories are extensively discussed and reviewed. The clinical importance of invasive methods, i.e., angiography and venography, has been reduced as far as the purely diagnostic evaluations are concerned, reflecting the wide availability and excellence of vascular ultrasonography. On the other hand, their value has markedly increased as a primary tool in periinterventional settings. Here in particular, the predominant role of computer-enhanced angiography has been highlighted. The present clinical role of these radiographic techniques and their direct impact on interventional therapy has been assessed and evaluated. In the final sections of the textbook, the search for better noninvasive and more advanced invasive visualization of the vascular system is documented.

We hope that the textbook will provide professionals in the field with a useful guide to modern vascular diagnostics and foster the much-needed interdisciplinary approach to vascular care. We wish to thank all our colleagues and co-authors, as well as the staff of Springer-Verlag in Heidelberg, especially Dr. V. Gebhardt and Mr. W. Bischoff, for making this project possible.

Peter Lanzer
Josef Rösch

Contents

Section II: Computed Tomography

Section III: Intravascular Ultrasound

Section IV: Angioscopy

List of Contributors

C. J. G. Bakker
Department of Radiology
University Hospital Utrecht (E 01.132)
Heidelberglaan
3584 CX Utrecht
The Netherlands

R. E. Barton
Oregon Health Sciences University
School of Medicine
Charles Dotter Institute of Interventional
Therapy
3181 S. W. Sam Jackson Park Road, L605
Portland, OR 97201-3098
USA

G. Biamino
Abt. für Klinische und
Interventionelle Angiologie
Rudolf Virchow Universitätsklinikum
der Freien Universität Berlin
Augustenburger Platz 1
D-13353 Berlin 65, FRG

P. Boesiger
Universität und ETH Zürich
Institut für Biomedizinische Technik und
Medizinische Informatik
Gloriastraße 35
CH-8092 Zürich
Swizerland

E. G. Cape
University of Pittsburgh
Schools of Medicine and Engineering
1249 Benedum Hall
Pittsburgh, PA 15261
USA

J. Carreira
Unidad de Radiologia Vascular e
Intervencionista
Hospital Nuestra Senora del Pino
Angel Guimera 93
35005 Las Palmas de Gran Canaria
Espana

L.E. Crooks
University of California, San Francisco
UCSF Radiologic Imaging Laboratory
400 Grandview Drive
South San Francisco, CA 94080
USA

P. de Jaegere
Catheterization Laboratory
Thoraxcenter Bd 414
P.O. Box 1738
3000 DR Rotterdam
The Netherlands

P. J. Fitzgerald
Stanford University Medical Center
Center for Research in
Cardiovascular Interventions
300 Pasteur Drive
Stanford, CA 94305
USA

A. Fronek
University of California, San Diego
Department of Surgery, 0643
School of Medicine
Basic Science Building, Rm. 5028
La Jolla, CA 92093-0643
USA

E. T. Fry
Nasser, Smith & Pinkerton Cardiology, Inc.
St. Vincent Professional Building
8402 Hardcourt Road
Indianapolis, IN 46260
USA

C. Gervas
Unidad de Radiologia Vascular e
Intervencionista
Hospital Nuestra Senora del Pino
Angel Guimera 93
35005 Las Palmas de Gran Canaria
Espana

E. Gorriz
Unidad de Radiologia Vacular e
Intervencionista
Hospital Nuestra Senora del Pino
Angel Guimera 93
35005 Las Palmas de Gran Canaria
Espana

C. M. Gross
Abt. für Kardiologie, Angiologie und
Pulmonologie
Rudolf Virchow Universitätsklinikum der
Freien Universität Berlin
Augustenburger Platz 1
D-13353 Berlin 65, FRG

E. J. Gussenhoven
Erasmus Universiteit Rotterdam
Exp. Echocardiography (Ee2312)
P.O. Box 1738
3000 Dr Rotterdam
The Netherlands

K. Haag
Abteilung Innere Medizin II
Gastroenterology, Hepatologie
Albert-Ludwigs-Universität Freiburg
Hugstetterstraße 55
D-79106 Freiburg/Br., FRG

M. J. Hartkamp
Department of Radiology
University Hospital Utrecht (E 01.132)
Heidelberglaan 100
3584 CX Utrecht
The Netherlands

J. Haase
Kardiologische Gemeinschaftspraxis
am Roten Kreuz Krankenhaus
Alfred-Brehm-Platz 5–9
D-60132 Frankfurt/Main, FRG

D. Hausmann
University of California, San Francisco
Intravascular Ultrasound Research Group
Cardiovascular Research Institute
San Francisco, CA 94143-0124
USA

M. Hennerici
Ruprecht-Karls-Universität Heidelberg
Klinikum Mannheim
Neurologische Klinik
Theodor-Kutzer-Ufer 1
D-68167 Mannheim, FRG

J. Hennig
Klinikum der Albert-Ludwigs-Universität
Abt. Röntgendiagnostik
Hugstetterstraße 55
D-79106 Freiburg, FRG

J. B. Hermiller
Nasser, Smith & Pinkerton Cardiology, Inc.
St. Vincent Professional Building
8402 Hardcourt Road
Indianapolis, IN 46260
USA

R. T. Higaschida
UC Neurovascular Medical Group, Inc.
Department of Radiology
UCSF Medical Center
505 Parnassus Avenue, Room L352
San Francisco, CA 94143-0628
USA

N. Hylton
University of California, San Francisco
UCSF Radiologic Imaging Laboratory
400 Grandview Drive South
San Francisco, CA 94080
USA

D. Keane
Catheterization Laboratory
Thoraxcenter Bd 414
P.O. Box 1738
3000 DR Rotterdam
The Netherlands

F. S. Keller
Oregon Health Sciences University
School of Medicine
Charles Dotter Institute of
Interventional Therapy
3181 S. W. Sam Jackson Park Rod, L605
Portland, OR 97201-3098
USA

M. Kouwenhoven
MR Clinical Science
Philips Medical Systems
PO Box 10.000
NL-5680 DA Best
The Netherlands

W. Krause
Schering Aktiengesellschaft
Fachbereich Pharma, Forschung Röntgen-
kontrastmittel
Müllerstraße 178
Postfach 65 03 11
D-13342 Berlin, FRG

P. C. Lakin
Oregon Health Sciences University
School of Medicine
Charles Dotter Institute of
Interventional Therapy
3181S.W. Sam Jackson Park Road, L605
Portland, OR 97201-3098
USA

P. Lanzer
Kardiologisch-Angiologische
Gemeinschaftspraxis
Saalbaustraße 27
D-64283 Darmstadt, FRG

W. Li
Erasmus Universiteit Rotterdam
Exp. Echocardiography (Ee2312)
P.O. Box 1738
3000 NR Rotterdam
The Netherlands

W. März
Abt. für Labormedizin
Universitätsklinik Freiburg
Hugstetter Straße 55
D-79105 Freiburg, FRG

W. P. Th. M. Mali
Department of Radiology
University Hospital Utrecht (E 01.132)
Heidelberglaan 100
3584 CX Utrecht
The Netherlands

M. R. Malinow
Oregon Regional Private Research Center
505 NW 185th Avenue
Beaverton, OR 97006
USA

M. Maynar
Unidad de Radiologia Vascular e
Intervencionista
Hospital Nuestra Senora del Pino
Engel Guimera 93
35005 Las Palmas de Gran Canaria
Espana

K. Mizuno
Chiba Hokusoh Hospital
Nippon Medical School
1715 Kamakari, Inba, Inba, Chiba 270-16
Japan

G. L. Moneta
Oregon Health Sciences University
School of Medicine
Div. of Vascular Surgery
3181 S.W. Sam Jackson Park Road, OP11
Portland, OR 97201-3098
USA

M. Nauck
Abt. für Labormedizin
Universitätsklinik Freiburg
Hugstetter Straße 55
D-79106 Freiburg, FRG

J. Niepel
Siemens AG, RAM 4
Postfach 32 60
D-91050 Erlangen, FRG

J. Noordzij
Radiology Department, E.01.132
University Hospital Utrecht
Heidelberglaan 100
3584 CX Utrecht
The Netherlands

T. Peters
Nasser, Smith & Pinkerton Cardiology, Inc.
St. Vincent Professional Building
8402 Hardcourt Road
Indianapolis, IN 46260
USA

C. M. Orr
Nasser, Smith & Pinkerton Cardiology, Inc.
St. Vincent Professional Building
8402 Hardcourt Road
Indianapolis, IN 46260
USA

H. Pieterman
Erasmus Universiteit Rotterdam
Exp. Echocardiography (Ee2312)
P.O. ox 1738
3000 DR Rotterdam
The Netherlands

C. A. Pinkerton
Nasser, Smith & Pinkerton Cardiology, Inc.
St. Vincent Professional Building
8402 Hardcourt Road
Indianapolis, IN 46260
USA

L. J. Polman
Radiology Department, E.01.132
University Hospital Utrecht
Heidelberglaan 100
3584 CX Utrecht
The Netherlands

J. M. Porter
Oregon Health Sciences University
School of Medicine
Div. of Vascular Surgery
3181 S.W. Sam Jackson Park Road, OP11
Portland, OR 97201-3098
USA

J. M. Pulido-Duque
Unidad de Radiologia Vascular e
Intervencionista
Hospital Nuestra Senora del Pino
Angel Guimera 93
35005 Las Palmas de Gran Canaria
Espana

W. Rautenberg
Ruprecht-Karls-Universität Heidelberg
Klinikum Mannheim
Neurologische Klinik
Theodor-Kutzer-Ufer 1
D-68167 Mannheim, FRG

H. Refsum
University of Bergen
Clinical Pharmacological Unit
Central Laboratory Haukeland Hospital
N-5021 Bergen
Norway

N. Reifart
Kardiologische Gemeinschaftspraxis
Am Roten Kreuz Krankenhaus
Alfred-Brehm-Platz 5–9
D-60316 Frankfurt/Main, FRG

R. Reyes
Unidad de Radiologia Vascular e
Intervencionista
Hospital Nuestra Senora del Pino
Angel Guimera 93
35005 Las Palmas de Gran Canaria
Espana

J. Rösch
Oregon Health Sciences University
School of Medicine
Charles Dotter Institute of
Interventional Therapy
3181 S.W. Sam Jackson Park Road, L605
Portland, OR 97201-3098
USA

P. J. Rubio
Unidad de Radiologia Vascular e
Intervencionista
Hospital Nuestra Senora del Pino
Angel Guimera 93
35005 Las Palmas de Gran Canaria
Espana

R. R. Saxon
Oregon Health Sciences University
School of Medicine
Charles Dotter Institute of
Interventional Therapy
3181 S.W. Sam Jackson Park Road, L605
Portland, OR 97201-3098
USA

M. Scheidegger
Universität und ETH Zürich
Institut für Biomedizinische Technik und
Medizinische Informatik
Gloriastraße 35
CH-8092 Zürich
Swizerland

P. W. Serruys
Cardiac Catheterization Laboratory
Div. Cardiology, Thoraxcenter
Erasmus University
P.O. Box 1738
3000 DR Rotterdam
The Netherlands

W. Steinke
Ruprecht-Karls-Universität Heidelberg
Klinikum Mannheim
Neurologische Klinik
Theodor-Kutzer-Ufer 1
D-68167 Mannheim, FRG

B. H. Strauss
Catheterization Laboratory
Thoraxcenter Bd 414
P.O. Box 1738
3000 NR Rotterdam
The Netherlands

G. P. Teitelbaum
University of Southern California
School of Medicine
Los Angeles, CA 90033
USA

S. H. K. The
Erasmus Universiteit Rotterdam
Exp. Echocardiography (Ee2312)
P.O. Box DR Rotterdam
The Netherlands

P. M. Ueland
University of Bergen
Clinical Pharmacological Unit
Central Laboratory
Haukeland Hospital
N-5021 Bergen
Norway

V. A. W. M. Umans
Catheterization Laboratory
Thoraxcenter Bd 414
P.O. Box 1738
3000 DR Rotterdam
The Netherlands

A. van der Lugt
Erasmus Universiteit Rotterdam
Exp. Echocardiography (Ee2312)
P.O. Box 1738
3000 DR Rotterdam
The Netherlands

F. C. van Egmond
Erasmus Universiteit Rotterdam
Exp. Echocardiography (Ee2312)
P.O. Box 1738
3000 DR Rotterdam
The Netherlands

M. S. van Leeuwen
Radiology Department, E.01.132
University Hospital Utrecht
Heidelberglaan 100
3584 CX Utrecht
The Netherlands

J. van Tassel
Nasser, Smith & Pinkerton Cardiology, Inc.
St. Vincent Professional Building
8402 Hardcourt Road
Indianapolis, IN 46260
USA

H. van Urk
Erasmus Universiteit Rotterdam
Exp. Echocardiography (Ee2312)
P.O. Box 1738
3000 DR Rotterdam
The Netherlands

B. Velthuis
Radiology Department, E.01.132
University Hospital Utrecht
Heidelberglaan 100
3584 CX Utrecht
The Netherlands

I. Wendelhag
Wallenberg Laboratory
Sahlgren's Hospital
S-41345 Göteborg
Sweden

K. U. Wentz
Klinikum der Albert-Ludwigs-Universität
Abt. Röntgendiagnostik
Hugstetterstraße 55
D-79106 Freiburg, FRG

H. Wieland
Abt. für Labormedizin
Universitätsklinik Freiburg
Hugstetter Straße 55
D-79106 Freiburg, FRG

J. Wikstrand
Wallenberg Laboratory
Sahlgren's Hospital
S-41345 Göteborg
Sweden

P. G. Yock
Stanford University Medical Center
Center for Research in
Cardiovascular Interventions
300 Pasteur Drive
Stanford, CA 94305
USA

A. P. Yoganathan
Georgia Institute of Technology
Atlanta, Georgia 30332
USA

E. Zeitler
Abt. für Diagnostische und
Interventionelle Radiologie
Klinikum Nürnberg-Nord
D-90340 Nürnberg, FRG

Part I
Noninvasive Techniques

Section I
General Vascular Diagnostics

Vascular Physical Examination

P. Lanzer

Introduction

Even in the high technology era the physical examination remains the priciple means of assessing patients with vascular disease. Its primary objectives are to establish a tentative diagnosis and to design an efficient diagnostic plan. In peri-interventional settings acute complications and outcome should be assessed. The vascular examination provides a comprehensive evaluation of the entire cardiocirculatory system. Specifically, the individual vascular beds, their function and the functional state of the target end-organs are assessed. Similar to a standard examination it consists of oral (medical history) and physical evaluations. The individual steps and components are listed in Table 1.

Medical History (MH)

The main objective of the MH in the cardiovascular examination is to provide a comprehensive cardiovascular profile of an individual patient based on presenting symptoms, history of present illness, cardiovascular risk status, and prior cardiovascular diseases. Other objectives include establishment of a general rapport between the individual patient and the physician, and mutual agreement on the therapeutic objectives and means to achieve them.

Chief Complaints (CCs) and Current Symptoms (CSs)

The physician usually begins the patients interview with a detailed and thorough inquiry about the chief complaints (CCs) which have led the patient to seek medical advice. All CCs are explored; their severity, onset, duration, frequency, provoking factors, and response to the attempts to relieve them should be carefully assessed and documented. Additional and accompanying symp-

Table 1. Outline of the cardiovascular physical examination

I. Medical history

I.1	Chief complaints and current symptoms (detailed)
I.2	Present illness (detailed)
I.3	Past medical history (brief)
I.4	Current medications (detailed)
I.5	Cardiovascular risk (detailed)
I.6	Cardiovascular diseases (detailed)
I.7	Psychosocial history (brief)
I.8	Allergies (brief)
I.9	Other (e.g., review of systems) (optional)

II. Physical examination

II.1	General cardiovascular examination (symptom independent)
II.1.1	General survey
II.1.2	Vital signs
II.1.3	Body surface, skin
II.1.4	Thorax (heart and lungs)
II.1.5	General vascular examination
II.2	Specific cardiovascular/end-organ examination (symptom oriented)
II.2.1	Acute arterial syndromes
II.2.1.1	Cerebrovascular
II.2.1.2	Coronary
II.2.1.3	Visceral
II.2.1.4	Peripheral
II.2.2	Chronic arterial syndromes
II.2.2.1	Cerebrovascular
II.2.2.2	Coronary
II.2.2.3	Visceral
II.2.2.4	Peripheral
II.2.3	Acute venous syndromes
II.2.3.1	Cerebrovascular
II.2.3.2	Visceral
II.2.3.3	Peripheral
II.2.4	Chronic venous syndromes
II.2.4.1	Neurocerebral
II.2.4.2	Visceral
II.2.4.3	Peripheral
II.3	Specific nonvascular (symptom oriented), e.g., musculoskeletal, neurologic

toms (CSs) are also explored and documented. The patient's level of physical performance and its limiting factors should be stated.

Present Illness (PI)

After obtaining the CCs and CSs the physician proceeds to inquire about the history of the present illness, giving a full account of the chronological development of CC/CS. Avaiable medical records and results of previous CC/CS-related treatments are obtained and evaluated.

Past Medical History (PMH)

A brief account of major past medical problems such as illnesses requiring hostitalization, operations, and accidents is provided. An in-depth exploration of the general medical problems is usually not necessary.

Current Medications (CM)

A complete list of the patient's medications, their dosages, and regimens including timetables are obtained.

Cardiovascular Risk (CR)

A detailed evaluation of the cardiovascular risk profile allows estimates of the probability of the disease in risk persons and of new vascular events in patients with known cardiovascular disease. The risk level assists in determining the need for further diagnostic evaluations. For example, in patients with suspected ischemic disease the presence of arterial hypertension, disturbances of the carbohydrates (insulin-dependet and insulin-independent diabetes mellitus), lipoprotein (cholesterol-, triglycerides-, apolipoprotein-related dyslipoproteinemias), homocysteine, iron and uric acid metablism, tobacco use, genetic familial predisposition, obesity (feminine or masculine), presence of negative stressors (e.g., night shifts in hospital workers), and level of physical activity should be determined. Each risk factor should be individually documented, e.g., in cigarette smokers number of packs per day in years, secondary organ involvement in diabetic and hypertensive patients, and severity of familial predisposition.

The laboratory results of the latest metablic evaluations should be recorded. Similarly, in patients with suspected venous disorders, venous risk factors, such as familial predisposition, occupational hazards, in females pregnancies and oral contraceptives, as well as disturbances of the hemostatic functions such as coagulation abnormalities (e.g., platelet dysfunctions, dysfibrinogenemias, antithrombin III, protein C and S deficiencies, presence of abnormal phospholipid antibodies) should be known.

Cardiovascular Diseases (CD)

To complete the patient's cardiovascular profile all previous cardiovascular disease, in particular myocardial infarctions, cerebrovascular accidents, peripheral/visceral arterial and venous diseases, and pulmonary embolizations are listed. Each CD is thoroughly documented.

Psychosocial History (PSH)

A brief account of the patient's occupation, marital and family status usually suffices. In some patients, however, a more extensive PSH is needed.

Allergies (A)

History of previous allergies is given. In particular, adverse reactions to iodine contrast agents are noted.

Other components of the standard MH such as Review of Systems (ROS) and Current Health Status (CHS) are not always included and remain at the descretion of the attending physician. For more in-depth information the reader is referred to the standard literature [1, 2].

In peri-interventional settings detailed knowledge and understanding of the planned or performed intervention is essential to allow a detailed evaluation of the results including possible complications.

Physical Examination (PE)

In the PE the techniques of inspection, palpation, percussion, and asculation are integrated into a powerful diagnostic tool allowing a basic yet comprehensive assessment of the cardiovascular status of the individual patient. A systematic approach is necessary to maximize the diagnostic information while keeping patient discomfort and time requirements to a minimum. The examination is preferably performed after the patient has been well acclimatized in an adequately lit and quiet environment. The patient is comfortably resting in a supine position with a pillow supporting the neck. To allow a complete examination the patient should be undressed to the underwear. The cardiovascular PE consists of two parts, general and specific.

General Cardiovascular Examination (GCE)

A general cardiovascular examination is performed in all patients presenting with cardiovascular symptoms. A systematic step-by-step yet flexible approach is adopted.

General Survey (GS)

The patient's general appearance (habitus, posture, gait, nourishment, etc.) is recorded. Height and weight are measured.

Vital signs (VS)

Pulse and respirations are counted. Blood pressure in both arms is measured. To enable reproducible measurements to be taken a standardized protocol for blood pressure determination is followed [3]. Body temperature is taken, if indicated.

Skin, Body Surface (SBS)

Careful inspection and palpation of the entire body surface is an integral part of the GCE. General and regional status of the skin, skin appendages, and mucous membranes is thoroughly evaluated. In particular changes in color and temperature, edemas, and ulcerations are noted. In this chapter only two SBS changes, peripheral edemas and ulcerations, will be discussed. A comprehensive review is provided in the standard literature [4].

Peripheral Edemas. Edemas represent an inappropriate fluid accumulation in the interstitial space due to imbalance of the Starling's capillary

Table 2. Qualitative grading of the severity of peripheral edemas

Grade	Features
1 (mild)	Normal contour, slight pit
2 (mild to moderate)	Normal contour, deeper pit
3 (moderate)	Lighter swelling, deep pit
4 (severe)	Prominent swelling, deep pit

forces. Initially the interstitial fluid begins to accumulate within the subfascial space. Subfascial peripheral edema connot be detected by visual inspection; on palpation, however, the consistency of the musculature is increased. With further accumulation of the fluid the subfascial space become exhausted and the fluid begins accumulate also within the epifascial space. A mild epifascial edema may be revealed by a puffiness or by a gentle palpation of the retromalleolar, pretibial, and presacral regions. With increasing severity of fluid accumulation the surface morphology becomes distorted and the edema becomes clearly apparent. The severity of the peripheral edema can be estimated on a 4-point scale (Table 2). More commonly the circumference of the limbs at defined points is measured and compared with follow-up evaluations. In patients with a generalized edema the body weight should be routinely determined.

Important causes of peripheral edemas are listed in Table 3. In general, regional lower leg venous

Table 3. Principal causes of peripheral edemas

I. Decreased venous outflow
    I.1   Mechanical venous obstructions
    I.1.1 Intraluminal (e.g., thormbosis)
    I.1.2 Extraluminal (e.g., compressions by tumors)
    I.2   Functional venous disorders (e.g., valve insufficiency)
    I.3   Systemic venous hypertension (e.g., right heart failure, constrictive pericarditis)
    I.4   Portal venous hypertension
    I.5   Muscular insufficiency (e.g., hemiplegia)

II. Combined arteriolar and capillary membrane disorders (e.g., vasculitis, glomerulonephritis)

III. Lymphatic circulatory disorders

IV. Decreased oncotic transcapillary pressure
    IV.1 Albumin-losing disorders (e.g., nephrotic syndrome, protein-loosing enteropathy)
    IV.2 Albumin synthesis disorders (e.g., liver failure)

venous discorders are associated with unilateral edemas and in advances stages with accompanying dermal changes. In contrast, systemic edemas are bilateral, dermal changes being rare. Lymphedemas are nonpitting, often bilateral, involving the toes. Lipedemas are also nonpitting; however, the foot and the toes are spared. Secondary skin changes do not usually occur.

In contrast to peripheral edemas other end-organ edemas such as the pulmonary edema potentially represent life-threatening complications; the associated physical findings are discussed elsewhere [5].

Peripheral Ulcerations. The majority of ulcerations of the lower extremity are venous. Venous ulcers are usually localized at the lower calf most frequently behind the inner malleolus. Their borders are edematous and irregular, sometimes encircling the entire circumference of the calf („boot ulcers"). The demarcation is usually poor. The ulcus base is either filled with inflammatory purulent secretions or epithelial/granulation tissues. Occasionally, it is traversed by variose cushions/convolutes. Larger ulcerations tend to be shallow with a better healing tendency whereas small ulcerations particulary in the atrophic skin areas are often deeply undermined and poorly healing. Venous ulcers are often accompanied by hyperpigmentations, lymphedema, stasis dermatitis, indurations with a glossy appearance, thickening, and scarring of the surrounding skin areas. In advanced stages lymphedema, secondary skeletal changes, e.g., malleolar ankylosis, and mycotic and bacterial superinfection are seen. The venous ulcers are frequently painless; if pain is present it usually does not tend to be severe.

Ulcerations associated with chronic arterial insufficiency are frequently found at the pressure points, points of trauma, or following the principle of the „last meadow" at the limb periphery such as toes, finger tips, heels, and the lateral aspects of the foot. The arterial ulcers display irregular yet usually well demarcated borders and variable depth. They appear dark, are often dry, and are often filled with a necrotic tissue. Gangrenous „dry" or „wet" superinfections do occur. The surrounding skin is usually atrophic (arterophie blanche), hairless and pale, dusky, or cyanotic on dependency. A severe nagging rest pain is often present.

Combined ischemic and neuropathic ulcerations are encountered in patients with diabetes melli-tus. The diabetic ischemic ulcerations often develop at the toe tips, interdigitally, at the dorsum of the foot, over the head of metatarsus I and V, or at the heels. Starting from a small painful nodule, poorly demarcated deep tissue, often painless necrosis rapidly develops. Bacterial or mycotic superinfections are frequent. The borders are typically irregular and the demarcation is usually poor. The surrounding skin is often atrophic white or reddishly discolored sometimes with interspersed small scars. The neuropathic diabetic ulceration frequently develops at plantar locations, and presents with calluses and loss of sensation. The arterial pulses and the foot temperature are normal; the skin blood flow is increased.

Mechanical pressure ulcerations develop typically at the pressure points. Associated disturbances of arterial or venous hemodynamics may be present. Dissemited ulcerations and skin necrosis can accompany a number of other vasculitic, inflammatory, neoplastic, and hematologic disorders; their morphologic appearances are described elsewhere [4, 7].

Thorax (T)

A thorough examination of the lungs, heart, and central circulation is mandatory. The examination techniques are described elsewhere [1, 2, 6].

General Vascular Examination (GVE)

In all patients an orienting examination of the arterial and venous circulation is performed. When appropriate capillary and lymphatic examinations may be included.

Arterial Examination (AE). The complete pulse status is taken. Typical palpatory sites are given in Fig. 1; the pulse examination techniques are described elsewhere [1, 2]. The pulses may be classified simply as being present or absent or they may be evaluated on a scale from 0 to 4 (Table 4). Occasionally, an experienced observer is able to identify the individual components of the normally triphasic peripheral pulse. A deep gentle abdominal palpation to detect pulsatile masses follows the peripheral pulse palpation. Then, arterial ausculation at the standard sites at rest, and infrequently following exercise, is performed

Table 4. Qualitative grading of arterial pulse palpation

Grade	Pulse character
0	Pulse absent
1	Pulse markedly diminished
2	Pulse moderately diminished
3	Pulse slightly diminished
4	Normal pulse

(Fig. 1). If a stenotic arterial murmur is present, its character and duration should be noted. Typically, low-grade stenoses produce early systolic, moderate stenoses and mid-systolic and high-grade stenoses produce holosystolic or systolic/diastolic murmurs. Pancyclic murmurs may, however, also indicate arteriovenous shunts or malformations. High-grade or subtotal stenoses may be clinically silent due to the low volumetric flow or they may produce only a soft barely audible low-pitch murmur often missed on clinical examination. In some patients with a variable degree of stenoses no audible murmurs are produced. In contrast, accidental flow murmurs may accompany flow disturbances in morphologically normal but tortuous arteries or in systemic high-flow states accompanying, for example, anemia, severe aortic insufficiency, and hypothyreoidism. Care must also also be taken to apply the stethoscope gently to avoid artificial murmurs due to arterial compressions.

Venous Examiniation (VE). The veins of the limbs are inspected with the patient in the supine and dependent position. Skin infiltrations, rubor, venous filling state, and the presence and site of the varicose veins are noted [1]. Following inspection a gentle systematic palpation is performed and the skin temperature, presence of edemas, sensitivity to pressure, and consistency of the super-

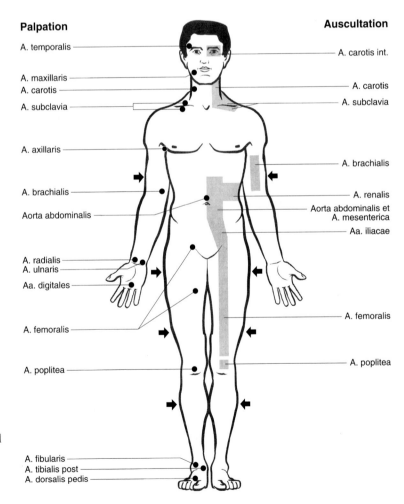

Fig. 1. Standard locations of arterial pulse palpation, auscultation, and segmental blood pressure measurements (*arrows*) are indicated. (Adapted from [8])

ficial tissues are assessed. The veins of the trunk are poorly visible in the normal state, but may engorge upon collateralization in patients with portocaval hypertension. The examination techniques to evaluate the central venous and right heart hemodynamics based on external and internal jugular vein evaluations are described in the literature [6].

Capillary and Lymphatic Examination (CLE). Capillary membrane dysfunction often manifests as a regional or generalized urticaria. An increased capillary fragility can be demonstrated clinically using the Rumpel-Leede or the suction bell test, described in the literature [8]. Gentle palpation of the major lymphatic pathways is performed, and the consistency, pressure sensitivity, and movability against the underlined tissues and skin of the enlarged lymph nodes is noted. With suspected lymphedema the movability of the skin at the dorsum of the feet is tested (Stemmer' skin fold sign of the lymphedema is positive when the skin firmly adheres to the underlined tissue and cannot be folded).

Specific Cardiovascular/End-organ Examination (SCVEE)

SCVEE is tailored to the individual patient and his symptoms. Its purpose is to assess the functional status of a specific vascular bed and that of the affected end-organ. Due to the great number of vascular beds and the even substantially greater number of corresponding pathologic vascular related end-organ abnormalities, different examination techniques are required to assess properly each of the dysfunctional states in the individual vascular territory [8, 9]. In this context only the principles of the peri-interventional examinations of patients presenting with occlusive diseases of the major arterial and venous beds will be provided. This subject is treated more extensively in the standard literature [4–9].

Acute Arterial (Ischemic) Syndromes

Acute ischemic syndromes are commonly due to systemic emboli. Less frequently local thrombotic complications of atherosclerosis, arterial wall injuries, or other arteriopathies are responsible. The systemic emboli originate most frequently from the left-sided heart chambers and are associated with ischemic and valvular heart disease, arrhythmias, in particular atrial fibrillation, intracardiac masses, endocarditis, or mitral valve prolapse. Other causes of systemic emboli include aneurysmatic and atherosclerotic lesions, vascular malformations, and deep venous thromboses in patients with a patent foramen ovale („paradox emboli"). Preferred sites of embolic occlusions are arterial bifurcations or branching points. In decreasing order of frequency occur intracerebral, lower and upper extremity, and visceral arterial embolizations. Thrombotic occlusions predominate in the coronary and in the carotid arteries. Acute thromboembolic occlusions typically result in acute-organ ischemia. However, the severity of the ischemia and the systemic hemodynamic response depend on the functional state of the collateral circulation, the end-organ's anaerobic capacity, its functional state, and plasma coagulability [10]. Therefore, an „identical" vascular pathology may be associated with a wide spectrum of clinical syndromes and physical findings.

In general, in acutely ischemic patients the physical examination must be brief and focused. The vital signs, the ischemic end organ, the systemic circulation, and where accessible the affected vascular beds are assessed. Rapid yet thorough examinations are the key to successful management of patients with acute vascular syndromes.

Cerebrovascular. In all patients presenting with acute cerebrovascular symptoms a complete neurologic examination is mandatory. The examination is preferably performed by neurologists or other neurovascular specialists. If not available, the examination is performed by physicians familiar with the presenting neurologic symptoms and the management of cerebrovascular emergencies [11–13].

Acute cerebrovascular accidents may be divided into those resolving completely within 24, i.e., transient ischemic attacks (TIAs), or less than 3 weeks, i.e., prolonged reversible ischemic neurologic deficits (PRINDs), and those resolving incompletely leaving behind permanent neurologic deficits, i.e., progressive and completed strokes, respectively. The presenting symptoms vary depending on the affected vascular territory, status of the circle of Willis, and secondary intracerebral steal phenomenas.

The ischemic thromboembolic symptoms originating from the carotid artery territory are often associated with ipsilateral blindness (amaurosis fugax), monocular visual disturbances (oph-thalmic artery), contralateral hemiparesis and sensory losses, apraxia (anterior cerebral artery), expressive aphasia, contralateral hemianopsia, dysarthria (medial cerebral artery), anosognosia, bilateral hemianopsia, spatial disorientation, and dysphagia (posterior cerebral artery). With expert knowledge of the clinical neurophysiology, often quite precise identification of a specific involved vascular territory becomes feasible [14]. With developing brain edema and a threatening lateral or downward herniation, the clinical picture becomes dominated by signs of diffuse supra- or infratentorial mass lesions associated with changes in arousal (mild confusion, somnolence, stupor, coma). Depending on the presence or absence of reaction to pain stimuli, optic/stretch/gag reflexes, and respiratory/circulatory function, the depth of the coma can be further classified (stages I–V) [15, 16].

The ischemic symptoms originating from the vertebrobasilar vascular territory include dizziness, increased perspiration, nausea, emesis, binocular visual disturbances („foggy" or double vision, scotomas, transient blindness, visual field defects), amnesia, rotatory vertigo, dysarthria, variable sensorimotor disturbances of one limb, gait ataxia, headaches, tremor, „drop attacks," apraxia, and dysarthria [15]. Based on the clinical manifestations, brain stem and cerebellar lesions may often be identified [15].

Hemorrhagic subarachnoidal bleeding, most frequently due to ruptured aneurysms, may be clinically suspected based on prodromal signs such as severe beadache, nuchal rigidity, drowsiness, confusion, light-headedness, dizziness, syncope, parasthesias, restlessness preceding acute symptoms such as seizures, emesis, autonomic dysregulation with brady-/tachycardia, profuse perspiration, high temperature, psychosyndromes, and coma.

Focal intracerebral hemorrhages are mostly due to ruptured hypertensive atherosclerotic lesions and are associated with clinical symptoms often localizing the hemorrhages to the putamen (conjugate deviation) with the patient gazing towards the side of the lesion or sometimes ipsilateral gaze palsy (contralateral weakness, and hemiparesis), thalamus (contralateral hemiparesis, sensory changes, and homonymous hemianopsia), pons (early coma, quadriplegia, bilateral extensor posturing), or cerebellum (occipital headache, ataxia, nausea, and vomiting). Cisternal bleeding usually results in a deep coma, initially narrow later wide fixed pupils, loss of stretch muscle reflexes, positive bilateral Babinski reflexes, and extensor posturing [15, 17].

The proper recognition and interpretation of neurologic symptoms in patients presenting with acute cerebrovascular accidents are a key to optimum managment. In the majority of patients, however cranial CT or MR scans are required to establish definite diagnosis.

Coronary. Acute myocardial ischemia in the vast majority of patients is due to ruptured coronary artery atheroma and superimposed thrombosis. Typically these patients present with unstable angina, acute myocardial infarction or sudden arrhythmogenic death. In some patients, however, the symptoms of a stable exertional angina are present. Occasionally the ischemia remains clinically silent. Typically, the clinical picture is dominated by an anginal retrosternal, or precordial chest or abdominal pain often radiating in the neck, back, or into the arms. In the course of physical examination the vital signs, the left and right ventricular function, the heart rhythm, the systemic an pulmonary hemodynamic are evaluated. The principles of the cardiac examination in coronary syndromes are described elsewhere and will not be repeated here [18]. Although the physical examination is helpful in assessing these critically ill cardiac patients, early ECG and serial enzymatic measurements are mandatory for definite diagnostics.

Visceral. Thromboembolic atherosclerotic disease is the major cause of acute visceral ischemia. The majority of patients presents with nonspecific symtoms and signs. Patients with acute superior mesenteric embolic occlusions may present with an acute abdomen. The sharp abdominal pain is located periumbilically or in the right lower quadrant and is accompanied by nausea and vomiting. The abdomen is soft and tender; bowel sounds are present. Bloody diarrhea and systemic circulatory compromise may be present. Splenic artery occlusions may be accompanied by epigastric or left upper quadrant discomfort, sometimes radiating to the left scapula. Hepatic artery occlusions are either asymptomatic or may be associated with visceral pain in the right upper quadrant, occasionally radiating to the back. The intestinal artery occlusions may be accompanied by periumbilical or lower quadrant pain. Renal artery occlusions are frequently initially silent.

Later in the course sharp flank or back pain, costovertebral angle or paravertebral tenderness, nausea, vomiting, and hematuria may develop [19]. The main objective of the examination is to raise suspicion of vascular causes of the symptomatology, not to establish definite diagnosis.

Peripheral. The majority of patients, approximately 70%–80%, presenting with acute peripheral syndromes have suffered an embolic event. Less frequently, acute thrombosis or other causes are responsible. The clinical presentation depends on the level and localization of the arterial obstruction, the preexisting collateral circulation, and the patient's hemodynamic status. In general, more distal obstructions produce more severe ischemia. Usually however, the most severe symptoms accompany acute obstructions of the bifurcation of the femoral artery.

The patients with acute peripheral syndromes typically present with a sharp, stabbing ischemic muscular pain at rest or on minimum exertion in the lower or upper extremity distal to the arterial obstruction. The limb appears pale and cold, the venous filling is diminished, the pulses distal to the obstruction are absent, and paraesthesia and muscular weakness are common. With the exception of acute abdominal aortic obstructions, symptoms are unilateral. The examination includes a careful evaluation of the extremity involved. To assess the severity of the ischemia the ankle/brachial index (ABI) and the elevation test are useful. In the latter the extremity is elevated to 60° from horizontal and the time for pallor to occur is measured. Subsequently, the time for venous filling and color to return are measured at dependency. An ABI lower than 0.15 invariably indicates severe lower limb ischemia. Similarly, pallor in the horizontal position, the return of color, and of the venous filling return after more than 40s are consistent with severe limb ischemia (Tables 5, 6) [20]. In patients with severe ischemia the limb viability must be assessed. The limb is thought to be threatened when the capillary return is slow

Table 5. Qualitative assessment of peripheral ischemia by the elevation test (modified from [20])

Grading of elevation pallor	
Grade	Duration of elevation
0	No pallor in 60 s
1	Pallor at 60 s
2	Pallor at less than 60 s
3	Pallor at less than 30 s
4	Pallor on the level

Table 6. Qualitative assessment of peripheral ischemia by the elevation test (modified from [20])

Color return and venous filling time		
Degree of ischemia	Time (s) for color to return	Venous filling time (s)
None	10	15
Moderate	15–20	20–30
Severe	40+	40+

and muscle weakness and a sensory loss are incomplete. In these patients an emergency revascularization is mandatory. Irreversible tissue damage is characterized by an absent capillary return, profound paralysis, and complete anesthesia (Table 7) [20]; limb loss and amputation are an obligatory outcome. A careful physical examination of the extemity completed with Doppler evaluations provides a reliable assessment of the underlying arterial obstruction and the resulting end-organ, i. e., limb tissue, ischemia. Based on the results periinterventional selective angiography and revascularization strategy can be planned.

Occasionally, multiple occlusions of the small arteries, arterioles, and capillaries of the extremities or the parenchymatous organs secondary to embolizations of cholesterol crystal, and debris from ruptured atheromas are encountered. The

Table 7. Qualitative assessment of tissue viability in peripheral ischemia (modified from [20])

Tissue viability	Capillary return	Paralysis	Paresthesia
Viable	Intact	None	None
Threatened imcomplete	Intact, slow	Mild, partial	Mild
Irreversible	Absent (marbling)	Profound (rigor)	Profound (anesthesia)

clinical picture in the extremities is dominated by sharply demarcated cyanotic skin lesions and often quite severe ischemic pain.

Chronic Arterial Syndromes

Chronic ischemic syndromes in the majority of patients are due to occlusive atherothrombosis. Usually the symptoms develop slowly and progress gradually. The physical findings reflect the degree of the resulting end organ and if present of the systemic hemodynamic compromise. Due to the great variability in collateral function and end organ adaptation to chronic ischemia, the correlations between the underlying vascular status, the resulting endorgan dysfunction, and the physical findings are poor, making further laboratory evaluations mandatory in the majority of patients.

Cerebrovascular. In patients with a chronic cerebrovascular insufficiency or multi-infarct dementia the cerebral perfusion decreases below level required for maintaining a normal metabolism, causing a variety of symptoms and psychosyndromes variably associated with dementia. In the vertebrobasilar territory the cerebral underperfusion is characterized in lacunar state by bulbar dysarthria, dysphagia, gaze paresis, increased stretch and present pathologic reflexes, and facial nerve pareses. Sometimes respiratory and circulatory disturbances are present [15]. Due to the as yet limited role of vascular medicine in patients with chronic cerebrovascular insufficiency the physical examination is primarily performed by neurologists, geriatricians, and other physicians.

Coronary. Chronic coronary syndromes are due to occlusive coronary artery atherosclerosis. With the coronary blood flow supply droping below the demand level, patients typically develop stenocardic chest pains. In more advanced stages the symptoms of cardiac dysfunction may prevail with full-blown left and/or right heart failure resulting from severe ischemic episodes in patients with multiple-vessel disease or end-staged ischemic cardiomyopathies. Occasionally, cardiac symtoms are more subtle or they are completely lacking. The techniques of the cardiocirculatory examination in patients with chronic coronary syndromes are discussed elsewhere [6, 18, 21, 22].

Visceral. Chronic visceral arterial syndromes are mostly due to occlusive atherosclerosis of the abdominal aorta and/or its visceral branches. The physical findings in these usually elderly patients are often nonspecific. Chronic obstructions of the superior mesenteric artery may present with intestinal malabsorbtion, weight loss, periumbilical or epigastric pain sometimes radiating to the back. The abdominal anginal pain is usually dull or colicky occurring during meals often lasting up to 1 hour after the meal is completed. Changes in bowel habits with obstipation/diarrhea cycles are frequent. Generalized atherosclerosis is frequently manifest in these patients. The physical examination of the abdomen may reveal nonspecific tenderness on palpation or arterial bruits on auscultation. Patients with chronic renal artery stenosis present typically with arterial hypertension, signs of chromic renal failure and abdominal bruits. In patients with abdominal aorta aneurysms a pulsatile tumor may be felt or in slender patients seen on inspection. To establish the diagnosis of a chronic visceral arterial insufficiency, however, a selective arteriography is nearly always required. In planning revascularizations a close collaboration between gastroenterologists or nephrologists and vascular specialists is required [19].

Peripheral. Chronic peripheral syndromes are in the majority of patients due to occlusive atherosclerotic disease. Patients typically present with ischemic muscular pain at a variable level of exercise or in advanced stages at rest. In the early stages the ischemic pain is reproducible, sharp, cramping or paralyzing exercise induced, resolving quickly at rest, and involving identical muscle groups in a given patient. In the advanced stages the ischemic pain at rest appears. It is aggravated in the horizontal and alleviated in the dependent position. According to the principle of the „last meadow" the most peripheral muscle groups are usually the most severely involved. The pain invariably occurs in the limb musculature distal to the blood flow limiting lesion. Based on the localization of the obstructing lesions, the peripheral (lower leg), upper thigh, pelvic, aortic arch (including shoulder-arm, cervical-carotid, and vertebrobasilar) and combined types can be differentiated. A more specific differentiation is based on the involvement of the individual vascular beds. Here, a number of corresponding ischemic syndromes and accompanying physical findings have been described [8].

In lower limb ischemia the physical examination includes segmental blood pressure measurements to determine the approximate level of critical stenosis (Fig. 1). The severity of chronic lower limb ischemia may be assessed using the Fontaine classification with exercise-induced pain corresponding to stages I and II and rest pain corresponding to stages III and IV. Using the modified Fontaine classification a further differentiation of stage II based on the length of pain-free walking distance (PFWD) and of stage III based on height of systolic ankle and/or toe blood pressure is possible. A PFWD greater than 200 m corresponds to stage IIa, and a PFWD of less than 200 m corresponds to stage IIb. Similarly, an ankle pressure of greater than 50 mmHg corresponds to stage IIIa, and an ankle pressure lower than 50 mmHg corresponds to stage IIIb (Table 8). Ankle pressures below 50 mmHg along with toe systolic pressures lower than 30 mmHg and continuous requriements for analgesia for more than 2 weeks characterize critical chronic limb ischemia [23]. The elevation test (Ratschow) and assessment of the tissue viability complement the physical examination in patients presenting in Fontaine stages IIb, III, and IV.

Special attention must be paid to diabetic patients frequently presenting with signs and symptoms of arterial (marcroangiopathic) as well as arteriolar and capillary (microangiopathic) involvement. In these patients the vascular disease is usually more severe, more distal, and frequently occurring at an earlier age. The diabetic arteriopathy is frequently complicated by sensory, motor, and autonomic polyneuropathy as well as neuropathic and ischemic ulcertions. The corresponding physical findings are described elsewhere [4, 7–9, 23].

In the relatively rare chronic occlusive arterial disease of the upper limb, occlusive atherosclerosis plays a less dominant role, whereas arteriitis, compression syndromes, and systemic collagenoses become more prominent causes. The physical findings of exercise-induced claudication, rest pain, pulselessness distal to the arterial obstructions, stenotic bruits, and tissue loss are similar to the lower extremities. However, compared with the lower extremity stages of the upper limb ischemia are clinically less well defined. To estimate the severity of ischemia the clenched fist test may be applied. Here, the patient elevates the arm and performs approximately 60 fist squeezes in 2 min. Similarly to the elevation test of the legs the pallor and hyperemic response to dependency are semiquantitatively evaluated. In patients with suggested occlusion of the radial or ulnar artery the clenched fist test may be repeated with one of the lower arm arteries being compressed (Allen's test). Diffuse pallor of the palms is indicative of an obstruction of the noncompressed artery.

The compression syndromes of the upper extremity are due to extraluminal arterial compressions. The most frequent causes are accessory ribs, inappropriate insertion of the tendons of the anterior, medial, minimus scalenus or minor pectoralis muscles and a narrow gap between the clavicle and the first rib causing compression of the subclavian artery, ischemic pain and parasthesias. A right-left upper arm blood pressure difference of greater than 20 mmHg is typically found. Employing the provocation tests, the arterial compression symptoms may often be reproduced. Thus, in Adson's test dorsal flexion of the head with turning to the suspected side may produce disappearance of the radial pulse and/or occurrence of the stenotic bruit in patients with scalenus syndromes. Similarly, elevation and hyperabduction of the flexed arm supported by a deep inspiration or the adduction against resistance of the arm elevated over the head may reduce the radial pulse in patients with the costoclavicular and the minor pectoralis syndromes, respectively [7, 8].

In patients presenting with chronic limb ischemia the physical examination provides a relatively accurate estimate of limb tissue ischemia and serves as an important guide to the entire clinical management in these patients.

Table 8. Qualitative assessment of chronic peripheral ischemia by the Fontaine classification (modified from [20])

Modified Fontaine classification	
Stage	Symtpoms
I	Absent
II	Intermittent claudication
IIa	Pain-free walking more than 200 m
IIb	Pain-free walking less than 200 m
III	Rest/nocturnal pain
IV	Tissue loss

Acute Venous Syndromes

In contrast to the arterial circulation, venous hemodynamics are more complex, the driving pressures and blood flow velocities are low. Whereas atherosclerosis plays only an important role in veins only following arterialization such as in aortocoronary bypasses and AV fistulas, the major venous pathogenetic principles remain slow flow, endothelial damage, and hypercoagulable states. The acute venous syndromes are typically related to venous thromboses. The physical findings reflect the tissue changes secondary to the venous outflow obstructions. Occasionally venous embolic complications may develop. Due to the multiple venous drainage of the same area, obstructions of smaller veins may remain clinically undetected.

Pathogenesis. The acute venous pathogenesis is complex involving numerous systemic disorders. In this context, discussion will be limited to the physical findings associated with acute venous thrombotic occlusions. For a more comprehensive review the reader is referred to the standard literature [4, 7–9, 24].

Cerebrovascular. The cerebral venous outflow obstructions are related to infectious or aseptic thromboses of the intracerebral veins or the extracerebral sinuses. In the course of the thrombotic occlusions ischemic or hemorrhagic infarcts and rarely pulmonary embolizations may develop. The examiner should be aware of frequent associations with inflammations of the skull and face, in particular of the sinuses, mastoids, and middle ear, and also with systemic in particular hematologic disorders. In females, a disproportionate number of cerebral venous thromboses occur postpartum and with intake of oral contraceptives. The symptoms usually develop in a protracted undulating fashion. A slow rise in intracerebral pressure accompanied by headaches, changes in arousal, organic cerebral psychosyndromes, nuchal rigidity, nausea, emesis, venous neck congestions, waxing and waning pareses occasionally involving cranial nerves III, IV, VI, and VII, epileptic seizures, extrapyramidal signs, and hyperpyrexia are frequently encountered. Due to the greater variability of the venous outflow, well-defined focal neurologic deficits are not typical in these patients. Based on presenting neurologic deficits syndromes of the transverse and cavernous sinus, of the ascending and descending cortical veins and of the internal cerebral veins may be differentiated [15]. Although the physical examination may raise suspicions of an acute cerebral venous thrombotic event, CT or MR scans of the brain are always required to confirm or to refute the diagnosis. To avoid permanent cerebral damage an early diagnosis is essential allowing timely intervention.

Visceral. Visceral vein thromboses are frequently associated with portal hypertension, inflammatory bowel diseases, malignancies, and trauma. In females an association with the intake of oral contraceptives and pregnancies is found. The symptoms and physical findings are nonspecific. In patients with an acute superior mesenteric vein occlusion an undulating poorly localized abdominal pain lasting days to weeks prior to examination is usually present. Also, abdominal distension secondary to fluid loss into the bowel lumen and ascites, general abdominal tenderness, and low-grade temperatures may be present. Isolated splenic, renal, or portal vein thrombosis particularly in patients with preexisting portal hypertension may remain clinically silent. Hepatic veins obstructions in patients with Budd-Chiari syndrome are related to membranous webs of the lower caval vein, parasitic infections, tumors, or hematologic disorders. In females intake of oral contraceptives and pregnancy may be causal. Clinically ascites, progressive hepatic dysfunction, and portal hypertension may be manifest. Although the physical examination may raise the suspicion of venous abdominal disease, Doppler flow or selective angiographic studies are required to confirm the diagnosis [19].

Peripheral. The acute peripheral venous syndromes are due mostly to thrombotic venous obstructions. The physical findings are dependent on the extent, level, and localization of the obstruction. Differentiation between the involvement of the superficial, deep, or transfascial venous system on clinical grounds alone is rarely possible. When an acute peripheral venous syndrome is suspected, the examiner should be aware of the predisposing conditions including immobilization, venous compression and trauma, radiation therapy, heart failure, malignancies, and hematologic disorders. Typically patients complain about a dull aching pain and heaviness in the limb, occasionally reporting muscular cramps worsening in a dependent positon and inability to stand. In patients with pelvic vein thrombosis, additionally limb swelling and cyanosis are frequently present. General symptoms such as a rise in temperature, anxiety, depressive mood, and fatigue may complete the clinical picture. Patients are examined in the recumbent and standing position. Both legs are evaluated in comparison. Inspection may reveal no abnormalities, or it may reveal edema, increased filling of the superficial veins (collateral circulation), increased consistency of the skeletal muscles, and cyanosis. In all patients the circumferences of the upper and lower extremities at defined points should be measured. Differences of more than 1.0 cm in the former, and of more than 1.5 cm in the latter, are considered significant. The following thrombotic signs lack specificity, and in general, do not increase the diagnostic accuracy of the examination [70]: tenderness along the adductor canal and the groin (Rieland's), pain in the calf (Tschermack's), pain in the calf on plantar flexion (Homan's), retromalleolar pain (Bisgaard's), pain following blood pressure cuff obstruction (Lowenberg's), pain following coughing (Louvel's), pain in the feet following pressure and plantar flexion (Payr's), spontaneous pain of the feet (Denecke's), pain following calf compression (Moses') or cuff inflation (Ramirez'), pain of the knee on leg elevation and patella compression (Sigg's), calf spasms following leg elevation and feet extension (Peabody's), and pretibial vein dilatation on the level (Pratt's). Therefore, in the majority of patients further laboratory studies are mandatory to confirm or to exclude the diagnosis and if positive to determine accurately the level of the venous obstruction.

Although similarly to acute arterial occlusions the majority of venous thrombotic occur in the legs, the frequency of upper extremity thrombotic occlusions is increasing due to the placement of the indwelling catheters and pacemaker electrodes. The clinical findings are similar to those described in the legs. Due to the less well developed collateral circulation, occlusion of the upper extremity veins is frequently accompanied by marked peripheral edema.

In patients with superficial thrombophlebitis the presenting signs include painful and hardened varicose veins with a local increased in temperature and reddish discoloration. In addition to common thrombophlebitis, a number of specific venous conditions such as migratory, infectious, and embolic occlusions and superficial vein occlusions should be recognized [8].

Table 9. Qualitative assessment of chronic peripheral ischemia by clinical classification (modified from [20])

Clinical classification

Grade	Category	Clinical description
I	0	Asymptomatic
	1	Mild claudication
	2	Moderate claudication
	3	Severe claudication
II	4	Ischemic rest pain
	5	Minor tissue loss, nonhealing ulcer, focal gangrene with diffuse pedal ischemia
III	6	Major tissue loss extending above transmetatarsal level, foot not salvageable

Patients with phlegmasia cerulea dolens due to an present acute venous and arterial obstruction with pronounced cyanotic limb discoloration, glistening skin, skin distension, necroses overlying massive peripheral edema, and reduced peripheral pulses.

Chronic Venous Syndromes

Chronic venous syndromes are frequent in the lower extremities, but are seen with progressively decreasing frequency in the visceral and cerebral venous circulation.

Cerebrovascular. Following resolution of intracranial, i.e., intracerebral vein or sinus thromboses, neurologic deficits may remain. Besides focal neurologic deficits in patients with ischemic brain infarcts, less specific symptoms such as headaches and various autonomic and hypophyseal dysfunctions can be encountered. In selected patients, hydrocephalus internus may result from resolved superior sagittal or transversal sinus thrombosis. In these patients the physical findings are nonspecific and brain imaging studies are required to establish the diagnosis [15].

Visceral. Chronic occlusions of intestinal veins may cause hypoxemia and eventually end-organ infarction. In these patients clinical findings are usually nonspecific and vascular imaging studies are needed to establish the diagnosis. In the portal circulation portal hypertension represents the common pathogenic pathway of intra- and extrahepatic chronic flow obstructions or of those conditions associated with increased hepatic perfusion. Increased flow resistance and/or volume load causes secondary hepatomegaly, formation of ascites, and secondary engorgement of the preformed numerous portocaval collateral circulations [26]. The recruitment of the umbilicoepigastric, splenoparietal, and mesentericorectal veins, becomes clinically apparent the former becoming evident as venous ectasias and varicosities at the frontal aspects of the trunk, the latter as internal hemorrhoids on rectal examination. Specific vascular studies are always required to define the underlying vascular pathology. Although in the past chronic visceral venous disorders and in particular portal hypertension represented a domain of abdominal surgery, the introduction of percutaneous implantation of the portocaval stents has heightened the interest of interventionalists in this important vascular territory.

Peripheral. Chronic peripheral venous syndromes are among the most frequently encountered disorders in clinical medicine. The recognition of the clinical findings and physical signs accompanying these disorders belongs to the standard knowledge of each vascular specialist. Primary varicosis occurs frequently in patients with a familial or occupational predisposition or those with specific peripheral orthopedic and/or vascular abnormalities. In females, additionally, intake of oral contraceptives and multiple pregnancies play a predisposing role. The venous distension is due to increased compliance of the venous walls associated with valvular insufficiency. The varicosities are recognized as ectasias and convolutions of the subcutaneous epifascial veins. The varicose veins may be asymptomatic or they may cause heaviness, dull pain or other less specific complaints. The patients are examined in the standing, sitting, and recumbent position. The inspection confirms the presence, extension, and localization of the varicose veins; signs of inflammation, edema, or secondary dermatologic changes are sought. The formerly used functional tests (Trendelenburg's I and II, Mahoner-Ochsner, Perthes', Linton's) [8], have become obsolete with the advent of Doppler/duplex sonography.
Complete varicosis of the greater saphenous vein is due to magna valve insufficiency typically located several centimeters below the groin. Based on the distal extent of the varicosities, stages I–IV can be differentiated (Table 10). Leg fatique, heaviness, calf tension, and cramps worsening on

Table 10. Qualitative assessment of peripheral varicosis (modified from [7])

Complete greater saphenous vein varicosis	
Stage	Extension of varicosities
I	isolated insufficiency of the magna valve
II	Proximal to the knee
III	Distal to the knee
IV	Up to the ankle

long standing and in the course of the day occur only in advanced stages and are enhanced by an associated insufficiency of the perforating veins („blowouts"). Dermal changes of advanced chronic venous insufficiency such as hyperpigmentation, paraplanter corona, white atrophy, ulcerations, and scars are relatively rare. Partial varicosis of the greater saphenous vein is characterized by varicosities in the magna territory in the presence of an intact magna valve. This disorder is due to valvular incompetence of one or several of the perforating veins. Lesser saphenous vein varicosis is due to parva valve insufficiency typically located at the knee joint level. Based on the distal extension of the varicosities clinical stages I–III can be differentiated (Table 11).
Incompetence of the perforating veins is frequently associated with varicosis of the major superficial veins. Clinically in addition to the „blowouts" gaps in the superficial fascia and changes secondary to chronic venous insufficiency are present.
In some patients isolated varicosis of one or several of the branches of the intact greater and lesser saphenous vein are evident. Neither these nor the reticular or the „spider's-web-like" telangiectatic cutaneous are of hemodynamic relevance.
Varicose vein complications, rupture, and phlebitis are clinically recognized based on the development of hematomas and of the inflammatory signs (reddening, pain, tenderness), respectively. Sec-

Table 11. Qualitative assessment of peripheral varicosis (modified from [7])

Lesser saphenous vein varicosis	
Stage	Extension of varicosities
I	Isolated insufficiency of the parva valve
II	Proximal to the ankle
III	Including ankle region

Table 12. Qualitative assessment of chronic venous insufficiency (modified from [7])

Severity of chronic venous insufficiency	
Stage	Physical findings
I	Reversible edema, minor dermal changes including cutaneous telangiectases
II	Persistent edema, hyperpigmentation, sclerofibrosis, eczema, dermal atrophy
III	Stage II plus florid or healed ulcerations

ondary varicosis results from venous valve destruction occurring in the course of recanalization of a deep vein thrombosis. The distinction between the primary and secondary varicosis is clinically important in particular in regard to venous surgery and prevention. However, based on the physical findings alone usually the primary and secondary varicosis cannot be distinguished and venous imaging studies are required to establish the diagnosis.

Various chronic venous pathologies involving the deep venous system, compromise the venous hemodynamics clinically resulting in a syndrome of the chronic venous insufficiency. In this syndrome the venous return is decreased resulting in venous congestion, edema and associated dermal and/or skeletal changes. Based on the severity stages I–III can be distinquished (Table 12).

Summary and Conclusions

Traditionally the examination of vascular patients has aimed at differentiation between the presurgical and surgical stages of the peripheral vascular disease. More recently, with advances in vascular biology, prevention and intervention the focus shifted towards an earlier and more subtle definition of the systemic vascular pathology and the target's end-organ function. Whereas in the past, the physical examination often represented the only stage of vascular evaluations, it represents today the basic level of a complex diagnostic pyramid. A thorough knowledge of the systemic vascular and vascular related end-organ pathology along with focused diligence in eliciting and interpreting the physical findings are important prerequisites to expeditious and efficacious diagnostics required in modern vascular care.

References

1. Bates B (1983) A guide to physical examination and history taking. JB Lippincott, Philadelphia
2. Judge RD, Zuidema GD, Fitzgerald Ft (eds) (1989) Clinical diagnosis. Little, Brown, Boston
3. Perloff D, Grim C, Flack J, Frohlich ED, Hill M, McDonald M, Morgenstern BZ (1993) Human blood pressure determintion by sphygmomanometry. Circulation 88: 2460–2470
4. Rudofsky G (ed) (1992) Kompaktwissen Angiologie. Perimed, Erlangen
5. Ingram RH, Braunwald E (1992) E Braunwald (ed) Heart Disease. Pulmonary edema: cardiogenic and noncardiogenic. In: WB Sauders, Philadelphia
6. Perloff JK (1982) Physical examination of the heart and circulation. WB Saunders Philadelphia
7. Rieger H (ed) (1993) Angiologie, Hypotonie, Hypertonie. Urban & Schwarzenberg, Munich
8. Kappert A (ed) (1987) Lehrbuch und Atlas der Angiologie. Hans Huber, Bern
9. Alexander K (ed) (1994) Gefäßkrankheiten. Urban & Schwarzenberg, Munich
10. Arnold G, Kübler W, Lichtlen PR, Loogen F (eds) (1993) Organ-Ischämien. Z Kardiol 82 [Suppl 5]: 1–168
11. De Jong RN (1979) The neurologic examination. Harper and Row, New York
12. Massey EW, Pleet AB, Scherokman B (1985) Diagnostic test in neurology. Year Book Medical Publishers, Chicago
13. Finke J (1968) Die neurologische Untersuchung. JF Lehmanns, Munich
14. Gilman S, Newman SW (1987) Manter and Gatz's essential of clinical neuroanatomy and neurophysiology. FA Davis, Philadelphia
15. Paal G (1984) Klinik der Hirndurchblutungsstörungen. In: Paal G (ed) Therapie der Hirndurchblutungsstörungen. Edition Medizin, Weinheim
16. Plum F (1992) Sustained impairments of consciousness. In: Cecil textbook of medicine. Wyngaarden JB, Smith LH Jr, Benett JC (eds) WB Saunders, Philadelphia
17. Pulsineli WA, Levy DE (1992) Wyngaarden JB Cerebrovascular diseases. In: Cecil textbook of medicine. Smith LH Jr, Benett JC (eds) WB Saunders, Philadelphia
18. Rutherford JD, Braunwald E (1992) Chronic ischemic heart disease. In: Branwald E (ed) Heart disease. WB Sanders, Philadelphia
19. Rutherford RB (ed) (1989) Vascular surgery. WB Saunders, Philadelphia
20. Pentecost MJ, Criqui MH, Dorros G, Goldstone J, Johnston W, Martin EC, Ring EJ, Spies JB (1994) Guidelines for peripheral percutaneous transluminal angioplasty of the abdominal aorta and lower extremity vessels. Circulation 89: 511–531
21. Braunwald E, Grossman W (1992) Clinical aspects of heart failure. In: Branwald E (ed) Heart disease. WB Saunders, Philadelphia
22. Weil MH, von Planta M, Rackow EC (1992) Acute circulatiory failure. In: Braunwald E (ed) Heart disease. WB Saunders, Philadelphia

23. Consensus Document (1991) Chronic critical leg ischemia. Circulation [Suppl IV] 84: IV 2-IV 22
24. Weber J, May R (1989) Funktionelle Phlebologie. Thieme, Stuttgart
25. Altenkämper H, Felix W, Gericke A, Gerlach HE, Hartmann M (1991) Phlebologie für die Praxis. de Gruyter, Berlin
26. Lusza G (1969) X-ray anatomy of the vascular system. JB Lippincott, Philadelphia

Laboratory Examinations

A. Fronek

Introduction

There are several reasons for performing vascular laboratory examinations: to identify the presence or absence of flow obstruction, to assess the severity of disease, and to ascertain the location of the disease. The suspicion of venous disease adds to these the determination of possible venous valvular insufficiency. In the past three decades a number of modalities have found wide acceptance that now form the backbone of noninvasive examination of the peripheral vascular system. The following discussion considers methodological principles common to several application areas.

Plethysmography encompasses by definition all methods which record changes in limb volume. A variety of underlying principles are used: water or air-filled plethysmography, strain gauge plethysmography, photoplethysmography, impedance plethysmography, and capacitance plethysmography. Only the most widely used systems are discussed below.

Air plethysmography uses air as transmitting medium to minimize the technical difficulties encountered with water plethysmography (leakage, etc.). Interest in air plethysmography has increased with the introduction of the pulse volume recorder by Raines and coworkers [1985], using the principle earlier described by Winsor [1950]. Volume changes, either synchronous with the heart beat or slow changes induced by increased outflow pressure (pressure cuff inflation), are registered by a thin-walled cuff and monitored either by a differential manometer [Winsor, 1953] or by a similarly responding semiconducting transducer [Raines et al, 1972]. Recent reports favor the use of air plethysmography in the diagnosis of venous disease and have revived interest in this technique [Nicolaides et al, 1989].

Regarding strain gauge plethysmography, Whitney [1949] introduced mercury – filled silastic tubing, which responds very sensitively to minute changes in limb volume because its electrical resistance increases by extending its length and simultaneously diminishing its cross-section. This double effect explains its high sensitivity. Its relative simplicity and ruggedness have contributed to its fast acceptance. This is potentiated by the introduction of electrical calibration [Brakkee & Vendrik, 1966; Hokanson et al, 1975] which has become a permanent part of these plethysmographs.

Impedance plethysmography is based on the effect of increasing or decreasing blood volume on the electrical impedance between two electrodes which create a very weak but uniform electrical field. Increased blood volume lowers the electrical impedance between two additional sensing electrodes, and decreased volume heightens it. Although the method was originally developed for the diagnosis of arterial occlusive disease [Nyboer et al, 1944; Holzer et al, 1945], it has found wider acceptance as a diagnostic method for detecting venous disease [Wheeler and Anderson, 1985].

Photoplethysmography uses a light source (now usually a light – emitting diode) which illuminates a limited portion of the tissue, and an adjacent photoelectric sensor registers the reflected light [Hertzman and Spealman, 1937]. Increased local blood volume increases the absorption, and therefore less light is picked up by a photosensitive sensor. The advantages of this detection system are its ruggedness and small size. This is counterbalanced to some extent by difficulties related to its calibratability. This, however, does not diminish its great utility for recording relative changes (arterial and venous diagnosis).

Doppler ultrasound velocity determination represents one of the most important methods in the vascular laboratory. This method is discussed in detail by others in this volume (Part I, Section III), and only its application to the peripheral arterial and venous system is discussed below.

Transcutaneous Po_2 measurement is based on the ability of a modified Clark-type platinum electrode to detect partial oxygen tension on the surface of the skin. The necassary precondition is local vasodilation, which is usually accomplished by a built-in heater [Huch et al, 1972] and set to 43° or 44 °C. This method continuously monitors oxygen availability in the skin, and although its sensitivity in detecting peripheral arterial occlusive disease is inferior to that of other currently used methods, it is superb in quantifying skin viability especially when searching for the optimal amputation level.

Arterial System

The most helpful hemodynamic parameters in examining the arterial system of the lower or upper extremities are segmental pressure, flow velocity (Doppler), and pulse volume.

Segmental Pressure Examination

Measurement Principles

The single most important noninvasive test for diagnosing arterial occlusive disease is the measurement of segmental pressure. This is based on the detection of peripheral oscillations after the cuff pressure is slowly reduced from suprasystolic levels. The appearance of oscillations indicates the systolic pressure. The pressure is measured at several sites, most frequently above the ankle (AA), but it is also very useful to place the cuff at the following measurement sites: upper thigh (UT), above the knee (AK), below the knee (BK), and the base of the great or second toe [Fronek 1989 a]. In most cases the Doppler flow signal is used to detect the reappearing perfusion [from the posterior tibial or dorsalis pedis artery) after reducing the cuff pressure. However, it is more expedient to use the toe pulse signal by strain gauge plethysmography or photoplethysmography because these permit recording of the pres-

sure from both legs simultaneously. This not only reduces the time needed for the study but also increases the accuracy of measurement in view of the spontaneuous pressure fluctuations (10 %–15 %). The advantage of Doppler signal monitoring on the other hand, is the fact that it can be performed with a hand-held portable system and does not require a recording device, which is necessary for the toe pulse monitoring.

It is important to pay attention to the size of the cuffs used because narower cuffs result in overestimation of the pressure. Although a cuff width of 15 cm at UT, AK, and BK levels and one of 13 cm at the AA level results in a segment/arm pressure of 1.0±0.15, most laboratories currently use a uniform cuff width of 12 cm for all four segments and for the arm. This is due mainly to practical considerations (uniform size of cuffs) and to the evidently increased accuracy in identifying the site of arterial obstruction in the thigh when narrower cuffs are used. The results are usually expressed as a segmental/arm pressure ratio (index). The average ratio is about 1.0±0.10 with the uniform 12-cm cuffs, and an index 0.85 or lower is considered pathological. A 2.5-cm-wide cuff is used to measure toe pressure, and the onset of oscillations is recorded with either a strain gauge or photoplethysmographic transducer connected to the respective plethysmograph. Doppler velocity monitoring is not suitable for measurement of toe pressure because of the small signal output from digital arteries. A toe/arm pressure index of 0.65 or lower should be considered pathological.

Clinical Use

UT/Arm Pressure Index. A reduced index indicates iliac artery obstruction; usually the lower the index, the more significant the obstructions. However, proximal obstruction of the superficial femoral artery may also cause a decrease in the UT/arm pressure index. It is therefore very useful to add a common femoral artery Doppler velocity examination (see below) to confirm or exclude iliac artery obstruction. A normal common femoral artery Doppler signal combined with a reduced UT/arm index virtually rules out hemodynamically significant iliac artery obstruction.

AK/Arm Pressure Index. A reduced AK/arm index in the presence of a normal UT/arm pressure index is strongly suggestive of superficial femoral artery stenosis. In the presence of an already reduced UT/arm index an additional reduction by at least 0.1 again points to an additional superficial femoral artery stenosis. A positive popliteal artery Doppler velocity finding (see below) represents strong confirmation of this conclusion. An AK/arm index of 0.6 or lower (with a normal UT/arm index) is usually the result of superficial femoral artery occlusion.

BK/Arm Pressure Index. Although a reduced BK/arm index (in the presence of a normal AK/arm index) should theoretically be an expression of popliteal artery obstruction, in reality it is usually caused by distal superficial femoral artery obstruction.

AA/Arm Pressure Index. As mentioned above, this is the most widely used pressure parameter. A normal ratio virtually rules out significant arterial occlusive disease, with three caveats, however: (a) there is no increase in arterial wall stiffness (e.g., in diabetes mellitus) which could cause erroneously normal pressure readings in the presence of decreased ankle pressure, (b) ankle pressure is normal at rest but drops with any type of stress test (e.g., exercise), and (c) ankle pressure ist normal, while toe pressure is reduced.

Toe/Arm Pressure Indes. A toe/arm pressure index of 0.65 or lower in the pressence of a normal AA/arm index suggests some obstructive disease either in the foot or the toes. A uniformly reduced toe/arm pressure index points to the former, but some toes yielding normal pressure and others reduced pressures suggests obstructive disease limited to specific toes.

Penile Arterial Blood Pressure Measurement. Impotence is believed to be related in more than 50 % of cases to impaired pelvic blood supply, especially to the penile arteries. In addition, information regarding penile hemodynamics, especially penile arterial blood pressure, helps in situations in which the intactness of the common iliac artery is questioned. The basic principle is, again, the oscillometric principle using either the photophlethysmographic or Doppler velocity signal as an oscillation monitor. Usually a 2.5-cm-wide bladder cuff is placed at the base of the penis, and the same criteria are used as described for segmental pressures (while decreasing the cuff pressure the first reliably identifiable signal corresponds to the systolic pressure). A penile/arm index of 0.8 or higher is considered normal, one of 0.6 or lower pathological, and one between these limits borderline. Kempczinski [1979] reported an age-related correlation and considered an index of 0.75 or higher to be normal in subjects aged over 40 years.

Potential Difficulties

The difficulties that man be encountered in measuring segmental pressures include the following:

- Increased arterial wall stiffness (Moenkenberg's disease): As mentioned above, this can cause falsely elevated pressure readings. Measurement at additional sites may help (BK and/or toe) because increased arterial wall stiffness is found most often at the ankle level.
- Cuff width: Strict adherence to a standard cuff size is very important; smaller cuff width results in erroneuously higher pressure readings.
- Rate of cuff pressure reduction: Too rapid reduction may lead to erroneously lower pressure readings. A rate of 3 mmHg/heartbeat offers reliable results.
- Inadequate accuracy of the manometer: The mercury manometer remains the most accurate pressure gauge, and if an aneroid type of gauge is used, it is advisable to compare it about every 6 months with a mercury manometer. If an electronic sensing device is used, the manufacturer's recommendations as to quality control should be strictly observed.
- Environmental temperature: Low ambient temperature leads to vasoconstriction, and this may affect particularly the smallest vessels and arteries of the toes. It is recommended that room temperature be kept as close as possible to 24 °C.

Flow Velocity (Doppler) Examination

Measurement Principles

As discussed in more detail in part I, section III. Doppler velocity determination uses the Doppler effect on reflected ultrasonic energy. The advantage of this method is its noninvasiveness. The relationship of the Doppler signal to flow velocity expressed by the well-known formula:

$$\Delta F = \frac{2\,f\,v\,\cos\varnothing}{c}$$

where $\triangle F$ is the Doppler-shifted frequency (difference between the transmitted and received frequency), f the transmitted frequency, v the blood flow velocity, $\varnothing$ the angle of the ultrasonic beam, and c the propagation speed of ultrasonic energy in biological tissues. This equation has several practical implications:

- $\triangle F$: Fortunately this frequency difference is within the ear's sensitivity range and is therefore easily detected.
- f: The higher the frequency, the higher is the attenuation, but the better the resolution. For peripheral arterial diagnostic the most useful frequencies are between 5 and 9 MHz.
- cos $\varnothing$: The angle of insonation is very important, and for all practical purposes the best results are obtained with a probe angle of about $60° \pm 10$. Although cos $0° = 1$, reducing the angle beyond a certain value causes a reduction in the recovered signal because less energy reaches the examined vessel.
- c: Propagation of ultrasonic energy is extremely reduced by air, and therefore water containing contrast gel is mandatory to secure optimal transmission conditions.

As a technical note it should be added that the Doppler-shifted signal is usually processed by using either the „zero-crossing" system or frequency analysis. Although a detailed analysis is beyond the scope of this chapter, it should be said that despite the many deficiencies of the zero-crossing method, because of its simplicity it is still the most widely used detection mode in most Doppler instruments. Frequency analysis is used mainly in the more expensive instruments, specifically in the duplex system.

Clinical Use

Doppler velocity signals are used on the basis of either acoustic response or recording the velocity signals. These are most often evaluated on the basis of qualitative changes – „pattern recognition," semiquantitatively or quantitatively.

Acoustic Analysis. Although the least reliable mode of evaluation, the simplest and therefore a still widely used mode is acoustic analysis. The absence of a Doppler velocity signal largely confirms the diagnosis of an occluded artery, with the exception of the dorsalis pedis artery, which is missing in about 10 % of young normal subjects.

A strong and a triphasic signal from the femoral and popliteal artery may rule out a hemodynamically significant obstruction in the respective arteries, while the posterior tibial artery may present with an adequate intensity and frequency (pitch) but with a missing negative component and can still be considered normal. The proper frequency (pitch), intensity, and presence or absence of the negative component can be judged with some training and is very helpful for a quick orientation under outpatient clinic conditions or at the bedside. Otherwise the recorded signal is always preferred, evaluated either semiquantitatively or quantitatively.

Semiquantitative Evaluation. Gosling and King [1974] introduced the pulsatility index which is the peak/mean velocity ratio. The advantage of this evaluation method is related to the fact that it does not require calibration since the numerator and denominator have the same units. The range of pulsatility index values for the common femoral artery is 5–10, and for the posterior tibial artery 7–15. The pulsatility index is useful in advanced cases of arterial occlusive disease, but its sensitivity is disappointing in light and moderate degrees of the disease. Inspection of the Doppler tracing (pattern recognition) is, again, helpful in advanced cases but is not informative enough in light cases of arterial occlusive disease. A triphasic common femoral and popliteal artery tracing (with a well-developed negative component) usually rules out significant obstruction in these arteries. On the other hand, biphasic and especially reduced tracing are strongly suggestive of significant obstruction in the respective arteries.

Quantitative Evaluation. The most accurate flow velocity determination can be accomplished with the duplex system, which takes into account the actual insonation angle and uses Fast Fourier Transform processing. The less expensive zero-crossing systems (see above), however, are most widely used for routine Doppler evaluation of the peripheral arterial system. The equipment can be calibrated using a 0.5 % Sephadex suspension or comparing the results with a duplex system. Since the actual angle of insonation is unknown, the principle of „maximum amplitude search" is recommended. The artery to be examined is first scanned horizontally (right to left and back) until the maximum amplitude is reached. At this point the angle of the Doppler probe is changed, again, until a maximum amplitude is reached. The same procedure is used during the calibration. In this case, after the maximum amplitude has been obtained, the position of the probe is locked in, and the flow velocity is controlled either by a screw clamp (if hydrostatic difference is used as a driving force) or by changing the pump speed [Thangavelu et al 1977]. Normal values have been established using an 8-MHz zero-crossing Doppler velocity system [Fronek et al 1976]. The most informative parameters seem to be peak velocity, decay time, and deceleration. Decay time has the advantage of not being dependent on calibration, being only time dependent (Fig. 1). A common femoral artery decay time longer than 200 ms can be considered borderline, while one longer than 230 ms reflects significant obstruction (Table 1). It should be noted that the velocity values obtained with the duplex system are significantly higher than those reported in Table 1. There are several reasons for this discrepancy. First, peak velocities obtained with the duplex system are usually expressed in „peak" values at the time of peak systole, while peak values obtained with nonimaging systems are the result of so-called zero-crossing systems which yield lower values. In addition, duplex devices usually employ a pulsed system, while most nonimaging instruments use the continuous wave system. It must be added, however, that these circumstances do not fully explain the difference. Systematic research is under way to clarify this discrepancy. In the meantime, two recommendations can be made: (a) use decay time, which is independent of calibration, and (b) determine normal control values with the equipment used in the respective laboratory.

Venous System

Noninvasive evaluation of the venous system is more complex than that of the arterial system because of the more complex functional anatomy. While the principal question in arterial pathology is generally the presence or absence of obstruction, the additional question of venous valvular insuffiency must be clarified in venous pathology. The combination of two methods is therefore recommended: one that examines outflow, i.e., to determine the presence or absence of outflow obstruction (deep venous thrombosis), and a second that determines the absence or presence of reflux in the venous system. In the past only a combination of Doppler velocity examination with some type of plethysmography could fulfill this requirement, but in recent years duplex venous scanning, as pioneered by Talbot [1982], competes very effectively. Duplex scanning of the venous system is discussed by Moneta and Porter (p. 163); the description below focuses on venous Doppler and venous plethysmography. Clinical indications for noninvasive evaluation of the venous system are the determination of the hemodynamic significance of varicose veins, incompetence of communicating veins, identification of venous valvular insufficiency, and thrombosis of the deep venous system.

Table 1. Normal values

	Peak forward velocity (cm/s)	Peak reverse velocity (cm/s)	Mean velocity (cm/s)	Decay time (ms)	Acceleration (cm/s^2)	Deceleration (cm/s^2)	Peak vel./ mean vel.	Accel./ Decel.
Femoral artery (n=78) extremities	40.7±10.9	6.5±3.6	9.8±5.3	163.8±40	353.0±113.1	250.0±60.0	4.8±1.6	1.4±0.2
Popliteal artery (n=72)	29.3± 5.9	10.2±2.9	4.4±2.3	157.3±48	263.1± 93	186.3±47.0	8.6±6.3	1.3±0.3
Posterior tibial artery (n=78)	16.0±10.0	2.0±2.3	4.0±3.5	124.0±52	145.0± 73.7	129.8±75.7	4.8±2.5	1.2±0.1
Dorsalis pedis artery	16.8± 5.7	1.3±2.2	3.4±1.6	127.6±45	160.5± 55.3	137.9±54.5	6.0±4.1	1.3±0.5

Mean ± SD; *n*, number of extremities.

Ultrasonic Arterial Velocity Profile

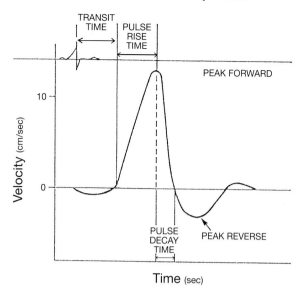

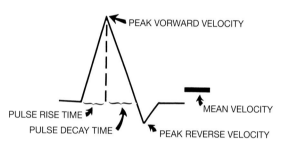

$$\text{ACCELERATION} = \frac{\text{PEAK VELOCITY}}{\text{PULSE RISE TIME}}$$

$$\text{DECELERATION} = \frac{\text{PEAK VELOCITY}}{\text{PULSE DECAY TIME}}$$

Fig. 1. Ultrasonic flow velocity pulse (typical for the femoral artery)

Doppler Examination

The method of venous Doppler examination is simple as to the equipment, but the learning curve is rather long (at least a few months) before reliable results can be expected. The absence of imaging represents, a significant drawback, which is compensated to some extent by the portability of the system. The most frequently used sites for this examination [Fronek 1989 b] are (a) the deep venous system: common femoral vein, popliteal vein, and posterior tibial vein; and (b) the superficial venous system: greater saphenous vein, lesser saphenous vein, and perforating (communicating) veins.

Test for Venous Obstructive Disease (Deep Vein Thrombosis)

Under normal conditions respiratory fluctuations of flow velocity in the common femoral vein are very pronounced, while significant outflow obstruction (e.g., iliac vein obstruction) diminishes these oscillations. Under extreme conditions there is a high-pitched, continuous velocity signal which usually indicates small collateral vessels. Absence of a velocity signal in the area of the assumed site of the common femoral vein of course confirms the diagnosis of common femoral vein occlusion.

Compression of the examined vein distal to the Doppler probe position (Fig. 2 b) elicits an increase in venous flow velocity, and it is helpful in all three veins representing the deep venous system: compression of the foot while monitoring the posterior tibial vein, compression of the calf while monitoring the popliteal vein, and compression of the thigh while monitoring the common femoral vein.

Test for Venous Valvular Insuffciency

Increased intra-abdominal pressure induced by the Valsalva maneuver is one of the most sensitive tests for examining the competency of the proxi-

a

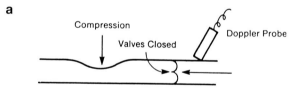

Test for Reflux

b

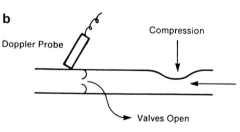

"Augmentation" Test

Fig. 2 a,b. Venous velocity signals and external compression. **a** Compression above the probe (valves closed, no reflux, normal). **b** Compression below the probe (augmentation, high velocity, no obstruction)

mal venous system. A continuous backflow during the Valsalva maneuver is a reliable sign of venous valvular insufficiency. Disappearance of backflow while compressing the long saphenous vein or thigh cuff inflation (18 cm wide and 20 mmHg pressure) or while applying a tourniquet suggests insufficiency of the long saphenous vein.

Figure 2a depicts the position of the Doppler probe and site of compression for examining the venous valvular system. In contrast to the test for venous obstructive disease, the site of compression is proximal to the position of the Doppler probe, i.e., the compression site is the calf if the posterior tibial vein is monitored, and the thigh is compressed while the popliteal vein is examined.

Plethysmography

Several types of plethysmography are currently available: air plethysmography, strain gauge plethysmography, photoplethysmography, impedance plethysmography, and foot volumetry.

Air Plethysmography

The old method of air plethysmography was given new impetus by the results of a series of studies from the St. Mary's Hospital group in London [Nicolaides et al 1989] which showed a high correlation with invasive venous pressure measurements. A combination of exercise and position tests documents both the capacity of the venous system and its efficiency in displacing blood from legs using a standardized exercise protocol. The test consists of two parts: (a) calf volume change due to orthostatics (90 % VV; from supine to erect position) and the time required to reach 90 % of calf filling (VFT 90). The average filling rate (venous filling index: VFI=90 % VV/VFT 90) is expressed in milliliters per second. In the second part of the test the patient is asked to tiptoe first one time and then ten times. The amount of displaced (or ejected) blood volume (EV) is recorded during the single tiptoe movement, and the ejection fraction is calculated as: EF=(EV/VV) x 100. The displacement after ten tiptoe movements yields the residual volume (RV). Finally, the residual volume fraction can be calculated as: RVT=(RV/VV) x 100. Both normal values and values for different degrees of venous insufficiency have been established, and it is recom-

mended to peruse, for details, the respective literature [Nicolaides et al, 1989]. Briefly, a VFT 90 of less than 20 confirms venous valvular insufficiency, which can be confirmed by a FVI greater than 3 while an RVF of more than 25 % reflects an inadequate venomuscular pump.

Strain Gauge Plethysmography

A silicon rubber tubing, originally filled with mercury [Whitney 1949] but now with gallium and indium, is used to record changes in calf volume induced by changes in leg position and exercise, similar to the tests described above. The ability to quantify the results is the major advantage of the method: however, the limited shelf-life of the older mercury-filled gauges and restriction of its use to the calf level have limited its widespread use.

Impedance Plethysmography

As noted above, impedance plethysmography is based on the close relationship of local blood volume and electrical impedance. Its application to diagnosis of the venous system is based on the relationship of venous capacitance measured by blocking the venous outflow for about 2 min and measuring the rate of outflow (after sudden cuff release), generally using the volume 2 or 3 s after cuff release [Wheeler and Anderson 1985]. This method has found wide acceptance principally in the United States and is highly sensitive to venous obstructive disease above the knee. Its main deficiency is in its lack of information regarding the venous valvular system.

Photoplethysmography

In contrast to its application in the arterial system, photoplethysmography in diagnosis of the venous system is used in the so-called d.c. (direct current) mode, i.e., recording the slow events induced by position and exercise tests, as described above. Photoplethysmography, popularized in recent years as „light reflection rheography", is used mainly to record local blood volume changes at the medial aspect of the ankle. The advantages of the method are the ruggedness of its sensors, ease of application, and high sensitivity to venous valvular insufficiency. The difficulty of signal calibration has until now been a significant drawback, but this has been overcome by the introduction of quantitative photoplethysmography either by manual calibration (changing the light intensity of the light source) or by using a computer-assisted compensation light of light-emitting diode intensity at a predetermined level at which the amplifying system begins to operate [Blazek et al 1989, Fronek et al 1992].

Foot Volumetry

Foot volumetry measures changes in foot volume induced by exercise (knee bending). These changes are recorded by monitoring the water level in an open container (the feet are immersed up to the ankle in a water bath). The relative ease of calibration and its ruggedness are significant advantages; however, one must accept an hygienic compromise when immersing the unprotected feet in a water bath.

Summary

The most practical of the above methods for detecting venous valvular insufficiency is the simple venous Doppler examination. Its combination with a tourniquet permits the approximate localization of incompetence, i.e., superficial or deep venous system. Plethysmography remains the method of choice for diagnosing deep venous thrombosis, and in view of the fact that air plethysmography also permits evaluation of venous valvular insufficiency, this method can be recommended for an overall evaluation of venous disease in a laboratory environment as long as the exact identification of the involved vein is not required. In the latter case, venous duplex scanning is the method of choice.

Cerebrovascular System

The most widely used method for examining the cerebrovascular system is duplex scanning using both B-mode and the Doppler system, as discussed in detail Steinke et al. (p. 97). In the past, before introduction of the duplex system, several methods were used, most of which can now be considered obsolete, with the exception of oculopneumoplethysmography, which offers some

quantitative hemodynamic information unique to this technique. The clinical indication is evaluation of the hemodynamic significance of contralateral collateral circulation.

Oculopneumoplethysmography is basically an oscillometric method for indirectly measuring ophthalmic artery pressure. This is achieved by recording the reappearance of eye volume pulses during a gradual reduction in intraocular pressure which is transiently increased by suction applied to the eyeball [Gee et al, 1982]. The lesion (generally internal carotid artery stenosis) is most likely of hemodynamic significance if the pressure difference is greater than 15 mmHg, or if the ophthalmic artery/brachial artery pressure ratio is under 0.66 [McDonald et al, 1979]. Although the method is noninvasive, the patient must be warned that at the height of suction a transient dimming of vision will occur. Failure to explain this can jeopardize the cooperation of the patient. The method was originally developed for use in conjuction with carotid artery compression in documenting the efficacy of collateral circulation, thus representing a substitute for preoperatively measured stump pressures [Gee et al, 1975]. Currently the method is most often used without compression to help in deciding whether to use a shunt during carotid endarterectomy.

Clinical Microcirculation

Clinical microcirculation has recently gained attention due to the adoption of methods previously used only in experimental microcirculation. It should be pointed out that some of these methods have not yet attained wide acceptance because of low correlation with pathological findings. The following discussion is therefore limited to methods of proven clinical diagnostic value. The clinical indications are evaluation of the state of perfusion of the skin with special reference to skin viability, optimal amputation level determination, collagen disease, Raynaud's syndrome, and vasodilator or vasoconstrictor effect of drugs.

Skin Thermometry

Skin temperature is a proven clinical indicator of skin perfusion. There is a virtually linear relationship between skin temperature and low or moderate skin blood flow. However, this relationship becomes nonlinear when high blood flows are evaluated (>28 °C skin temperature) [Felder et al. 1954].

Direct (Contact) Thermometry

In the past mainly thermocouples were used, placed in direct contact with the skin. Thermocouples consist of two different metals (e.g., copper and constantan) joined together; an increase in temperature causes increased voltage. The main disadvantage of thermocouples has been its relatively low sensitivity, which requires the addition of a stable DC amplifier, but the introduction of highly sensitive thermistors has made the high amplification superfluous. The principle of temperature sensitivity of thermistors is based on the temperature dependence of certain alloys. In contrast to most metals which have a positive thermal coefficient, thermistors are composed of mixtures of different metallic oxides that have a negative thermal coefficient, i.e., with increasing temperature the resistance decreases.

Liquid Crystals

Mixtures of certain cholesteric substances change color as a function of temperature [Selawry et al, 1966]. Sheets of plastics impregnated with these substances offer an inexpensive overview of temperature distribution in the examined area. This method is suited especially to monitoring, perfusion changes in the upper and lower extremities as a function of medical or surgical therapy.

Laser Doppler Flux Measurement

The selection of a narrow, monochromatic light source (laser) has made it possible to monitor red blood cell movement in the cutaneous capillary system. Similarly, as with the Doppler-shifted signals obtained by insonation of relatively large vessels with ultrasound, the network of cutaneous microvessels is the target of laser light, and the resulting Doppler-shifted signals are fairly highly related to flow velocities in the cutaneous microcirculation [Stern 1975, Watkins and Holloway 1978, Nilsson et al 1980]. The output from the commercially available systems, however is related to the product of average velocity and local hematocrit, termed flux. Although the variability (in sites and time) is not insignificant [Tenland et al 1983], this method is superbly suited to monitoring relative changes in skin perfusion due to its noninvasiveness, ease of operation, and continuous (uninterrupted) output. The absence of calibratability may be a negative factor under some conditions; however changes during postocclusive reactive hyperemia or due to temperature changes can be conveniently recorded [Ninet and Fronek 1985 a, b].

Capillaroscopy

Static Capillaroscopy

Static capillaroscopy is performed best with the subject in the sitting position and the hand positioned at heart level (to minimize the effects of phlebostatics). The nailfold of the finger or toe is the best site of observation, and the examination is conducted first with a microscope at low magnification (x 12) and then with a wide-field lens [Maricq 1970]. This permits a rapid overview of the microvascular pattern and is usually followed by a more detailed evaluation using a higher magnification (x 25 or 50). Fagrell has emphasized the potential importance of this method by introducing a classification of the microscopic pattern [Fagrell 1973, Bollinger and Fagrell 1990]. Mahler [1981] recommends the use of a conventional ophthalmoscope, and a magnification of x 10 can be achieved with a 40-diopter built-in lens. While this method does not permit detailed analysis of red blood cell movement, the optical field provides an overview of the microvascular network and the qualitative changes in capillary blood flow, which can help in some diagnostic alternatives, such as Raynaud's syndrome.

Dynamic Capillaroscopy

The combination of video monitoring and microscopy in conjunction with electronic evaluation of recorded red blood cell movement makes it possible to record red blood cell velocity and flow rate (including capillary dimensions) [Bollinger et al 1974, Fagrell et al 1977]. The introduction of computer analysis has brought this technique closer to clinical application [Fagrell et al 1988].

Transcutaneous Po₂ Measurement

Although reduced transcutaneous Po_2 may be observed in patients with significant peripheral arterial occlusive disease [Franzeck et al 1982, Matsen et al 1980], the most useful application of this method is in optimizing the level of amputation. It has been shown that transcutaneous Po_2 values below a certain level preclude a per primam amputation stump healing. Some authors set the critical value at 30 mmHg [Burgess et al 1982] and others at 10 mmHg [Franzeck et al 1982]. The response to oxygen inhalation [Harward et al, 1985, Oishi et al 1988] seem to increase the reliability of this test: a failure of transcutaneous Po_2 to increase above 10 mmHg after 5 min of 100 % O_2 exposure reflects very poor skin viability, incompatible with an amputation stumpf healing.

Summary

Of the methods described above, transcutaneous Po_2 determination is the method of choice for optimal amputation level determination. Laser Doppler flux measurement is the most practical one for evaluating the efficacy of vasoactive drugs, while skin temperature measurement offers the most convenient method for documenting inflammation.

References

Blazek V, Schmitt HJ, Schultz-Ehrenburg U, Kerner J: Digitale Photoplethysmographie (D-PPG) fur die Beinvenendiagnostik. Phlebol und Proktol 18: 91, 1989.

Bollinger A, Fagrell B: Clinical capillaroscopy. Huber Publisher, Toronto, 1990.

Bollinger A, Butti P, Barras JP, Trachsler H, Siegenthaler W: Red blood cell velocity in nailfold capillaries of man measured by a television microscopy technique. Microvasc Res 7: 61, 1974.

Brakkee AJM, Vendrik AJH: Strain-gauge plethysmography: theoretical and practical notes on a new design. J Appl Physiol 21: 701, 1966.

Burgess Em, Matsen FA, Wyss CR, Simmons CW: Segmental transcutaneous measurements of Po₂ in patients requiring below-the-knee amputation for peripheral vascular insufficiency. J Bone Joint Surg 64A: 378, 1982.

Fagrell B: Vital capillary microscopy. Scand J Clin Lab Invest (Suppl) 133, 1973.

Fagrell B, Eriksson SE, Malmstrom S, Sjolund A: Computerized data analysis of capillary blood cell velocity. Int J Microcirc Clin Exp 7: 276, 1988.

Fagrell B, Fronek A, Intaglietta M: A microscope television system for studying flow velocity in human skin capillaries. Am J Physiol 233: H318, 1977.

Felder D, Russ E, Montgomery H, Horwitz O: Relationship in the toe of skin surface temperature to mean blood flow measured with a plethysmograph. Clin Sci 12: 251, 1954.

Franzeck U, Talke P, Bernstein EF, Golbranson FL, Fronek A: Transcutaneous Po₂ measurements in health and peripheral arterial occlusive disease. Surgery 91: 156, 1982.

Fronek A: Noninvasive diagnostics in vascular disease. Mc Graw-Hill, New York, pp 88 a, 129 b, 1989.

Fronek A, Coel M, Bernstein EF: Quantitative ultrasonographic studies of lower extremity flow velocities in health and disease. Circulation 53: 953, 1976.

Fronek A, Blazek V, Bundens WP: Quantitative photoplethysmography, physiologic and clinical implications. IN: Fortschritte in der computerunterstützten nichtinvasiven Gefäßdiagnostik. 3rd Intl Symp CNVD 1991, VDI Verlag Publ. Düsseldorf, 1992.

Gee W: Ocular pneumoplethysmography. IN Noninvasive diagnostic techniques in vascular disease. 2nd edition, (EF Bernstein ed), Mosby, St. Louis, pg 220, 1982.

Gee W, Mehigan JT, Wylie EJ: Measurement of collateral cerebral hemispheric blood pressure by ocular pneumoplethysmography. Am J Surg 130: 121, 1975.

Harward T, Volny J, Goldbranson F, Bernstein EF, Fronek A: Oxygen inhalation-induced transcutaneous Po₂ changes as a predictor of amputation level. J Vasc Surg 2: 220, 1985.

Hertzman AB, Spealman CR: Observations on the finger volume pulse recorded photoelectrically. Am J Physiol 119: 334, 1937.

Hokanson DE, Sumner DS, Strandness DE Jr: An electrically calibrated plethysmograph for direct measurement of limb blood flow. IEEE Trans Biomed Engr BME 22: 25, 1975.

Holzer W, Polzer K, Marko A: Rheokardiographie. W Maudrich, Vienna 1945.

Huch A, Lübbers DW, Huch R: Quantitative continuous measurement of partial oxygen pressure on the skin of adults and newborn babies. Pflüg Arch Ges Physiol 337: 185, 1972.

Kempczinski RF: Role of the vascular diagnostic laboratory in the evaluation of male impotence. Am J Surg 138: 278, 1979.

Mahler F: Kapillarmikroskopie mit dem Augenspiegel. VASA 10: 180, 1981.

Maricq HR: „Wide-field" photography of nailfold capillary bed and a scale of plexus visualization scores (PVS). Microvasc Res 2: 335, 1970.

Matsen FA III, Wyss CR, Pedegana LR, Kruguire RB Jr, Simmons CW, King RV, Burgess EM: Transcutaneous oxygen tension measurement in peripheral vascular disease. Surg Gynecol Obstet 150: 525, 1980.

McDonald KM, Gee W, Kaupp HA, Bast RG: Screening for significant carotid stenosis by ocular pneumoplethysmography. Am J Surg 137: 1441, 1979.

Nicolaides AN, Christopoulos D, Vadekis S: Progress in the investigation of chronic venous insufficiency. Ann Vasc Surg 3: 278, 1989.

Nilsson GE, Tenland T, Oberg PA: A new instrument for continuous measurement of tissue blood flow by light beating spectroscopy. IEEE Trans Biomed Engr BME 27: 12, 1980.

Ninet J, Fronek A: Laser Doppler flux monitored cutaneous response to local cooling and heating. VASA 14: 38, 1985 a.

Ninet J, Fronek A: Cutaneous post-occlusive reactive hyperemia monitored by laser Doppler flux metering and skin temperature. Microvasc Res 30: 125, 1985 b.

Nyboer J: Electrical impedance plethysmograph. IN: Medical physics. (O Glaser ed), Year Book, Chicago p. 340, 1994.

Oishi C, Fronek A, Goldbranson F: The role of noninvasive vascular studies in determining levels of amputation. J Bone Join Surg 70: 1520, 1988.

Raines JK: The pulse volume recorder in peripheral arterial disease. IN: Noninvasive Diagnostic techniques in vascular disease. 3rd ed. (EF Bernstein ed), Mosby, St. Louis, p 563, 1985.

Raines JK: Diagnosis and analysis of arteriosclerosis in the lower limbs from the arterial pressure pulse. Doctoral Thesis MIT, Cambridge MA, 1972.

Selawry OS, Selawry HS, Holland JF: Use of liquid cholesteric crystals for thermographic measurement of skin temperature in man. Mol Cryst 1: 495, 1966.

Stern MD: In vivo evaluation of microcirculation by coherent light scattering. Nature 524: 46, 1975.

Talbot SR: Use of real-time imaging in identifying deep venous obstruction. A preliminary report. Bruit 6: 41, 1982.

Tenland T, Salerud EG, Nilsson GE, Oberg PA: Spatial and temporal variations in human skin blood flow. In J Microcirc Clin Exp 2: 81, 1983.

Thangavelu M, Fronek A, Morgan R: Simple calibration of doppler velocity metering. Proc San Diego Biomed Symp 16: 1, 1977.

Watkin DW, Holloway GA Jr: An instrument to measure cutaneous blood flow using the doppler shift of laser light. IEEE Trans Biomed Engr BME 25: 28, 1978.

Wheeler HB, Anderson FA Jr: The diagnosis of venous thrombosis by impedance plethysmography. IN: Noninvasive diagnostic techniques in vascular disease. 3rd ed. (EF Bernstein ed), Mosby, St. Louis, p 805, 1985.

Whitney RJ: The measurement of changes in human limb volume by means of a mercury-in-rubber strain gauge. J Physiol (London) 109: 5, 1949.

Winsor T: Clinical plethysmography. I. An improved direct writing plethysmograph. Angiology 4: 134, 1953.

Section II
Metabolic Vascular Diagnostics

Diagnostics of Lipids and Lipoproteins

H. Wieland, W. März, and M. Nauck

Introduction

Lipid diagnostics are primarily concerned with the major serum lipids, cholesterol, and triglycerides. Since these molecules are highly hydrophobic, they are transported in the serum in macromolecular complexes of lipids and proteins, called lipoproteins. The principle lipoproteins are low-density lipoprotein (LDL), high-density lipoprotein (HDL), very low density lipoprotein (VLDL), and chylomicrons.

Serum lipoproteins differ with regard to their composition, size, and physicochemical properties (Table 1). All lipoproteins contain triglycerides, cholesterol, cholesteryl esters, and phospholipids. The relative amounts of these lipids, however, vary considerably. During protein electrophoresis the serum lipoproteins do not migrate with the same mobility but form three distinct bands. The HDLs migrate with α-1 mobility, the VLDLs exhibit α-2 mobility, and the LDLs are the β-lipoproteins. Only the albumin fraction and the γ-globulins are lipid free.

These differences in electrophoretic mobility served some 25 years ago as the basis for the new classification system of hyperlipidemias introduced by Fredrickson et al. [120–124]. To each hyperlipidemia it was possible to assign a specific electrophoretic serum lipoprotein pattern. The increased lipoprotein could be clearly identified by an unusually intensely stained band (chylomicrons, β-lipoproteins, and pre-β-lipoproteins) or by unusual elecrophoretic mobility (β-VLDL).

The lipid concentration in the serum repesents the sum of concentrations of the individual lipoprotein classes. Different lipoproteins differ considerably in their atherogenicity. The serum concentrations of lipoproteins provide only a static picture, and do not reflect the complex dynamics of lipoprotein metabolism. Both proteins and lipids are exchanged between the different lipoprotein fractions; therefore the structure of serum lipoproteins is subject to constant metabolic remodeling [109, 171].

Why Perform Lipoprotein Determinations?

Serum lipids and lipoproteins are causally related to the development of atherosclerotic lesions [59, 61, 208]. Successful attempts to arrest or even reverse atherogenesis have been documented in a number of interventional studies. Since lipopro-

Table 1. Characteristics of lipoproteins

	Density (kg/l)	Electrophoretic mobility	Particle diameter (nm)	Composition (% mass)				
				TG	FC	CE	PL	Pr
Chylomicrons	<0.95	–	>1000	90	1	3	4	2
VLDL	<1.006	Pre-β	55	55	7	12	18	8
IDL	1.006–1.019	Pre-β to β	25	29	6	23	24	18
LDL	1.019–1.063	β	20	5	9	41	24	21
Lp(a)[a]	1.080–1.100	Pre-β	24	2	9	38	15	24
HDL₂	1.063–1.125	α	11	3	4	19	28	46
HDL₃	1.125–1.210	α	9	2	2	14	20	62

TG, triglycerides; FC, free cholesterol; CE, cholesterol esters; PL, phospholipids; Pr, protein.
[a] Carbohydrate content of 12%.

tein disorders can be effectively treated, lipoprotein diagnostics have become an essential component of vascular diagnostics.

Biochemistry of Lipids and Lipoproteins

Structure and Function of Serum Lipids (Cholesterol and Triglycerides)

The diagnostically relevant lipids are cholesterol and the triglycerides. Cholesterol occurs in the serum mostly as cholesteryl esters (70 % – 89 %), and the cells contain mostly free cholesterol (Fig. 1). In the cholesteryl esters the free OH-group of cholesterol is esterified to a long-chain fatty acid. The esters are insoluble in water and can be transported in the serum only if they are protected from the water by a coat of phospholipid molecules. The polar head groups of phospholipids form hydrogen bonds with the water molecules. The fatty acid chain interacts hydrophobically with the unpolar lipids in the core. By these mechanisms a spherical particle is formed which presents its outer polar surface to the serum water and contains a core of water-insoluble lipids. Unesterified cholesterol has similar physicochemical properties to phospholipids and becomes part of the surface monolayer, the hydroxyl group being exposed to the water.

Cholesterol and other isoprenoids are essential cell components. Nearly all animal tissues are able to synthesize cholesterol from activated acidic acid (acetyl CoA). A 70-kg man produces about 1 g cholesterol/day. The rate-limiting step of cholesterol biosynthesis is the reduction of β-hydroxy-β-methyl-glutaryl CoA (HMG CoA) into mevalonate, catalyzed by the HMG CoA-reductase located in the smooth endoplasmic reticulum.

In the triglycerides the long-chain fatty acids are esterified with the three free hydroxyl groups of glycerol (Fig. 1). Of the biomolecules triglycerides have the highest energy content per mole. Therefore their major purpose is storage and transport of energy. In order to utilize the energy the fatty acids have to be enzymatically released by different lipases. The lipase present in the adipose tissue is activated by phosphorylation via a cAMP-dependent protein kinase and is therefore called hormone-sensitive lipase. The lipase active in the blood is normally not present in the blood but immobilized at the surface of blood capillaries in muscle and adipose tissue. A special lipase is attached to the sinusoids of the liver (see below). The lipoprotein lipases can be released from the capillaries by heparin.

These so-called lipoprotein lipases (LPLs) „catch" passing triglyceride-rich particles, punch a little hole in the phospholipid monolayer and then hydrolyze the triglycerides in the core of the particles. In order to be caught and attacked by the lipase of the capillaries, the particles have to be equipped with special surface proteins. These proteins, present in the particles, are called apolipoproteins or apoproteins.

Structure and Function of Lipoproteins

The major apolipoproteins of triglyceride-rich lipoproteins are apo-C, apo-E, and apo-B. The

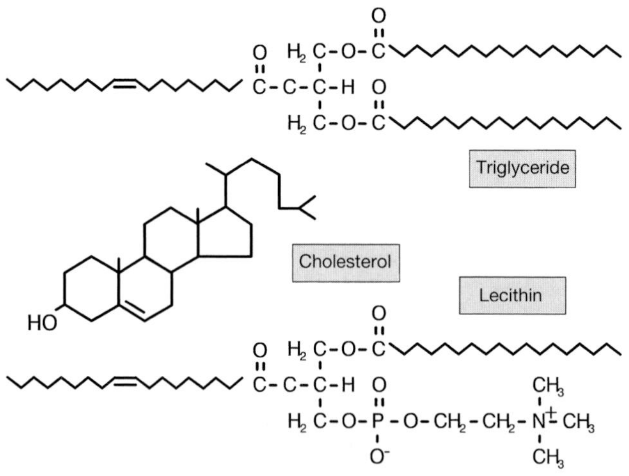

Fig. 1. Structure of serum lipids

chylomicrons contain a truncated apo-B. Apo-C consists of three different small peptides. Only the biological role of one of them is firmly established (apo-C-II, see below).

Without the apolipoproteins the „little fatballs" of lipoproteins would be metabolized only randomly mainly by the reticuloendothelial system. Apolipoproteins regulate the constant remodeling of the lipoprotein particles by activation or inhibition of enzymes (apo-C-II activates the LPL). This remodeling exposes ligands to specific cell surface receptors or changes their conformation in such a way that they can be recognized by the receptor and taken up by the cell. Most lipoproteins are eliminated from the circulation at a specific state of their metabolism by cellular uptake. The triglyceride component of the particles originates either from the intestine or it is synthesized by the liver. Intestinal triglycerides are formed from dietary lipids and become part of the chylomicrons, the liver synthesizing triglycerides preferentially from long-chain fatty acids. These reach the liver from the adipose tissue bound to albumin and leave it as components of VLDL. Chylomicrons and VLDLs are both triglyceride-rich but also contain cholesterol. Therefore marked hypertriglyceridemia is always accompanied by hypercholesterolemia. Chylomicrons consist of up to over 90 % triglycerides, VLDL only up to 50 %. The LDL lipids are mainly cholesteryl esters, and 20 % of the LDL is protein. Hypercholesterolemia without hypertriglyceridemia is almost always due to elevated LDL. One-half of the HDL is protein; the core lipids triglycerides and cholesteryl esters make up 5 % and 10 %, respectively. The contribution of the HDL concentration to the serum cholesterol level is about 20 % – 30 %.

Low-density lipoproteins contain mostly apo-B-100. The major apolipoproteins of HDL are A-I (ligand for receptors and activator of LCAT) and A-II (function still unknown). In addition, the HDLs contain most other apolipoproteins, even traces of apo-B.

In the fasting state the concentration of serum triglycerides reflects mainly the concentration of VLDLs. The contribution of LDLs and HDLs is about 40 mg/dl. Postprandially the triglycerides of a healthy person increase not more than about 100 mg/dl, even after an oral fat load. The triglyceride level is the result of both absorptive (rather complicated production of chylomicrons in the mucosal cell) and catabolic processes (LPL activity). Both activities last several hours. Only 12 h

after the last meal, the blood is free of chylomicrons, therefore triglycerides should be determined only after fasting for 12 h. Since the chylomicrons contain very little cholesterol (2 % – 3 %), the blood cholesterol can be determined at any time.

Lipoprotein Metabolism

In Figs. 2 and 3 an overview of lipoprotein metabolism has been presented. The half-life of chylomicrons in the blood is approximately 1 h [155]. After prolonged exposure to LPL the core of a chylomicron shrinks considerably and the surface becomes much too large and loses some of its components [102]. These components are lipids together with proteins and are considered to be lipoproteins (HDL-2, see below). They are devoid of triglycerides and contain mostly protein and phospholipids, a characteristic feature of HLDs. These split products associate again with nascent triglyceride-rich lipoproteins from the ductus thoracicus or the liver [171] and are cleaved off again after the processing of the particle by the LPL. Their major function is the activation of LPL (C-II [344]) and the protection of the nascent particle against premature elimination by the liver (C-III) [446].

After hydrolysis of the core and loss of surface constituents the chylomicron is called a remnant particle (CM remnant). It still contains all of the cholesterol of the chylomicron and is further enriched with cholesteryl esters [63, 103, 299, 333]. The CM remnants are removed rapidly from the circulation by the liver, most probably via a specific receptor [51, 193, 195, 358].

Inside the liver cell the taken up cholesterol causes a series of intracellular reactions all designed to keep the intracellular free cholesterol content low. These reactions include the inactivation of β-hydroxy-β-methyl (HMG-)CoA reductase, the key enzyme of cholesterol biosynthesis, the reesterification of the free cholesterol (acyl-CoA-cholesterol-acyltransferase, ACAT; [386]), and, most importantly, the down-regulation of cell surface receptors responsible for elimination of LDLs from the bloodstream (LDL-R, see below). This negative feedback regulation is achieved at the transcriptional level and can be visualized as follows: If the cholesterol content of the cell is low, an unknown transcription factor binds to the gene and facilitates transcription. If the cholesterol content is high, sterols bind to a

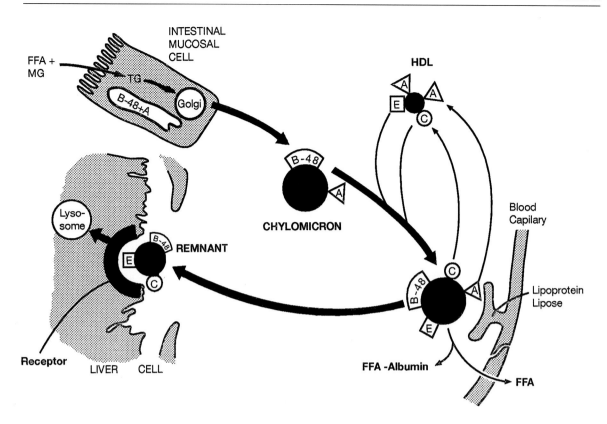

Fig. 2. Pathway for transport of dietary triglyceride and cholesterol, showing the two steps in chylomicron metabolism following secretion of nascent chylomicrons from intestinal mucosal cells. (Modified from [172a], with permission from W.B. Saunders, Philadelphia)

sterol-binding protein (SBP), change its conformation, and cancel the effect of the positive transcription factor, resulting in a blocked transcription of the gene [149, 279, 298].

In Western societies normally approximately 140 g fat/day is ingested. All this fat reaches the bloodstream in the form of chylomicrons, the amount of chylomicron cholesterol reaching the liver per day being equivalent to 9–14 eggs (2.8–4.2 g). It is easy to understand that the LDL-R of the liver is downregulated considerably by this daily cholesterol load. Dietary fat therefore blocks the uptake of blood cholesterol. Since the cholesterol of the nascent chylomicrons can be derived not only from dietary cholesterol but also from the biliary cholesterol already present in the intestinum or from de novo synthesis by the mucosal cells, it does not matter whether the dietary fat contains cholesterol at all. The mucosal cells also express LDL receptors and do not have to synthesize all the cholesterol.

Also the triglyceride-rich particles originating from the liver, the VLDLs, are processed by the LPL. In contrast to nascent chylomicrons, nascent VLDLs contain apo-B-100 and apo-C [388]. Their intravasal metabolism is similar to that of chylomicrons. Their half-life in the blood is about 4 h [202].

The metabolism of the VLDL remnants is somewhat more complicated than that of the CM remnants. They are either taken up by the liver or converted to LDLs [44, 52, 128, 140, 172, 357, 371]. This conversion is not well understood. Most probably it occurs in the bloodstream by the action of another LPL (hepatic triglyceride hydrolase, HTGL), situated in sinusoids of the liver. This enzyme deprives the VLDL remnants or intermediate density lipoproteins (LDLs) further of their triglycerides on their way to LDLs. This conversion is supposedly facilitated by apolipoprotein-E [254, 405]. A deficiency of HTGL leads to an impaired catabolism of IDL and to the formation of β-VLDLs (see below) [76]. In this case IDLs and HDLs contain more triglycerides than usual [14, 77]. It is not clear whether all LDL particles are derived from the triglyceride-rich precursors. A direct secretion of LDL particles

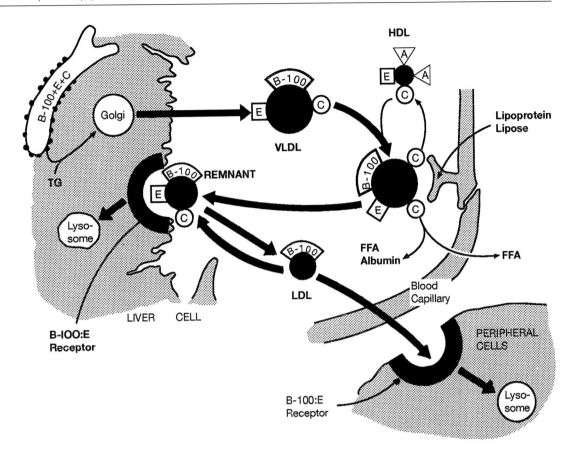

Fig. 3. Summary of the steps of VLDL metabolism, showing the similarity of the first step between VLDL and chylomicron metabolism and the partial divergence of the subsequent processing of VLDL remnants to form LDL, which, unlike CM remnants, is catabolized both in the liver and in peripheral cells. (From [172a], with permission from W.B. Saunders, Philadelphia)

from the liver is possible [43, 191, 192, 280, 288, 343, 371, 396, 442].

Intermediate density lipoproteins are, however, not the only substrate of the hepatic lipase. Also relatively light and triglyceride-rich HDLs interact with HTGL. Their triglycerides have been transferred to them by an intravasal modeling process catalyzed by a special cholesteryl ester transfer protein (CETP) [22, 88, 102, 110, 294, 315]. This protein delivers triglycerides in exchange for cholesteryl esters between lipoproteins. The cholesteryl esters have been formed on HDL particles as a workbench as a component of a metabolic pathway designated „reverse cholesterol transport" (Fig. 4).

The liver is the only organ designed to excrete cholesterol from the body [49]. It does so by excreting cholesterol into the bile either unchanged or transformed into bile acids. Cholesterol therefore has to be transported from the peripheral tissues to the liver. The first step is the transfer of free cholesterol from endothelial cell membranes to HDLs [142, 295, 339, 354]. The HDL particles are either spherical HDLs or disk-like HDLs synthesized in the intestinal mucosa or derived from the constituents of triglyceride-rich particles. Following the uptake the cholesterol is esterified and the HDL particles increase in size and decrease in density [294]. For the esterification, lecithin:cholesterol acyltransferase (LCAT) is responsible, activated by apolipoprotein A-I [18, 276, 370]. LCAT transfers to the hydroxyl group of the free cholesterol fatty acids from the HDL phospholipids. The newly formed cholesteryl esters are then removed from the surface of the particle. This is achieved either by hiding them in the core or transferring them to triglyceride-rich particles [23, 103, 110]. During the incorporation of cholesteryl esters the disks are converted into spheres [143, 164]. The „blown-up" HDL particles acquire

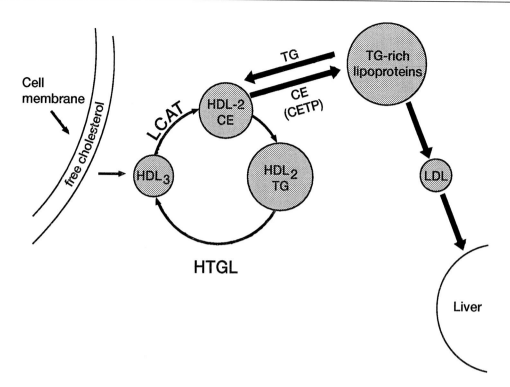

apo-E and travel rather slowly to the liver [264]. CETP transfers cholesteryl esters from and delivers triglycerides to the HDL particle. These triglyceride-enriched particles are regenerated by HTGL, in order to be able to accommodate another cholesterol molecule from endothelial cells or macrophages. The ability to accept cholesterol is also present in disk-like particles, precursors of HDL [47]. The intestinal mucosa may be a major source of HDL precursors but cannot synthesize A-II [194].

The mechanisms by which the disks and the regenerated HDL particles absorb free cholesterol from the membranes of peripheral cells are poorly understood. The particles probably interact with the presumptive HDL receptors (HDL-Rs). These receptors also bind apo-E-free HDL and therefore can be distinguished from the LDL-Rs and the LRP (see below). The expression of these receptors can be stimulated by preincubation with cholesterol [294]. Their major function is the translocation of free cholesterol from intracellular pooles to the cell surface. They presumably work via G proteins and protein kinase C [274, 275, 397]. The transfer of cholesterol to extracellular acceptors follows a concentration gradient [207].

The processes mediated by LCAT, HTGL, and CETP lead to two main HDL fractions: HDL-2 and HDL-3. The difference between HDL-2 and

Fig. 4. Reverse cholesterol transport

HDL-3 is the smaller size and the higher content of apo-A-II of HDL-3. HDL-2s are generated from HDL-3s by the incorporation of cholesteryl esters (LCAT). The cholesteryl esters are then exchanged with triglycerides (CETP) and the triglyceride-rich HDL-2s are reconverted to HDL-3 by the hydrolysis of the triglycerides (HTGL). HDL-2s and HDL-3s differ possibly in their vasoprotective properties. Although HDL-3s remove cellular cholesterol more avidly than HDL-2s [294], epidemiological studies suggest that it is the HDL-2 fraction which exhibits protective effects [152, 252]. The HDL-2 concentration bears a direct relationship to the ability of an individual to metabolize triglyceride-rich particles [157, 315]. Therefore perhaps the HDL cholesterol concentrations mainly reflect the ability to dispose of triglyceride-rich particles, which may be rendered more atherogenic by CETP because of being in the blood for a longer time.

If CETP transfers the newly formed cholesteryl esters from HDL to CM remnants, the transferred cholesteryl esters usually immediately end up in the liver together with the remnants. If the acceptor is a VLDL particle, the cholesteryl esters become part of an IDL particle. The further fate of the IDL (conversion into LDL or uptake in the liver) depends on the nature and amount of specific apolipoproteins present on the particle (apo-E and apo-C-III) and on the degree of the expression of LDL-Rs on the surface of liver cells). Since the cholesteryl esters cannot leave the particle, the esterification provides an efficient way of cholesterol targeting to the liver for removal. The excretion of the steroid ring occurs as already mentioned either unchanged as cholesterol or as bile acid. Bile acids are reabsorbed in terminal ileum and reach the liver via the portal vein; cholesterol is reabsorbed after a fat-containing meal and returns as part of a chylomicron. The only tissues capable of utilizing cholesterol are those able to produce lipoproteins or bile acids and the gonad and adrenal glands. The half-life of LDL in the blood is approximately 2 days [202, 233, 359, 383].

Receptors and Ligands (Apolipoproteins)

The serum concentrations of lipoproteins depend critically on the extent of receptor-lipoprotein interactions. In this process not only the receptors play a critical role but also the ligands, especially apolipoprotein E and apolipoprotein B. In order to understand the processes regulating the concentrations of serum lipoproteins, we have to briefly discuss the ligands and then the receptors.

Ligands (Apolipoproteins)

The structure and function of the major apolipoproteins is presented in Table 2. The most important ligands of atherogenic lipoproteins are apo-B and apo-E. Since it is not clear whether apo-A is also a ligand and the HDL receptor is still putative, they will not be discussed in this context.

Apolipoprotein E. Triglyceride-rich lipoproteins contain in addition to apo-C and apo-B an additional apolipoprotein, apo-E. This multifunctional protein greatly facilitates the hepatic uptake of particles too small to be further attacked by the LPL. It interacts with two diffeent receptors, the LDL receptor and the LDL receptor related protein (see later). Apo-E is a well-characterized 34-kDa glycoprotein [327]. cDNA and the structure of the gene are known [305]. Apo-E is responsible for the uptake of CM remnants in the liver and for the catabolism of VLDL remnants [27, 222, 235, 384]. It facilitates the intravasal conversion of IDLs to LDLs and plays a major role in the uptake of apo-E-containing HDLs in the liver. More than 90% of the apo-E found in the blood originates from the liver [224]. Apo-E mRNA is found in many different tissues and cell types.

Apo-E occurs in three different forms which fulfill their tasks quite differently. This is due to the different distribution of arginine and cysteine residues to different positions of the polypeptide chain. The interaction with cell surface receptors

Table 2. Structure and function of apolipoproteins

Apo	M_r (kDa)	Synthesis	Function
A-I	28 331	Intestine, liver	LCAT activation, receptor binding
A-II	8 707	Liver	Cofactor of HTGL and LCAT (?)
A-IV	46 000	Intestine	LCAT activation
(a)	250–700		?
B-100	512 937	Liver	Receptor binding
B-48	275 000	Intestine	Structural protein
C-I	6 550	Liver	Cofactor of LCAT and LPL
C-II	8 837	Liver	Activation of LPL
C-III	8 240	Liver	Inhibitor of LPL and clearance remnant
D	32 500	?	?
E	34 145	Liver	Receptor binding, LCAT activation

LCAT, lecithin, cholesterol, acyltransferase; LPL, lipoprotein lipase; HTGL, hepatic triglyceride lipase.

is most effective when position 112 and position 156 are also occupied by arginine (E4). Cysteine at both positions abolishes the interaction (E2). The most common situation is cysteine at position 112 and arginine at position 156 (E3). Since all three allele genes of the apo-E locus are expressed, six different phenotypes can arise. For each isoform of apo-E there are homozygous and heterozygous individuals. Homozygosity for the inefficient ligand is a prerequisite for type III hyperlipoproteinemia (see below). The serum cholesterol concentration correlates with the sum of the suffixes of apo-E (the concentration is highest at E4/E4).

Apolipoprotein B. Apolipoprotein B is the major structural protein of LDLs. Since these are mainly derived from VLDLs via IDLs, these lipoproteins also contain apo-B. Lp(a) (see below) also contains apo-B. The primary structure of apo-B has been established by several groups [68, 72, 214, 247]. The gene for apo-B is 43 kb long and consists of 29 exons [37, 213]. The mRNA for apo-B is found in both the liver and the intestine. The apo-B from the intestine is, however, truncated, lacking the C-terminal half, which is necessary for the interaction with the LDL-Rs. In contrast to the hepatic apo-B (apo-B-100), the truncated apo-B is called apo-B-48. Its mRNA is derived from the mRNA of apo-B-100 by a modification of an already existing mRNA for apo-B-100 by posttranslational modification [42, 69, 86, 95, 321]. In humans this editing takes place only in the intestine and not in the liver. Triglyceride-rich lipoproteins from the gut (chylomicrons and CM remnants) are therefore recognized by the LDL-Rs if at all via their apo-E content. Differences in the sequence have so far been found for more than 75 positions. Some of these polymorphisms are possibly connected with the concentration of LDL cholesterol or even with coronary artery disease (CAD) (see below) [1, 2, 34, 175, 246, 285, 326, 393, 401, 448].

Of clinical importance is the position 3500. A mutation at this position leads to an autosomal dominant condition with a markedly lower (80%) affinity of apo-B to the LDL-Rs (familial defective apo-B-100, FDB) [197, 262]. The low affinity is due to a substitution of glutamine for arginine at position 3500.

Lipoprotein Receptors

The first lipoprotein receptor, the LDL receptor (LDL-R), was described in the early 1970s by Brown and Goldstein [51]. Since then more members of the gene family of the LDL-Rs have been identified: the *gp* 330 [204, 296, 330], an extrahepatic receptor for β-VLDL [398], and the LDL-R-related protein (LRP) [178]. Scavenger receptors are responsible for the elimination of modified lipoproteins.

Low-Density Lipoprotein Receptor. Brown and Goldstein demonstrated that LDLs are bound with a high affinity to the surface of cultured fibroblasts and subsequently internalized and degraded by these cells. The interaction of LDLs with the cell surface showed all the characteristics of a receptor-mediated binding: specificity, high affinity, and saturability.

The LDL-R plays the most important role in the regulation of the LDL cholesterol level. Since it recognizes apo-B-100 as well as apo-E it is more precisely called apo-B-100:E-receptor. It is one of the best-characterized receptors [387]. Defects of the apo-B-100:E-receptor lead to the classical form of familial hypercholesterolemia. Our detailed knowledge of the structure of the apo-B-100:E-receptor stems from cell biological research, the investigation of many naturally occurring mutants, and most recently from experiments based on site-directed mutagenesis.

The LDL-R consists of five different domains. The amino terminus is the ligand-binding domain. It is cysteine rich and consists of seven homologous stretches (complement-type repeats). The positions of the cysteines have been well conserved during evolution. All cystein residues are involved in intramolecular disulfide bridges. Binding of apo-B and apo-E to the repeats is achieved through a cluster of negatively charged amino acids (glutamate and aspartate). Receptor and ligands are internalized into endosomes via coated pits. Within the endosomes a proton pump lowers the pH. This decreases the negative charge of these amino acids (protonization) and the ligand is set free. The receptor is mostly sent back to the cell surface via vesicular transport and the internalized lipoproteins are further degraded after fusion of the endosome with a lysosome.

The second domain possesses a high homology to the precursor of the epidermal growth factor (EGF precursor). It contains three cysteine-rich repeats (growth factor repeats). This region also participates in the pH-dependent uncoupling of the receptor and ligand. The third domain contains 18 threonine and serine residues, an ideal scaffold for *O*-glycosidic binding of oligosaccharide chains. These chains serve possibly as supporters for the receptors to assume an upright position on the cell surface. The membrane-spanning region is made up from a stretch of 22 hydrophobic amino acids. It anchors the protein in the membrane. The C-terminus protrudes into the cytoplasm and is responsible for the clustering of the receptor molecules in the coated pits at the cell surface.

Low-density lipoprotein receptors can be found in varying numbers on nearly all cells. In vivo only liver, intestine, adrenals, and gonads express LDL-Rs [373]. Fibroblasts in culture can express up to 70 000 receptors/cell.

As already mentioned not only apo-B but also apo-E binds to the receptor. Apo-E containing lipoproteins possess an almost tenfold higher affinity to the receptor and nevertheless the binding capacity for these lipoproteins is only 25 % of that for apo-B-100-containing lipoproteins. This is explained by the fact that one single LDL-R can bind several LDL particles since apo-B contains only one receptor-binding site per molecule and apo-E-containing lipoproteins are equipped with several molecules of apo-E per particle. One single particle can therefore occupy several of the multiple binding sites of the receptor molecules. The expression of the LDL-Rs is subject to feedback regulation by the content of the cell of free cholesterol. A decreased expression of LDL-Rs on the surface of the liver causes an impaired elimination of LDL precursors (IDLs) with a concomitant increased production rate of LDLs. Thus the expression of the LDL-Rs influences the LDL cholesterol concentration not only by modifying the catabolic rate of LDLs but also their production rate.

Remnant Receptor. Even if the LDL-R is completely nonfunctional (as in the homozygous form of familial hypercholesterolemia) there is no accumulation of CM remnants. In one clinical entity this is explained by a structural defect of the LDL-R which only impairs the binding of apo-B but not of apo-E (allele FH626: deletion of the fifth exon of the sixth coplement type repeat of the ligand-binding domain [183]). Most binding defects affect, however, both apolipoproteins.

Other mutations cause a failure of the LDL-Rs to reach the cell surface (class 2 defects) or impair receptor synthesis (class 1 defects).

It was therefore reasonable to assume that CM remnants are taken up by the liver via a specific receptor distinct from the LDL-R. This receptor has not yet been unequivocally identified, but a likely candidate is the 1988 cloned LDL-R-related protein (LRP) [178, 179]. It is one of the largest integral membrane proteins known so far (600 kDa). It shows a considerable homology with the LDL-Rs. Instead of seven complement type repeats and three growth factor repeats it contains 31 copies of the former and 22 copies of the latter [178]. LRP binds not only apo-E [27] but also LPL [28, 443], α2-macroglobulin [235, 384], and other proteins. Among many different cells it is also expressed in neuronal tissues (neurons and astrocytes) [283, 447]. Its biological function probably extends far beyond the clearance of CM remnants. Its activity is regulated not by its expression on the cell surface but rather most probably by its association with a regulatory protein (39 kDa; receptor-associated protein, RAP), which inhibits its interaction with the different ligands [192, 294].

Scavenger Receptor. After the receptor-mediated uptake of lipoproteins, the cells are enriched with cholesteryl esters. These are newly formed by the cells after the intralysosomal cholesteryl esters of the lipoproteins have been cleaved by an acid lipase and the free cholesterol has escaped in the cytoplasma. Some cells (macrophages, smooth muscle cells) produce considerable amounts of cholesteryl esters, which are then stored as lipid droplets. Foam cells have accumulated many such droplets. The macrophage cannot be converted in vitro into a foam cell by uptake of normal LDL via the the LDL-R. This conversion can, however, be achieved by incubation with chemically modified LDL (acetyl-LDL). The macrophage recognizes these particles as foreign to the organism and takes them up avidly via a specific receptor (acetyl-LDL-receptor, scavenger receptor) [50, 146]. Unlike LDL-R, the expression of the scavenger receptor is not regulated by negative feedback by cholesterol, a condition allowing an unchecked uptake of lipoproteins and foam cell formation.

The biologically occurring equivalent to acetyl-LDL could be oxidized LDL ([311], see below).

Lipoprotein(a)

We have now mentioned all the diagnostically relevant lipoproteins (chylomicrons, CM remnants, VLDLs, IDLs, LDLs, HDL-2s, and HDL-3s) in the context of their metabolism except one. This is lipoprotein(a) [„LP little a", Lp(a)]. Lp(a) is a modified LDL particle. This modification consists in the association of the particle with another very large protein, the apo(a). This association consists of a covalent bond via one disulfide bridge between apo(a) and apo-B. It is sufficient to change almost all the characteristic properties of LDL particles (hydrated density, elecrophoretic mobility, and interaction with receptors).

The structure of an apo(a) molecule can be derived from the corresponding cDNA. It is closely related to that of plasminogen [206, 248] and specifies a characteristic montonous protein. It consists of a variable number (up to 40) kringle-4 domains, one kringle-5 domain, and a protease domain of the plasminogen molecule. Kringles 1–3 of plasminogen are not found in Lp(a). The apo(a) gene has probably arisen by duplication of the plasminogen gene [99, 225, 272].

Lipoprotein(a) was first described by Berg [30] and considered to be a genetic variant of LDLs. Its hydrated density is slightly higher than that of LDLs [4, 100, 130, 351, 360, 435] and it electrophoretically migrates considerably faster than the β-migrating LDLs (β-lipoproteins). It shares its pre-β mobility with the VLDLs but in contrast to these sediments during ultracentrifugation at serum density. This led to the designation „sinking pre-β-lipoprotein". As might be expected, it dissociates under reducing conditions spontaneously in apo(a) and an LDL particle [101, 405, 406]. Recently it has been shown that a certain fraction of the Lp(a) particles in the blood contain not only apo(a) and apo-B but also apo-E [21].

The Lp(a) catabolism in vivo proceeds somewhat slower than that of LDL [228–232]. The different concentrations found in different individuals are presumably mainly due to different rates of synthesis [231, 233]. The site in the organism where Lp(a) is catabolized is not known. The major route of catabolism is certainly not via the apo-B-100:E-receptor, since therapeutic increases of its expression do not lead to a decreased Lp(a) level in the blood. Lp(a) has a much lower affinity to the apo-B-100:E-receptor than LDL [114, 233]. It seems possible that apo(a) partially masks the receptor-binding domain of apo-B-100 [8, 11].

Lp(a) was considered as an autosomal dominant trait as long as only quantitative methods were available for its detection [31, 336]. The advent of more sensitive methods led to the conclusion that Lp(a) is ubiquitous. However, interindividually strikingly different levels are genetically determined [4, 6, 167, 286, 352]. Caucasians exhibit a distribution which is strongly skewed toward the left [4]. It is assumed that the Lp(a) concentration is regulated by the apo(a) locus on chromosome 6 [94]. Today at least 20 allelic forms of apo(a) are known, ranging between 320 kDa and 838 kDa [132, 412–414]. The major difference between the isoforms is the number of copies homologous to the kringle 4 of plasminogen [221]. The apo(a) isoforms can be differentiated by polyacrylamide gel electrophoresis. They are associated with the serum concentrations of Lp(a) [412–415]. The higher the molar mass of the isoform the lower the concentration. The underlying mechanism of this correlation of isoform and serum concentration is largely unknown.

Lp(a) has no well-defined hydrated density but is found over a relatively wide density range. It can be found together with the dense LDLs and also with the light HDLs [158, 318, 345]. The size of naturally occurring Lp(a) particles varies between 2000 and 10 000 kDa.

Metabolism of Lp(a)

The metabolism of Lp(a) in man is largely unknown. Except for the rhesus monkey [111, 112] and the quinea pig [329] an animal model is lacking. Interestingly, almost all lipoproteins of the hedgehog are made up of Lp(a) [244]. Lp(a) is possibly synthesized by the liver [224, 269]. In vitro it is possible to reconstitute Lp(a) from recombinant apo(a) and LDL.

Diagnostics of Lipoproteins

For the translation of hyperlipemia into hyperlipoproteinemia methods are required to separate and quantitate serum lipoproteins. Serum lipoproteins differ in the following physicochemical properties: size, density, electrical charge at a given pH, and relative amount and nature of the protein part. These differences are exploited for their separation, using molecular sieves, ultracentri-

fugation, electrophoresis, and immunological assessment of the apoproteins. In addition, differing affinities to polyanions (dextrane sulfate, he-
paran sulfate, sodium phosphotungstic acid) or
differences in the solubility in organic solvents
(Cohn fractionation) can be used for the separation of lipoproteins.

Ultracentrifugation

Lipoproteins have a lower hydrated density than
all other serum proteins. Even if the density of
the serum is increased to 1.21 g/ml (the approximate density of the Dead Sea), the lipid-free proteins sediment at forces of more than $100 \times g$
employed for 24 h. All lipoproteins stay concentrated at the top of the tube. The HDL sediment
at $d = 1.063$ g/ml, the LDL sediment at serum
density $d = 1.006$ g/ml, and it is impossible to
achieve a sedimentation of the VLDLs by ultracentrifugation except at the density of pure water,
1 g/ml.
Using analytical ultracentrifugation the concentrations of lipoproteins sedimenting or floating at a certain density of the aqueous medium
can be determined. In this way the distribution of
lipoproteins over a density spectrum could be established. It was found that at certain densities
the concentration of lipoproteins is very low
whereas at other densities concentration peaks
could be observed. In this manner the above-
mentioned cutoff points for the so-called density
classes were established. Analytical ultracentrifugation is carried out at the density $d = 1.063$ g/
ml. This is the cutoff point between the still sedimenting HDLs and all other lipoproteins. Since
these lipoproteins float at this density, flotation
constants (Sf values) were assigned to them. The
VLDLs have Sf values between Sf 400 and Sf 20,
and the LDL density class contains all lipoproteins with Sf values between Sf 20 and Sf 0. It is
further sudivided into LDL-2s (Sf 12-0) and LDL-
1s (Sf 20-12).
The preparative version of ultracentrifugation
gave rise to the most commonly used nomenclature of serum lipoproteins. Ultracentrifugation is
still the most important method for the separation
of all types of lipoproteins.
Chylomicrons (Sf >400) float even at the density
of water. At serum density ultracentrifugation is
not necessary to make them float. If left undisturbed in the refrigerator for at least 10 h, the chy-

lomicrons concentrate at the top of the serum
tube and can easily be detected in this way. IDLs
sediment at the serum density and float at $d =$
1019 g/ml. The LDL fraction still sedimenting at
this density is LDL-2. The cutoff point between
HDL-2 and the more dense HDL-3 is $d = 1.12$ g/
ml. Since the LDL fraction resides between the
density of the serum and $d = 1.063$, it is evident
that LDL cannot be prepared by a single-step procedure.
Each density class can theoretically be fraction-
ated into an indefinite number of density subclasses. This is achieved by zonal ultracentrifugation or density gradient centrifugation. Only in
rare cases does this yield biologically distinct lipoprotein fractions. An important exception is the
triglyceride-rich less dense LDL-1s, the IDLs,
and the small dense LDLs. The latter particles accumulate in FDB (apo-B-3500 defect).
The density classes (HDL, LDL, and VLDL) differ considerably qualitatively as well as quantitatively in their apoprotein content. The fact that,
using sensitive immonological methods for their
detection, almost all existing apolipoproteins can
be found in every density class, indicates that the
density classes are hardly biologically and meta-
bolically homogeneous entities. They rather comprise a polydisperse system of partially different
lipoprotein particles which exhibit marked differences in their metabolism.
Within the VLDL density class the apoproteins
cluster together mostly on the same particle, although not all particles are uniformly equipped
with the same apoprotein and also not in the same
relative amounts. The apolipoproteins of the
HDL density class are part of a variety of different particles and are sometimes even the sole
apoprotein of a distinct particle. The LDL-2 density class is mostly made up of particles containing
exlusively apo-B-100. Some particles additionally
contain apo-E or apo-C or both [3, 217, 218]. This
is regularly the case for the IDLs. The presence of
C-II or C-III or apo-E influences the biological
properties of lipoproteins considerably [70]. The
apo-B-100-containing lipoproteins usually contain
only one molecule of apo-B per particle [400, 440].

Lipoprotein Electrophoresis

The origins of lipoprotein diagnostics can be
dated back to the late 1960s, when Fredrickson
and Lees introduced the electrophororetic separa-

tion of lipoproteins on paper in order to classify the different hyperlipemias according to the prevailing lipoprotein [120–124, 251]. In this system the lipoproteins of interest are not the nonmigrating chylomicrons, but the migrating VLDLs (pre-β-lipoproteins) with α-2 mobility and the β-lipoproteins (LDLs). HDLs stain only weakly. The IDLs migrate with a slightly increased β-mobility [108, 313, 314, 437]. Incompletely degraded chylomicrons, VLDLs, and IDLs migrate partially more slowly than VLDLs and cause a broad β-band. This is a characteristic feature of type-III hyperlipoproteinemia. Another name for these lipoproteins, exhibiting the density of LDLs but an electrophoretic mobility close to VLDLs, is „β-VLDLs", which are probably a potent atherogenic lipoproteins [13, 56, 173, 270, 314, 324]. The diagnosis can be establisehd by the demonstration of homozygosity for E-2 [407–410].

Lipoprotein electrophoresis found its first clinical use as the basis of the typing system of Fredrickson. This system was mainly used for the differential diagnosis of a turbid serum sample. It became even more useful with the advent of a quantitative form [291]. This is still today the only method for direct quantitation of LDLs and in addition it allows the easy determination of the ratio of atherogenic lipoproteins to non-atherogenic lipoproteins (β-lipoprotein/α-lipoprotein ratio) [24, 438]. All the different isoforms of Lp(a) exhibit pre-β mobility. Lipoprotein electrophoresis is a single-step procedure for the separation of all relevant lipoproteins. This is a considerable advantage over ultracentrifugation.

Precipitation Methods

In order to determine HDL cholesterol by means of the ultracentrifuge, the density of the sample has to be adjusted to $d = 1.063$ g/ml using NaBr. At this density the VLDLs and LDLs can be removed by flotation and subsequent aspiration from the tube. This type of separation can more easily be achieved by polyanion precipitation [26, 53, 168].

Polyanions (heparin, sodium phosphotungstic acid, dextran sulfate, etc.) bind to the surface of the corresponding lipoproteins and convey a strong negative electrical charge to the particle. This can be used for the formation of an insoluble complex with some divalent cations (Mg^{2+}, Mn^{2+}, Ca^{2+}, etc.) [70] and subsequent removal of the complexed undesired lipoproteins by centrifugation. This can be achieved much more easily in the case of VLDLs and LDLs than with HDLs [16, 53].

Lipoproteins can also be precipitated specifically using polyethylene glycol (PEG) [71, 199, 319, 417]. Using PEG as well as dextran sulfate conditions can be found under which, in addition to VLDLs and LDLs, HDL-2s also precipitate [139, 220]. This is the basis of commercially available kits for the determination of HDL-2 and HDL-3 cholesterol.

Most prospective studies have employed the precipitation of VLDLs and LDLs by the combination of heparin and $MnCl_2$. HDL cholesterol was then determined by a chemical colorometric method (e.g., Liebermann-Burchard). The phosphate ions present in most buffers of enzymatic test kits for cholesterol determination form insoluble complexes with manganese ions. This causes turbidities and leads to falsely elevated values. Therefore the European standard procedure for the determination of HDL cholesterol uses the sodium salt of phosphotungstic acid as the polyanion, which in combination with the appropriate amount of magnesium ions (Mg^{2+}) causes a complete precipitation of VLDLs and LDLs [258]. Mg^{2+} does not form interfering complexes with phosphate.

Since at present the single most important parameter is LDL cholesterol, an easy and specific method for the determination of LDL cholesterol is required. One possibility is the direct precipitation of LDLs without coprecipitation of VLDLs from native serum. In the past decade several methods have been developed [7, 9, 12, 25, 439]. The examination of the precipitated fraction shows, however, that these „LDLs" are heavily contaminated by VLDLs. Even the best method yields LDL triglyceride concentrations twice as high as those determined by ultracentrifugation.

The usual procedure for the determination of LDL cholesterol is the precipitation of LDLs in a serum sample which has been freed from VLDLs by ultracentrifugation at serum density for at least 18 h. This is achieved by subtraction of the cholesterol concentration in the fraction that is left after precipitation (supernatant) from the cholesterol concentration of the sample after removal of the VLDLs by ultracentrifugation [53, 54]. This is in theory a highly specific method; however, the „LDL" are necessarily contaminated with Lp(a). This is not the case with electrophoretically determined LDL, since Lp(a) exhibits not β- but pre-β mobility. Therefore in this case the VLDLs are contaminated with Lp(a). The ultracentrifugal procedure has the major advantage is that not only the concentration of cholesterol but also of any other LDL constituent in the serum can be determined (e.g., LDL triglycerides, see below).

The most common way for the assessment of LDL cholesterol is not the determination by ultracentrifugation but calculation by means of the Friedewald formula [126]. It is based on the following considerations: The major cholesterol-containing fractions are VLDLs, LDLs, and HDLs. When the HDL cholesterol concentration can be reliably measured, the VLDL cholesterol reliables approximated, then the LDL cholesterol can be calculated. VLDL-cholesterol can be estimated since VLDL are the major carriers of the triglycerides in the fasting plasma. If one assumes that the composition of VLDLs with regard to cholesterol and triglycerides is fairly constant, one can calculate a VLDL cholesterol equivalent from the serum triglycerides. Division by five yields a VLDL cholesterol which together with HDL cholesterol is substracted from the total cholesterol. The difference is the „Friedewald-LDL-cholesterol". This calculation is not applicable in patients with serum triglyceride levels greater than 400 mg/dl.

Since the serum triglycerides are not exclusively sequestered in the VLDL fraction and also the composition of VLDL is not constant to a high degree from individual to individual, this is a rather crude procedure, but it works surprisingly well. Since HDL cholesterol has to be determined in any case, this is an economic way to approach the true LDL cholesterol value. The presence of chylomicrons leads to an underestimation of LDL cholesterol, since they contain far more than five times more triglycerides than cholesterol.

Determination of IDLs

There is no easy way to quantitate IDLs. As rather triglyceride-rich lipoproteins they contribute considerably to the concentration of triglycerides present in LDL (normally 30 mg/dl). In some of our clinical studies the concentration of triglycerides in LDL has been found to be even more closely associated with the presence of CAD than the LDL cholesterol. It is not simple to determine the LDL triglyceride concentration accurately and precisely since steps identical to those for determination of LDL cholesterol are required. It is, however, much more critical to avoid contamination with the ultracentrifugally separated VLDLs. Since the normal range lies between 20 and 35 mg/dl, and 40 mg/l has to be considered an elevated value, the precision is crucial. The determination of IDLs requires two ultracentrifugation steps. In the first step, the VLDLs are removed at serum density and then the density of the infranatant is adjusted to 1.019 g/ml. At this density the IDLs can be separated by flotation and quantitated in the supernatant.

Determination of Lp(a)

The determination of Lp(a) presents some specific difficulties.

Initially Lp(a) was determined qualitatively using immuno-double diffusion [80–83, 423] and electrophoretically as „sinking pre-β-lipoprotein" [46, 82, 334] or as pre-β1-lipoprotein [80–83, 198, 234, 320]. The antisera were obtained by immunization with Lp(a)-positive human sera, with subsequent absorption of all the undesired antibodies using Lp(a)-negative sera. At this time an individual was either Lp(a) positive or Lp(a) negative. Later, quantitative immunological methods were employed such as radial immunodiffusion (RID) [4, 5, 81], electroimmunoassay [64, 100, 130, 131, 160, 219, 230, 304, 423], immunonephelometry [64], latex-immunoassay [421], radioimmunoassay [6, 97, 352], and enzyme immunoassay [98, 131, 239, 422].

The immunological quantitation of lipoprotein(a) only measures the apo(a) part. Since the size of this component of the particle can vary considerably, it is impossible to base any conclusion concerning the amount of Lp(a) particles in any material on the apo(a) value [132, 413]. In addition all limitations regarding the determination of apolipoproteins have to be taken in account. Since there is a strong cross-reactivity of older antisera against Lp(a) with plasminogen, older reports in the literature concerning the quantitation of Lp(a) must be interpreted with caution.

At present Lp(a) is mostly determined by electroimmunoassay (EIA, rocket electrophoresis), ELISA, and RIA. All methods are commercially available. Recently turbidimetric assays have developed, which can be performed on any modern clinical chemical analyzer. The cutoff point con-

---

sidered to be associated with increased risk for atherosclerosis is 30 mg/dl Lp(a). As outlined above it is difficult to assign to this value a certain number of Lp(a) particles for two reasons: the amount of apo(a) per particle is variable and no analytical method has been standardized sufficiently thus far.

Lipoprotein Particles

The most complete quantification of lipoproteins would be the determination of the concentrations of all the individual lipoprotein particles. This could be achieved by a series of sandwich ELISAs. These methods would at least yield the information of what amount of which apolipoprotein is associated with what amount of another apolipoprotein on the same particle. This method has been used to determine what percentage of A-I is associated with A-II and the proportion of A-I with A-II to A-I without A-II [127, 292, 323]. However, these techniques have not yet been sufficiently established to become routinely used in clinical laboratories.

Diagnostics of Lipoproteins of the Postprandial Serum

Paradoxically lipoprotein diagnostics is almost exclusively performed on samples taken after an overnight fast. This is certainly not the most representative metabolic condition in most individuals. Rather it represents an exception since one is almost never a fasting state for 12 h. It is therefore conceivable that atherogenic postprandial lipoproteins may escape detection. Possible candidates for atherogenesis are CM remnants [362]. These particles can be induced and labeled by an oral fat load with concomitant oral administration of retinyl esters. Retinyl esters are incorporated in the chylomicrons and can be subsequently found in the remnants. They can be quantitated by fluorescence spectrometry in the lipoprotein fraction of the serum sample. Since uptake of the CM remnants in the liver destroys the esters, their measurement is specific for intact chylomicrons or their remnants. Ten hours after an oral fat load the chylomicrons have usually disappeared from the circulation and are also no longer produced by the intestine. The detectable fluorescence in the VLDL fraction therefore reflects quantitatively the concentration of CM remnants. Preliminary results from our laboratory indeed indicate that CAD patients are distinguished by a longer residence time of CM remnants in their circulation.

Diagnostics of Apolipoproteins

As all apoproteins are present in all density classes and as no single density class exclusively contains only one apolipoprotein species, the determination of apolipoproteins should give different results from the determination of lipoproteins. Apo-B, for instance, is a constituent of chylomicrons, CM remnants, VLDLs, IDLs, β-VLDLs, LDL-2s, and Lp(a). Therefore its concentration in the serum is not equivalent to the concentration of LDLs. The concentration of apo-A-I correlates sufficiently well with the concentration of HDL cholesterol [429]. Despite this fact and the scope for determining A-I and other apolipoproteins turbidimetrically on clinical chemical analyzers, A-I has not been able to replace HDL cholesterol mainly because of the lack of prospective data regarding the diagnostic significance of apo-A-I. Apo-B appears to be a useful parameter since in contrast to cholesterol its serum concentration reflects the amount of potentially atherogenic lipoproteins. In the cord blood only 40 % of the cholesterol is transported by apo-B-containing lipoproteins [14, 15, 19, 21, 77]. This makes it a useful parameter for screening newborns for hypercholesterolemia, which in this case is most likely familial. By compulsory determination of apo-B from dried blood spots one could provide „case finding" and „early detection" of familial hypercholesterolemia in the unsuspecting parents. In VLDL-free serum the apo-B concentration is a direct measure of the amount of apo-B-containing particles, since one particle contains only one molecule of apo-B [400, 440]. Since we have no prospective data for apo-B either, its determination has so far not found widespread use despite the above-mentioned advantages.

An additional reason for the reluctance towards routinely performed determinations of apolipoproteins is the theoretical and practical difficulties of standardization. On the one hand it is a prerequisite of all immunological determinations of a protein in biological samples that the protein to be determined and the standard be in the same physicochemical condition (the standards can therefore not be stabilized by freezing or lyophilization, since these procedures alter the lipoproteins, the matrix of the apolipoproteins); on the other hand, a stable standard is a condition sine qua non for any comparability of apolipoprotein values between laboratories.

It is reasonable to assume that the inclusion of the determination of apolipoproteins in the diagnostic panel will have a positive impact on the diagnostic usefulness of lipidologic examinations of the serum. There are, for instance, indications that the magnitude of the ratio of apo-C-III in the serum to apo-C-III in the supernatant after heparin/MnCl$_2$ precipitation may play a role in the progression of coronary artery disease [39]. The diagnosis of inborn or acquired deficiencies of apolipoproteins is of course best made by the immunological determination of the corresponding apolipoprotein.

Besides simple information about their concentration, apolipoproteins sometimes also bear clinically useful qualitative information. A prominent example is the polymorphism of apolipoprotein-E. Demonstration of E-2 homozygosity is the safest way to diagnose type III hyperlipoproteinemia. Apo-E polymorphism is most easily investigated by isoelectric focusing of the serum in agarose. In order to bring about the charge differences in apo-E the sample has to be delipidized using non-ionic detergents. The apo-E bands have to be identified among the thousands of other bands through immobilization in the gel by a specific antiserum (immunoblot) [269]. Recently, it has become clear that the ε4 allele is overrepresented in patients suffering from Alzheimer's disease. Since E4 is most readily taken up by cells in comparison with the other isoforms, it seems likely that a hypercholesterolemic E4 individual will benefit more than the E3 homozygote from a reduction in dietary fats, since its CM remnants are the most effective ones in the downregulation of the LDL-Rs.

Clinical Significance of Serum Lipoproteins

The concentrations of lipoproteins are usually determined in the context of the diagnosis and treatment of dyslipoproteinemias connected with atherosclerosis. Therefore, a short excursion into the present theories about the connection of atherosclerosis with serum lipoproteins seems to be adequate. The amorphous material which has accumulated in the atherosclerotic plaques is mainly cholesterol and cholesteryl esters [445]. The esters are present almost exclusively in the blood and it seemed therefore very likely that the esters of the plaque originate from the bloodstream and reach the vessel wall by perfusion [91]. Besides the lipids, atherosclerotic lesions contain necrotic material, cells, and connective tissue. This led Virchow to the view that atherosclerosis is basically the consequence of chronic inflammation [418–420]. The presence of fibrin, hemoglobin, and iron in the atherosclerotic lesion led to the assumption that the incorporation of platelets may also play a significant role [92, 93].

Atherosclerosis can be considered a lipid-rich scar of a focally occurring inflammatory process of the arterial wall. The single stages of the development of the atherosclerotic lesion can be demonstrated in animal experiments. It is questionable, however, if atherogenesis takes place in a similar fashion in man. The atherosclerosis of cholesterol-fed animals and of humans has in common the occurrence of foam cells. These cells were first thought to originate from macrophages [249]. The origin was later extended also to the smooth muscle cells of the arterial wall [78, 129, 163, 169, 170, 182, 389] and is today transferred back to the macrophages [7, 20, 118, 119, 134, 135, 301, 348, 378]. These cells can be identified in the lesions using monoclonal antibodies [7]. The key to the understanding of atherogenesis lies in the early phase of the conversion of macrophages into foam cells.

Initially certain patches of the endothelium attract monocytes which bind to the endothelial cells and migrate between these cells into the intima. There they become macrophages and in a progressive atherosclerotic lesion they are immobilized in the subintimal space [107, 133]. The conversion of the macrophages into foam cells requires the uptake of lipoproteins. Within the foam cells the cholesteryl esters of the lipoproteins are hydrolyzed and the free cholesterol is subsequently reesterified by the ACAT enzyme [146]. The uptake of these lipoproteins occurs via specific receptors. The apo-B-100:E-receptor is not expressed significantly on these macrophages; therefore the macrophage cannot be converted in vitro into a foam cell by normal LDLs taken up this way, by only by chemically modified LDLs (acetyl-LDLs) via the scavenger receptor.

As mentioned before, the biologically occurring equivalent to acetyl-LDLs could be oxidized LDLs. In these lipoproteins the fatty acid moieties of the phospholipids and cholesteryl esters have undergone oxidations, apo-B has been cleaved by an unknown mechanism, and lysin residues of the protein have formed bonds with aldehydes (4-hydroxynonenal, malone dialdehyde). Such modifications can be performed by endothelial cells, smooth muscle cells, macrophages, and even foam cells [117, 176, 177, 186, 310, 311, 338, 379, 380]. The atherosclerotic plaque indeed contains oxidized LDLs. These modified lipoproteins can be eluted from the plaque but are also detectable by immunofluorescence [307, 452]. Oxidized LDLs often occur in the lesion together with mRNA for the acetyl-LDL-Rs [453]. This underlines the possible atherogenetic role of oxidized LDLs.

Macrophages are also endowed with a receptor for β-VLDLs [146, 147, 263, 416]. Foam cells can also be generated by β-VLDLs [189, 312]. The β-VLDL-receptor recognizes apo-E [196, 441]. It is possible that this receptor is identical with the LDL-Rs [215, 216].

The modification of lipoproteins in the arterial wall gives rise to neo-antigens [308] potentially eliciting characteristic autoimmune reactions documented by the presence of T-suppressor cells in the atherosclerotic plaque. Recent evidence exists that indeed in patients with angiographically proven coronary artery disease (CAD) the titers of antibodies against modified LDLs are higher than in normal controls [436].

Significance of Serum Cholesterol

The positive association of the serum cholesterol concentration with atherosclerotic diseases has been firmly established [208, 223, 250, 277, 278, 316, 325, 341, 376, 377, 451]. Of heterozygous patients suffering from familial hypercholesterolemia, 96% die from CAD [278]. The incidence rate of CAD is also strongly influenced by the serum cholesterol concentration [162, 188, 237, 242, 322, 451]. An autopsy study has revealed that the differences in the prevalence of severe coronary lesions between Norway and Japan can be explained solely by differences in the serum cholesterol concentration [369] and that the size of atheromatous plaques also depends significantly on the serum cholesterol concentration [368].

Significance of Serum Triglycerides

That increases in serum triglycerides and atherosclerosis are correlated is more controversial. However, the evidence is mounting that a similar positive correlation indeed exists. For example, prospective studies from Scandinavia with long observation times have revealed strong correlations between the concentration of triglycerides in fasting serum and CAD mortality [57, 317, 403]. A similar clear prospective relationship could also be observed in Scotland [257] and in the Japanese population of Hawaii [29]. In Framingham in the United States such a connection could only be observed among elderly persons (60–70 years) [62] and women [60]. Serum triglycerides are also a good predictor of future coronary events for Swedish women [245].

Serum triglycerides also apparently influence the progression of CAD in diabetics [349] and are of predictive significance also regarding restenosis of a vessel used for coronary bypass [306]. Men suffering from a significantly premature myocardial infarction (before 50 years of age) exhibit in their serum higher concentrations of both triglycerides and cholesterol [340]. Increased triglycerides are also found in patients having undergone coronary bypass operations [253] and other patients with CAD [279, 434].

In the United States hypertriglyceridemia has not for a long time been regarded as an independent risk factor. The fact that hypertriglyceridemia was associated with a high CAD incidence rate [58] was usually explained by the presence of other accompanying risk factors such as low HDL, high LDL, obesity, and glucose intolerance in the multifactorial analytical model. Hypertriglyceridemia was regarded as clinically insignificant since populations with CAD incidence rates lower than in industrialized Western nations exhibited higher triglyceride concentrations [205].

In summary it appears rather doubtful that the atherogenicity of triglyceride-rich lipoproteins can be explained by low HDL cholesterol levels. At least three clinical studies have demonstrated an independent effect of the high triglyceride concentration on the incidence rate of CAD [19, 356, 455]. This independent effect is modified by the prevailing serum cholesterol concentration [356].

As mentioned previously the concentration of triglycerides is the sum of the concentrations of triglyceride-containing lipoproteins, mainly the VLDLs, chylomicrons, β-VLDLs, IDLs, and remnant particles. In our view and in the opinion of others the IDLs or CM remnants are undoubtedly atherogenic [347, 381].

Significance of Lipoproteins

Low-Density Lipoproteins

The incidence rate of CAD in hypercholesterolemic men is strong influenced by the LDL cholesterol concentration [255].

Prospective studies also including determining the concentrations of LDLs have only been undertaken recently. Recently in terms of prospective studies means less than 12 years [79] (GRIPS), [355] (PROCAM). Since these studies will be confounded in the future by the widespread use of lipid-lowering agents our most important information regarding LDL cholesterol must be either derived from its close correlation with the serum cholesterol concentration or from the results of interventional regression studies [38, 48]. In these studies the best results were achieved in the groups of patients where the decrease in LDL cholesterol was accompanied by a marked increase in HDL cholesterol under drug therapy.

High-Density Lipoproteins

In contrast to LDL cholesterol, HDL cholesterol has been included in prospective studies ongoing for more than 12 years [209, 444, 449]. The Framingham study provides the largest amount of person-years observed to date. HDL cholesterol unfortunately was only included to the time when all the observed persons were older than 50 years. In this study a negative correlation was found between the incidence of atherosclerotic disease and the HDL cholesterol concentration. In the Framingham study the methodology was quite different from today's methods (heparin/$MnCl_2$ precipitation combined with colorometric determination of HDL cholesterol). In two recent German studies modern technology was employed. Despite the fact that identical methodology was employed, the prevalence of low HDL cholesterol levels in men (below 35 mg/dl) differed between the two studies (PROCAM, 17%; GRIPS, 11%). Although the follow-up periods are still relatively short (5 years), it is already evident that at least in persons older than 50 years HDL cholesterol has

a considerable predictive significance (PROCAM study). An increase in HDL cholesterol levels seems to lower the incidence rate of CAD. An increase of 1 mg/dl appears to lower the risk for future CAD by 4%, and preferentially in women [150, 151].

Significance of IDL/LDL Triglycerides

In all cases of familial hypercholesterolemia there is also an increased concentration of IDL. The persons at the highest risk of premature myocardial infarction, the homozygotes, invariably have high IDL concentrations [201, 226, 372]. This fact is confirmed by the Watanabe rabbits suffering from genetic hypercholesterolemia (internalization defect) and CAD (leading to breeding difficulties) [210]. The most convincing example of the atherogenicity of high levels of IDL is, however, type III hyperlipoproteinemia. The premature atherosclerosis involves not only the coronary arteries but also the femoral and carotid arteries. Even in the absence of type III hyperlipoproteinemia, IDLs have been found to be closely correlated with CAD [381, 390].

In a young population of myocardial infarction survivors, the IDL-equivalent LDL triglycerides have been shown to be better discriminators than LDL cholesterol [165]. The IDL concentration correlates better with the extent and severity of CAD than any other lipid parameter in men and women [256, 332]. In a Japanese study where total cholesterol levels showed no difference between CAD patients and controls, it was possible to differentiate between patients and controls using IDL cholesterol levels [203]. Of all the lipid parameters, IDL concentration correlates most closely with the progression or regression of CAD [227].

In addition, the increased susceptibility to atherosclerosis of patients with secondary hypertriglyceridemia such as patients undergoing hemodialysis or diabetics could be explained by the increased concentration of LDL triglycerides [190, 290].

Clinical Significance of Lipid and Lipoprotein Ratios

Since VLDLs and LDLs can be regarded as atherogenic lipoproteins and HDLs are neutral if not protective, the ratio of VLDL+LDL cholesterol or only LDL cholesterol to HDL cholesterol reflects the risk of premature CAD. The total cholesterol/HDL cholesterol ratio can be used similarly. The latter ratio is increased either by a decrease in protective lipoproteins or by an increase in atherogenic lipoproteins [VLDLs, IDLs, LDLs, Lp(a)]. The ratio is less influenced by factors of the preanalytical phase such as position of the body and venous congestion by the turniquet during and before drawing of the blood [212]. In contrast to the Friedewald-LDL-cholesterol concentration this ratio is insensitive to the presence of chylomicrons.

Comparative epidemiological studies have concluded that differences in this ratio can explain up to 50% of the differences in the incidence rate of CAD between populations including women [361]. In preference to the recommendations of the European Atherosclerosis Society, in Switzerland an increased risk of CAD is assumed if the ratio of serum cholesterol to HDL cholesterol exceeds 5 [159]. The only drawback of using this ratio is the relatively low comparability because of methodological variations of the HDL-cholesterol methods together with the strong influence of HDL-cholesterol in this ratio.

Significance of Polymorphisms of Apolipoprotein E

Apo-E2 only weakly binds to apo-B-100:E-receptors [241, 350, 431]. This leads to a delayed in vivo clearance and accumulation in the blood of remnants of chylomicrons and VLDLs. This decreased cholesterol flux into the liver causes an augmentation of LDL-Rs on the liver surface, leading to decreased concentrations of apo-B and LDL cholesterol in the serum of E2/E2 homozygotes. Because of its association with low cholesterol levels, the E2 allele is considered to be cardioprotective.

In contrast to the E2 allele, the E4 allele is for unknown reasons associated with rather high concentrations of LDL cholesterol [87]. In vitro apo-E4 and apo-E3 exhibit the same affinities to LDL-Rs; in vivo, however, apo-E4 is catabolized more efficiently than apo-E3 [154]. This has been attributed to a different distribution of apo-E among lipoproteins. Apo-E3 associates preferentially with HDLs, and apo-E4 has a higher affinity for triglyceride-rich lipoproteins [382].

Apo-E2 and apo-E3 both contain a cysteine residue at position 112. This enables them to form in the serum multimers stabilized by disulfide bridges [430]. These multimers have lower affinities to the LDL-Rs [433]. Apo-E4 cannot be part of a multimer and is therefore catabolized at a faster rate than apo-E3. This increases the hepatic cholesterol pool and suppresses the LDL-Rs.

Since apo-E polymorphism has been included in prospective studies only recently, the relative risk of the different isoforms of atherosclerotic disease has not yet been established. Perhaps it can be estimated from its influence on the LDL cholesterol concentration. The data from clinical angiography studies are still conflicting.

Significance of Lp(a)

Every human has a given serum level of Lp(a). This concentration is genetically determined [5]. The increased risk for CAD appears to be associated with concentrations greater than 20–30 mg/dl [30, 84, 113, 125, 236, 335]. The connection of Lp(a) with CAD was established in the early 1970s [6, 15, 30, 31, 81–84, 254, 300, 303, 309, 320, 334]. Despite this overwhelming evidence and a thorough study of the Lp(a) problem by Kostner and coworkers [219], this connection has largely been ignored. Starting in the mid-1980s, the number of publications documenting the connection of Lp(a) with CAD increased dramatically [10, 85, 90, 97, 136, 335, 342, 353, 454]. The presence of Lp(a) in atheromas [187] had already been demonstrated much earlier by Walton [424] and was also confirmed later in the guinea pig [329]. The serum concentration of Lp(a) correlates well with the extent of CAD [85] and is of predictive significance also regarding a restenosis of a vessel used for a coronary bypass [174, 185]. Whereas only 13% of a normal population exceed the cutoff point, in children of sufferers from myocardial infarction it is exceeded by 32%. Lp(a) seems to be much more closely associated with peripheral atherosclerosis than LDL [55, 281]. How Lp(a) exerts its atherogenic effect is still a matter of much speculation. Interfering influences on the fibrinolytic system have to be considered as well as the special affinity of Lp(a) to glycosaminoglycans of the vessel wall [36, 104].

Hyperlipoproteinemias

Classification of lipoprotein disorders started with the typing system of Fredrickson. It soon became clear that the different phenotypes only rarely represented genotypes and that hyperlipoproteinemias can also be secondary to other diseases. Since a classification of dyslipoproteinemias should lead to clear therapeutic concepts and therapy must often start with lipid concentrations not yet characteristic of a distinct hyperlipoproteinemia, other classification systems have evolved. The hyperlipoproteinemias can be differentiated into primary and secondary hyperlipoproteinemias. The primary hyperlipoproteinemias can either be traced back to a single gene defect (monogenic hyperlipoproteinemias) or must be considered as polygenic. For practical therapeutic purposes in recent years several consecutive classification systems have evolved which have also considered not only lipid disturbances but also the accompanying risk factors. The latest was published in March 1994 [289].

Primary hyperlipoproteinemia is present when secondary causes of hyperlipoproteinemia, such as diabetes mellitus, renal insufficiency, hypothyroidism, cholestasis, and drugs have been excluded. The most common monogenic forms are the familial deficiency of LPL, familial C-II deficiency, familial type III hyperlipoproteinemia. familial hypercholesterolemia, familial defective apo-B-100, familial hypertriglyceridemia, and familial combined hyperlipoproteinemia.

Familial Lipoprotein Lipase Deficiency

The autosomal recessive deficiency of LPL leads to a defect in the catabolism of triglyceride-rich lipoproteins and to excessive hypertriglyceridemia (type I and V) [116]. This condition is very rare except in some parts of Canada (prevalence of heterozygotes, 2.5 %). The fasting serum contains chylomicrons, VLDLs are slightly elevated, and HDLs are markedly decreased. Heterozygotes have decreased LPL activity but mostly normal serum lipid levels. Diagnosis is established by determining the postheparin lipolytic activity (injection of heparin and subsequent examination of the ability of the serum to hydrolyze an artificial substrate). The concentration of C-II is normal. The disease is clearly not associated with an in-

creased risk of atherosclerotic disease. The major symptoms are abdominal cramps. These can be avoided by omitting fat from the diet almost completely or by substituting triglycerides consisting of long-chain fatty acids with those containing only medium-chain fatty acids. These are not re-esterified to triglycerides but are transported to the liver via the portal vein.

Familial Apo-C-II Deficiency

A deficiency of C-II, one of the three peptides of apo-C, can also lead to the persistence of chylomicrons [45, 115]. VLDL concentration is also increased. The disease is inherited as an autosomal recessive trait. Since the disease is extremely rare, no information regarding the atherogenicity of this condition has been obtained so far. Heterozygotes have normal lipids but decreased C-II levels. The treatment consists of the infusion of normal serum (containing sufficient quantities of C-II). Best known mutations cause a decrease or a complete lack of C-II. Only one missense mutation at the C-II locus is known so far (*Thr*50). It is associated with chylomicronemia [116]. The clinical symptoms are indistinguishable from those of lipoprotein lipase deficiency.

Familial Type III Hyperlipoproteinemia

In familial type III hyperlipoproteinemia, triglyceride and cholesterol levels are both elevated to values up to 600 mg/dl, reflecting the accumulation of remnants of chylomicrons and of VLDLs (IDLs) [35, 65, 66, 202, 302, 331]. The disorder becomes apparent in early adulthood and is considered highly atherogenic [265, 266]. About two-thirds of patients present with widespread atherosclerotis at the time of diagnosis. More than 90 % of these patients are homozygous for apo-E2. Although the prevalence of E2 homozygotes in the population is about 1 %, only 5 % of these persons develop type III hyperlipoproteinemia. The overall prevalence is therefore 0.05 %. Therefore it appears that in addition to the E2 homozygosity there must be other metabolic conditions predisposing the patient to the full-blown disease [87, 153, 154, 265, 407, 408, 411]. Such conditions may either be other genetic defects of lipoprotein metabolism (e.g., familial combined hyperlipemia, see below) or secondary causes such as obesity, diabetes mellitus, hypothyroidism, or oral contraceptives. The diagnosis is performed by measuring VLDLs, which have a characteristically altered cholesterol/triglyceride ratio of higher than 0.45. The remnants migrate electrophoretically faster than LDLs but slower than VLDLs; this abolishes the separation of β- and pre-β-lipoprotein („broad beta disease"). A major feature of the disease is the rapid disappearance of the remnants after drug therapy with clofibrate or its derivatives. This together with the homozygosity for apo-E2 is sufficient proof.

The correct diagnosis has important therapeutic implications, since it is possible to normalize the lipids completely by drug treatment (mainly clofibrate and its derivatives) and elimination of the precipitating conditions. After this has been achieved the risk of atherosclerosis may even be lower than normal (E2 homozygosity).

There are, however, some exceptions to the rule of obligate E2 homozygosity. Rarely type III patients can be found without this genetic trait. It appears that in these patients apo-E is abnormal and has a decreased affinity to the receptors [138, 260, 261, 267, 271, 328, 391, 425–427, 432, 450]. In addition to these rare mutants, two families have been found exhibiting a complete absence of apo-E [137, 259, 346].

Familial Hypercholesterolemia

Familial hypercholesterolemia (FH) is one of the most common inherited metabolic diseases (frequency of heterozygotes: 1/500) [51]. It is inherited as an autosomal dominant trait. The defect lies in a malfunction of the LDL receptor [145]. About 5 % of all patients with myocardial infarction before the age of 60 years are heterozygous for FH. This corresponds to a 25-fold increased risk for premature CAD. On the other hand, 85 % of the heterozygotes have already had one myocardial infarction before the age of 60 years. The LDL cholesterol level in homozygotes is usually greater than 600 mg/dl, and the LDL cholesterol level in heterozygotes lies between 230 and 450 mg/dl. The concentration of triglycerides is normal (Fredrickson type IIa). The defect leads to an impaired catabolism of LDL and to an increased production rate.

Today about 100 [184] different mutations are known. Besides structural mutations of the receptor protein impairing the binding of lipoproteins,

every stage of the metabolism of the receptor can be defective (synthesis, migration to the cell surface, anchoring in the cell membrane, and internalization) [148]. This large number of possible defects is the reason that most „homozygotes" are in reality „compound" heterozygotes [148, 287].

In the homozygous patient the severity of the disease is mostly a consequence of the nature of the mutation at the LDL-R locus [375, 398]. In the heterozygous patient many exogenous factors (age, gender, diet) as well as genetic polymorphisms of the two ligands of the receptor, apo-E [105, 161, 411] and apo-B [2, 261], exert additional effects.

Familial hypercholesterolemia is likely if serum cholesterol concentration lies between 350 and 450 mg/dl; xanthomas of the tendons are present and half of the first-degree relatives suffer from hypercholesterolemia. The diagnosis can be definitively established by studying the interaction of LDLs with cultivated skin fibroblasts from the patient. The heterogeneity of the disease and the complex structure of the gene make DNA diagnosis difficult.

In heterozygotes the treatment consists of increased expression of the remaining LDL receptors in the liver. This is achieved by interruption of the enterohepatic circulation of bile acids by an ion-exchange resin. The increased need for sterols, the precursors of bile acids, leads to an increased expression of hepatic LDL receptors but also to an increased cholesterol biosynthesis by the liver. This can be overcome by the additional administration of inhibitors of HMG-CoA-reductase. These inhibitors also cause a further increase in the number of LDL receptors at the surface of liver cells. This combined treatment usually leads to a reduction of LDL cholesterol by 50 %. In some cases the therapeutic goal of 120 mg/dl LDL cholesterol cannot be reached. In combination with clinical symptoms of atherosclerotic disease this is an indication of extracorporeal LDL elimination. The latter procedure is the method of choice for the treatment of homozygotes.

Familial Defective Apo-B-100

A mutation at the 3500 position of apo-B-100 leads to an autosomal dominant condition with a markedly lower (80 %) affinity of apo-B to the LDL-Rs (familial defective apo-B-100, FDB)

[197, 262, 404]. The low affinity is due to a substitution of glutamine for arginine at this position. FDB is one of the most common point mutations with metabolic consequences (prevalence, 2 : 1000). Heterozygotes have only a moderate hypercholesterolemia (between 250 and 350 mg/dl). The serum cholesterol level o the few so far described homozygotes is not much higher. Apparently as long as the particles contain apo-E they are recognized by the LDL-Rs, and the LDL precursors are eliminated with a speed sufficient to avoid increased LDL production. This is in contrast to that form of FH which is due to a receptor dysfunction. Correspondingly, at present the condition is regarded as far less atherogenic than FH. Studies regarding the prevalence in survivors of myocardial infarction are currently being undertaken. Although the hepatic LDL receptors are sufficiently expressed if not even overexpressed, the condition can be successfully treated with HMG-CoA reductase inhibitors.

Familial Hypertriglyceridemia

Familial hypertriglyceridemia is inherited as an autosomal dominant trait. It appears most frequently in the form of Fredrickson type IV and rarely type V hyperlipoproteinemia. Its frequency is about the same as that of FH (1/500). The VLDLs of the patients are enriched with triglycerides. This is probably due to an overproduction of triglycerides not accompanied by an overproduction also of apo-B. This condition is frequently associated with impaired glucose tolerance, hyperuricemia, and arterial hypertension. The pathomechanism and genetic defect have not yet been determined. The diagnosis of familial hypertriglyceridemia is established only after exclusion of a secondary hypertriglyceridemia together with a corresponding family history. Since in these families hyperlipoproteinemias of Fredrickson type IIa and IIb are absent, it is considered to be a separate entity and not a form of combined familial hyperlipemia. The risk of CAD is increased. Besides a low-fat diet the common antihypertriglyceridemic drugs such as nicotinic acid and clofibrates and its derivatives are effective. In severe cases fish oils to decrease the synthesis of triglycerides may be helpful.

Familial Combined Hyperlipemia

A characteristic feature of combined familial hyperlipemia is the simultaneous occurrence of different phenotypes of hyperlipoproteinemia (usually Fredrickson types IIa, IIb, and IV) in the same family. It is associated with an increased risk of premature CAD and it is found in about 10 % of all survivors of myocardial infarction. Obesity, impaired glucose tolerance, and hyperuricemia are common. The disease is inherited as an autosomal dominant trait; however, the underlying cause is not known. Perhaps an increased secretion of VLDLs plays an important role. The diagnosis is established by family examination. Xanthomas almost never occur. The treatment is that of the corresponding Fredrickson phenotype. Type IIb is best treated by a combination of ion exchange resins with antihypertriglyceridemic drugs. According to present knowledge, these drugs should not be combined with HMG-CoA reductase inhibitors.

Polygenic („Common") Hyperlipoproteinemia

In most cases of hypercholesterolemia (80 %), it is impossible to establish a molecular cause for the disease. Although it is called polygenic hypercholesterolemia, the underlying cause may still be an unknown monogenic one with a low expressivity. More likely, however, is a condition in which several genetic factors interact to produce the hypercholesterolemia, each of which alone is not sufficiently strong to increase the LDL cholesterol concentration, but together they are successful. Most of these factors are still unknown. Probable candidates are variations of all the proteins involved with synthesis, secretion, and catabolism of lipoproteins. The relative contributions of these factors to the hypercholesterolemia may vary from individual to individual. There is no sharp distinction between normocholesterolemia and polygenic hypercholesterolemia. The risk for premature coronary heart disease starts to incline markedly in both instances at serum cholesterol levels of 200 mg/dl [377].

Hyperapobetalipoproteinemia

There is a strong possibility that not only the concentration of lipoproteins but also their quality, i.e., their composition may be of clinical and therefore diagnostic significance. According to reports in the literature, patients with CAD often exhibit LDL particles with an unusually high content of apo-B in comparison to their cholesterol content. This condition is called hyperapobetalipoproteinemia [156, 238, 240, 364, 365, 367]. According to our current knowledge, these particles have to be either lipid-poor or the cholesterol must have been replaced by another lipid, most probably triglycerides. This condition can be induced by a hypertriglyceridemia [365, 394], by continuous ambulatory pertoneal hemodialysis (CAPD) [366, 395], or by diabetes mellitus [156]. The underlying cause is presumably an overproduction of the corresponding lipids [156]. This is believed to be a rather common condition and is presumably then main feature of familial combined hyperlipemia.

Despite several attempts using several patient groups from several hospitals from several parts of Germany, we were never able to demonstrate this condition as being overrepresented in patients with CAD. On the contrary this rare condition was found more often in normal controls than in CAD patients.

Classification Systems

The Fredrickson Classification

The Fredrickson classification has been declared obsolete several times. The fact that it has found a firm place in the clinic can be attributed to its scope for describing with a simple roman numeral a complex metabolic situation and its treatment. The phenotypes (I–V) identified by lipid measurements and visual evaluation of an electrophoretic pattern are by no means all genetic entities, but type I (chylomicrons present because of a hereditary lack of the LPL or the activating C-II) and type III (broad beta-band caused by delayed catabolism of chylomicron and VLDL remnants and hence their accumulation in the serum due to homozygosity of E-2 and an unknown additional condition) come close to it.

What remains is type II, type IV, and type V. In type II the slowest migrating lipoproteins accumulate (β-lipoproteins, LDLs). This of course causes hypercholesterolemia. Additional accumulation of VLDLs leads also to hypertriglyceridemia (type IIb in contrast to the normotriglyceridemic type IIa). Type IV is an accumulation solely of

VLDLs (pre-β-lipoproteins migrating one step further than β-lipoproteins) and type V is a combination of type IV and type I.

Classification Systems for Therapeutic Guidelines

Even in normal populations the concentrations of lipoproteins cover a wide range. The normal range is usually defined as cholesterol values less or greater than a maximum and minimum 2.5 % of all the values determined in an apparently healthy population, respectively. Based on this definition, a serum cholesterol level of 260 mg/dl is still normal in our society. In contrast the majority of the factory workers in Wuhan (Peoples Republic of China) would „suffer" from abnormally low cholesterol values (the upper limit there is 150 mg/dl).

Since it is not the cholesterol concentration but the concentration of LDL cholesterol which carries the risk of CAD, a threshold value for LDL cholesterol of 155 mg/dl has been established by the experts of the European Atherosclerosis Society (1988) [106]. An increased risk of CAD is also due to an HDL cholesterol concentration of below 35 mg/dl (for women 45 mg/dl) [106]. This LDL cholesterol value is exceeded by about 40 % of the 40- to 60-year-old German population (male and female). All exceed a serum cholesterol level of 200 mg/dl. The combination of increased LDLs and decreased HDLs is rare. A concomitant low HDL cholesterol concentration is found in an additional 7 %. This makes the prevalence of dyslipoproteinemias about 45 %.

The most recent guidelines regarding lipid disorders has been published in the United States within the second report of the expert panel on detection, evaluation, and treatment of high blood cholesterol levels in adults of the National Cholesterol Education Program [289]. The guidelines are based on the determination of cholesterol triglycerides and HDL cholesterol. The subsequent determination of LDL cholesterol is recommended for HDL cholesterol levels of below 35 mg/dl or total cholesterol levels above 240 mg/dl („high blood cholesterol"). The desirable LDL cholesterol concentration should be below 130 mg/dl, „high-risk" LDL cholesterol levels start at 160 mg/dl. Depending on the accompanying risk factors (two or more), an LDL cholesterol concentration between 130 and 160 mg/dl is also considered to require lipid-lowering therapy. For symptomatic patients the optimal LDL cholesterol concentration is below 100 mg/dl. The triglyceride concentration is considered normal if it is below 200 mg/dl, very high triglyceride levels start at 1000 mg/dl, with 400 mg/dl being the border between high triglycerides and borderline to high triglycerides. If a patient with elevated triglycerides has established CAD, the associated lipid abnormality is probably a contributing factor to CAD and deserves specific therapy.

Based on current recommendations it is evident that the Fredrickson types reside in the regions of „high-risk" LDL cholesterol and high triglycerides and that the recent guidelines also extend to lower-level lipid disorders not included in the typing system.

Genetic Influences on the Lipoprotein System

The concentrations of lipoproteins in the serum should be regarded as quantitative phenotypes, being the result of the effects of measurable genetic traits (measurable genotypes), of a pool of not yet measurable polygenic components and of the sum of nongenetic factors. Systematic investigations show that about 50 % of the variability of the serum concentrations of lipoproteins can be explained by hereditary factors [32, 74, 75, 144, 284, 363]. Similar estimates have been made for the concentrations of apolipoproteins [32, 166] and for the overall risk of atherosclerosis [32, 33, 293].

It is conceivable that there are slight variations in the structure of proteins involved in the regulation of lipid metabolism. So far only for very few genetic markers has an influence on serum lipoprotein concentrations been established.

Presumably the information provided by genetic parameters exceeds that which can be derived from lipoprotein concentrations alone. Certain alleles at the loci for apolipoproteins may not influence the concentration of the gene products but rather their quality, i.e., their atherogenic potency. For instance, so far only discrepant results have been obtained for one genetic marker of apo-B, the *Xba*I polymorphism in the codon for *Thr* 2488 (cDNA position 7674). The base exchange does not affect the primary structure of apo-B. The allele *(X2)* which lacks the cutting site for the restriction enzyme has been found to be associated with increased concentrations of cholesterol and apo-B [1, 35, 246, 393]. The allele without the cutting site *(X1)* was found in some studies to be as-

sociated with the prevalence of CAD [175, 285]. Other studies could not confirm this association [89, 108]. Both alleles are equally common among Caucasians. Another example of a polymorphism at the apo-B locus is the *ins/del* polymorphism. The two alleles differ with respect to an insertion or deletion of nine base pairs coding for the amino acids –16 to –14 (leucine-alanine-leucine) of the signal peptide of apo-B. The *ins-* allele is found in 60 % – 70 % of the population [40]. It is associated with somewhat higher concentrations of apo-B and triglycerides [448]. Neither polymorphism influences the structure of apo-B of Lipoproteins. The *X2* allele of the *Xba* polymorphism is associated with a delayed clearance of apo-B-containing lipoproteins. It is therefore somehow connected („linkage dysequilibrium") with a functionally relevant mutation. This mutation has not yet been identified [96].

The *ins/del* polymorphism influences the length of the signal peptide of apo-B [40]. It could therefore exert a direct influence on the intracellular processing and the secretion of apolipoprotein-B. On the other hand, this polymorphism could also be linked to another sequence variation of apo-B without any functional consequences.

The overall significance of a genetic variation is not based on the expressivity in a single individual. If it is sufficiently common, its significance can be fairly high even at a low level of expressivity. A good example is the polymorphism of apolipoprotein-E. The presence of the E4 allele increases the LDL cholesterol concentration up to 15 mg/dl. Since the apo-E polymorphism is fairly common, it explains a significant part of the total variability of the LDL cholesterol concentration. In contrast, defects of the LDL-Rs lead to markedly elevated LDL concentrations in the affected individuals, but since these defects are relatively rare, they explain only 1 % of the variability of the LDL concentration.

Clinical-Chemical Comments

Lipid and lipoprotein diagnostics are based on the quality, i.e., accuracy and precision of the chemical determination of the cholesterol and triglyceride concentrations in the serum and within the individual lipoprotein fractions. The serum cholesterol concentration of an individual is subject to considerable variation. The precision and accuracy of cholesterol determination depend critically on the pipetting stage, the reaction mechanism of the method, the composition of the reagents, interfering substances (drugs or biological substances), the control material, standardization, and last but not least the person who does the work.

Cholesterol values which have been obtained by a chemical method (Liebermann-Burchard) without extraction directly from the serum are on average 20 mg/dl higher than the results from enzymatic methods [278]. But also the colorimetric determination after extraction gives higher values than enzymatic methods (10 mg/dl) [211]. Even enzymatic methods differ within a range of 10 mg/dl. Since all prospective studies with observation times of longer than 10 years were not using enzymatic methods, our current interpretations of cholesterol values are possibly based on erroneously high values.

In addition to methodological influences, we should also consider the influences of the preanalytical phase, which are of at least the same magnitude. These influences include the position of the body before and during the drawing of the blood, the site from where the sample is obtained, and the extent and duration of venous congestion before venipuncture. Also certain properties of the sample such as anticoagulant content and inhomogeneous specimens because of freezing and thawing without adequate mixing and evaporation of water may play an important role. The cholesterol concentration in the serum is 4 % lower than that of the corresponding plasma [73]. The cholesterol level in the serum of capillary blood is about 5 % higher [17]. The position of the body (upright or lying) together with venous congestion can lead to deviations from the „true" cholesterol concentration either direction of 5 % – 10 %.

The biological variation includes diurnal monthly and annual rhythms, hormonal influences, and the influences of nutrition diseases.

The determination of HDL cholesterol is especially sensitive to differences in methodology [273, 337]. HDL cholesterol concentration is determined by 90 % of laboratories within a range of ±7 mg/dl. Results from commercial laboratories vary by up to 18 % from the true value. Laboratories involved in screening programs have missed the target value by up to 18 % and generally find lower values. These results reflect the worldwide differences in methodology in HDL cholesterol determination. For example, in the United States a different precipitation method is used than in

Europe. The HDL cholesterol cutoff points are derived with a different method (heparin/MnCl$_2$ followed by a colormetric determination of cholesterol).

Because of the variations in HDL cholesterol values, it is difficult to judge the risk of CAD from the ratio of total cholesterol to HDL cholesterol. However, the accuracy of the quantitative measurement has considerably improved at least in Europe by the introduction of enzymatic methods and sodium phosphotungstate as polyanion.

Even if analytical and preanalytical variations can be kept to a minimum, biological variations remain considerable. Day-to-day variations are about 15 % for cholesterol, 20 % for triglycerides, 10 % for HDL cholesterol, and 8 % for „Friedewald LDL" [41]. This raises serious questions about the reliability of any cholesterol value. Only if it does not exceed 185 mg/dl can one be sure that the true cholesterol level does not exceed 200 mg/dl. A measured value of 255 mg/dl certainly reflects a true cholesterol level of over 240 mg/dl. An LDL cholesterol level of below 116 mg/dl is certainly below 130 mg/dl and a LDL cholesterol level of over 174 mg/dl lies reliably over 160 mg/dl. If a cholesterol value lies close to a cutoff point, the determination should be repeated. For example, to be able to decide whether a change of at least 10 % has occurred at least six determinations are necessary at each time [428].

In view of the difficulties regarding accuracy and precision of cholesterol determination and the marked influences of the biological variation, one may ask whether a single cholesterol determination is of any value at all. From prospective studies we know that single cholesterol determinations are better than expected [181]. The coefficient of correlation between initial values and control values after 2 years is 0.66 in men [402]. In the Lipid Research Prevalence Study two-thirds of the persons remained in the upper quintile [200].

Since dyslipoproteinemias are a serious problem and their sequelae can nowadays be prevented, the question arises at what age of the individual should the first cholesterol determination be undertaken. In order to detect familial hypercholesterolemia at an early age, the apo-B level in the cord blood should be determined. As already mentioned, familial hypercholesterolemia is about 200 times less frequent than polygenic hypercholesterolemia. This type of dyslipoproteinemia can certainly not be detected in children before puberty. Hypercholesterolemic children have only a 50 % chance of becoming hypercholesterolemic adults [385]. At the time of puberty the lowest cholesterol values in their entire life except for the 1st year are found [141, 374].

Recommendations

In each person over 30 years of age at least total cholesterol, triglyceride, HDL cholesterol, and Lp(a) levels should be determined. If HDL cholesterol concentration is below 35 mg/dl or if total cholesterol concentration is above 240 mg/dl, lipoprotein diagnostics must follow. LDL cholesterol must be evaluated according to the most recent guidelines of the National Cholesterol Education Program [289]. Lipoprotein diagnostics is most easily performed using the Friedewald formula, since most necessary information is already at hand. Elevated Lp(a) level needs to be considered as one additional risk factor. Marked hypercholesterolemias or hypertriglyceridemias should be characterized at the molecular level if possible. The lipoprotein system also deserves attention in cases of familial dyslipoproteinemias or increased incidence of cardivascular events in the family. The therapy should be monitored at short intervals in order to detect clearly increases or decreases in lipoprotein concentrations. An interval of 6 months is not sufficient.

Summary

Today lipoprotein diagnostics are an essential component of evaluations of patients with clinical vascular disease and those at high risk. Additionally, with an increasing role of vascular prevention lipoprotein screening is justified in wide segments of adult population. Up-to-date recommendations regarding the management of dyslipoproteinemias are vailable and should be followed [289]. More specific diagnostics regarding the determination of atherogenicity of the individual lipoprotein classes will become available in the future.

References

1. Aalto-Setälä K, Tikkanen MJ, Taskinen MR, Nieminen M, Holmberg P, Kontula K (1988) XbaI and c/g polymorphism of the apolipoprotein B gene locus are associated with serum cholesterol and LDL-cholesterol levels in Finland. Atherosclerosis 74: 47–54
2. Aalto-Setälä K, Gylling H, Helve E, Kovanen P, Miettinen TA, Turtola H, Kontula K (1989) Genetic polymorphism of the apolipoprotein B gene locus influences serum LDL cholesterol level in familial hypercholesterolemia. Hum Genet 82: 305–307
3. Alaupovic P, Lee DM, McConathy WJ (1972) Studies on the composition and structure of plasma lipoproteins. Distribution of lipoprotein families in major density classes of normal human plasma lipoproteins. Biochim Biophys Acta 260: 689–707
4. Albers JJ, Hazzard WR (1974) Immunochemical quantification of human plasma Lp(a) lipoprotein. Lipids 9: 15–26
5. Albers JJ, Wahl P, Hazzard WR (1974) Quantitative genetic studies of the human plasma Lp(a) lipoprotein. Biochem Genet 11: 475–486
6a. Albers JJ, Adolphson JL, Hazzard WR (1977) Radioimmunoassay of human plasma Lp(a) lipoprotein. J Lipid Res 18: 331–338
6b. Alcindor LG, Aalam H, Piot MC (1983) Practical value of the selective precipitation of LDL, LDL-phospholipids and the molar ratio of cholesterol to LDL-phospholipids in lecithin-cholesterol-acyltransferase deficiency. Ann Biol Clin 41: 311–314
7. Aqel N, Ball RY, Waldmann H, Mitchinson MJ (1985) Identification of macrophages and smooth muscle cells in human atherosclerosis using monoclonal antibodies. J Pathol 146: 197–204
8. Armstrong VW, Walli AK, Seidel D (1985) Isolation, characterization, and uptake in human fibroblasts of an apo(a)-free lipoprotein obtained on reduction of lipoprotein(a). J Lipid Res 26: 1314–1323
9. Armstrong VW, Seidel D (1985) Evaluation of a commercial kit for the determination of LDL cholesterol in serum based on precipitation of LDL with dextran sulfate. Ärztl Lab 31: 325–330
10. Armstrong VW, Cremer P, Eberle E, Manke A, Schulze F, Wieland H, Kreuzer H, Seidel D (1986) The association between serum Lp(a) concentrations and angiographically assessed coronary atherosclerosis. Dependence on serum LDL levels. Atherosclerosis 62: 249–257
11. Armstrong VW, Harrach B, Robenek H, Helmhold M, Walli AK, Seidel D (1990) Heterogeneity of human lipoprotein Lp(a): cytochemical and biochemical studies on the interaction of two Lp(a) species with the LDL receptor. J Lipid Res 31: 429–441
12. Assmann G, Jabs HU, Nolte W, Schriewer H (1984) Precipitation of LDL with sulphopolyanions: a comparison of two methods for LDL cholesterol determination. J Clin Chem Clin Biochem 22: 781–785

13. Aubry F, Lapierre YL, Noel C, Davignon J (1971) Ultracentrifugal demonstration of floating beta lipoproteins in type 3 hyperlipoproteinemia. Diagnostic value. Ann Intern Med 75: 231–237

14. Auwerx JH, Marzetta CA, Hokanson JE, Brunzell JD (1989) Large buoyant LDL-like particles in hepatic lipase deficiency. Arteriosclerosis 9: 319–325

15. Avogaro PA, Cazzolato G (1975) „Sinking" lipoprotein in normal, hyperlipoproteinaemic and atherosclerotic patients. Clin Chim Acta 61: 239–246

16. Bachorik PS, Wood PD, Albers JJ, Steiner P, Dempsey M, Kuba K, Warnick R, Karlsson L (1976) Plasma high-density lipoprotein cholesterol concentrations determined after removal of other lipoproteins by heparin/-manganese precipitation or by ultracentrifugation. Clin Chem 22: 1828–1834

17. Bachorik PS, Cloey TA, Finney CA, Lowry DR, Becker DM (1991) Lipoprotein-cholesterol analysis during screening: accuracy and reliability. Ann Intern Med 114: 741–747

18. Banka CL, Bonnet DJ, Black AS, Smith RS, Curtiss LK (1991) Localization of an apolipoprotein A-I epitope critical for activation of lecithin-cholesterol acyltransferase. J Biol Chem 266: 23886–23892

19. Barrbir M, Wile D, Trayner I, Aber VR, Thompson GR (1988) High prevalence of hypertriglyceridaemia and apolipoprotein abnormalities in coronary artery disease. Br Heart J 60: 397–403

20. Barbolini G, Scilabra GA, Botticelli A, Botticelli S (1969) On the origin of foam cells in cholesterol-induced atherosclerosis of the rabbit. Virchows Arch 3: 24–32

21. Bard JM, Delattre-Lestavel S, Clavey V, Pont P, Derudas B, Parra HJ, Fruchart JC (1992) Isolation and characterization of two sub-species of Lp(a), one containing apo E and one free of apo E. Biochim Biophys Acta 1127: 124–130

22. Barter PJ, Lally JI (1979) The metabolism of esterified cholesterol in rabbit plasma low density lipoproteins. Biochim Biophys Acta 572: 510–518

23. Barter PJ (1984) HDL metabolism in relation to plasma cholesteryl ester transport. In: Miller NE, Miller GJ (eds) Clinical and metabolic aspects of high density lipoproteins. Elsevier, Amsterdam, p 167–186

24. Bartholomé M, Wieland H, Seidel D (1980) Quantification of plasma lipoprotein cholesterol: a simple procedure for enzymatic determination of cholesterol in electrophoretically separated lipoproteins. Clin Chim Acta 104: 101–105

25. Bartl K, Ziegenhorn J, Steitberger I, Assmann G (1983) Turbidimetric kinetic method for serum low density lipoprotein quantitation. Clin Chim Acta 128: 199–208

26. Beaumont JL, Carlson LA, Cooper GR, Fejfar Z, Fredrickson DS, Strasser T (1970) Classification of hyperlipidaemias and hyperlipoproteinaemias. Bull WHO 43: 891–915

27. Beisiegel U, Weber W, Ihrke G, Herz J, Stanley KK (1989) The LDL-receptor-related protein, LRP, is an apolipoprotein E-binding protein. Nature 341: 162–164

28. Beisiegel U, Weber W, Bengtsson-Olivecrona G (1991) Lipoprotein lipase enhances the binding of chylomicrons to low density lipoprotein receptor-related protein. Proc Natl Acad Sci USA 88: 8342–8346

29. Benfante RJ, Reed DM, MacLean CJ, Yano K (1989) Risk factors in middle age that predict early and late onset of coronary heart disease. J Clin Epidemiol 42: 95–104

30. Berg K (1968) Serum lipoproteins. Bibl Haematologica 29: 21–32

31. Berg K, Dahlen G, Frick MH (1974) Lp(a) lipoprotein and pre-beta1-lipoprotein in patients with coronary heart disease. Clin Genet 6: 230–238

32. Berg K, Dahlen G, Borresen AL (1979) Lp(a) phenotypes, other lipoprotein parameters, and a family history of coronary heart disease in middle-aged males. Clin Genet 16: 347–352

33. Berg K (1983) Genetics of coronary heart disease. Prog Med Genet 5: 35–90

34. Berg K (1984) Twin studies of coronary heart disease and its risk factors. Acta Genet Med Gemellol (Roma) 33: 349–361

35. Berg K, Powell LM, Wallis SC, Pease R, Knott TJ, Scott J (1986) Genetic linkage between the antigenic group (Ag) variation and the apolipoprotein B gene: assignment of the Ag locus. Proc Natl Acad Sci USA 83: 7367–7370

35a. Berman M, Hall M, Levy RI, Eisenberg S, Bilheimer DW, Phair RD, Goebel RH (1978) Metabolism of apo B and apo C lipoproteins in man. Kinetic studies in normal and hyperlipoproteinaemic subjects. J Lipid Res 19: 38–56

36. Berg K (1986) DNA polymorphism at the apolipoprotein B locus is associated with lipoprotein level. Clin Genet 30: 515–520

36a. Bihari-Varga M, Gruber E, Rotheneder M, Zechner R, Kostner GM (1988) Interaction of lipoprotein Lp(a) and low density lipoprotein with glycosaminoglycans from human aorta. Arteriosclerosis 8: 851–857

37. Blackhart BD, Ludwig EM, Pierotti VR, Caiati L, Onasch MA, Wallis SC, Powell L, Pease R, Knott TJ, Chu ML, et al. (1986) Structure of the human apolipoprotein B gene. J Biol Chem 261: 15364–15367

38. Blankenhorn DH, Nessim SA, Johnson RL, Sanmarco ME, Azen SP, Cashin-Hemphill L (1987) Beneficial effects of combined colestipol-niacin therapy on coronary atherosclerosis and coronary venous bypass grafts. JAMA 257: 3233–3240

39. Blankenhorn DH, Alaupovic P, Wickham E, Chin HP, Azen SP (1990) Prediction of angiographic change in native human coronary arteries and aortocoronary bypass grafts. Lipid and non-lipd factors. Circulation 81: 470–476

40. Boerwinkle E, Chan L (1989) A three codon insertion/deletion polymorphism in the signal peptide region of the human apolipoprotein B

(APOB) gene directly typed by the polymerase chain reaction. Nucleic Acids Res 17: 4003

41. Bookstein L, Gidding SS, Donovan M, Smith FA (1990) Day-to-day variability of serum cholesterol, triglyceride, and high-density lipoprotein cholesterol levels. Impact on the assessment of risk according to the National Cholesterol Education Program guidelines. Arch Intern Med 150: 1653–1657

42. Boström K, Lauer SJ, Poksay KS, Garcia Z, Taylor JM, Innerarity TL (1989) Apolipoprotein B48 RNA editing in chimeric apolipoprotein EB mRNA. J Biol Chem 264: 15701–15708

43. Bouma ME, Pessah M, Renaud G, Amit N, Catala D, Infante R (1988) Synthesis and secretion of lipoproteins by human hepatocytes in culture. In Vitro Cell Dev Biol 24: 85–90

44. Bradley WA, Gianturco SH (1986) Apo E is necessary and sufficient for the binding of large triglyceride-rich lipoproteins to the LDL receptor; apoB is unnecessary. J Lipid Res 27: 40–48

45. Breckenridge WC, Little JA, Steiner G, Chow A, Poapst M (1978) Hypertriglyceridemia associated with deficiency of apolipoprotein C-II. N Engl J Med 298: 1265–1273

46. Breckenridge WC, Maquire GF (1981) Quantification of sinking pre beta lipoprotein in human plasma. Clin-Biochem 14: 82–86

47. Breslow JL (1989) Familial disorders of high density lipoprotein metabolism. In: Scriver RC, Beaudet AL, Sly WS, Valle D (eds) The metabolic basis of inherited disease. McGraw-Hill, New York, p 1253

48. Brown G, Albers JJ, Fisher LD, Schaefer SM, Lin JT, Kaplan C, Zhao XQ, Bisson BD, Fitzpatrick VF, Dodge HT (990) Regression of coronary artery disease as a result of intensive lipid-lowering therapy in men with high levels of apolipoprotein B (see comments). N Engl J Med 323: 1289–1298

49. Brown MS, Goldstein JL (1983) Lipoprotein receptors in the liver. Control signals for plasma cholesterol traffic. J Clin Invest 72: 743–747

50. Brown MS, Goldstein JL (1983) Lipoprotein metabolism in the macrophage: implications for cholesterol deposition in atherosclerosis. Annu Rev Biochem 52: 223–261

51. Brown MS, Goldstein JL (1986) A receptor-mediated pathway for cholesterol homeostasis. Science 232: 34–47

52. Brown SA, Via DP, Gotto AM Jr, Bradly WA, Gianturco SH (1986) Apolipoprotein E mediated binding of hypertriglyceridemic VLDL to isolated LDL-receptors detected by ligand blotting. Biochem Biophys Res Commun 139: 333–340

53. Burstein M, Scholnick HR, Morfin R (1970) Rapid method for the isolation of lipoproteins from human serum by precipitation with polyanions. J Lipid Res 11: 583–595

54. Burstein M, Scholnick HR (1973) Lipoprotein-polyanion-metal interactions. Adv Lipid res 11: 67–108

55. Cambillau M, Simon A, Amar J, Giral P, Atger V, Segond P, Levenson J, Merli I, Megnien JL, Plainfosse MC, et al. (1992) Serum Lp(a) as a discriminant marker of early atherosclerotic plaque at three extracoronary sites in hypercholesterolemic men. The PCVMETRA group. Arterioscler Thromb 12: 1346–1352

56. Carlson K, Carlson LA (1975) Comparison of behaviour of very low density lipoproteins of type-III hyperlipoproteinaemia on electrophoresis on paper and on agarose gel with a note on a late (slow) pre-beta VLDL lipoprotein. Scand J Clin Lab Invest 35: 655–660

57. Carlson LA, Bottiger LE (1985) Risk factors for ischaemic heart disease in men and women. Results of the 19-year follow-up of the Stockholm Prospective Study. Acta Med Scand 218: 207–211

58. Castelli WP, Doyle JT, Gordon T, Hames CG, Hjortland MC, Hulley SB, Kagan A, Zukel WJ (1977) HDL cholesterol and other lipids in coronary heart disease. The cooperative lipoprotein phenotyping study. Circulation 55: 767–772

59. Castelli WP (1984) Epidemiology of coronary heart disease: the Framingham study. Am J Med 76: 4–12

60. Castelli WP (1988) Cardiovascular disease in women. Am J Obstet Gynecol 158: 1553–1560

61. Castelli WP (1988) Cholesterol and lipids in the risk of coronary artery disease – the Framingham Heart Study. Can J Cardiol 4, Suppl. A: 5A–10A

62. Castelli WP, Wilson PW, Levy D, Anderson K (1989) Cardiovascular risk factors in the elderly. Am J Cardiol 63: 12H–19H

63. Castro GR, Fiedling CJ (1985) Effects of postprandial lipemia on plasma cholesterol metabolism. J Clin Invest 75: 874–882

64. Cazzolato G, Prakasch G, Green S, Kostner GM (1983) The determination of lipoprotein Lp(a) by rate and endpoint nephelometry. Clin Chim Acta 135: 203–208

65. Chait A, Brunzell JD, Albers JJ, Hazzard WR (1977) Type-III hyperlipoproteinaemia („remnant removal disease"). Lancet II: 1176–1178

66. Chait A, Hazzard WR, Albers JJ, Kushwaha RP, Brunzell JD (1978) Impaired very low density lipoprotein and triglyceride removal in broad beta disease. Comparison with endogenous hypertriglyceridaemia. Metabolism 27: 1055–1066

67. Cham BE (1976) Nature of the interaction between low-density lipoproteins and polyanions and metal ions, as exemplified by heparin and Ca^{++}. Clin Chem 22: 1812–1816

68. Chen SH, Yang CY, Chen PF, Setzer D, Tanimura M, Li WH, Gotto AM Jr, Chan L (1986) The complete cDNA and amino acid sequence of human apolipoprotein B-100. J Biol Chem 261: 12918–12921

69. Chen SH, Habib G, Yang CY, Gu ZW, Lee BR, Weng SA, Silberman SR, Cai SJ, Deslypere JP, Rosseneu M, et al. (1987) Apolipoprotein B-48 is the product of a messenger RNA with an organ-specific in-frame stop codon. Science 238: 363–366

70. Cheng Q, Blackett P, Jackson KW, McConathy, WJ, Wang CS (1990) C-terminal domain of apolipoprotein C II as both activator and competitive

lipaseinhibitor of lipoprotein lipase. Biochem J 269: 403–407

71. Chesebro B, Svehag SE (1968) Precipitation of human serum proteins by polyethylene glycol. Clin Chim Acta 20: 527–529

72. Cladaras C, Hadzopoulou-Cladaras M, Nolte RT, Atkinson D, Zannis VI (1986) The complete sequence and structural analysis of human apolipoprotein B-100: relationship between apoB-100 and apoB-48 forms. EMBO J 5: 3495–3507

73. Cloey T, Bachorik PS, Becker D, Finney C, Lowry D, Sigmund W (1990) Reevaluation of serum-plasma differences in total cholesterol concentration. JAMA 263: 2788–2789

74. Christian JC, Cheung SW, Kang K, Harmath FP, Huntzinger DJ, Powell RC (1976) Variance of plasma free and esterified cholesterol in adult twins. Am J Hum Genet 28: 174–178

75. Christian JC, Feinleib M, Hulley SB, Castelli WP, Fabsitz RR, Garrison RJ, Borhani NO, Rosenman RH, Wagner J (1976) Genetics of plasma cholesterol and triglycerides: a study of adult male twins. Acta Genet Med Gemellol (Roma) 25: 145–149

76. Connelly PW, Ranganathan S, Maguire GF, Lee M, Myher JJ, Kottke BA, Kuksis A, Little JA (1988) The beta very low density lipoprotein present in hepatic lipase deficiency competitively inhibits low density lipoprotein binding to fibroblasts and stimulates fibroblast acyl-Co-A cholesterol acyltransferase. J Biol Chem (Canada) 263: 14184–14188

77. Connelly PW, Maguire GF, Lee M, Little JA (1990) Plasma lipoproteins in familial hepatic lipase deficiency. Arteriosclerosis 10: 40–48

78. Cooke PH, Smith SC (1968) Smooth muscle cells: the source of foam cells in atherosclerotic white Carneau pigeons. Exp Mol Pathol 8: 171–189

79. Cremer P, Elster H, Labrot B, Kruse B, Muche R, Seidel D (1988) Incidence rates of fatal and nonfatal myocardial infarction in relation to the lipoprotein profile: first prospective results from the Göttingen Risk, Incidence, and Prevalende Study (GRIPS). Klin Wochenschr 66 [Suppl 11]: 42–49

80. Dahlén G, Ericson C, Furberg C, Lundkvist L, Svardsudd K (1972) Studies on an extra pre-beta lipoprotein fraction. Acta Med Scand [Suppl] 531: 1–29

81. Dahlén G (1974) The pre-beta lipoprotein phenomenon in relation to serum cholesterol and triglyceride levels, the Lp(a) lipoprotein and coronary heart disease. Acta Med Scand [Suppl] 570: 1–45

82. Dahlén G, Berg K, Gillnas T, Ericson C (1975) Lp(a) lipoprotein/pre-beta1-lipoprotein in Swedish middle-aged males and in patients with coronary heart disease. Clin Genet 7: 334–341

83. Dahlén G, Frick MH, Berg K, Valle M, Wiljasalo M (1975) Further studies of Lp(a) lipoprotein/pre-beta1-lipoprotein in patients with coronary heart disease. Clin Genet 8: 183–189

84. Dahlén G, Berg K, Frick MH (1976) Lp(a) lipoprotein/pre-beta1-lipoprotein, serum lipids and atherosclerotic disease. Clin Genet 9: 558–566

85. Dahlén GH, Guyton JR, Attar M, Farmer JA, Kautz JA, Gotto AM Jr (1986) Association of levels of lipoprotein Lp(a), plasma lipids, and other lipoproteins with coronary artery disease documented by angiography. Circulation 74: 758–765

86. Davies MS, Wallis SC, Driscoll DM, Wynne JK, Williams GW, Powell LM, Scott J (1989) Sequence requirements for apolipoprotein B RNA editing in transfected rat hepatoma cells. J Biol Chem 264: 13395–13398

87. Davignon J, Gregg RE, Sing CF (1988) Apolipoprotein E polymorphism and atherosclerosis. Arteriosclerosis 8: 1–21

88. Deckelbaum RJ, Eisenberg S, Oschry Y, Granot E, Sharon I, Bengtsson-Olivecrona G (1986) Conversion of human plasma high density lipoprotein-2 to high density lipoprotein-3. Roles of neutral lipid exchange and triglyceride lipases. J Biol Chem 261: 5201–5208

89. Deeb S, Failor A, Brown BG, Brunzell JD, Albers JJ, Motulsky AG (1986) Molecular genetics of apolipoproteins and coronary heart disease. Cold Spring Harbor Symp Quant Biol 51: 403–409

90. de Faire U, Dahlen G, Liljefors I, Lundman T, Theorell T (1981) Pre-beta1-lipoprotein in patients with ischemic heart disease. Genetic determination and relation to early insulin response. Acta Med Scand 209: 65–68

91. Doerr W (1963) Theorie der Perfusion. In: Bergmann W, Doerr W (eds) Zwanglose Abhandlungen aus dem Gebiete der normalen und pathologischen Anatomie. Perfusionstheorie der Arteriosklerose. Thieme, Stuttgart, 91–97

92. Duguid JB (1946) Thrombosis as a factor in the pathogenesis of coronary atherosclerosis. J Path Bact 58: 207–212

93. Duguid JB (1948) Thrombosis as a factor in the pathogenesis of aortic atherosclerosis. J Path Bact 60: 57–61

94. Drayna DT, Hegele RA, Hass PE, Emi M, Wu LL, Eaton DL, Lawn RM, Williams RR, White RL, Lalouel JM (1988) Genetic linkage between lipoprotein(a) phenotype and a DNA polymorphism in the plasminogen gene. Genomics 3: 230–236

95. Driscoll DM, Wynne JK, Wallis SC, Scott J (1989) An in vitro system for the editing of apolipoprotein B mRNA. Cell 58: 519–525

96. Dunning AM, Houlston R, Frostegard J, Revill J, Nilsson J, Hamsten A, Talmud P, Humphries S (1991) Genetic evidence that the putative receptor binding domain of apolipoprotein B (residues 3130 to 3630) is not the only region of the protein involved in interaction with the low density lipoprotein receptor. Biochim Biophys Acta 1096: 231–237

97. Durrington PN, Ishola M, Hunt L, Arrol S, Bhatnagar D (1988) Apolipoproteins (a), AI, and B and parental history in men with early onset ischaemic heart disease. Lancet 1: 1070–1073

98. Duvic CR, Smith G, Sledge WE, Lee LT, Murray MD, Roheim PS, Gallaher WR, Thompson JJ

(1985) Identification of a mouse monoclonal antibody, LHLP-1, specific for human Lp(a). J Lipid Res 26: 540–548

99. Eaton DL, Fless GM, Kohr WJ, McLean JW, Xu QT, Miller CG, Lawn RM, Scanu AM (1987) Partial amino acid sequence of apolipoprotein(a) shows that it is homologous to plasminogen. Proc Natl Acad Sci USA 84: 3224–3228

100. Ehnholm C, Garoff H, Simons K, Aro H (1971) Purification and quantitation of the human plasma lipoprotein carrying the Lp(a) antigen. Biochim Biophys Acta 236: 431–439

101. Ehnholm C, Garoff H, Renkonen O, Simons K (1972) Protein and carbohydrate composition of Lp(a) lipoprotein from human plasma. Biochemistry 11: 3229

102. Eisenberg S (1980) Plasma lipoproteins interconversion. Ann NY Acad Sci 348: 30–47

103. Eisenberg S (1985) Preferential enrichment of large-sized very low density lipoprotein populations with transferred cholesteryl esters. J Lipid Res 26: 487–494

104. Ericson C, Dahlen G, Berg K (1977) Interaction of isolated Lp(a) lipoprotein with calcium ions and glycosaminoglycans in vitro. Clin Genet 11: 433–440

105. Eto M, Watanabe K, Chonan N, Ishii K (1988) Familial hypercholesterolemia and apolipoprotein E4. Atherosclerosis 72: 123–128

106. Carmena R, Crepaldi G, De Backer G, de Gennes JL, Eisenberg S, Galton D, Gotto AM, Goodwin JF, Greten H, Hanefeld M, Huttunen JK, Jacotot B, Katan MB, Mann JL, Miettionen TA, Norum KR, Oganov RG, Olsson AG, Paoletti R, Pometta D, Pyorala K. Schettler G, Shepherd J, Schwandt P, Tikkanen MJ (1988) The recognition and management of hyperlipidaemia in adults: policy statement of the European Atherosclerosis Society. Eur Heart J 9: 571–600

107. Fagiotto A, Ross R, Harker L (1984) Studies of hypercholesterolemia in the nonhuman primate. I. Changes that lead to fatty streak formation. Arteriosclerosis 4: 323–340

108. Ferns GA, Robinson D, Galton DJ (1988) DNA haplotypes of the human apoprotein B gene in coronary atherosclerosis. Hum Genet 1988, 81: 76–80

109. Fielding CJ (1984) The origin and properties of free cholesterol potential gradients in plasma, and their relation to atherogenesis. J Lipid Res 25: 1624–1628

110. Fielding CJ (1987) Factors affecting the rate of catalyzed transfer of cholesteryl esters in plasma. Am Heart J 113: 532–537

111. Fless GM, Scanu AM (1979) Isolation and characterization of the three major low density lipoproteins from normolipidemic rhesus monkeys (Macaca mulatta). J Biol Chem 254: 8653–8661

112. Fless GM, Fischer-Dzoga K, Juhn DJ, Bates S, Scanu AM (1982) Structural and functional changes of rhesus serum low density lipoproteins during cycles of diet-induced hypercholesterolemia. Arteriosclerosis 1982, 2: 475–486

113. Fless GM, ZumMallen ME, Scanu AM (1986) Physiochemical properties of apolipoprotein(a) and lipoprotein(a-) derived from the dissociation of human plasma lipoprotein(a). J Biol Chem 261: 8712–8718

114. Floren CH, Albers JJ, Bierman EL (1981) Uptake of Lp(a) lipoprotein by cultured fibroblasts. Biochem Biophys Res Commun 102(2): 636–639

115. Fojo SS, de Gennes JL, Beisiegel U (1991) Molecular genetics of apoC-II and lipoprotein lipase deficiency. Adv Exp Med Biol 285: 329–333

116. Fojo SS, Brewer HB (1992) Hypertriglyceridaemia due to genetic defects in lipoprotein lipase and apolipoprotein C-II. J Intern Med 231: 669–677

117. Fong LG, Parthasarathy S, Witztum JL, Steinberg D (1987) Nonenzymatic oxidative cleavage of peptide bonds in apoprotein B-100. J Lipid Res 28: 1466–1477

118. Fowler S, Shio H, Haley NJ (1979) Characterization of lipid-laden aortic cells from cholesterolfed rabbits. IV. Investigation of macrophage-like properties of aortic cell populations. Lab Invest 41: 372–378

119. Fowler S (1980) Characterization of foam cells in experimental atherosclerosis. Acta Med Scand [Suppl] 642: 151–158

120. Fredrickson DS, Levy RI, Lees RS (1967) Fat transport in lipoproteins – an integrated approach to mechanisms and disorders. N Engl J Med 276: 34–42

121. Fredrickson DS, Levy RI, Lees RS (1967) Fat transport in lipoproteins – an integrated approach to mechanisms and disorders. N Engl J Med 276: 94–103

122. Fredrickson DS, Levy RI, Lees RS (1967) Fat transport in lipoproteins – an integrated approach to mechanisms and disorders. N Engl J Med 276: 148–156

123. Fredrickson DS, Levy RI, Lees RS (1967) Fat transport in lipoproteins – an integrated approach to mechanisms and disorders. N Engl J Med 276: 215–225

124. Fredrickson DS, Levy RI, Lees RS (1967) Fat transport in lipoproteins – an integrated approach to mechanisms and disorders. N Engl J Med 276: 273–281

125. Frick MH, Dahlen G, Berg K, Valle M, Hekali P (1978) Serum lipids in angiographically assessed coronary atherosclerosis. Chest 73: 62–65

126. Friedewald WT, Levy RJ, Fredrickson DS (1972) Estimation of the concentration of low density lipoprotein cholesterol in plasma, without use of preparative ultracentrifuge. Clin Chem 18: 499–509

127. Fruchart JC, Ailhaud G (1992) Apolipoprotein A-containing lipoprotein particles: physiological role, quantification, and clinical significance. Clin Chem 38: 793–797

128. Gabelli C, Gregg RE, Zech LA, Manzato E, Brewer BH (1986) Abnormal low density metabolism in apolipoprotein E deficiency. J Lipid Res 27: 326–333

129. Gaton E, Wolman M (1977) The role of smooth muscle cells and hematogenous macrophages in atheroma. J Pathol 123: 123–128

130. Gaubatz JW, Heideman C, Gotto AM Jr, Morrisett JD, Dahlen GH (1983) Human plasma lipoprotein(a). Structural properties. J Biol Chem 258: 4582–4589

131. Gaubatz JW, Cushing GL, Morrisett JD (1986) Quantitation, isolation, and characterization of human lipoprotein(a). Methods Enzymol 129: 167–186

132. Gaubatz JW, Ghanem KI, Guevara J Jr, Nava ML, Patsch W, Morrisett JD (1990) Polymorphic forms of human apolipoprotein(a): inheritance and relationship of their molecular weights to plasma levels of lipoprotein(a). J Lipid Res 31: 603–613

133. Gerrity RG, Naito HK, Richardson M, Schwartz CJ (1979) Dietary induced atherogenesis in swine. Am J Pathol 95: 775–793

134. Gerrity RG, Naito HK (1980) Ultrastructural identifications of monocyte-derived foam cells in fatty streak lesions. Artery 8: 208–214

135. Gerrity RG, Naito HK (1980) Lipid clearance from fatty streak lesions by foam cell migration. Artery 8: 215–219

136. Ghilain JM, Parfonry A, Kozyreff V, Heller FR (1988) Lipoprotein(a), cholesterol, and coronary heart diseases. Lancet II: 963

137. Ghiselli G, Schaefer EJ, Gascon P, Breser HB Jr (1981) Type-III hyperlipoproteinemia associated with apolipoprotein E deficiency. Science 214: 1239–1241

138. Ghiselli G, Gregg RE, Brewer HB Jr (1984) Apolipoprotein E Bethesda. Isolation and partial characterization of a variant of human apolipoprotein E isolated from very low density lipoproteins. Biochim Biophys Acta 794: 333–339

139. Gidez LI, Miller GJ, Burstein M, Slagle S, Eder HA (1982) Separation and quantitation of subclasses of human plasma high density lipoproteins by a simple precipitation procedure. J Lipid Res 23: 1206–1223

140. Ginsberg HN, Le NA, Gibson JC (1985) Regulation of the production and catabolism of plasma low density lipoproteins in hypertriglyceridemic subjects. J Clin Invest 75: 614–623

141. Ginsburg BE, Zetterström R (1980) Serum cholesterol concentrations in early infancy. Acta Paediatr Scand 69: 581–585

142. Glomset JA (1968) The plasma lecithin: cholesterol acyltransferase reaction. J Lipid Res 9: 155–167

143. Glomset JA, Norum KR, Nichols AV, King WC, Mitchell CD, Applegate KR, Gong EL, Glone E (1975) Plasma lipoproteins in familial lecithin: cholesterol acyltransferase deficiency. Scand J Clin Lab Invest [Suppl] 35: 1–55

144. Goldbourt U, Neufeld HN (1986) Genetic aspects of arteriosclerosis. Arteriosclerosis 6: 357–377

145. Goldstein JL, Brown MS (1973) Familial hypercholesterolaemia: identification of a defect in the regulation of 3-hydroxy-3-methylglutaryl coenzyme A reductase activity associated with overproduction of cholesterol. Proc Natl Acad Sci USA 70: 2804–2808

146. Goldstein JL, Ho YK, Basu SK, Brown MS (1979) Binding site on macrophages that mediates uptake and degradation of acetylated low density lipoprotein, producing massive cholesterol deposition. Proc Natl Acad Sci USA 76: 333–377

147. Goldstein JL, Ho YK, Brown MS, Innerarity TL, Mahley RW (1980) Cholesteryl ester accumulation in macrophages resulting from receptor-mediated uptake and degradation of hypercholesterolemic canine beta-very low density lipoproteins. J Biol Chem 255: 1839–1848

148. Goldstein JL, Brown MS (1984) Progress in understanding the LDL receptor and HMG-CoA reductase, two membrane proteins that regulate the plasma cholesterol. J Lipid Res 25: 1450–1461

149. Goldstein JL, Brown MS (1990) Regulation of the mevalonate pathway. Nature 343: 425–430

150. Gordon DJ, Knoke J, Probstfield JL, Superko R, Tyroler HA (1986) High-density lipoprotein cholesterol and coronary heart disease in hypercholesterolemic men: the Lipid Research Clinics Coronary Primary Prevention Trial. Circulation 74: 1217–1225

151. Gordon DJ, Probstfield JL, Garrison RJ, Neaton JD, Castelli WP, Knike JD, Jacobs DR Jr, Bangdiwala S, Tyroler HA (1989) High-density lipoprotein cholesterol and cardiovascular disease. Four prospective American studies. Circulation 79: 8–15

152. Gotto AM Jr (1983) High-density lipoproteins: biochemical and metabolic factors. Am J Cardiol 52: 2B–4B

153. Gregg RE, Zech LA, Schaefer EJ, Brewer HB Jr (1981) Type-III hyperlipoproteinemia defective metabolism of an abnormal apolipoprotein E. Science 211: 584–586

154. Gregg RE, Brewer HB Jr (1988) The role of apolipoprotein E and lipoprotein receptors in modulating the in vivo metabolism of apolipoprotein B-containing lipoproteins in humans. Clin Chem 34: B28–32

155. Grundy SM, Mok HYI (1976) Chylomicron clearance in normal and hyperlipidemic man. Metabolism 25: 1225–1239

156. Grundy SM, Vega GL, Kesianiemi YA (1985) Abnormalities in metabolism of low density lipoproteins associated with coronary heart disease. Acta Med Scand [Suppl] 701: 23–37

157. Gunby P (1983) High HDL2 levels lower postprandial lipids [news]. JAMA 249: 1250

158. Guo HC, Chapman MJ, Bruckert E, Farriaux JP, De Gennes JL (1991) Lipoprotein Lp(a) in homozygous familial hypercholesterolemia: density profile, particle heterogeneity and apolipoprotein(a) phenotype. Atherosclerosis 86: 69–83

159. Gutzwiller F, Bertel O, Darioli R, Epstein FH, Hartmann G, Keller U, Kummer H, Mordasini R, Noseda G, Pometta D, Rickenbach M, Riesen W, Rutishauser W, Stähelin HB (1989) Lipide und die Prävention der koronaren Herzkrank-

heit: Diagnostik und Massnahmen. Schweiz Ärztezeitung 70: 1279–1292

160. Guyton JR, Dahlen GH, Patsch W, Kautz JA, Gotto AM Jr (1985) Relationship of plasma lipoprotein Lp(a) levels to race and to apolipoprotein B. Arteriosclerosis 5: 265–272

161. Gylling H, Aalto-Setälä K, Kontula K, Miettionen TA (1991) Serum low density lipoprotein cholesterol level and cholesterol absorption efficiency are influenced by apolipoprotein B and E polymorphism and by the FH-Helsinki mutation of the low density lipoprotein receptor gene in familial hypercholesterolemia. Arterioscler Thromb 11: 1368–1375

162. Hagman M, Wilhelmsen L, Wedel H, Pennert K (1987) Risk factors for angina pectoris in a population study of Swedish men. J Chronic Dis 40: 265–275

163. Haley NJ, Shio H, Fowler S (1977) Characterization of lipid-laden aortic cells from cholesterol-fed rabbits. I. Resolution of aortic cell populations by metrizamide density gradient centrifugation. Lab Invest 37: 287–296

164. Hamilton RL, Williams MC, Fielding CJ, Havel RJ (1976) Discoidal bilayer structure of nascent high density lipoproteins from perfused rat liver. J Clin Invest 58: 667–683

165. Hamsten A, Wallidus G, Dahlen G, Johansson B, de Faire U (1986) Serum lipoproteins and apolipoproteins in young male survivors of myocardial infarction. Atherosclerosis 59: 223–235

166. Hamsten A, Iselius L, Dahlen G, De Faire U (1986) Genetic and cultural inheritance of serum lipids, low and high density lipoprotein cholesterol and serum apolipoproteins A-I, A-II and B. Atherosclerosis 60: 199–208

167. Harvie NR, Schultz JS (1973) Studies on the heterogeneity of human serum Lp lipoproteins and on the occurrence of double Lp lipoprotein variants. Biochem Genet 9: 235–245

168. Hatch FT (1968) Practical methods for plasma lipoprotein analysis. Adv Lipid Res 6: 1–68

169. Haust MD, More RH (1963) Significance of the smooth muscle cell in atherogenesis. In: Jones RJ (ed) Evolution of the atherosclerotic plaque. University of Chicago Press, Chicago, pp 51–63

170. Haust MD (1977) Myogenic foam cells in explants of fatty dots and streaks from rabbit aorta. Morphological studies. Atherosclerosis 26: 441–464

171. Havel RJ, Kane JP, Kashyap ML (1973) Interchange of apolipoproteins between chylomicrons and high density lipoproteins during alimentary lipemia in man. J Clin Invest 52: 32–38

172. Havel RJ (1984) The formation of LDL: mechanisms and regulation. J Lipid Res 25: 1570–1576

172a. Havel RJ (1982) Med Clin North Am 66: 319–333

173. Hazzard WR, Bierman EL (1975) The spectrum of electrophoretic mobility of very low density lipoproteins: role of slower migrating species in endogenous hypertriglyceridemia (type IV hyperlipoproteinemia) and broad-beta disease (type-III). J Lab Clin Med 86: 239–252

174. Hearn JA, Donohue BC, Ba'albaki H, Douglas JS, King SB, Lembo NJ, Roubin GS, Sgoutas DS (1992) Usefulness of serum lipoprotein(a) as a predictor of restenosis after percutaneous transluminal coronary angioplasty. Am J Cardiol 69: 736–739

175. Hegele RA, Huang LS, Herbert PN, Blum CB, Buring JE, Hennekens CH, Breslow JL (1986) Apolipoprotein B-gene DNA polymorphisms associated with myocardial infarction. N Engl J Med 315: 1509–1515

176. Henriksen T, Mahoney EM, Steinberg E (1981) Enhanced macrophage degradation of low density lipoprotein previously incubated with cultured endothelial cells: recognition by receptors for acetylated low density lipoproteins. Proc Natl Acad Sci USA 78: 6499–6503

177. Henriksen T, Mahoney EM, Steinberg D (1982) Enhanced macrophage degradation of biologically modified low density lipoprotein. Arteriosclerosis 3: 149–159

178. Herz J, Hamann U, Rogne S, Myklebost O, Gausepohl H, Stanley KK (1988) Surface location and high affinity for calcium of a 500-kd liver membrane protein closely related to the LDL-receptor suggest a physiological role as lipoprotein receptor. EMBO J 7: 4119–4127

179. Herz J, Kowal RC, Ho YK, Brown MS, Goldstein JL (1990) Low density lipoprotein receptor-related protein mediates endocytosis of monoclonal antibodies in cultured cells and rabbit liver. J Biol Chem 265: 21355–21362

180. Herz J, Goldstein JL, Strickland DK, Ho YK, Brown MS (1991) 39-kDa protein modulates binding of ligands to low density lipoprotein receptor-related protein/alpha 2-macroglobulin receptor. J Biol Chem 266: 21232–21238

181. Hetland ML, Haarbo J, Christiansen C (1992) One measurement of serum total cholesterol is enough to predict future levels in healthy postmenopausal women. Am J Med 92: 25–28

182. Hinek A, Rosnowski A (1975) Comparison of morphology of isolated cells obtained from aortas of normal and cholesterol fed rabbits. Paroi Arterielle 3: 17–29

183. Hobbs HH, Brown MS, Goldstein JL, Russell DW (1986) Deletion of exon encoding cysteine-rich repeat of low density lipoprotein receptor alters its binding specificity in a subject with familial hypercholesterolemia. J Biol Chem 261: 13114–13120

184. Hobbs HH, Brown MS, Goldstein JL (1992) Molecular genetics of the LDL receptor gene in familial hypercholesterolemia. Hum Mutat: 445–466

185. Hoff HF, Beck GJ, Skibinski CI, Jurgens G, O'Neil J, Kramer J, Lytle B (1988) Serum Lp(a) level as a predictor of vein graft stenosis after coronary artery bypass surgery in patients. Circulation 77: 1238–1244

186. Hoff HF, O'Neil J, Chisolm GM 3d, Cole TB, Quehenberger O, Esterbauer H, Jurgens G (1989) Modification of low density lipoprotein with 4-hydroxynonenal induces uptake by macrophages. Arteriosclerosis 9: 538–549

187. Hoff HF, O'Neil J, Yashiro A (1993) Partial characterization of lipoproteins containing apo[a] in human atherosclerotic lesions. J Lipid Res 34: 789–798

188. Holme I, Helgeland A, Hjermann I, Leren P, Lund-Larsen PG (1980) Four and two-thirds years incidence of coronary heart disease in middle-aged men: the Oslo study. Am J Epidemiol 112: 149–160

189. Horrigan S, Campbell JH, Campbell GR (1991) Oxidation of beta-very low density lipoprotein by endothelial cells enhances its metabolism by smooth muscle cells in culture. Arteriscler Thromb 11: 279–289

190. Howard BV, Knowler WC, Vasquez B, Kennedy AL, Pettitt DJ, Benett PH (1984) Plasma and lipoprotein cholesterol and triglyceride in the Pima Indian population. Comparison of diabetics and nondiabetics. Arteriosclerosis 4: 462–471

191. Huff MW, Telford DE (1985) Direct synthesis of low-density lipoprotein apoprotein B in the miniature pig. Metabolism 34: 36–42

192. Huff MW, Telford DE, Woodcroft K, Strong WL (1985) Mevinolin and cholestyramine inhibit the direct synthesis of low density lipoprotein apoprotein B in miniature pigs. J Lipid Res 26: 1175–1186

193. Hui DY, Innerarity TL, Mahley RW (1984) Defective hepatic lipoprotein receptor binding of beta-very low density lipoproteins from type-III hyperlipoproteinemic patients. Importance of a prolipoprotein E. J Biol Chem 259: 860–869

194. Hussain MM, Zannis VI (1990) Intracellular modification of human apolipoprotein AII (apoAII) and sites of apoAII mRNA synthesis: comparison of apoAII with apoCII and apoCIII isoproteins. Biochem 29: 209–217

195. Innerarity TL, Friedlander EJ, Rall SC, Weisgraber KH, Mahley RW (1983) The receptor binding domain of human apolipoprotein E. Binding of apolipoprotein E fragments. J Biol Chem 258: 12341–12347

196. Innerarity TL, Arnold KS, Weisgraber KH, Mahley RW (1986) Apolipoprotein E is the determinant that mediates the receptor uptakes of beta-very low density lipoproteins by mouse macrophages. Arteriosclerosis 6: 114–122

197. Innerarity TL, Mahley RW, Weisgraber KH, Bersot TP, Krauss RM, Vega GL, Grundy SM, Friedl W, Davignon J, McCarthy BJ (1990) Familial defective apolipoprotein B-100: a mutation of apolipoprotein B that causes hypercholesterolemia. J Lipid Res 31: 1337–1349

198. Iselius L, Dahlen G, de Faire U, Lundman T (1981) Complex segregation analysis of the Lp(a)/pre-beta 1-lipoprotein trait. Clin Genet 20: 147–151

199. Iverius PH, Laurent TC (1967) Precipitation of some plasma proteins by the addition of dextran or polyethylene glycol. Biochim Biophys Acta 133: 371–373

200. Jacobs DR Jr, Barrett-Connor E (1982) Retest reliability of plasma cholesterol and triglyceride. The Lipid Research Clinics Prevalence Study. Am J Epidemiol 116: 878–885

201. James RW, Martion B, Pometta D, Fruchart JC, Duriez P, Puchois P, Farriaux JP, Tacquet A, Demant T, Clegg RJ (1989) Apolipoprotein B metabolism in homozygous hypercholesterolaemia. J Lipid Res 30: 159–169

202. Janus ED, Nicoll AM, Turner PR, Magill P, Lewis B (1980) Kinetic bases of the primary hyperlipidaemias: studies of apolipoprotein B turnover in genetically defined subjects. Eur J Clin Invest 10: 161–172

203. Kameda K, Matsuzawa Y, Kubo M, Ishikawa K, Maejima I, Yamamura T, Yamamoto A, Tarui S (1984) Increased frequency of lipoprotein disorders similar to type-III hyperlipoproteinemia in survivors of myocardial infarction in Japan. Atherosclerosis 51: 241–249

204. Kanalas JJ, Makker SP (1991) Identification of the rat Heymann nephritis autoantigen (GP330) as a receptor site for plasminogen. J Biol Chem 266: 10825–10829

205. Kannel WB (1980) Influence of blood lipids on risk in hypertension. Hypertension update. In: Hunt JC (ed) Dialogoes in Hypertension. Heart Learning System Inc., Bloomfield, New York

206. Karädi I, Kostner GM, Gries A, Nimpf J, Romics L, Malle E (1988) Lipoprotein(a) and plasminogen are immunochemically related. Biochim Biophys Acta 960: 91–97

207. Karlin JB, Johnson WJ, Benedict CR, Chacko GK, Phillips MC, Rothblat GH (1987) Cholesterol flux between cells and high density lipoprotein. Lack of relationship to specific binding of the lipoprotein to the cell surface. J Biol Chem 262: 12557–12564

208. Keys A, Menotti A, Aravanis C, Blackburn H, Djordevic BS, Buzina R, Dontas AS, Fidanza F, Karvonen MJ, Kimura N (1984) The seven countries study: 2289 deaths in 15 years. Prev Med 13: 141–154

209. Keys A (1988) High density lipoprotein cholesterol and longevity. J Epidemiol Community Health 42: 60–65

210. Kita T, Brown MS, Bilheimer DW, Goldstein JL (1982) Delayed clearence of very low density and intermediate density lipoproteins with enhanced conversion to low density lipoprotein in WHHL rabbits. Proc Natl Acad Sci USA 79: 5693–5607

211. Kitamura M (1991) Historical aspects of cholesterol value by various analytical methods. Rinsho Byori 39: 495–500

212. Kjeldsen SE, Eide I, Leren P, Foss OP (1983) Effects of posture on serum cholesterol fractions, cholesterol ratio and triglycerides. Scand J Clin Lab Invest 43: 119–121

213. Knott TJ, Rall SC Jr, Innerarity TL, Jacobson SF, Urdea MS, Levy-Wilson B, Powell LM, Pease RJ, Eddy R, Nakai H, et al. (1985) Human apolipoprotein B: structure of carboxyl-terminal domains, sites of gene expression, and chromosomal localization. Science 230: 37–43

214. Knott TJ, Pease RJ, Powell LM, Wallis SC, Rall SC Jr, Innerarity TL, Blackhart B, Taylor WH, Marcel Y, Milne R, et al. (1986) Complete protein sequence and identification of structural domains of human apolipoprotein B. Nature 323: 734–738

215. Koo C, Wernette-Hammond ME, Innerarity TL (1986) Uptake of canine beta-very low density lipoproteins by mouse peritoneal macrophages is mediated by a low density lipoprotein receptor. J Biol Chem 261: 11194–11201

216. Koo C, Wernette-Hammond ME, Garcia Z, Malloy MJ, Uauy R, East C, Bilheimer DW, Mahley RW, Innerarity TL (1988) Uptake of cholesterol-rich remnant lipoproteins by human monocyte-derived macrophages is mediated by low density lipoproteins receptors. J Clin Invest 81: 1332–1340

217. Kostner G, Alaupovic P (1972) Studies of the composition and structure of plasma lipoproteins. Separation and quantification of the lipoprotein families occurring in the high density lipoproteins of human plasma. Biochemistry 11: 3419–3428

218. Kostner GM, Patsch JR, Sailer S, Braunsteiner H, Holasek A (1974) Polypeptide distribution of the main lipoprotein density classes separated from human plasma by rate zonal ultracentrifugation. Eur J Biochem 45: 611–621

219. Kostner GM, Avogaro P, Cazzolato G, Marth E, Bittolo-Bon G, Qunici GB (1981) Lipoprotein Lp(a) and the risk for myocardial infarction. Atherosclerosis 38: 51–61

220. Kostner GM, Molinari E, Pichler P (1985) Evaluation of a new HDL2/HDL3 quantitation method based on precipitation with polyethylene glycol. Clin Chim Acta 148: 139–147

221. Koschinsky ML, Beisiegel U, Henne-Bruns D, Eaton DL, Lawn RM (1990) Apolipoprotein(a) size heterogeneity is related to variable number of repeat sequences in its mRNA. Biochemistry 29: 640–644

222. Kowal RC, Herz J, Goldstein JL, Esser V, Brown MS (1989) Low density lipoprotein receptor-related protein mediates uptake of cholesterol esters derived from apoprotein E-enriched lipoproteins. Proc Natl Acad Sci USA 86: 5810–5814

223. Kozarevic D, McGee D, Vojvodic N, Gordon T, Racic Z, Zukel W, Dawber T (1981) Serum cholesterol and mortality: the Yugoslavia Cardiovascular Disease Study. Am J Epidemiol 114: 21–28

224. Kraft HG, Menzel HJ, Hoppichler F, Vogel W, Utermann G (1989) Changes of genetic apolipoprotein phenotypes caused by liver transplantation. Implications for apolipoprotein synthesis. J Clin Invest 83: 137–142

225. Kratzin H, Armstrong VW, Niehaus M, Hilschmann N, Seidel D (1987) Structural relationship of an apolipoprotein(a) phenotype (570 kDa) to plasminogen: homologous kringle domains are linked by carbohydrate-rich regions. Biol Chem Hoppe Seyler 368: 1533–1544

226. Krauss RM (1987) Relationship of intermediate and low-density lipoprotein subspecies to risk of coronary artery disease. Am Heart J 113: 578–582

227. Krauss RM, Lindgren FT, Williams PT, Kelsey SF, Brensike J, Vranizan K, Dete KM, Levy RI (1987) Intermediate-density lipoproteins and progression of coronary artery disease in hypercholesterolaemic men. Lancet II: 62–66

228. Krempler F, Kostner G, Bolzano K, Sandhofer F (1978) Studies on the metabolism of the lipoprotein Lp(a) in man. Atherosclerosis 30: 57–65

229. Krempler F, Kostner G, Bolzano K, Sandhofer F (1979) Lipoprotein(a) is not a metabolic product of other lipoproteins containing apolipoprotein B. Biochim Biophys Acta 575: 63–70

230. Krempler F (1980) Stoffwechsel und klinische Bedeutung des Lipoproteins Lp(a). Acta Med Austriaca 7: 101–103

231. Krempler F (1980) Metabolism of lipoprotein Lp(a). Artery 8: 151–156

232. Krempler F, Kostner GM, Bolzano K, Sandhofer F (1980) Turnover of lipoprotein(a) in man. J Clin Invest 65: 1483–1490

233. Krempler F, Kostner GM, Roscher A, Haslauer F, Bolzano K, Sandhofer F (1983) Studies on the role of specific cell surface receptors in the removal of lipoprotein(a) in man. J Clin Invest 71: 1431–1441

234. Krempler F (1984) Untersuchungen über Stoffwechsel und mögliche Mechanismen der Atherogenität von Lipoprotein(a). Wien Klin Wochenschr [Suppl] 151: 1–12

235. Kristensen T, Moestrup SK, Gliemann J, Bendtsen L, Sand O, Sottrup-Jensen L (1990) Evidence that the newly cloned low-density-lipoprotein receptor related protein (LRP) is the alpha 2-macroglobulin receptor. FEBS Lett 276: 151–155

236. Kreuzer H, Seidel D (1986) The association between serum Lp(a) concentration and angiographically assessed coronary atherosclerosis. Atherosclerosis 62: 249–257

237. Kuprionite JA (1983) Incidence of ischaemic heart disease in relation to blood cholesterol level, and the influence on non-medicamentous preventive measures on the cholesterol level in an open population. Cor Vasa 25: 413–421

238. Kwiterovich PO Jr (1988) HyperapoB: a pleiotropic phenotype characterized by dense low-density lipoproteins and associated with coronary artery disease. Clin Chem 34: B71–77

239. Labeur C, Michiels G, Bury J, Usher DC, Rosseneu M (1989) Lipoprotein(a) quantified by an enzyme-linked immunosorbent assay with monoclonal antibodies. Clin Chem 35: 1380–1384

240. Ladias JA, Kwiterovich PO Jr, Smith HH, Miller M, Bachorik PS, Forte T, Lusis AJ, Antonarakis SE (1989) Apolipoprotein B-100 Hopkins (arginine 4019 – tryptophan). A new apolipoprotein B-100 variant in a family with premature atherosclerosis and hyperapobetalipoproteinemia. JAMA 262: 1980–1988

241. Lalazar A, Weisgraber KH, Rall SC Jr, Giladi H, Innerarity TL, Levanon AZ, Boyles JK, Amit B, Gorecki M, Mahley RW, et al. (1988) Site-specific mutagenesis of human apolipoprotein E. Receptor binding activity of variants with single amino acid substitutions. J Biol Chem 263: 3542–3545

242. Lamm G, Csukas M, Gyarfas J, Ostor E (1985) Risk factors for coronary heart disease in rural Hungary. Int J Epidemiol 14: 327–329

243. Landis BA, Rotolo FS, Meyers WC, Clark AB, Quarfordt SH (1987) Influence of apolipoprotein E on soluble and heparin-immobilized hepatic lipase. Am J Physiol 252: 805–810

244. Laplaud PM, Beaubatie L, Rall SC Jr, Luc G, Saboureau M (1988) Lipoprotein(a) is the major apoB-containing lipoprotein in the plasma of a hibernator, the hedgehog (Erinaceus europaeus). J Lipid Res 29: 1157–1170

245. Lapidus L (1985) Ischaemic heart disease, stroke and total mortality in women – results from a prospective population study in Götheburg, Sweden. Acta Med Scand 705 [Suppl] 14K: 1–42

246. Law A, Wallis SC, Powell LM, Pease RJ, Brunt H, Priestley LM, Knott TJ, Scott J, Altman DG, Miller GJ, et al. (1986) Common DNA polymorphism within coding sequence of apolipoprotein B gene associated with altered lipid levels. Lancet I: 1301–1303

247. Law SW, Grant SM, Higuchi K, Hospattankar A, Lackner K, Lee N, Brewer HB Jr (1986) Human liver apolipoprotein B-100 cDNA: complete nucleic acid and derived amino acid sequence. Proc Natl Acad Sci USA 83: 8142–8146

248. Lawn R (1987) cDNA sequence of human apolipoprotein(a) is homologous to plasminogen. Nature 330: 132–137

249. Leary T (1941) The genesis of atherosclerosis. Arch Path 32: 507–555

250. Leaverton PE, Sorlie PD, Kleinman JC, Dannenberg AL, Ingster-Moore L, Kannel WB, Cornoni-Huntley JC (1987) Representativeness of the Framingham risk model for coronary heart disease mortality: a comparison with a national cohort study. J Chronic Dis 40: 775–784

251. Lees RS, Fredrickson DS (1965) The differentiation of exogenous and endogenous hyperlipemia by paper electrophoresis. J Clin Invest 44: 1968–1977

252. Lewis B (1983) Relation of high-density lipoproteins to coronary artery disease. Am J Cardiol 52: 5B–8B

253. Leszczynski DE, Cleveland JC, Kummerow FA (1980) Plasma lipoprotein patterns in patients hospitalized for coronary artery bypass surgery. Clin Cardiol 3: 252–259

254. Linden L, Kallberg M, Gustafson A, Dahlen G (1976) Studies on an additional pre-beta-lipoprotein, sinking pre-beta (SPB). I. Isolation and characterization. Scand J Clin Lab Invest 36: 51–58

255. Lipid Research Clinics Program (1984) The Lipid Research Clinics Coronary Primary Prevention Trial results. II. The relationship fo reduction in incidence of coronary heart disease to cholesterol lowering. JAMA 251: 365–374

256. Lipinska I, Gurewich V, Meriam CM, Kosowsky BD, Ramaswamy K, Philibin E, Losordo D (1987) Lipids, lipoproteins, fibrinogen and fibrinolytic activity in angiographically assessed coronary heart disease. Artery 15: 44–60

257. Logan RL, Riemersma RA, Oliver MF, Olsson AG, Rossner S, Wallidus G, Kaijser L, Carlson LA, Locherbie L, Lutz W, The Edinburgh-Stockholm-Study of coronary heart disease risk factors: a summary. In: Kritchevcky D, Paoletti R, Holmes WL (eds) Drugs, lipid metabolism and atherosclerosis. Plemun, New York, pp 287–294

258. Lopes-Virella MF, Stone P, Ellis S, Colwell JA (1977) Cholesterol determination in high-density lipoproteins separated by three different methods. Clin Chem 23: 882–884

259. Mabuchi H, Itoh H, Takeda M, Kajinami K, Wakasugi T, Koizumi J, Takeda R, Asagami C (1989) A young type-III hyperlipoproteinemic patient associated with apolipoprotein E deficiency. Metabolism 38: 115–119

260. Maeda H, Nakamura H, Kobori S, Okada M, Niki H, Ogura T, Hiraga S (1989) Molecular cloning of a human apolipoprotein E variant: E5 (Glu3----Lys3). J Biochem (Tokyo) 105: 491–493

261. Maeda H, Nakamura H, Kobori S, Okada M, Mori H, Niki H, Ogura T, Hiraga S (1989) Identification of human apolipoprotein E variant gene: apolipoprotein E7 (Glu244,245----Lys244,245). J Biochem (Tokyo) 105: 51–54

262. März W, Ruzicka C, Pohl T, Usadel KH, Gross W (1992) Familial defective apolipoprotein B-100: mild hypercholesterolaemia without atherosclerosis in a homozygous patient [letter]. Lancet II, 340: 1362

263. Mahley RW, Innerarity TL, Brown MS, Ho YK, Goldstein JL (1980) Cholesterol ester synthesis in macrophages: stimulation by beta-very low density lipoproteins from cholesterol-fed animals of several species. J Pipid Res 21: 970–980

264. Mahley RW, Hui DY, Innerarity TL, Weisgraber KH (1981) Two independent lipoprotein receptors on hepatic membranes of dog, swine, and man. Apo-B, E and apo-E receptors. J Clin Invest 68: 1197–1206

265. Mahley RW (1988) Apolipoprotein E: cholesterol transport protein with expanding role in cell biology. Science 240: 622–630

266. Mahley RW, Hui DY, Innerarity TL, Beisiegel U (1989) Chylomicron remnant metabolism. Role of hepatic lipoprotein receptors in mediating uptake. Atherosclerosis 9: I14–18

267. Mailly F, Xu CF, Xhignesse M, Lussier-Cacan S, Talmud PJ, Davignon J, Humphries SE, Nestruck AC (1991) Characterization of a new aolipoprotein E5 variant detected in two French-Canadian subjects. J Lipid Res 32: 613–620

268. Mann WA, Gregg RE, Sprecher DL, Brewer HB Jr (1989) Apolipoprotein E-1Harrisburg: a new variant of apolipoprotein E dominantly associated with type-III hyperlipoproteinemia. Biochim Biophys Acta 1005: 239–244

269. Marth E, Cazzolato G, Bittolo Bon G, Avogaro P, Kostner GM (1982) Serum concentrations of Lp(a) and other lipoprotein parameters in heavy alcohol consumers. Ann Nutr Metab 26: 56–62

270. Masket BH, Levy RI, Fredrickson DS (1973) The use of polyacrylamide gel electrophoresis in differentiating type 3 hyperlipoproteinemia. J Lab Clin Med 81: 794–802

271. McLean JW, Elshourbagy NA, Chang DJ, Mahley RW, Taylor JM (1984) Human apolipoprotein E mRNA, cDNA cloning and nucleotide sequencing of a new variant. J Biol Chem 259: 6498–6504

272. McLean JW, Tomlinson JE, Kuang WJ, Eaton DL, Chen EY, Fless GM, Scanu AM, Lawn RM (1987) cDNA sequence of human apolipoprotein(a) is homologous to plasminogen. Nature 330: 132–137

273. McQueen MJ, Henderson AR, Patten RL, Krishnan S, Wood DE, Webb S (1991) Results of a province-wide quality assurance program assessing the accuracy of cholesterol, triglycerides, and high-density lipoprotein cholesterol measurements and calculated low-density lipoprotein cholesterol in Ontario, using fresh human serum. Arch Pathol Lab Med 115: 1217–1222

274. Mendez AJ, Oram JF, Bierman EL (1991) Role of the protein kinase C signaling pathway in high-density lipoprotein receptor-mediated efflux of intracellular cholesterol. Trans Assoc Am Physicians 104: 48–53

275. Mendez AJ, Oram JF, Bierman EL (1991) Protein kinase C as a mediator of high density lipoprotein receptor-dependent efflux of intracellular cholesterol. J Biol Chem 266: 10104–10111

276. Meng QH, Calabresi L, Fruchart JC, Marcel YL (1993) Apolipoprotein A-I domains involved in the activation of lecithin: cholesterol acyltransferase. Importance of the central domain. J Biol Chem 268: 16966–16973

277. Menotti A, Seccareccia F (1987) Blood pressure, serum cholesterol and smoking habits predicting different manifestations of arteriosclerotic cardiovascular diseases. Acta Cardiol 42: 91–102

278. Menzinger P, Sitzmann FC (1979) Vergleich zweier Cholesterinbestimmungsmethoden bei Kindern (Liebermann-Burchard und vollenzymatischer Farbtest). Klin Padiatr 191: 61–65

278a. Miettinen TA, Gylling H (1988) Mortality and cholesterol metabolism in familial hypercholesterolemia. Long-term follow-up of 96 patients. Arteriosclerosis 8: 163–167

279. Metherall JE, Goldstein JL, Luskey KL, Brown MS (1989) Loss of transcriptional repression of three sterol-regulated genes in mutant hamster cells. J Biol Chem 264: 15634–15641

279a. Miller NE, Hammett F, Saltissi S, Rao S, van Zeller H, Coltart J, Lewis B (1981) Relation of angiographically defined coronary artery disease to plasma lipoprotein subfractions and apolipoproteins. Br Med J 282: 1741–1744

280. Moberly JB, Cole TG, Alpers DH, Schonfeld G (1990) Oleic acid stimulation of apolipoprotein B secretion from HepG2 and Caco-2 cells occurs post-transcriptionally. Biochem Biophys Acta 1042: 70–80

281. Molgaard J, Klausen IC, Lassvik C, Faergeman O, Gerdes LU, Olsson AG (1992) Significant association between low-molecular-weight apolipoprotein(a) isoforms and intermittent claudication. Arterioscler Thromb 12: 895–901

282. Moestrup SK, Gliemann J (1991) Analysis of ligand recognition by the purified alpha 2-macroglobulin receptor (low density lipoprotein receptor-related protein). Evidence that high affinity of alpha 2-macroglobulin-proteinase complex is achieved by binding to adjacent receptors. J Biol Chem 266: 14011–14017

283. Moestrup SK, Gliemann J, Pallesen G (1992) Distribution of the alpha 2-macroglobulin receptor/low density lipoprotein receptor-related protein in human tissues. Cell Tissue Res 269: 375–382

284. Moll PP, Powsner R, Sing CF (1979) Analysis of genetic and environmental sources of variation in serum cholesterol in Tecumseh, Michigan. V. Variance components estimated from pedigrees. Ann Hum Genet 42: 343–354

285. Monsalve MV, Young R, Jobsis J, Wiseman SA, Dhamu S, Powell JT, Greenhalgh RM, Humphries SE (1988) DNA polymorphisms of the gene for apolipoprotein B in patients with peripheral arterial disease. Atherosclerosis 70: 123–129

286. Morton NE, Gulbrandsen CL, Rhoads GG, Kagan A (1978) The Lp lipoprotein in Japanese. Clin Genet 14: 207–212

287. Myant NB (1990) Current approaches to the genetics of coronary heart disease (CHD) including an account of work done at Hammersmith Hospital. Boll Soc Ital Biol Sper 66: 1015–1041

288. Nakaya N, Chung BH, Patsch JR, Taunton OD (1977) Synthesis and release of low density lipoproteins by the isolated perfused pig liver. J Biol Chem 252: 7530–7533

289. National Cholesterol Education Program (1994) Detection, evaluation, and treatment of high blood cholesterol in adults (adult treatment panel II). Circulation 89: 1330–1445

290. Nestel PJ, Fifge NH, Tan MH (1982) Increased lipoprotein-remnant formation in chronic renal failure. N Engl J Med 307: 329–333

291. Neubeck W, Wieland H, Habenicht A, Muller P, Baggio G, Seidel D (1977) Improved assessment of plasma lipoprotein patterns. III. Direct measurement of lipoproteins after gel-electrophoresis. Clin Chem 23: 1296–1300

292. Nichols AV, Gong EL, Blanche PJ, Forte TM, Shore VG (1987) Pathways in the formation of human plasma high density lipoprotein subpopulations containing apolipoprotein A-I without apolipoprotein A-II. J Lipid Res 28: 719–732

293. Nora JJ, Lortscher RH, Spangler RD, Nora AH, Kimberling WJ (1980) Genetic-epidemiologic study of early-onset ischemic heart disease. Circulation 61: 503–508

294. Oram JF, Brinton EA, Bierman EL (1983) Regulation of high density lipoprotein receptor activity in cultured human skin fibroblasts and human arterial smooth muscle cells. J Clin Invest 72: 1611–1621

295. Oram JF, Johnson CJ, Brown TA (1987) Interaction of high density lipoprotein with its receptor on cultured fibroblasts and macrophages: evidence for reversible binding at the cell surface without internalization. J Biol Chem 262: 2405–2410

296. Orlando RA, Kerjaschki D, Kurihara H, Bie-mesderfer D, Farguhar MG (1992) gp330 associ-ates with a 44-kDa protein in the rat kidney to form the Heymann nephritis antigenic complex. Proc Natl Acad Sci USA 89: 6698–6802

298. Osborne TF (1991) Single nucleotide resolution of sterol regulatory region in promoter for 3-hydroxy-3-methylglutaryl coenzyme A reductase. J Biol Chem 266: 13947–13951

299. Oschry Y, Olivecrona T, Deckelbaum RJ, Eisen-berg S (1985) Is hypertriglyceridemic very low density lipoprotein a precursor of normal low density lipoprotein? J Lipid Res 26: 158–167

300. Ose L, Kalager T, Grundt IK (1976) Serum beta-lipoprotein subfractions in polyacrylamide gel electrophoresis associated with coronary heart disease. Scand J Clin Lab Invest 36: 75–79

301. Pachauri SP, Jacotot B, Beaumont JL (1976) Cir-culating lipophages and aortic foam cells in ex-perimental atherosclerosis of rabbits under al-tered reticuloendothelial activity. Nutr Metab 20: 14–26

302. Packard CJ, Clegg RJ, Dominiczak MH, Lori-mer AR, Shepherd J (1986) Effects of bezafibrate on apolipoprotein B metabolism in type-III hy-perlipoproteinaemic subjects. J Lipid Res 27: 930–938

303. Pagnan A, Donadon W, Tonolli E (1974) Corona-ropatia e banda pre-beta „accessoria": una relazi-one causale? Minerva Med 65: 3123–3126

304. Pagnan A, Kostner G, Braggion M, Ziron L, Bittolo-Bon G, Avogaro P (1983) Familial study on „sinking pre-beta", the Lp(a) lipoprotein, and its relationship with serum lipids, apolipoprotein A-I and B and clinical atherosclerosis. J Clin Chem Clin Biochem 21: 267–272

305. Paik YK, Chang DJ, Reardon CA, Davies GE, Mahley RW, Taylor JM (1985) Nucleotide se-quence and structure of the human apolipopro-tein E gene. Proc Natl Acad Sci USA 82: 3445–3449

306. Palac RT, Meadows WR, Hwang MH, Loeb HS, Pifarre R, Gunnar RM (1982) Risk factors re-lated to progressive narrowing in aortocoronary vein grafts studies 1 and 5 years after surgery. Cir-culation 66: 140–144

307. Palinski W, Rosenfeld ME, Yla-Herttuala S, Gurtner GC, Socher SS, Butler SW, Parthasara-thy S, Carew TE, Steinberg D, Witztum JL (1989) Low density lipoprotein undergoes oxida-tive modification in vivo. Proc Natl Acad Sci USA 86: 1372–1376

308. Palinski W, Yla-Herttuala S, Rosenfeld ME, But-ler SW, Socher SA, Parthasarathy S, Curtiss LK, Witztum JL (1990) Antisera and monoclonal anti-bodies specific for epitopes generated during oxidative modification of low density lipoprotein. Arteriosclerosis 10: 325–335

309. Papadopoulos NM, Bedynek JL (1973) Serum li-poprotein patterns in patients with coronary atherosclerosis. Clin Chim Acta 44: 153–157

310. Parthasarathy S, Steinbrecher UP, Barnett J, Witztum JL, Steinberg D (1985) Essential role of phospholipase A2 activity in endothelial cell-

induced modification of low density lipoprotein. Proc Natl Acad Sci USA 82: 3000–3004

311. Parthasarathy S, Printz DJ, Boyd D, Joy L, Steinberg D (1986) Macrophage oxidation of low density lipoprotein generates a modified form re-cognized by the scavenger receptor. Arterioslero-sis 6: 505–510

312. Parthasarathy S, Quinn MT, Schwenke DC, Ca-rew TE, Steinberg D (1989) Oxidative modifica-tion of beta-very low density lipoprotein. Poten-tial role in monocyte recruitment and foam cell formation. Arteriosclerosis 9: 398–404

313. Patsch JR, Sailer S, Kostner G, Sandhofer F, Ho-lasek A, Braunsteiner H (1974) Separation of the main lipoprotein density classes from human plasma by rate-zonal ultracentrifugation. J Lipid Res 15: 356–366

314. Patsch JR (1975) Lipoprotein of the density 1.006–1.020 in the plasma of patients with type-III hyperlipoproteinaemia in the postabsorptive state. Eur J Clin Invest 5: 45–55

315. Patsch JR, Prasad S, Gotto AM Jr, Bengtsson-Olivecrona G (1984) Postprandial lipemia: a key for the conversion of HDL2 into HDL3 by he-patic lipase. J Clin Invest 74: 2017–2023

316. Pekkanen J, Nissinen A, Puska P, Punsar S, Kar-vonen MJ (1989) Risk factors and 25 year risk of coronary heart disease in a male population with a high incidence of the disease: the Finnish co-horts of the seven countries study. Br Med J 299: 81–85

317. Persson B, Johansson BW (1984) The Kockum study: twenty-two-year follow-up. Coronary heart disease in a population in the south of Swe-den. Acta Med Scand 216: 485–493

318. Pfaffinger D, Schuelke J, Kim C, Fless GM, Scanu AM (1991) Relationship between apo(a) isoforms and Lp(a) density in subjects with diffe-rent apo(a) phenotype: a study before and after a fatty meal. J Lipid Res 32: 679–683

319. Polson A, Potgieter GM, Largier JF, Mears GEF, Joubert FJ (1964) The fractionation of protein mixtures by linear polymers of high molecular weight. Biochim Biophys Acta 82: 463–475

320. Postle AD, Darmady JM, Siggers DC (1978) Double pre-beta lipoprotein in ischaemic heart disease. Clin Genet 13: 233–236

321. Powell LM, Wallis SC, Pease RJ, Edwards YH, Knott TJ, Scott J (1987) A novel form of tissue-specific RNA processing produces apolipoprote-in-B48 in intestine. Cell 50: 831–840

322. Prokhorskas RP, Grabauskas VI, Baubinene AV, Glazunov IS, Domarkene SB (1987) Chief risk factors of ischemic heart disease and mortality of the middle-aged male population of Kaunas. Kardiologiia 27: 14–19

323. Puchois P, Kandoussi A, Fievet P, Fourrier JL, Bertrand M, Koren E, Fruchart JC (1987) Apoli-poprotein A-I containing lipoproteins in coronary artery disease. Atherosclerosis 68: 35–40

324. Quarfordt S, Levy RI, Fredrickson DS (1971) On the lipoprotein abnormality in type 3 hyperlipo-proteinemia. J Clin Invest 50: 754–761

325. Ragland DR, Brand RJ (1988) Coronary heart disease mortality in the Western Collaborative Group Study. Follow-up experience of 22 years. Am J Epidemiol 127: 462–475

326. Rajput-Williams J, Knott TJ, Wallis SC, Sweetnam P, Yarnell J, Cox N, Bell GI, Miller NE, Scott J (1988) Variation of apolipoprotein-B gene is associated with obesity, high blood cholesterol levels, and increased risk of coronary heart disease. Lancet II: 1442–1446

327. Rall SC Jr, Weisgraber KH, Mahley RW (1982) Human apolipoprotein E. The complete amino acid sequence. J Biol Chem 257: 4171–4178

328. Rall SC Jr, Newhouse YM, Clarke HR, Weisgraber KH, McCarthy BJ, Mahley RW, Bersot TP (1989) Type-III hyperlipoproteinemia associated with apolipoprotein E phenotype E3/3. Structure and genetics of an apolipoprotein E3 variant. J Clin Invest 83: 1095–1101

329. Rath M, Pauling L (1990) Immunological evidence for the accumulation of lipoprotein(a) in the atherosclerotic lesion of the hypoascorbemic guinea pig. Proc Natl Acad Sci USA 87: 9388–9390

330. Raychowdhury R, Niles JL, McCluskey RT, Smith JA (1989) Autoimmune target Heymann nephritis is a glycoprotein with homology to the LDL receptor. Science 244: 1163–1165

331. Reardon MF, Poapst ME, Steiner G (1982) The independent synthesis of intermediate density lipoproteins in type-III hyperlipoproteinaemia. Metabolism 31: 421–427

332. Reardon MF, Nestel PJ, Craig IH, Harper RW (1985) Lipoprotein predictors of the severity of coronary artery disease in men and women. Circulation 71: 881–888

333. Rodgrave TG (1970) Formation of cholesteryl ester-rich particulate lipid during metabolism of chylomicrons. J Clin Invest 49: 465–471

334. Rhoads GG, Morton NE, Gulbrandsen CL, Kagan A (1978) Sinking pre-beta lipoprotein and coronary heart disease in Japanese-American men in Hawaii. Am J Epidemiol 108: 350–356

335. Rhoads GG, Dahlén G, Berg K, Morton NE, Dannenberg AL (1986) Lp(a) lipoprotein as a risk factor for myocardial infarction. JAMA 256: 2540–2544

336. Rittner C, Wichmann D (1967) Zur Genetik des Lp-Systems. Nachweis der erblichen quantitativen Merkmalsprägung sowie einer pranatalen Selektion. Humangenetik 5 (1): 43–53

337. Rivin AU (1989) Total and high-density lipoprotein cholesterol measurements. Hazards in clinical interpretation. West J Med 15: 289–291

338. Rosenfeld ME, Khoo JC, Miller E, Parthasarathy S, Palinski W, Witztum JL (1991) Macrophage-derived foam cells freshly isolated from rabbit atherosclerotic lesions degrade modified lipoproteins, promote oxidation of low-density lipoproteins, and contain oxidation-specific lipid-protein adducts. J Clin Invest 87: 90–99

339. Rothblat GH, Bamberger M, Phillips MC (1986) Reverse cholesterol transport. In: Albers JJ, Segrest JP (eds) Methods in enzymology, vol 129. Academic, London, pp 628–644

340. Rubba P, Faccenda F, Iorio D, Pauciullo P, Cortese C, Spampinato N, Mancini M (1987) Lipoprotein abnormalities and extracoronary atherosclerosis in patients with premature ischemic heart disease. Int Angiol 6: 331–337

341. Samuelsson O, Wilhelmsen L, Elmfeldt D, Pennert K, Wedel H, Wikstrand J, Berglund G (1985) Predictors of cardiovascular morbidity in treated hypertension: results from the primary preventive trial in Götheborg, Sweden. J Hypertens 3: 167–176

342. Sandkamp M, Funke H, Schulte H, Kohler E, Assmann G (1990) Lipoprotein(a) is an independent risk factor for myocardial infarction at a young age. Clin Chem 36: 20–23

343. Sato R, Imanaka T, Takano T (1990) The effect of HMG-CoA reductase inhibitor (cs-514) on the synthesis and secretion of apolipoproteins B and A-1 in the human hepatoblastoma Hep G2. Biochim Biophys Acta 1042: 36–41

344. Saxena U, Goldberg IJ (1990) Interaction of lipoprotein lipase with glycosaminoglycans and apolipoprotein C-II: effects of free-fatty-acids. Biochim Biophys Acta 1043 (2): 161–168

345. Scanu AM (1990) Lipoprotein(a): a genetically determined cardiovascular pathogen in search of a function. J Lab Clin Med 116: 142–146

346. Schaefer EJ, Gregg RE, Ghiselli G, Forte TM, Ordovas JM, Zech LA, Brewer HB JR (1986) Familial apolipoprotein E deficiency. J Clin Invest 78: 1206–1219

347. Schaefer EJ, McNamara JR, Genest J Jr, Ordovas JM (1988) Clinical significance of hypertriglyceridemia. Semin Thromb Hemost 14: 143–148

348. Schaffner T, Taylor K, Bartucci EJ, Fischer-Dzoga K, Beeson JH, Glagov S, Wissler RW (1980) Arterial foam cells with distinctive immunomorphologic and histochemical features of macrophages. Am J Pathol 100: 57–80

349. Schauer UJ, Pissarek D, Panzram G (1989) Association of coronary heart disease with serum lipid and apolipoprotein concentrations in long-term diabetes. Results of the Erfurt study. Acta Diabetol 26: 35–42

350. Schneider WJ, Koyanen PT, Brown MS, Goldstein JL, Utermann G, Weber W, Havel RJ, Kotite L, Kane JP, Innerarity TL, Mahley RW (1981) Familial dysbetalipoproteinemia. Abnormal binding of mutant apoprotein E to low density lipoprotein receptors of human fibroblasts and membranes from liver and adrenal of rats, rabbits, and cows. J Clin Invest 68: 1075–1085

351. Schultz JS, Shreffler DC, Harvie NR (1968) Genetic and antigenic studies and partial purification of a human serum lipoprotein carrying the Lp antigenic determinant. Proc Natl Acad Sci USA 61: 963–970

352. Schultz JS, Schreffler DC, Sing CF, Harvie NR (1974) The genetics of the Lp antigen. I. Its quantitation and distribution in a sample population. Ann Hum Genet 38: 39–46

353. Seed M, Hoppichler F, Reaveley D, McCarthy S, Thompson GR, Boerwinkle E, Utermann G (1990) Relation of serum lipoprotein(a) concentration and apolipoprotein(a) phenotype to coronary heart disease in patients with familial hypercholesterolemia. N Engl J Med 322: 1494–1499

354. Schmitz G, Robenek H, Lohmann U, Assmann G (1985) Interaction of high density lipoproteins with cholesterylester laden macrophages: biochemical and morphological characterization of cell surface binding, endocytosis and resecretion of high density lipoproteins by macrophages. EMBO J 4: 613–622

355. Schulte H, Assmann G (1988) Results of the „Munster Prospective Cardiovascular" study. Soz Präventivmed 33: 337–345

356. Scott DW, Gotto AM, Cole JS, Gorry GA (1978) Plasma lipids as collateral risk factors in coronary artery disease – a study of 371 males with chest pain. J Chronic Dis 34: 337–345

357. Sheperd J, Packard CJ (1987) Metabolic heterogeneity in very low density lipoproteins. Am Heart J 113: 503–507

358. Sherrill BC, Innerarity TL, Mahley RW (1980) Rapid hepatic clearance of the canine lipoproteins containing only the E-apoprotein by high affinity receptor. Identity with the chylomicron remnant transport process. J Biol Chem 255: 1804–1807

359. Sigurdsson G, Nicoll A, Lewis B (1976) The metabolism of low density lipoprotein in endogenous hypertriglyceridaemia. Eur J Clin Invest 6: 151–158

360. Simons K, Ehnholm C, Renkonen O, Bloth B (1970) Characterization of the Lp(a) lipoprotein in human plasma. Acta Pathol Microbiol Immunol Scand [B] 78: 459–466

361. Simons LA (1986) Interrelations of lipids and lipoproteins with coronary artery disease mortality in 19 countries. Am J Cardiol 57: 5G–10G

362. Simons LA, Dwyer T, Simons J, Bernstein L, Mack P, Poonia NS, Balasubramaniam S, Baron D, Branson J, Morgan J (1987) Chylomicrons and chylomicron remnants in coronary artery disease: a case-control study. Artherosclerosis 65: 181–189

363. Sing CF, Orr JD (1978) Analysis of genetic and environmental sources of variation in serum cholesterol in Tecumseh, Michigan. IV. Separation of polygene from common environment effects. Am J Hum Genet 30: 491–504

364. Sniderman A, Shapiro S, Marpole D, Skinner B, Teng B, Kwiterovich PO Jr (1980) Association of coronary atherosclerosis with hyperapobetalipoproteinemia (increased protein but normal cholesterol levels in human plasma low density (beta) lipoproteins). Proc Natl Acad Sci USA 77: 604–608

365. Sniderman AD, Wolfson C, Teng B, Franklin FA, Bachorik PS, Kwiterovich PO Jr (1982) Association of hyperapobetalipoproteinemia with endogenous hypertriglyceridemia and atherosclerosis. Ann Intern Med 97: 833–839

366. Sniderman A, Cianflone K, Kwiterovich PO Jr, Hutchinson T, Barre P, Prichard S (1987) Hyperapobetalipoproteinemia: the major dyslipoproteinemia in patients with chronic renal failure treated with chronic ambulatory peritoneal dialysis. Atherosclerosis 65: 257–264

367. Solakivi T, Salo MK, Puska P, Nikkari T (1988) Plasma apolipoprotein B in middle-aged Finnish men. Evidence for a regional gradient of apo B and lack of negative correlation between apo B and dietary linoleate in hyperapobetalipoproteinemia. Atherosclerosis 72: 55–61

368. Solberg LA, Strong JP, Holme I, Helgeland A, Hjermann I, Leren P, Mogensen SB (1985) Stenoses in the coronary arteries. Relation to atherosclerotic lesions, coronary heart disease, and risk factors. The Oslo Study. Lab Invest 53: 648–655

369. Solberg LA, Ishii T, Strong JP, Guzman MA, Hosoda Y, Tsugane S, Newman WP, Tracy RE (1987) Comparison of coronary atherosclerosis in middle-aged Norwegian and Japanese men. An autopsy study. Lab Invest 56: 451–456

370. Soutar AK, Garner CW, Baker HN, Sparrow JT, Jackson RL, Gotto AM, Smith LC (1975) Effect of the human plasma apolipoproteins and phosphatidylcholine acyl donor on the activity of lecithin: cholesterol acyltransferase. Biochemistry 14: 3057–3064

371. Soutar AK, Myant NB, Thompson GR (1977) Simultaneous measurement of apolipoprotein B turnover in very-low- and low-density lipoproteins in familial hypercholesterolaemia. Atherosclerosis 28: 247–256

372. Soutar AK, Myant NB, Thompson GR (1982) The metabolism of very-low-density and intermediate-density lipoproteins in patients with familial hypercholesterolaemia. Atherosclerosis 43: 217–231

373. Spady DK, Turley SD, Dietschy JM (1985) Receptor-independent low density lipoprotein transport in the rat in vivo. Quantitation, characterization, and metabolic consequences. J Clin Invest 76: 1113–1122

374. Sporik R, Johnstone JH, Cogswell JJ (1991) Longitudinal study of cholesterol values in 68 children from birth to 11 years of age. Arch Dis Child 66: 134–137

375. Sprecher DL, Hoeg JM, Schaefer EJ, Zech LA, Gregg RE, Lakatos E, Brewer HB Jr (1985) The association of LDL receptor activity, LDL cholesterol level, and clinical course in homozygous familial hypercholesterolemia. Metabolism 34: 294–299

376. Stamler J, Wentworth D, Neaton JD (1986) Prevalence and prognostic significance of hypercholesterolemia in men with hypertension. Prospective data on the primary screenees of the Multiple Risk Factor Intervention Trial. Am J Med 80: 33–39

377. Stamler J, Wentworth D, Neaton JD (1986) Is relationship between serum cholesterol and risk of premature death from coronary heart disease continuous and graded? Findings in 356 222 primary screenees of the Multiple risk Factor Intervention Trial (MRFIT). JAMA 256: 2823–2828

378. Stary HC (1980) The intimal macrophage in atherosclerosis. Artery 8: 205–207

379. Steinbrecher UP, Parthasarathy S, Leake DS, Witztum JL, Steinberg D (1984) Modification of low density lipoprotein by endothelial cells involves lipid peroxidation and degradation of low density lipoprotein phospholipids. Proc Natl Acad Sci USA 81: 3883–3887

380. Steinbrecher UP, Lougheed M, Kwan WC, Dirks M (1989) Recognition of oxidized low density lipoprotein by the scavenger receptor of macrophages results from derivatization of apolipoprotein B by products of fatty acid peroxidation. J Biol Chem 264: 15216–15223

381. Steiner G, Schwartz L, Shumak S, Poapst M (1987) The association of increased levels of intermediate-density lipoproteins with smoking and with coronary artery disease. Circulation 75: 124–130

382. Steinmetz A, Jakobs C, Motzny S. Kaffarnik H (1989) Differential distribution of apolipoprotein E isoforms in human plasma lipoproteins. Arteriosclerosis 9: 405–411

383. Stewart JM, Packard CJ, Lorimer AR, Boag DE, Shepherd J (1982) Effects of bezafibrate on receptor-mediated and receptor-independent low density lipoprotein catabolism in type II hyperlipoproteinaemic subjects. Atherosclerosis 44: 355–365

384. Strickland DK, Ashcom JD, Williams S, Burgess WH, Migliorini M, Argraves WS (1990) Sequence identity between the alpha 2-macroglobulin receptor and low density lipoprotein receptor-related protein suggests that this molecule is a multifunctional receptor. J Biol Chem 265: 17401–17404

385. Stuhldreher WL, Orchard TJ, Donahue RP, Kuller LH, Gloninger MF, Drash AL (1991) Cholesterol screening in childhood; sixteen-year Beaver County Lipid Study. J Pediatr 119: 551–556

386. Suckling KE, Stange EF (1985) Role of acyl-CoA: cholesterol acyltransferase in cellular cholesterol metabolism. J Lipid Res 26: 647–671

387. Südhof TC, Goldstein JL, Brown MS, Russell DW (1985) The LDL receptor gene: a mosaic of exons shared with different proteins. Science 228: 815–822

388. Swift LL, Manowitz NR, Dunn GD, Lequire VS (1980) Isolation and characterization of hepatic Golgi lipoproteins from hypercholesterolemic rats. J Clin Invest 66: 415–425

389. Takebayashi S, Kubota I, Kamio A, Takagi T (1972) Ultrastructural aspects of human atherosclerosis; role of the foam cells and modified smooth muscle cells. J Electron Microsc (Tokyo) 21: 301–313

390. Tatami R, Mabuchi H, Ueda K, Ueda B, Haba T, Kametani T, Ito S, Koizumi J, Ohta M, Miyamoto S, Nakayama A, Kanaya H, Oiwake H, Genda A, Takeda R (1981) Intermediate-density lipoprotein and cholesterol-rich very low density lipoprotein in angiographically determined coronary artery disease. Circulation 64: 1174–1184

391. Tajima S, Yamamura T, Yamamot A (1988) Analysis of apolipoprotein E5 gene from a patient with hyperlipoproteinemia. J Biochem (Tokyo) 104: 48–52

392. Takahashi S, Kawarabayasi Y, Nakai T, Sakai J, Yamamoto T (1992) Rabbit very low density lipoprotein receptor: a low density lipoprotein receptor-like protein with distinct ligand specificity. Proc Natl Acad Sci USA 89: 9252–9256

393. Talmud PJ, Barni N, Kessling AM, Carlsson P, Darnfors C, Bjursell G, Galton D, Wynn V, Kirk H, Hayden MR, et al. (1987) Apolipoprotein B gene variants are involved in the determination of serum cholesterol levels: a study in normo- and hyperlipidaemic individuals. Atherosclerosis 67: 81–89

394. Teng B, Thompson GR, Sniderman AD, Forte TM, Krauss RM, Kwiterovich PO Jr (1983) Composition and distribution of low density lipoprotein fractions in hyperapobetalipoproteinemia, normolipidemia, and familial hypercholesterolemia. Proc Natl Acad Sci USA 80: 6662–6666

395. Teng B, Sniderman AD, Soutar AK, Thompson GR (1986) Metabolic basis of hyperapobetalipoproteinemia. Turnover of apolipoprotein B in low density lipoprotein and its precursors and subfractions compared with normal and familial hypercholesterolemia. J Clin Invest 77: 663–672

396. Teramoto T, Matsushima T, Horie Y, Watanabe T (1990) Production of apolipoprotein E-rich LDL by the liver. The effect of dietary cholesterol and some lipid lowering agents. Ann NY Acad Sci 598: 301–307

397. Théeret N, Delbart C, Aguie G, Fruchart JC, Vassaux G, Ailhaud G (1990) Cholesterol efflux from adipose cells is coupled to diacylglycerol production and protein kinase C activation. Biochem Biophys Res Commun 173: 1361–1368

398. Thompson GR, Seed M, Niththyananthan S, McCarthy S, Thorogood M (1989) Genotypic and phenotypic variation in familial hypercholesterolemia. Arteriosclerosis 9: I75–80

399. Thuren T, Weisgraber KH, Sisson P. Waite M (1992) Role of apolipoprotein E in hepatic lipase catalyzed hydrolysis of phospholipid in high-density lipoproteins. Biochemistry 31: 2332–2338

400. Tikkanen M, Schonfeld G (1985) The reconition domain for the low density lipoproteins cellular receptor is expressed only once on each lipoprotein particle. Biochem Biophys Res Commun 126: 773–777

401. Tikkanen MJ, Viikari J, Akerblom HK, Pesonen E (1988) Apolipoprotein B polymorphism and altered apolipoprotein B and low density lipoprotein cholesterol concentrations in Finnis children. Br Med J [Clin Res] 296: 169–170

402. Tornberg SA, Jakobsson KF, Eklund GA (1988) Stability and validity of a single serum cholesterol measurement in a prospective cohort study. Int J Epidemiol 17: 797–803

403. Tverdal A, Foss OP, Lern P, Holme I, Lund-Larsen PG, Bjartveit K (1989) Serum triglycerides as an independent risk factor for death from coronary heart disease in middle-aged Norwegian men. Am J Epidemiol 129: 458–465

404. Tybjaerg-Hansen A, Humphries SE (1992) Familial defective apolipoprotein B-100: a single mutation that causes hypercholesterolemia and premature coronary artery disease. Atherosclerosis 96: 91–107

405. Utermann G, Wiegandt H (1971) Comparative studies of the Lp(a)-lipoprotein and low density lipoproteins of human serum. Hoppe Seylers Z Physiol Chem 352: 938–946

406. Utermann G, Lipp K, Wiegandt H (1972) Studies on the Lp(a)-lipoprotein of human serum. IV. The disaggregation of the Lp(a)-lipoprotein. Humangenetik 14: 142–150

407. Utermann G, Hees M, Steinmetz A (1977) Polymorphism of apolipoprotein E and occurrence of dysbetalipoproteinaemia in man. Nature 269: 604–607

408. Utermann G, Canzler H, Hees M, Jaeschke M, Muhlfeller G, Schoenborn W, Vogelberg KH (1977) Studies on the metabolic defect in Broadbeta disease (hyperlipoproteinaemia type-III). Clin Genet 12 (3): 139–154

409. Utermann G, Vogelberg KH, Steinmetz A, Schoenborn W, Pruin N, Jaeschke M, Hees M, Canzler H (1979) Polymorphism of apolipoprotein E. II. Genetics of hyperlipoproteinemia type-III. Clin Genet 15: 37–62

410. Utermann G, Pruin N, Steinmetz A (1979) Polymorphism of apolipoprotein E. III. Effect of a single polymorphic gene locus on plasma lipid levels in man. Clin Genet 15: 63–72

411. Utermann G (1987) Apolipoprotein E polymorphism in health and disease. Am Heart J 113: 433–440

412. Utermann G, Menzel HJ, Kraft HG, Duba HC, Kemmler HG, Seitz C (1987) Lp(a) glycoprotein phenotypes. Inheritance and relation to Lp(a)-lipoprotein concentration in plasma. J Clin Invest 80: 458–465

413. Utermann G, Kraft HG, Menzel HJ, Hopferwieser T, Seitz C (1988) Genetics of the quantitative Lp(a) lipoprotein trait. I. Relation of Lp(a) glycoprotein phenotypes to Lp(a) lipoprotein concentrations in plasma. Hum Genet 78: 41–46

414. Utermann G, Duba C, Menzel HJ (1988) Genetics of the quantitative Lp(a) lipoprotein trait. II. Inheritance of Lp(a) glycoprotein phenotypes. Hum Genet 78: 47–50

415. Utermann G (1989) The mysteries of lipoprotein(a). Science 246: 904–910

416. van Lenten BJ, Fogelman AM, Hokom MM, Benson L, Haberland ME, Edwards PA (1983) Regulation of the uptake and degradation of beta-very low density lipoprotein in human monocyte macrophages. J Biol Chem 258: 5151–5157

417. Viikari J (1976) Precipitation of plasma lipoproteins by PED-6000 and its evaluation with electrophoresis and ultracentrifugation. Scand J Clin Lab Invest 36: 265–268

418. Virchow R (1852) Über parenchymatöse Entzündung. Virchows Arch Path Anat 4: 261–324

419. Virchow R (1859) Die Bindegewebsfrage. Virchows Arch Path Anat 16: 2–20

420. Virchow R (ed) (1867) Krankheiten der Blut- und Lymphgefäße. von Lebert, Erlangen, pp 335–353 (Handbuch der speciellen Pathologie und Therapie, vol V, 2)

421. Vu-Dac N, Chekkor A, Parra H, Duthilleul P, Fruchart JC (1985) Latex immunoassay of human serum Lp(a+) lipoprotein. J Lipid Res 26: 267–269

422. Vu-Dac N, Mezdour H, Parra HJ, Luc G, Luyeye I, Fruchart JC (1989) A selective bi-site immunoenzymatic procedure for human Lp(a) lipoprotein quantification using monoclonal antibodies against apo(a) and apoB. J Lipid Res 30: 1437–1443

423. Walton KW, Hitchens J, Magnani HN, Khan M (1974) A study of methods of identification and estimation of Lp(a) lipoprotein and its significance in health, hyperlipidaemia and atherosclerosis. Atherosclerosis 20: 323–346

424. Walton KW (1975) Factors affecting lipoprotein deposition in the arterial wall. In: Hautvast JG, et al. (eds) Blood and arterial wall in atherogenesis and arterial thrombosis. Brill, Leiden, pp 79–86

425. Wardell MR, Brennan SO, Janus ED, Fraser R, Carrell RW (1987) Apolipoprotein E2-Christchurch (136 Arg----Ser). New variant of human apolipoprotein E in a patient with type-III hyperlipoproteinemia. J Clin Invest 80: 483–490

426. Wardell MR, Weisgraber KH, Havekes LM, Rall SC Jr (1989) Apolipoprotein E3-Leiden contains a seven-amino acid insertion that is a tandem repeat of residues 121–127. J Biol Chem 264: 21205–21210

427. Wardell MR, Rall SC Jr, Schaefer EJ, Kane JP, Weisgraber KH (1991) Two apolipoprotein E5 variants illustrate the importance of the position of additional positive charge on receptor-binding activity. J Lipid Res 32: 521–528

428. Wasenius A, Stugaard M, Otterstad JE, Froyshov D (1990) Diurnal and monthly intra-individual variability of the concentration of lipids, lipoproteins and apoproteins. Scand J Clin Lab Invest 50: 635–642

429. Weinstock N, Bartholome M, Seidel D (1981) Determination of apolipoprotein A-I by kinetic nephelometry. Biochim Biophys Acta 663: 279–288

430. Weisgraber KH, Mahley RW (1978) Apoprotein (E--A-II) complex of human plasma lipoproteins. I. Characterization of this mixed disulfide and its identification in a high density lipoprotein subfraction. J Biol Chem 253: 6281–6288

431. Weisgraber KH, Innerarity TL, Mahley RW (1982) Abnormal lipoprotein receptor-binding activity of the human E apoprotein due to cysteine-arginine interchange at a single site. J Biol Chem 257: 2518–2521

432. Weisgraber KH, Rall SC Jr, Innerarity TL, Mahley RW, Kuusi T, Ehnholm C (1984) A novel electrophoretic variant of human apolipoprotein E. Identification and characterization of apolipoprotein E1. J Clin Invest 73: 1024–1033

433. Weisgraber KH, Shinto LH (1991) Identification of the disulfide-linked homodimer of apolipoprotein E3 in plasma. Impact on receptor binding activity. J Biol Chem 266: 12029–12034

434. Whayne TF, Alaupovic P, Curry MD, Lee ET, Anderson PS, Schechter E (1981) Plasma apolipoprotein B and VLDL-, LDL-, and HDL-cholesterol as risk factors in the development of coronary artery disease in male patients examined by angiography. Atherosclerosis 39: 411–424

435. Wiegandt H, Lipp K, Wendt GG (1968) Identifizierung eines Lipoproteins mit Antigenwirksamkeit im Lp-System. Hoppe Seylers Z Physiol Chem 349: 489–494

436. Wieland E (1994) Personal comminication

437. Wieland H, Seidel D (1973) Improved techniques for assessment of serum lipoprotein patterns. II. Rapid method for diagnosis of type 3 hyperlipoproteinemia without ultracentrifugation. Clin Chem 19: 1139–1141

438. Wieland H, Seidel D, Wiegand V, Kreuzer H (1980) Serum lipoproteins and coronary artery disease (CAD). Comparison of the lipoprotein profile with the results of coronary angiography. Atherosclerosis 36: 269–280

439. Wieland H, Seidel D (1983) A simple specific method for precipitation of low density lipoproteins. J Lipid Res 24: 904–909

440. Wiklund O, Dyer CA, Tsao BP, Curtiss LK (1985) Stoichiometric binding of apolipoprotein B-specific monoclonal antibodies to low density lipoproteins. J Biol Chem 260: 10956–10960

441. Williams KJ, Tall AR, Bisgaier C, Brocia R (1987) Phospholipid liposomes acquire apolipoprotein E in atherogenic plasma and block cholesterol loading of cultured macrophages. J Clin Invest 79: 1466–1472

442. Williams KJ, Brocia RW, Fisher EA (1990) The unstirred water layer as a site of control of apolipoprotein B secretion. J Biol Chem 265: 16741–16744

443. Willnow TE, Goldstein JL, Orth K, Brown MS, Herz J (1992) Low density lipoprotein receptor-related protein and gp330 bind similar ligands, including plasminogen activator-inhibitor complexes and lactoferrin, an inhibitor of chylomicron remnant clearance. J Biol Chem 267: 26172–26180

444. Wilson PW, Abbott RD, Castelli WP (1988) High density lipoprotein cholesterol and mortality. The Framingham Heart Study. Arteriosclerosis 8: 737–741

445. Windaus A (1910) Über den Gehalt normaler und atheromatöser Aorten und Cholesterin und Cholesterinestern. Hoppe Seylers Z Physiol Chem 67: 174–176

446. Windler E, Havel RJ (1985) Inhibitory effects of C apolipoproteins from rats and humans on the uptake of triglyceride-rich lipoproteins and their remnants by the perfused rat liver. J Lipid Res 26: 556–565

447. Wolf BB, Lopes MB, VandenBerg SR, Gonias SL (1992) Characterization and immunohistochemical localization of alpha 2-macroglobulin receptor (low-density lipoprotein receptor-related protein) in human brain. Am J Pathol 141: 37–42

448. Xu CF, Nanjee N, Tikkanen MJ, Huttunen JK, Pietionen P, Butler R, Angelico F, Del-Ben M, Mazzarella B, Antonio R, et al. (1989) Apolipoprotein B amino acid 3611 substitution from arginine to glutamine creates the Ag (h/i) epitope: the polymorphism is not associated with differences in serum cholesterol and apolipoprotein B levels. Hum Genet 82: 322–326

449. Yaari S, Goldbourt U, Even-Zohar S, Neufeld HN (1981) Associations of serum high density lipoprotein and total cholesterol with total, cardiovascular, and cancer mortality in a 7-year prospective study of 10 000 men. Lancet I: 1011–1015

450. Yamamura T, Yamamoto A, Sumiyoshi T, Hiramori K, Nishioeda Y, Nambu S (1984) New mutants of apolipoprotein E associated with atherosclerotic diseases but not to type-III hyperlipoproteinemia. J Clin Invest 74: 1229–1237

451. Yano K, Reed DM, McGee DL (1984) Ten-year incidence of coronary heart disease in the Honolulu Heart Program. Relationship to biologic and lifestyle characteristics. Am J Epidemio 119: 653–666

452. Yla-Herttuala S, Palinski W, Rosenfeld ME, Parthasarathy S, Carew TE, Butler S, Witztum JL, Steinberg D (1989) Evidence for the presence of oxidatively modified low density lipoprotein in atherosclerotic lesions of rabbit and man. J Clin Invest 84: 1086–1095

453. Yla-Herttuala S, Rosenfeld ME, Parthasarathy S, Sigal E, Särkioja T, Witztum JL, Steinberg D (1991) Gene expression in macrophage-rich human atherosclerotic lesions. 15-Lipoxygenase and acetyl low density lipoprotein receptor messenger RNA colocalize with oxidation specific lipid-protein adducts. J Clin Invest 87: 1146–1152

454. Zenker G, Koltringer P, Bone G, Niederkorn K, Pfeiffer K, Jürgens G (1986) Lipoprotein(a) as a strong indicator for cerebrovascular disease. Stroke 17: 942–945

455. Zampogna A, Luria MH, Manubens SJ, Luria MA (1980) Relationship between lipids and occlusive coronary artery disease. Arch Intern Med 140: 1067–1069

Diagnostics of Homocysteine Metabolism

P. M. Ueland, H. Refsum, and M. R. Malinow

Introduction

Homocysteine (Hcy) was discovered in 1932 by Du Vigneaud [27] as a product of demethylation of methionine, and in 1962, Carson and Neill [19] reported on to two siblings with the inborn error homocystinuria detected by a screening program of mentally retarded children. Since then about 600 patients with homocystinuria have been reported [64]. Deficiency of the enzyme cystathionine β-synthase is the most common cause, but other enzymic defects have been described in a minority of these patients. Notably, all forms of homocystinuria, irrespective of enzymic defect, are associated with a high incidence of cardiovascular disease that may occur in early adolescence and even in childhood [64]. The high incidence of vascular disease in these patients led to the Hcy theory of atherosclerosis, formulated by McCully in 1975 [62, 61] and later substantiated by epidemiological data [52, 88].

This chapter reviews the literature on clinical aspects of Hcy metabolism with emphasis on the methodology used for the determination of plasma Hcy levels.

Biochemistry

Hcy is a sulfur amino acid that is formed from methionine as a product of S-adenosylmethionine-dependent transmethylation (Fig. 1). Intracellular Hcy is salvaged to methionine by remethylation. The reaction is catalyzed in most tissues by the enzyme methionine synthase (EC 2.1.1.13) which requires methylcobalamin as cofactor and 5-methyltetrahydrofolate as methyl donor. Hcy is also remethylated by the enzyme betaine-homocysteine transmethylase, which is confined to the liver and possibly kidney. An alternative route of Hcy disposal is conversion to cysteine, and the first step of this pathway is catalyzed by the vitamin B_6-dependent enzyme cystathionine β-synthase, which completes the transsulfuration pathway [31].

Methionine synthase has low K_m for Hcy, and the activity increases at low dietary methionine intake. These features suggest that the enzyme conserves methionine. Cystathionine β-synthase has high K_m for Hcy; the activity increases in response to high intake of methionine, and the enzyme probably controls the catabolism of excess Hcy [31]. Cellular export of Hcy represents an additional mechanism regulating the intracellular Hcy content. This process becomes important under conditions of imbalance between Hcy production and metabolism [87]. Increased Hcy production (induced by methionine loading) or inhibition of Hcy metabolism (during folate or cobalamin deficiencies, or defect of cystathionine β-synthase) cause export of Hcy into the extracellular fluid. This is the biochemical basis for plasma Hcy as a marker of folate or cobalamin deficiency or inborn errors of Hcy metabolism [89].

Homocysteine Species and Concentrations in Plasma or Serum

Hcy is probably released into the extracellular fluid and plasma in its reduced form, and only trace amounts can be detected in plasma under physiological conditions [59, 60]. In plasma, Hcy undergoes oxidation and disulfide exchange reactions. In freshly prepared plasma, about 70 % of Hcy exists as albumin-Hcy mixed disulfide, and this fraction is refered to as protein-bound Hcy [48, 70]. When whole plasma or serum is deproteinized with acid, the soluble free Hcy is obtained, and most Hcy in this fraction has been identified as Hcy-cysteine mixed disulfide. The sum of all Hcy species in plasma/serum is termed total Hcy [87]. Total Hcy shows a skewed distribution toward higher values in healthy subjects. The me-

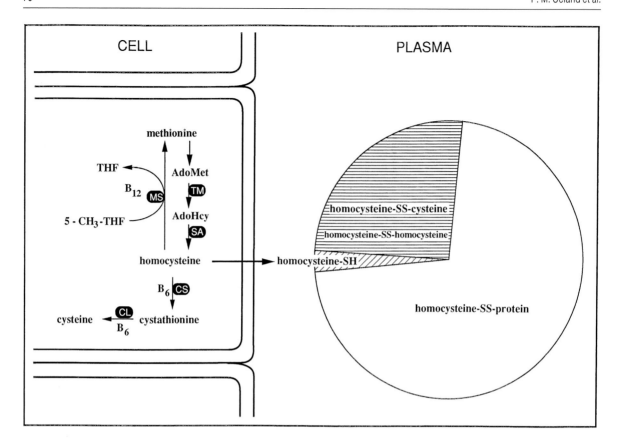

Fig. 1. Intracellular homocysteine metabolism and distribution of various homocysteine species in plasma. *AdoHcy, S*-Adenosylhomocysteine; *AdoMet, S*-adenosylmethionine; *CL*, cystathionine lyase (γ-cystathionase); *CS*, cystathionine β-synthase; *MS*, 5-methyl-THF-homocysteine methyltransferase (methionine synthase); *TM*, transmethylase; *SA, S*-adenosylhomocysteine hydrolase; *THF*, tetrahydrofolate

dian value has been reported as 10.7 µmol/l in 3000 healthy men aged 40–42 years, and the 95 th percentile as 17.6 µmol/l [89]. Total plasma Hcy seems to be dependent on age, gender, and in women possibly the menopausal status. The normal mean values are about 1 µmol/l lower in premenopausal women than in men or postmenopausal women, and there seems to be a significant increase (about 1–2 µmol/l) in the mean values as a function of age (from 20 to 70 years) in both sexes [3]. Good correlation between total Hcy measured in different laboratories and with different methods has been obtained, and values between 5 and 15 µmol/l are usually considered as normal [89].

Analytical Methods

There is a continuous redistribution of Hcy species in plasma/serum, so that after storage for days (at room temperature) or months (frozen), most Hcy becomes associated with plasma proteins. Reliable measurement of free Hcy therefore requires immediate deproteinization of plasma/serum, which is impractical in the clinical routine and has been largely abandoned [89]. Measurement of total Hcy is now widely recommended since the values remain stable during storage of plasma/serum. Total Hcy is measured by procedures including treatment of whole plasma/serum with a reductant. The Hcy disulfides are then quantitatively converted into reduced Hcy [89]. The methods used for separation and quantitation of reduced Hcy vary. The Hcy assays can be categorized into four types, according to the construction of the method: (a) radioenzymic assays, (b) gas chromatography-mass spectrometry, (c) assays based on precolumn derivatization, HPLC, and fluorescence detection, (d) HPLC and electrochemical detection, and (e) assays based on liquid chromatography and postcolumn derivatization, including the amino acid analyzer.

Radioenzymic Assays

These methods are based on the conversion of Hcy to S-adenosylhomocysteine catalyzed by the enzyme S-adenosylhomocysteine hydrolase. S-adenosylhomocysteine is quantitated by HPLC [70], paper [20] or thin-layer chromatography [21]. Low instrumental cost of the modification based on thin-layer chromatography separation is the main advantage of this assay. However, these assays are laborious, and the linearity may be limited by consumption of the cosubstrate (adenosine) used for the enzymic derivatization of Hcy.

Gas Chromatography-Mass Spectrometry

In this assay, the sample, supplemented with deuterated Hcy used as internal standard, is subjected to solid-phase extraction, and Hcy is derivatized with N-methyl-N(t-butyldimethylsilyl)trifluoroacetamide. The t-butyldimethylsilyl derivatives are separated and quantitated by capillary gas chromatography and selected ion monitoring [80, 79]. Attractive features of this method are codetermination of other metabolites such as methylmalonic acid [55]. The initial version of this technique has been simplified [79], but it still a cumbersome procedure. Furthermore, expensive equipment and technical skill are required.

Precolumn Derivatization, HPLC, and Fluorescence Detection

Hcy can be derivatized with the thiol-specific fluorogenic reagents monobromobimane (mBrB) [46, 72, 60, 32] or ammonium-7-fluoro-2,1,3-benzoxadiazole-4-sulfonate (SBD-F) [7, 85, 91], followed by separation of the adducts with HPLC. Both tags also label cysteine and cysteinylglycine, which are codetermined in these assays.

mBrB is a reactive agent, and the derivatization is completed within minutes. Assays based on this reagent can be fully automated [72]. The automatization results in high precision. The composition and pH of the mobile phase are critical for the separation of the Hcy adduct from hydrolysis products and other interfering material [32].

Experience in HPLC is necessary to operate this method.

SBD-F has low reactivity and derivatization is carried out at 60 °C for 30–60 min. This prevents automatization. The separation of thiol adducts is simple and fast since the reagent itself is not fluorogenic, and there is no interfering material [7, 85, 91].

Methods have recently been published which are based on derivatization with o-phthaldialdehyde [30, 44]. This agent is not a thiol-specific reagent but reacts with primary amino acids. These assays include several manual steps, and the presence of fluorescent material may cause chromatographic interference. They have not gained widespread use.

HPLC and Electrochemical Detection

In this assay, plasma/serum samples are subjected to HPLC immediately after treatment with reductant, and Hcy is detected with an electrochemical detector equipped with a gold-mercury electrode, which affords great specificity towards thiols. Simple sample processing, short run time, and high sample output are attractive features of this technique [78, 56]. However, particular attention must be paid to maintenance of flow cell and the gold-mercury electrode since deterioration of these parts of the detector system may cause baseline fluctuations and variable electrochemical response.

Amino Acid Analyzer and Postcolumn Derivatization

Hcy can be determined using an amino acid analyzer, either following reduction [2] or after the sulfhydryl group has been carboxymethylated using iodoacetic acid [51]. The free sulfhydryl is quantitated on a ion-exchange column eluted with the standard program [45] or with a mobile phase optimized for Hcy determination [2]. Even the optimized program results in long retention time (about 25 min) which is followed by column regeneration [2]. This seriously restricts sample output which is low compared to the HPLC methods. Other disadvantages include relatively high imprecision and formation of interfering ninhydrin-positive material upon storage of samples at –20 °C [89]. A method for total Hcy based on HPLC and postcolumn derivatization with thiol specific chromophor 4,4′-dithiodipyridine has recently been published [5]. Critical measures to reduce baseline noise have been worked out, and the method may turn out to be useful.

Procedures for Sample Collection and Processing

Total plasma Hcy increases slowly to a maximum increase of 15 %–20 % 6–8 h after a protein-rich meal. The increased Hcy level persists for several hours [89]. This effect from food intake is small relative to the high Hcy levels caused by some acquired or genetic diseases (see below, Table 1) and does not interfere with interpretation of data. However, a recent prospective study reported a 41 % increase in risk of myocardial infarction for each 4 µmol/l increase in Hcy level [9]. Thus, using plasma/serum Hcy as a parameter to evaluate cardiovascular risk, measurement of fasting levels is preferable.

Total Hcy is increased in plasma/serum when whole blood is left at room temperature. This is caused by a temperature and time-dependent release of Hcy from the blood cells. After 1 h at 22 °C there is a significant (10 %) increase in plasma Hcy [91, 6, 86, 32]. This artificial elevation is markedly reduced when the samples of whole blood are placed on ice. Under these conditions (0°–2 °C), plasma Hcy is stable for at least 4 h [32]. Therefore to stabilize plasma Hcy, it is recommended that whole blood is kept on ice and the blood cells removed from the plasma fraction within 1 h. Serum must be aspirated immediately after clot retraction. A release of Hcy from the blood cell before aspiration explains the observation that total Hcy in serum is slightly higher than in plasma [9].

Total Hcy in serum/plasma is stable for at least 4 days at room temperature, and for several weeks when stored at 0°–2 °C. In frozen samples kept at –20 °C, it is stable for years [89].

Table 1. Conditions or agents causing hyperhomocysteinemia

Condition/agent	Hyperhomocysteinemia	Cause of hyperhomocysteinemia
Genetic		
Homozygous for CS deficiency	I, S	Rare
Homozygous for MTFR deficiency	I, S	Rare
Cabalamin mutations (C, D, E, F, G)	I	Rare
Heterozygous for CS deficiency	M	Common
Heterozygous MTFR deficiency	M	Rare
Thermolabile MTFR	M	Probably common
Compound heterozygosity (MTFR deficiency and thermolabile MTFR)	I	–
Acquired		
Cobalamin deficiency	M, I, S	Fairly common
Folate deficiency	M, I	Common
Vitamin B_6 deficiency	(M)	Probably common
Renal failure	M, I	Common
Malignancy	M	Not common
Psoriasis	M	Fairly common
Hypothyroidism	M	Fairly common
Drugs	M	Fairly common
Methotrexate		
Nitrous oxide		
Antiepileptic agents		
Colestipol plus niacin		
Vitamin B_6 antagonists (azaribine, isoniazide)		

M, Moderate hyperhomocysteinemia, 15–30 µmol/l; I, intermediate hyperhomocysteinemia, 30–100 µmol/l; S, severe hyperhomocysteinemia, >100 µmol/l; CS, cystathionine β-synthase; MTFR, methylenetetrahydrofolate reductase.

Methionine Loading Test

The methionine loading test involves oral intake of a standard dose of methionine (0.1 g/kg or 3.8 g/m²), and total Hcy is measured after a fixed time interval, usually 4 or 6 h [13, 69, 4, 16, 88]. A typical Hcy response after a standard methionine load is shown in Fig. 2. The methionine loading test has been used to find possible defects in methionine metabolism in patients with cardiovascular disease [88]. Abnormal response has been defined as postload Hcy concentration or postload increase in Hcy exceeding the 95 th percentile, the mean plus 2 standard deviations for controls, or the highest control value [88]. Superfluous methionine is directed into the transsulfuration pathway via cystathionine β-synthase [31], and this agrees with the observation of abnormal response in homozygotes and most heterozygotes for cystathionine β-synthase deficiency [63]. Folate and cobalamin deficiency cause impaired Hcy remethylation, but data on the response to methionine loading in such patients are sparse and not conclusive [69; 16].

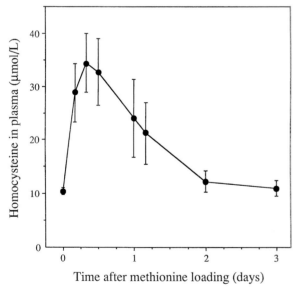

Fig. 2. Total homocysteine in plasma after methionine loading. Seven healthy postmenopausal women were given peroral methionine (0.1 g/kg). Data are given as mean ± standard deviation

Causes of Hyperhomocysteinemia

Hyperhomocysteinemia means elevated total Hcy in blood [56]; it is classified as moderate, intermediate, and severe. Mild hyperhomocysteinemia is defined as fasting total Hcy in plasma/serum of less than 30 μmol/l, moderate as concentrations between 30 and 100 μmol/l, and severe as concentrations higher than 100 μmol/l [52].

Hyperhomocysteinemia is caused by either genetic or acquired conditions (Table 1). Genetic diseases include the homozygous form of cystathionine β-synthase deficiency which is the most common cause of homocystinuria [64]. Rare forms are severe genetic defects of methylenetetrahydrofolate reductase, and inborn errors of cobalamin metabolism, classified as cblC, cblD, cblF, cblG, and cblE mutations [75]. Heterozygosity for cystathionine β-synthase deficiency is present in 0.3 %–1 %, or 2 % at the most, of the general population [64, 23], and 50 %–70 % of these subjects have moderate hyperhomocysteinemia [65, 77]. A mutation of the enzyme methylenetetrahydrofolate reductase, characterized by 50 % reduction in enzyme activity and thermolabile enzyme, occurs in 5 % of the general population, and these subjects have a tendency towards moderate hyperhomocysteinemia [49, 53]. Four subjects with compound heterozygosity of methylenetetrahydrofolate reductase deficiency and the thermolabile enzyme have been described; these had intermediate hyperhomocysteinemia [49]. Thus, heterozygosity for various forms of homocystinuria may explain the observation that total plasma Hcy is a genetic trait [68].

Among the acquired conditions causing elevated plasma Hcy, folate [47] or cobalamin deficiency [15, 1] are most often encountered. Folate deficiency is associated with moderate and intermediate hyperhomocysteinemia. In cobalamin-deficient patients, severe hyperhomocysteinemia is occasionally observed [89]. Elevation of plasma Hcy is also observed in disease states such as renal failure [93], acute leukemia, psoriasis, and hypothyroidism [88] and is induced by some drugs [71], i.e. methotrexate, nitrous oxide, antiepileptic agents, colestipol plus niacin [10], and some agent acting as vitamin B₆ antagonists [26, 71].

Hyperhomocysteinemia and Arterial Occlusive Diseases

Results from about 20 studies involving about 2 000 patients and a comparable number of controls have established that moderate hyperhomocysteinemia is an independent risk factor for vascular disease in the coronary, cerebral, and peripheral vessels [52, 88]. The overall increase in plasma Hcy in patients with premature cardiovascular disease is about 30 % compared to the level in healthy controls. The elevation shows some variability related to the site of the vascular lesions, and the incidence of hyperhomocysteinemia is highest in patients with cerebrovascular disease (about 40 %), intermediate in peripheral arterial disease (about 25 %) and lowest in coronary heart disease (about 15 %) [24, 58, 17, 66].

Coronary Artery Disease

Wilcken and Wilcken [94] reported elevation of cysteine-homocysteine mixed disulfide in coronary patients following methionine load, and this observation was confirmed by Murphy-Chutorian et al. [65] and by Clarke et al. [23] in a larger number of cases. Following the demonstration by Kang et al. [48] that a large proportion of total plasma homocysteine is bound to proteins, most investigators have measured basal total homocysteine. Thus, such levels were elevated in patients with myocardial infarction [45] and coronary artery disease established by coronary angiography [50]. These findings were confirmed by others [58, 34, 95, 84]. Most recently, prospective studies have confirmed that hyperhomocysteinemia is a risk factor for the coronary heart disease [82; 9]. Moreover, statistical analyses of the data demonstrated that hyperhomocysteinemia is independent of other common risk factors for atherosclerosis [23, 33, 82]. The influence of genetic factors in hyperhomocysteinemia in coronary patients was established by Williams et al. [95] and Genest et al. [33].

Cerebrovascular Disease

Brattström et al. [18], Boers et al. [12], and Clarke et al. [23] reported that patients with cerebrovascular disease attain higher levels of plasma homocysteine species after the methionine loading test. These studies were confirmed with measurements on basal plasma levels of total homocysteine [14, 8, 24, 17].

Peripheral Arterial Disease

Boers et al. [12] and Clark et al. [23] reported increased plasma levels of homocysteine species following methionine load in patients with peripheral arterial diseases. Studies on basal levels of total homocysteine confirmed these findings in patients with carotid, aortic, and ileofemoral arterial diseases [56] as well as in subjects with intermittent claudication [66]. Studies on thickness of carotid arteries by ultrasonography have yielded conflicting results. Clarke [22] found no increased frequency of carotid arteries plaques in 25 heterozygotes for cystathionine β-synthase deficiency whereas Rubba et al. [76] reported more frequent vascular lesions in the iliac and internal carotid arteries of 14 heterozygotes for cystathionine β-synthase than in 47 controls. Moreover, Malinow et al. [57] demonstrated that asymptomatic subjects with thickened carotid arteries have higher plasma total homocysteine levels than matched controls.

Mechanisms

Experimental studies have focused on a variety of mechanisms for the Hcy-induced atherogenesis. In vitro [35] and in vivo [39, 38] experiments suggest that Hcy promotes aggregation of platelets, but this conclusion has been contested [90; 43; 81]. Endothelial damage mediated by H_2O_2 production has been suggested by several authors, but most studies have been performed with high concentrations of D, L-Hcy or Hcy-thiolactone [92, 25, 37, 83]; cysteine induces similar effects, and the validity of these observations for the in vivo atherogenesis has been questioned [28]. Two reports have described oxidative modification of low-density lipoproteins by Hcy in vitro [42, 67], but increased lipid peroxidation has not been demonstrated in patients with hyperhomocysteinemia [11, 29].

Several recent reports describe stimulation of procoagulant activities and impairment of endothelial cell thromboresistance by Hcy. High concentrations of Hcy in vitro activate factor V [74], reduce protein C activation [73, 54], inhibit surface expression [54] and inactivate cofactor activity of thrombomodulin [41], and block tissue plasminogen activator binding to human endothelial cells [36]. The latter effect seems to be specific for Hcy, since the inhibition was reversed by cysteine. Harpel et al [40] recently demonstrated that physiological levels of Hcy enhance the binding of lipoprotein (a) to fibrin. Cysteine and other thiols have a similar effect. This indicates a link between sulfhydryl compounds and thrombosis and atherhogenesis. Stamler et al. [81] showed that low concentrations of Hcy also rapidly react with endothelium-derived relaxing factor/nitric oxide (NO) to form S-nitroso-Hcy, which acts as a potent antiplatelet agent and vasodilator. The formation of this adduct may attenuate H_2O_2 production from Hcy and thereby protect against the atherogenic properties of Hcy. According to this model, vascular injuries result under conditions of imbalance between NO production from dysfunctional endothelial cells and the levels of Hcy [81]. In conculusion, most experimental work on the adverse vascular properties of Hcy describes short-term effects provoked in the presence of very high concentrations of Hcy, and the effects are also produced by other thiols. Thus, no convincing or unifying hypothesis explaining the vascular injuries caused by hyperhomocysteinemia has yet been presented.

References

1. Allen RH, Stabler SP, Savage DG, Lindenbaum J (1990) Diagnosis of cobalamin deficiency. I. Usefulness of serum methylmalonic acid and total homocysteine concentrations. Am J Hematol 34; 90–98

2. Andersson A, Brattström L, Isaksson A, Israelsson B, Hultberg B (1989) Determination of homocysteine in plasma by ion-exchange chromatography. Scand J Clin Lab Invest 49: 445–450

3. Andersson A, Brattström L, Israelsson B, Isaksson A, Hamfelt A, Hultberg B (1992) Plasma homocysteine before and after methionine loading with regard to age, gender, and menopausal status. Eur J Clin Invest 22: 79–87

4. Andersson A, Brattström L, Israelsson B, Isaksson A, Hultberg B (1990) The effect of excess daily methionine intake on plasma homocysteine after a methionine loading test in humans. Clin Chim Acta 192: 69–76

5. Andersson A, Isaksson A, Brattström L, Hultberg B (1993) Homocysteine and other thiols determined in plasma by HPLC and a thiol-specific postcolumn derivatization. Clin Chem 39: 1590–1597

6. Andersson A, Isaksson A, Hultberg B (1992) Homocysteine export from erythrocytes and its implication for plasma sampling. Clin Chem 38: 1311–1315

7. Araki A, Sako Y (1987) Determination of free and total homocysteine in human plasma by high-performance liquid chromatography with fluorescene detection. J Chromatography 442: 43–52

8. Araki A, Sako Y, Fukushima Y, Matsumoto M, Asada T, Kita T (1989) Plasma sulfhydryl-containing amino acids in patients with cerebral infarction and in hypertensive subjects. Atherosclerosis 79: 139–146

9. Arnesen E, Refsum H, Bønaa KH, Ueland PM, Førde OH, Nordrehaug JE (1993) The Tromsø study; a population based prospective study of serum total homocysteine and coronary heart disease. (submitted)

10. Bankenhorn DH, Malinow MR, Mack WJ (1991) Colestipol plus niacin therapy elevates plasma homocysteine levels. Coron Art Dis 2: 357–360

11. Blom HJ, Engelen DPE, Boers GHJ, Stadhouders AM, Sengers RCA, De Abreu R, TePoele-Pothoff MTWB, Triebels JMF (1992) Lipid peroxidation in homocysteinaemia. J Inher Metab Dis 15: 419–422

12. Boers GHJ, Smals AGH, Trijbels FJM, Fowler B, Bakkeren JAJM, Schoonderwaldt HC, Kleijer WJ, Kloppenborg PWC (1985) Heterozygosity for homocystinuria in premature peripheral and cerebral occlusive arterial disease. N Engl J Med 313: 709–715

13. Brattström L, Israelsson B, Hultberg B (1988) Impaired homocysteine metabolism – a possible risk factor for arteriosclerotic vascular disease. In: Smith U, Eriksson S, Lindgärde F (eds) Genetic susceptibility to environmental factors a challenge for public intervention. Almqvist & Wiksell International, Stockholm, Sweden, pp 25–34

14. Brattström L, Israelsson B, Hultberg B (1988) Impaired homocysteine metabolism – a possible risk factor for arteriosclerotic vascular disease. In: Smith U, Eriksson S, Lindgärde F (eds) Genetic susceptibility to environmental factors a challenge for public intervention. Almqvist & Wiksell International, Stockholm, Sweden, pp 25–34

15. Brattström L, Israelsson B, Lindgärde F, Hultberg B (1988) Higher total plasma homocysteine in vitamin B12 deficiency than in heterozygosity for homocystinuria due to cystathionine β-synthase defiency. Metabolism 37: 175–178

16. Brattström L, Israelsson B, Norrving B, Bergqvist D, Thörne J, Hultberg B, Hamfelt A (1990) Impaired homocysteine metabolism in early-onset cerebral and peripheral occlusive arterial disease-effects of pyridoxine and folic acid treatment. Atherosclerosis 81: 51–60

17. Brattström L, Lindgren A, Israelsson B, Malinow MR, Norrving B, Upson B (1992) Hyperhomocysteinemia in stroke. Prevalence, cause and relationship to other risk factors or type of stroke. Eur J Clin Invest 22: 214–221

18. Brattström LE, Hardebo JE, Hultberg BL (1984) Moderate homocysteinemia – possible risk factor for arteriosclerotic cerebrovascular disease. Stroke 15: 1012–1016

19. Carson NAJ, Neill DW (1962) Metabolic abnormalities detected in a survey of mentally backward individuals in Northern Ireland. Arch Dis Child 37: 505–513

20. Chadefaux B, Coude M, Hamet M, Aupetit J, Kamoun P (1989) Rapid determination of total homocysteine in plasma. Clin Chem 35: 2002

21. Chu RC, Hall CA (1988) The total serum homocysteine as an indicator of vitamin B 12 and folate status. Am J Clin Pathol 90: 446–449

22. Clarke R (1990) The Irish experience. In: Robinson K (ed) Homocysteinaemia and vascular disease. Commission of the European Communities, Luxembourg, pp 41–48

23. Clarke R, Daly L, Robinson K, Naughten E, Cahalane S, Fowler B, Graham I (1991) Hyperhomocysteinemia: an independent risk factor for vascular disease. N Engl J Med 324: 1149–1155

24. Coull BM, Malinow MR, Beamer N, Sexton G, Nordt F, Garmo P (1990) Elevated plasma homocysteine concentration as a possible independent risk factor for stroke. Stroke 21: 572–576

25. De Groot PG, Willems C, Boers GHJ, Gonsalves MD, Van Aken WG, Van Mourik JA (1983) Endothelial cell dysfunction in homocystinuria. Eur J Clin Invest 13: 405–410

26. Drell W, Welch AD (1989) Azaribine-homocystinemia-thrombosis in historical perspectives. Pharmac Ther 41: 195–206

27. du Vigneaud V, Ressler C, Rachele JR (1950) The biological synthesis of „labile methyl groups." Science 112: 267–271

28. Dudman NPB, Hicks C, Wang J, Wilcken DEL (1991) Human arterial endothelial cell detachment in vitro – its promotion by homocysteine and cysteine. Atherosclerosis 91: 77–83

29. Dudman NPB, Wilcken DEL, Stocker R (1993) Circulating lipid hydroperoxide levels in human hyperhomocysteinemia – relevance to development of arteriosclerosis. Arterioscler Thromb 13: 512–516

30. Fermo I, Arcelloni C, Devecchi E, Vigano S, Paroni R (1992) High-performance liquid chromatographic method with fluorescence detection for the determination of total homocysteine in plasma. J Chromatography 593: 171–176

31. Finkelstein JD (1990) Methionine metabolism in mammals. J Nutr Biochem 1: 228–237

32. Fiskerstrand T, Refsum H, Kvalheim G, Ueland PM (1993) Homocysteine and other thiols in plasma and urine: automated determination and sample stability. Clin Chem 39: 263–271

33. Genest JJJr, McNamara JR, Upson B, Salem DN, Ordovas JM, Schaefer EJ, Malinow MR (1991) Prevalence of familial hyperhomocysteinemia in men with premature coronary artery disease. Arterioscler Thromb 11: 1129–1136

34. Genest JJJ, McNamara JR, Salem DN, Wilson PWF, Schaefer EJ, Malinow MR (1990) Plasma homocysteine levels in men with premature coronary artery disease. J Am Coll Cardiol 16: 1114–1119

35. Graeber JE, Slott JH, Ulane RE, Schulman JD, Stuart MJ (1982) Effect of homocysteine and homocystine on platelet and vascular arachidonic acid metabolism. Pediatr Res 16: 490–493

36. Hajjar KA (1993) Homocysteine-induced modulation of tissue plasminogen activator binding to its endothelial cell membrane receptor. J Clin Invest 91: 2873–2879

37. Harker LA, Harlan JM, Ross R (1983) Effect of sulfinpyrazone on homocysteine-induced endothelial injury and arteriosclerosis in baboons. Circ Res 53: 731–739

38. Harker LA, Ross R, Slichter SJ, Scott CR (1976) Homocysteine-induced arteriosclerosis. The role of endothelial cell injury and platelet response in its genesis. J Clin Invest 58: 731–741

39. Harker LA, Slichter SJ, Scott CR, Ross R (1974) Homocystinemia. Vascular injury and arterial thrombosis. N Engl J Med 291: 537–543

40. Harpel PC, Chang VT, Borth W (1992) Homocysteine and other sulfhydryl compounds enhance the binding of lipoprotein (a) to fibrin: a potential biochemical link between thrombosis, atherogenesis, and sulfhydryl compound metabolism. Proc Natl Acad Sci USA 89: 10193–10197

41. Hayashi T, Honda G, Suzuki K (1992) An atherogenic stimulus homocysteine inhibits cofactor activity of thrombomodulin and enhances thrombomodulin expression in human umbilical vein endothelial cells. Blood 79: 2930–2936

42. Heinecke JW, Rosen H, Suzuki LA, Chait A (1987) The role of sulfur-containing amino acids in superoxide production and modification of low density lipoprotein by arterial smooth muscle cells. J Biol Chem 262: 10098–10103

43. Hill-Zobell RL, Pyeritz RE, Scheffel U, Malpica O, Engin S, Camargo EE, Abbott M, Guilarte TR, Hill J, McIntyre PA, Murphy EA, Tsan M-F (1982) Kinetics and distribution of 111 indium-labeled platelets in patients with homocystinuria. N Engl J Med 307: 781–786

44. Hyland K, Bottiglieri T (1992) Measurement of total plasma and cerebrospinal fluid homocysteine by fluorescence following high-performance liquid chromatography and precolumn derivatization with orthophthaldialdehyde. J Chromatography 579: 55–62

45. Israelsson B, Brattström LE, Hultberg BJ (1988) Homocysteine and myocardial infarction. Atherosclerosis 71: 227–234

46. Jacobsen DW, Gatautis VJ, Green R (1989) Determination of plasma homocysteine by high-performance liquid chromatography with fluorescence detection. Anal Biochem 178: 208–214

47. Kang S-S, Wong PWK, Norusis M (1987) Homocysteinemia due to folate deficiency. Metabolism 36: 458–462

48. Kang S-S, Wong PWK, Becker N (1979) Protein-bound homocysteine in normal subjects and in patients with homocystinuria. Pediatr Res 13: 1141–1143

49. Kang S-S, Wong PWK, Bock H-GO, Horwitz A, Grix A (1991) Intermediate hyperhomocysteinemia resulting from compound heterozygosity of methylenetetrahydrofolate reductase mutations. Am J Hum Genet 48: 546–551

50. Kang S-S, Wong PWK, Cook HY, Norusis M, Messer JV (1986) Protein-bound homocysteine. A possible risk factor for coronary artery disease. J Clin Invest 77: 1482–1486
51. Kang S-S, Wong PWK, Curley K (1982) The effect of D-penicillamine on protein-bound homocysteine in homocystinurics. Pediatr Res 16: 370–372
52. Kang S-S, Wong PWK, Malinow MR (1992) Hyperhomocysteinemia as a risk factor for occlusive vascular disease. Annu Rev Nutr 12: 279–298
53. Kang S-S, Wong PWK, Susmano A, Sora J, Norusis M, Ruggie N (1991) Thermolabile methylenetetrahydrofolate reductase: an inherited risk factor for coronary artery disease. Am J Hum Genet 48: 536–545
54. Lentz SR, Sadler JE (1991) Inhibition of thrombomodulin surface expression and protein-C activation by the thrombogenic agent homocysteine. J Clin Invest 88: 1906–1914
55. Lindenbaum J, Stabler SP, Allen RH (1988) New assays for cobalamin defiency getting better spezificity. Lab Manag 26: 41–44
56. Malinow MR, Kang SS, Taylor LM, Wong PWK, Inahara T, Mukerjee D, Sexton G, Upson B (1989) Prevalence of hyperhomocysteinemia in patients with peripheral arterial occlusive disease. Circ Res 79: 1180–1188
57. Malinow MR, Nieto FJ, Szklo M, Chambless LE, Bond G (1993) Carotid artery intimal-medial wall thickening and plasma homocysteine in asymptomatic adults – the Atherosclerosis Risk in Communities study. Circulation 87: 1107–1113
58. Malinow MR, Sexton G, Averbuch M, Grossman M, Wilson DL, Upson B (1990) Homocysteinemia in daily practice: levels in coronary heart disease. Coron Art Dis 1: 215–220
59. Mansoor MA, Svardal AM, Schneede J, Ueland PM (1992) Dynamic relation between reduced, oxidized and protein-bound homocysteine and other thiol components in plasma during methionine loading in healthy men. Clin Chem 38: 1316–1321
60. Mansoor MA, Svardal AM, Ueland PM (1992) Determination of the in vivo redox status of cysteine, cysteinylglycine, homocysteine and glutathione in human plasma. Anal Biochem 200: 218–229
61. McCully KS (1992) Homocystinuria, arteriosclerosis, methylmalonic aciduria, and methyltransferase deficiency – a key case revisited. Nutr Rev 50: 7–12
62. McCully KS, Wilson RB (1975) Homocysteine theory of arteriosclerosis. Atherosclerosis 22: 215–227
63. McGill JJ, Mettler G, Rosenblatt DS, Scriver CR (1990) Detection of heterozygotes for recessive alleles. Homocysteinemia: paradigm of pitfalls in phenotypes. Am J Med Genet 36: 45–52
64. Mudd SH, Levy HL, Skovby F (1989) Disorders of transsulfuration. In: Scriver CR, Beaudet AL, Sly WS, Valle D (eds) The metabolic basis of inherited Disease. McGraw-Hill, New York, pp 693–734
65. Murphy-Chutorian DR, Wexman MP, Grieco AJ, Heininger JA, Glassman E, Gaull GE, Ng SKC, Feit F, Wexman K, Fox AC (1985) Methionine intolerance: a possible risk factor for coronary artery disease. J Am Coll Cardiol 6: 725–730
66. Mölgaard J, Malinow MR, Lassvik C, Holm A-C, Olsson AG (1992) Hyperhomocysteinemia: an independent risk factor for intermittent claudicatio. J Intern Med 231: 273–279
67. Parthasarathy S (1987) Oxidation of low density lipoprotein by thiol compounds leads to its recognition by the acetyl-LDL receptor. Biochim Biophys Acta 917: 337–340
68. Reed T, Malinow MR, Christian JC, Upson B (1991) Estimates of heritability for plasma homocysteine levels in aging adult male twins. Clin. Pharmacol. Ther. Genetics 39: 425–428
69. Refsum H, Helland S, Ueland PM (1989) Fasting plasma homocysteine as a sensitive parameter to antifolate effect. A study on psoriasis patients receiving low-dose methotrexate treatment. Clin Pharmacol Ther 46: 510–520
70. Refsum H, Helland S, Ueland PM (1985) Radioenzymic determination of homocysteine in plasma and urine. Clin Chem 31: 624–628
71. Refsum H, Ueland PM (1990) Clinical significance of pharmacological modulation of homocysteine metabolism. Trends Pharmacol Sci 11: 411–416
72. Refsum H, Ueland PM, Svardal AM (1989) Fully automated fluorescence assay for determining total homocysteine in plasma. Clin Chem 35: 1921–1927
73. Rodgers GM, Conn MT (1990) Homocysteine, an atherogenic stimulus, reduces protein-C activation by arterial and venous endothelial cells. Blood 75: 895–901
74. Rodgers GM, Kane WH (1986) Activation of endogenous factor V by a homocysteine-induced vascular endothelial cell activator. J Clin Invest 77: 1909–1916
75. Rosenblatt DS, Cooper BA (1990) Inherited disorders of vitamin-B12 utilization. BioEssays 12: 331–334
76. Rubba P, Faccenda F, Pauciullo P, Carbone L, Mancini M, Strisciuglio P, Carrozzo R, Sartorio R, Delgiudice E, Andria G (1990) Early signs of vascular disease in homocystinuria – a noninvasive study by ultrasound methods in eight families with cystathionine-beta-synthase deficiency. Metabolism 39: 1191–1195
77. Sartorio R, Carrozzo R, Corbo L, Andria G (1986) Protein-bound plasma homocysteine and identification of heterozygotes for cystathionine-synthase deficiency. J Inher Metab Dis 9: 25–29
78. Smolin LA, Benevenga NJ (1982) Accumulation of homocysteine in vitamin B-6 deficiency: a model for the study of cystathionine β-synthase deficiency. J Nutr 112: 1264–1272
79. Stabler SP, Lindenbaum J, Savage DG, Allen RH (1993) Elevation of serum cystathionine levels in patients with cobalamin and folate deficiency. Blood 81: 3404–3413
80. Stabler SP, Marcell PD, Podell ER, Allen RH (1987) Quantitation of total homocysteine, total cysteine, and methionine in normal serum and urine using capillary gas chromatography-mass spectrometry. Anal Biochem 162: 185–196
81. Stamler JS, Osborne JA, Jaraki O, Rabbani LE, Mullins M, Singel D, Loscalzo J (1993) Adverse vascular effects of homocysteine are modulated by endothelium-derived relaxing factor and related oxides of nitrogen. J Clin Invest 91: 308–318

82. Stampfer MJ, Malinow MR, Willett WC, Newcomer LM, Upson B, Ullmann D, Tishler PV, Hennekens CH (1992) A prospective study of plasma homocysteine and risk of myocardial infarction in United States physicians. J Am Med Ass 268: 877–881

83. Starkebaum G, Harlan JM (1986) Endothelial cell injury due to copper-catalyzed hydrogen peroxide generation from homocysteine. J Clin Invest 77: 1370–1376.

84. Ubbink JB, Vermaak WJH, Bennett JM, Becker PJ, van Staden DA, Bissbort S (1991) The prevalence of homocysteinemia and hypercholesterolemia in angiographically defined coronary heart disease. Klin Wochenschr 69: 527–534

85. Ubbink JB, Vermaak WJH, Bissbort S (1991) Rapid high-performance liquid chromatographic assay for total homocysteine levels in human serum. J Chromatography 565: 441–446

86. Ubbink JB, Vermaak WJH, Vandermerwe A, Becker PJ (1992) The effect of blood sample aging and food consumption on plasma total homocysteine levels. Clin Chim Acta 207: 119–128

87. Ueland PM, Refsum H (1989) Plasma homocysteine, a risk factor for vascular disease: plasma levels in health, disease, and drug therapy. J Lab Clin Med 114: 473–501

88. Ueland PM, Refsum H, Brattström L (1992) Plasma homocysteine and caardiovascular disease. In: Francis RB Jr (ed) Atherosclerotic cardiovascular disease, hemostasis, and endothelial function. Marcel Dekker, New York, pp 183–236

89. Ueland PM, Refsum H, Stabler SP, Malinow MR, Andersson A, Allen RH (1993) Total homocysteine in plasma or serum. Methods and clinical applications. Clin Chem 39: 1764–1779

90. Uhlemann ER, TenPas JH, Lucky AW, Schulman JD, Mudd SH, Shulman NR (1976) Platelet survival and morphology in homocystinuria due to cystathionine synthase deficiency. N Engl J Med 295: 1283–1286

91. Vester B, Rasmussen K (1991) High performance liquid chromatography method for rapid and accurate determination of homocysteine in plasma and serum. Eur J Clin Chem Clin Biochem 29: 549–554

92. Wall RT, Harlan JM, Harker LA, Striker GE (1980) Homocysteine-induced endothelial cell injury in vitro: a model for the study of vascular injury. Thrombosis Res 18: 113–121

93. Wilcken DEL, Gupta VJ, Betts AK (1981) Homocysteine in the plasma of renal transplant recipients: effects of cofactors for methionine metabolism. Clin Sci 61: 743–749

94. Wilcken DEL, Wilcken B (1976) The pathogenesis of coronary artery disease. A possible role for methionine metabolism. J Clin Invest 57: 1079–1082

95. Williams RR, Malinow MR, Hunt SC, Upson B, Wu LL, Hopkins PN, Stults BN, Kuida H (1990) Hyperhomocysteinemia in Utah siblings with early coronary disease. Coron Artery Dis 1: 681–685

Section III
Vascular Ultrasonography

Imaging Technology

E. G. Cape and A. P. Yoganathan

State-of-the-art ultrasonic imaging technology for vascular studies consists of three modalities of velocity measurement which can be used in combination with the basic B-mode image of solid structures: (a) continuous wave spectral Doppler (b) pulsed wave spectral Doppler, and (c) color Doppler flow imaging of blood velocities. As indicated, the first two modalities provide spectral display of velocities and are selected depending on the quantities of interest for the problem at hand. The third modality uses the same Doppler principles of velocity measurement as the second but in practice is more of an "imaging" technique than a quantitative velocity tool. This chapter discusses each of these tools so that the advantages and limitations associated with various examination techniques in the following chapters can be understood. Also included is a description of available transducer configurations.

mined in regions of interest. In the spectral Doppler modality the transducer detects a number of returning signals and displays each calculated velocity in spectral format, as shown in Fig. 1. The expanded vertical strip explains the concept of spectral display. A single vertical strip may be thought of as a histogram, with increasing intensity of shading representing more particles traveling within that velocity interval. These "strips" are updated rapidly and, when inspected over time, produce a time-dependent display of flow velocity. The information content of these spectra, with regard to the *origin* of the information, depends on the choice of continuous or pulsed wave modality.

Angle of Incidence Issues. Regardless of the modality of Doppler velocity measurement (each is discussed below) it is critical to recognize the im-

Spectral Doppler Velocity Measurements

Velocities of moving targets in the body may be obtained by interrogating regions of interest with ultrasound waves [1]. Waves which strike moving targets are reflected back to the transducer with a frequency shift which is proportional to the velocity of the target. Target velocities can then be calculated by the well established Doppler equation:

$$v = cf_d/2f_o\cos\theta \qquad (1)$$

where c = speed of sound in the medium (approximately 1540 m/s for blood and tissue), f_o = the frequency of ultrasound emitted from the transducer, f_d = the Doppler shift, which equals the returning frequency minus the emitted frequency, and θ = the angle between the ultrasound beam path and the blood cell velocity vector.

Flowing blood is filled with moving targets in the form of red blood cells, thus with a properly designed transducer cell velocities can be deter-

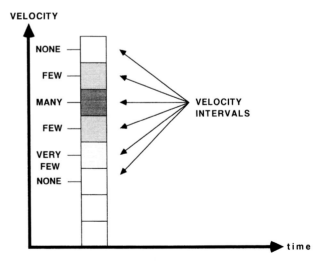

Fig. 1. Spectral Doppler velocimetry. Particles traveling within small intervals of velocity are represented by *shading* within that interval on a vertical spectrum which is rapidly updated. Actual spectral data to support this schematic is shown in the lower panel of Figure 7

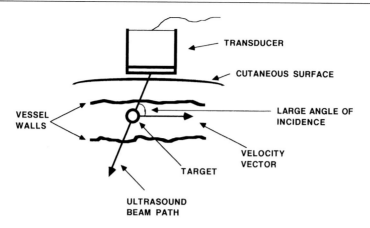

Fig. 2. Orthogonality of near-surface blood vessels. Vascular applications of ultrasound often involve interrogation of vessels near the cutaneous surface on which the transducer is placed. This necessarily introduces large angles of incidence between the ultrasound beam paths and flowing blood

portance of the angular term in the Doppler equation above. Unless requested to correct, most instruments default to an assumption that the angle of interrogation is zero. In vascular imaging it is rarely the case that the angle is actually zero. Blood vessels lie near the surface and approach a perpendicular orientation to the transducer (Fig. 2) [2]. Thus the angle of interrogation, measurable on the two-dimensional image, must be input to the instrument. Alternatively the velocity data must be manually corrected after acquisition. If the angle of interrogation is severe, the user must recognize that the signal to noise ratio of the data is very low, and correction for the angle by the Doppler equation may result in correction of noise, producing artifacts.

Careful angulation of the transducer can reduce the angle of incidence a priori, but the user must note that in some applications such as ophthalmologic or carotid imaging, the very slightest pressures applied to reduce the angle of incidence can alter resistance in the vessels of interest and change the flow itself.

Continuous Wave Spectral Doppler

In the continuous wave spectral modality the transducer continuously emits and receives ultrasound. All returning sound is analyzed for frequency shifts, velocities are calculated by the Doppler equation, and the resulting spectrum is displayed. Due to the continuous monitoring of returning sound in this configuaration it is impossible to determine from what distance the signals returned. In other words, for a given calculated velocity it is possible to state that a target was traveling at that speed, but it is not possible to state the location of the target. There is no range resolution. Despite the fact that range resolution is not available, continuous wave Doppler does offer a quick and convenient acquisition of the maximum velocity along a line of interest.

Pulsed Wave Spectral Doppler

While it is often convenient to obtain the maximum velocity along a line of interest, in many applications the velocity at a specified location is desired (for example, upstream or downstream of a stenosis), and this velocity may not be the maximum along any obtainable line of interrogation. In this case pulsed wave Doppler is applied. In this modality the transducer emits a burst of ultrasound, waits a time Δt, and then opens a "window" to catch the returning signal. The time, Δt, between emission of the burst and opening of the window to catch the returning signal determines the "depth" of the analyzed sample by the following equation:

$$depth = (c\Delta t)/2 \qquad (2)$$

where c = the speed of sound in the medium. The factor of 2 accounts for the fact that received sound must have traveled to and back from the target, or a total distance of two times the sample depth. This concept is further illustrated in Fig. 3.

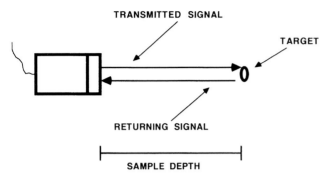

Fig. 3. Sample depth in pulsed wave Doppler. The ultrasound transducer sends a burst of ultrasound, waits a time Δt, then monitors the returning signal. If the speed of sound in the medium is c, the total distance traveled by the sound between emission and reception is $c(\Delta t)$, thus the distance between the transducer and sample volume is $c(\Delta t)/2$, as shown

Note that the length of time the window stays open determines the axial length of the resulting *sample volume*. Focusing considerations in the transducer determine the lateral dimensions of the sample volume for a given configuration.

While the pulsed wave modality allows for range resolution, it introduces a limitation called aliasing. The Nyquist principle, which is common to all frequency-dependent sampling processes, states that sampling must be done at a frequency at least twice as high as the frequency being detected. In the context of blood cell velocity measurement by ultrasound, the frequency of pulsing of the transducer must be at least twice as high as the Doppler shift, f_d, being used to calculated velocity. The pulsing frequency of the transducer is commonly referred to as the pulse repetition frequency (PRF; see "Instrument Settings"). If the transducer attempts to measure a cell velocity

which would, in principle, produce a shift more than twice the PRF, the signal *aliases*. This is best illustrated using the example depicted in Fig. 4. If the true cell velocity is 60 cm/s and the PRF has been selected so that a maximum velocity of 50 cm/s can be detected, the resulting signal "wraps" around to the corresponding negative value. In the pulsatile flow shown in Fig. 4 this scenario would produce a normal profile up to the point of aliasing, at which it would take on a chopped character with the aliased velocities appearing on the negative scale. On deceleration the spectrum would then appear normal as the true peak velocities fall below the aliasing level.

Continuous Versus Pulsed Wave Doppler

In the setting of vascular imaging, pulsed wave Doppler is usually the modality of choice since velocities are relatively low (<2 m/s) even in pathologic conditions, and the aliasing limitation can be easily overcome by increasing the PRF. Increasing the PRF as a rule requires depth reductions, but in most vascular imaging configurations these depths are already very short (1–7 cm). Thus, the use of continuous wave Doppler is very limited in the vascular setting.

Fig. 4. Aliasing. In the schematic example, blood cells accelerate and decelerate in pulsatile flow. The peak velocity is 60 cm/s, which exceeds the maximum detectable velocity (Nyquist limit) by 10 cm/s. On the spectral display, the signals exceeding 50 cm/s are truncated and displayed on the negative portion of the scale, as shown. In principle, these aliased signals can be "unwrapped," but high-velocity flows can be wrapped multiple times and diminish rapidly, eliminating the feasibility of unwrapping

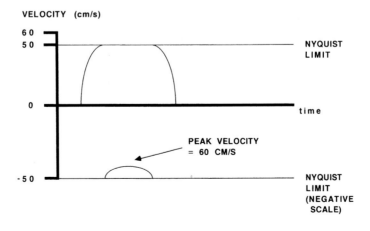

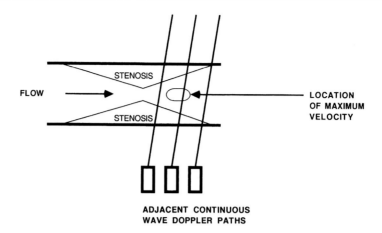

Fig. 5. Continuous wave error in maximum velocity. In nonvascular applications (cardiac, for example) it is correctly assumed that maximum velocities within certain chambers can be obtained by placing a continuous wave Doppler cursor along the axis of flow. This is not so easily achieved in vascular applications where vessels lie near and parallel to the surface. As shown in this schematic, the angle of incidence is large, and the continuous wave cursor must therefore intersect the desired flow in a volume of space not much larger than a pulsed wave sample volume. In summary, the convenience of maximum velocity acquisiton by continuous wave Doppler, which is taken for granted in other applications, is not readily achieved in vascular applications

Furthermore, the basic assumption of using continuous wave Doppler to obtain a maximum velocity along a line of interest cannot be confidently applied since it is rare that ultrasound beam can be placed along significant lengths of vascular vessels. Indeed, these vessels often approach orthogonality with the ultrasound beam, as shown in Fig. 5. Although the peak of the spectral envelope obtained by continuous wave Doppler corresponds to the maximum velocity along the beam, this fact is of limited use when the beam does not lie along the vessel as illustrated in Fig. 5. In short, the maximum velocity can still be easily missed using continuous wave Doppler, and it is therefore usually advisable to select pulsed wave Doppler and steer the sample volume to the desirable location on the two-dimensional B-mode image.

In summary, pulsed wave Doppler overcomes the limitation of range ambiguity present in continuous wave Doppler but introduces a maximum detectable velocity which, when violated, results in the confusing phenomenon of aliasing. However,

for the low velocities and high angles of incidence found in vascular applications pulsed wave Doppler is usually the modality of choice for all spectral velocity measurements.

Color Doppler Flow Mapping

The modality of color Doppler flow mapping allows two-dimensional "images" of blood flow to be superimposed on the tomographic B-mode images [3]. While B-mode imaging of the solid structures has been available for some time, color flow mapping has achieved widespread use only within the past decade. Although it uses Doppler velocity measurement principles, it is generally applied and interpreted as an "imaging" tool rather than a "velocimetry" method such as spectral Doppler. This controversial point is addressed in more detail below ("color Doppler 'Imaging' vs 'velocimetry'").

Color Doppler flow mapping is in principle an extension of pulsed wave Doppler [4]. Figure 6 shows the basic anatomy of a color Doppler image. The ultrasound transducer emits a burst of sound just as it does for the basic spectral pulsed wave technique. However, the first step in constructing a color Doppler image is to catch the returning signals by opening the window in a sequential manner. By the same pulsed wave principle as above, this process leads to a series of sample depths: depth $= n \, (c\Delta t)/2$; with the integer n representing the multiple sample volumes obtained by the sequential opening of the window. This configuration in which a string of sample volumes is obtained is called multigating [5].

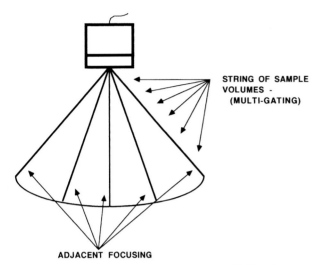

STRING OF SAMPLE
VOLUMES -
(MULTI-GATING)

ADJACENT FOCUSING

Fig. 6. Color Doppler image anatomy. Multigating processing algorithms allow strings of sample volumes to be obtained. Refocusing of these strings along adjacent paths allow construction of two-dimensional matrices of velocity information which are subsequently color coded. This figure shows a pie-shaped image which would be derived using a phased array transducer. Other available shapes are shown in Figure 8

Having obtained a string of sample volumes, the beam is refocused to an adjacent path, producing a second string of sample volumes, as shown in Fig. 6. This process is repeated until a pie-shaped sector, a vector array, or a linear array of sample volumes is constructed (depending on transducer configuration; see "Transducers"). These arrays of measured velocities are then updated at frame rates approaching those for B-mode imaging. (In color flow mapping, the increased data processing load generally causes some decrease in available frame rate compared to B-mode alone. For vascular imaging, however, due to the small depths of interrogation, this decrease is not as severe as for modalities using greater depths – cardiac imaging, for example).

Since it is impossible to examine spectra for each of the sample volumes simultaneously even for a single frame, color encoding is used. On the left side of Fig. 7 (see p. 94) a color bar is shown. This bar shows velocities ranging from zero to the aliasing velocity as increasing hues of red or blue, depending on direction toward or away from the transducer, respectively. Average pixel velocity magnitudes determined by the method described above are color coded in accordance with the color bar. The result is a two-dimensional image of solid structure (B-mode) and blood velocity (color

Doppler). It is important to note two critical limitations of the color Doppler method. First, limitations of pulsed wave Doppler (aliasing) are also found in color flow mapping since it is an extension of that modality. Second, the high data-processing requirements allow only a relatively small number of samples to be averaged for a single pixel in a single frame. A typical value might be 15. For highly turbulent flows or those flows with a high frequency of pulsation, these small sample sizes can render resulting velocity magnitudes meaningless, leaving the technique as simply a qualitative picture of the flow (see below).

Instrument Settings

Several instrument settings critically affect the resultant image on a color flow map.

Gain. The gain setting refers to the amplification of the basic Doppler signal. Depending on attenuation of sound gain should typically be adjusted to a level high enough to produce a clear image, but below the level which produces extraneous noise.

Pulse Repetition Frequency. As described above, in order to obtain range resolution in the modality of pulsed wave Doppler, the transducer must deliver bursts of ultrasound at high frequency. This pulsing frequency is commonly referred to as PRF.

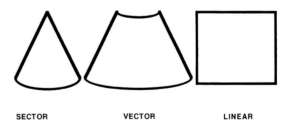

SECTOR   VECTOR   LINEAR

Fig. 8. Array shapes. Depending on transducer configuration, various shapes of velocity arrays can be obtained for subsequent color encoding. Sector arrays are pie shaped, with sample volume "strings" meeting in an apex at the top of the array. These arrays are produced by phased array and mechanical transducers. Vector arrays are similar but the bases of each scan line are arranged around a semicircular or elliptical shape in the near field as shown. Linear arrays are constructed of parallel scan lines, which may be more intuitively interpreted by the user but require a larger transducer footprint (area of interface between transducer and skin) to implement

Wall Filter. Solid structures have low velocities in the setting of vascular imaging, but combined with slight movements of the transducer on the cutaneous surface, high amplitude noise can obliterate important low-velocity signals. Therefore, high-pass filters are generally incorporated into the system to eliminate these low-frequency, high-amplitude signals.

Multivariate Motion Discriminators. Despite the fact that filters are quite low in vascular imaging, they can still obliterate important low velocities in many cases. To overcome this problem some manufacturers have implemented multivariate motion discriminators [6]. These algorithms in principle allow display of low velocity blood flow signals while still eliminating low-frequency signals from solid structures. These algorithms analyze signal characteristics in addition to velocity, such as power. By cutting off high-power signals of low velocity but retaining low-power signals, useful blood velocity information can be retained while structure noise is eliminated.

Carrier Frequency. The frequency of emitted ultrasound is used in the Doppler equation to calculate velocities. Carrier frequency is generally chosen by considering a trade-off between image quality and velocity detection. High-frequency transducers produce better image quality while low-frequency ones produce higher velocity limits.

Frame Rate. Regardless of the transducer configuration (see section below) image "frames" must be constructed which can be viewed in a fast sequential manner to produce the real-time imaging effect. Frame rates are considerably reduced when color Doppler is superimposed on the B-mode image due to the increased data processing demands, and decreased frame rates can be problematic in patients with elevated pulse frequencies (heart rates). This problem is more pronounced in applications with greater depth settings (cardiac) than vascular imaging.

Transducers

Transducers can be classified according to the "shape" image they produce and fall generally into the following three categories: sector (phased array and mechanical), vector (phased array and mechanical), and linear (phased array).

These shapes are shown in Fig. 8. Vector and sector arrays allow large tomographic slices to be obtained for relatively small transducer "footprints" (the area interfaced with the skin) due to the fanning nature of the beam focussing. The newer vector arrays provide greater fields of view without loss of resolution when compared to traditional sector arrays. For shorter depths and widths the linear arrays provide an image constructed of parallel lines which allow for more consistent angle correction than the multiangled beam configuration of vector or sector arrays.

Phased array transducers consist of an arrangement of crystals which focus the ultrasound beam in different directions to produce the final image. No components of the transducer head physically move. Mechanical transducers consist of an oscillating head which physically moves in accordance with the prescribed frame rate.

Color Doppler „Imaging" Versus „Velocimetry"

After initial enthusiasm associated with the introduction of color Doppler flow mapping for cardiac applications in the mid-1980s, it has largely remained a qualitative tool, serving as a guide for placement of spectral Doppler cursors or sample volumes and as a semiquantitative indicator of obstructions, restrictive orifices, regurgitant lesions, and high-velocity flows. Pitfalls accompany use of color Doppler either as (a) an imaging modality or (b) a velocity measurement method.

(a) Since physical entities such as jets are accompanied, almost defined, by strong velocity fields, images of these sources of energy naturally correspond to the composite shape of fluid particle paths. Since these lesions have traditionally been assessed by angiographic means, it is tempting to interchange the analysis of these images with time-honored means of assessing angiograms. If this approach is taken by the user, however, it is important to keep in mind that velocity fields can be easily interrupted by physical or technical factors, while the total passage of radio-opaque contrast in an angiographic image remains the same.

(b) Methods for assessing various lesions based on fluid mechanical principles have been proposed in various settings. In optimistic principle, color Doppler flow mapping is a panacea since it provides velocity maps throughout any lesion of interest. It must be remembered, however, that due to instrument limitations color flow mapping is still highly qualitative at this point in time. The extent of quantitative versus qualitative information is dependent on the nature of the flow field. (For example, color Doppler pixels within a turbulent jet are virtually useless beyond indicating that the flow is "there.") Minimal advances have been made in the past 5 years in terms of elevating color Doppler flow mapping to true velocimetry status due to marketing and user inertia.

Both (a) and (b) are affected by angle of incidence difficulties. By definition, Doppler calculations of velocity obtain components of velocity parallel only to the ultrasound beam. Thus, due to the two-dimensional array of sample volumes obtained for a single transducer location, the extent of error in velocity measurement due to angle of incidence effects varies at different points within the sector. The velocity measurement is therefore directly compromised, and any color images constructed using the Doppler principle are variable depending on the angle of incidence. In the vascular setting, since the angle of incidence often approaches 90° for vessels near the body surface, angle of incidence effects are much more pronounced than in other applications such as cardiac imaging.

Other Sources of Error

Despite the usefulness of ultrasound as a clinical tool the technology is relatively new, and many problems must still be overcome in the laboratories of the ultrasound companies. Two of these technical difficulties are discussed as follows.

Acoustic Impedance Mismatch. An acoustic impedance mismatch exists between blood and vessel walls. This mismatch can result in multiple spectral peaks and modify the shape of the resultant spectrum.

Spectral Broadening (Transit Time). Jones [7] gives a detailed explanation of this phenomenon. In principle, the Fourier transform of a sine wave is a delta function. However, for sine waves that are turned on, then off, such as in pulsed wave Doppler, the Fourier transform is a "broadened" delta function. Increased broadness in the Fourier transform makes it more difficult to locate the maximum frequency of the spectrum.

Clinical Examples

Having discussed the various components of a color Doppler image and the accompanying quantitative capabilities of spectral Doppler, this chapter concludes with four clinical images described in the context of the previous discussion.

1. Figure 7 shows a color Doppler image of flow through a stenosis with the spectral trace of pulsed wave Doppler in the lower panel. The first noticeable characteristic of this figure is the remarkable spatial resolution of the vessel structure. This is true not only for the cross-section of the vessel but for the morphology of the obstruction itself. Superimposed on this image is color Doppler which allows detailed insight into the flow field. The Nyquist limit in this case is 34 cm/s. Since the vessel is oriented almost perpendicular to the ultrasound beams emanating from this linear array transducer, the color Doppler window is angled at approximately 30° and tilted so that the beam follows flow moving away from the transducer. To account for this proximal image the color bar has been inverted to show blue as flow toward the transducer and red for flow away from the transducer. Thus, in this image, flow approaching the stenosis is displayed in shades of red. Fine gradations in red are notable as the flow approaches the stenosis in this excellent image, reflecting variations in velocity across the lumen of the vessel. As flow passes through the constriction, blood cells accelerate, producing a jet distal to the obstruction with velocities which greatly exceed the Nyquist limit (these peak velocities are approximately 1.5 m/s, as shown in the spectral envelopes below the image). Since these velocities exceed the Nyquist limit, the color image aliases, and we observe blue and mosaic patterns distal to the obstruction. A low velocity vortex (still in red) is detected just distal and inferior to the obstruction. The pulsed wave sample volume is shown just distal to the origin of the jet producing the quantitative spectral envelopes of velocity below.

2. Figure 9 shows a color image of a femoral artery bifurcation, with central flow along the bifurcation accelerating past the ailiasing velocity of 32 cm/s. The color window is, again, angled so that flows passing away from the transducer are red and the aliased ones are blue. This choice of angle here, as in the previous example, serves to

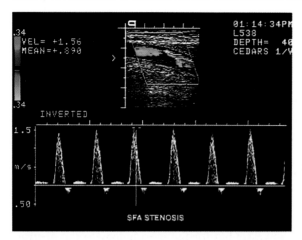

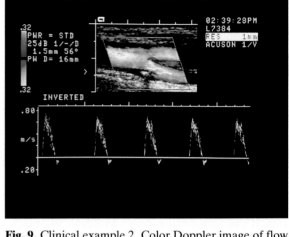

Fig. 7. Clinical example 1. Color Doppler image of flow through a vascular stenosis. Smoothly distributed flow is led into the stenosis where it accelerates and aliases on the color flow map. *Left*, color encoding bar. *Below*, spectral Doppler data

Fig. 9. Clinical example 2. Color Doppler image of flow in a femoral artery bifurcation.

Color figures are courtesy of Acuson Computed Sonography, Mountain View, CA

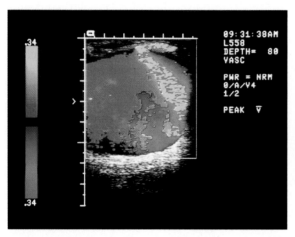

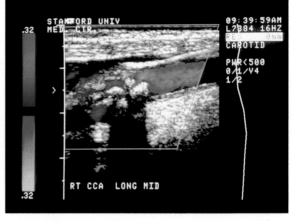

Fig. 10. Clinical example 3. Color Doppler image of superficial femoral artery pseudoaneurysm

Fig. 11. Clinical example 4. Color Doppler image of internal carotid artery lesion

maintain the convention of forward physiologic flow being red. Aliased or reversed flows are blue.

3. Figure 10 shows a color Doppler image of a superficial femoral artery pseudoaneurysm. Bulk flow toward the transducer is shown in red over most of the cross-section of the chamber. A mosaic jet is clearly detected on the right side of the image.

4. Figure 11 shows an internal carotid artery lesion. Smooth flow coded in red leads into the obstruction. Flow is characterized by a disturbed chaotic color pattern distal to the obstruction.

Summary

This chapter has described the principles of spectral and color Doppler flow mapping, with attention to limitations presented in the setting of vascular imaging. Individual instrument settings were discussed, as well as transducer configurations and accompanying imaging geometries. The usefulness of color Doppler imaging as a velocimetric tool was considered, with the conclusion that it remains for the time being an "imaging" modality, with little quantitative value. More technical sources of error resulting from acoustic impedance mismatch and spectral broadening effects were introduced. The chapter concluded with four clinical examples discussed in the context of principles presented in the chapter.

References

1. Kremkau FW (1990) Doppler ultrasound: principles and instruments. Saunders, Philadelphia.
2. Goldberg BB (1984) Abdominal ultrasonography. Wiley, New York.
3. Feigenbaum H (1986) Two-dimensional echocaradiography.
4. Bommer WJ, Miller L (1982) Real-time two-dimensional color flow Doppler: enhanced Doppler flow imaging in the diagnosis of cardiovascular disease. Am J Cardiol 49: 944 (abstract).
5. Lee R (1989) Physical priciples of flow mapping in cardiology. In: Nanda NC (ed) Textbook of color Doppler echocardiography. Lea and Febiger, Philadelphia.
6. Maslak SH, Freund JG (1991) Color Doppler instrumentation. In Lanzer P, Yoganathan AP (eds) Vascular imaging by color Doppler and magnetic resonance. Springer-Verlag Berlin.
7. Jones SA (1993) Fundamental sources of error and spectral broadening in Doppler ultrasound signals. CRC Critical Reviews in Biomedical Engineering 21: 399–483.

Cerebrovascular Ultrasonography

W. Steinke, W. Rautenberg, and M. Hennerici

Technology

A variety of noninvasive ultrasound techniques have been developed during recent years for the detection of both extracranial and intracranial arterial diseases [51, 59]. Continuous-wave (CW) and pulsed-wave (PW) Doppler sonography assess the hemodynamics according to the Doppler shift, whereas real-time B-mode sonography images tissue and vessel structures in a two-dimensional gray-scale display. These ultrasound techniques provide complementary information which can be used for the diagnosis of various stages of cerebrovascular diseases. In particular, since all these techniques are noninvasive, they have been used increasingly in studying the natural history of obstructive and dilatative atherosclerosis, transient and peristent disorders of the cerebral circulation due to vasospasm, and arteriovenous malformations [3, 59].

Combined B-mode and Doppler-mode technologies are used for subsequent or simultaneous imaging of both tissue and flow characteristics in cerebral vessels by means of duplex system or color-coded Doppler flow imaging (CDFI) [35, 50, 90, 128].

This chapter discusses the clinical applications of these methods with respect to the extra- and intracranial circulation.

Doppler Sonography

Both CW and PW Doppler methods are used for examining the intra- and extracranial brain-supplying arteries. Interpretation of the Doppler signals is based on analysis of the audio signals and the frequency spectrum.

Indirect tests marked the inital period of ultrasound evaluations in the study of cerebral circulation [89]. This periorbital method still provides useful and rapidly available information regarding the existence of collateral pathways. In the presence of severe stenosis or occlusion of the internal carotid artery retrograde blood supply from the external carotid artery via the ophthalmic anastomosis can be easily defected with CW Doppler (Fig. 1). With sufficient collateralization from the contralateral carotid or the vertebrobasilar systems orthograde perfusion of the ophthalmic artery is observed. However, this indirect test fails to detect even hemodynamically significant ipsilateral carotid obstructions in up to 20 % of patients. Thus, it should be understood that the detection of retrograde perfusion in the ophthalmic artery is a strong indicator of a severe pathology within the ipsilateral extracranial carotid system (good sensitivity). However, if the ophthalmic branches are normally perfused, even severe carotid stenosis or occlusion can not be excluded (poor specificity).

Direct tests of the carotid system in the neck are used to detect various degrees of obstruction. According to the distribution of abnormal blood flow patterns within, proximal to, or distal to a narrowed arterial segment, they provide information on the extent, site, and degree of lesions of more than 40 % lumen narrowing. In such lesions the sensitivity (92 %–100 %) and specificity (93–100 %) of various Doppler techniques have been shown to be similar to those of arteriography in large series studied [20, 59]. The reliability of the diagnosis of carotid artery plaques producing less than 40 % stenosis is considerably smaller. This is true for both the CW Doppler technique and the conventional PW Doppler analysis incorporated in duplex systems. Neither method can separate normal conditions from initial stages of atherosclerosis on the basis of hemodynamic measurements alone. Small plaques in the carotid artery producing less than 40 % lumen narrowing usually remain undetectable for hemodynamic tests such as Doppler sonography. Sometimes the audio signal in such cases is altered due to local turbulences, and spectral broadening may be de-

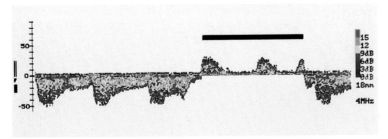

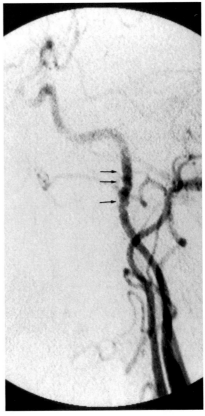

Fig. 1. Retrograde flow direction in the supratrochlear artery (branch of the ophthalmic artery). The flow signal is directed towards the probe and shows inversion during compression of branches of the external carotid artery (facial and superficial temporal arteries)

Fig. 2. Dopplersonography (**a**) and Angiography (**b**) of a distal ICA lesion (fibromuscular dysplasia) in a female patient. The Doppler examination was performed using a PW system and a submandibular approach. Recording depth was 51 mm. Note the low frequency signals indicating a significant stenosis

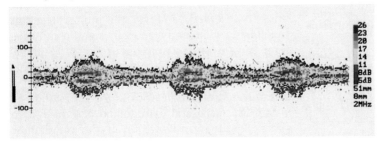

a   b

monstrated in spectrum analysis. For the detection of these small plaques, either simultaneous or complementary use of high-resolution B-mode imaging devices is necessary.

Low-frequency PW Doppler devices are used to assess the proximal supraaortic vessel segments [innominate artery, origin of common carotid artery (CCA) and vertebral arteries] by a supraclavicular approach [49]. This is also the method of choice in patients with *extracranial distal lesions of the internal carotid artery (ICA); e.g., carotid dissections, fibromuscular dysplasia, atypical atherosclerosis, aneurysms).* Adequate positioning of the probe in the submandibular region allows recording of flow velocity in the ICA up to the base of the skull (recording depth, 50–80 mm; Fig. 2).

Several stages of *carotid stenosis* are to be separated: (a) *Mild stenosis* (40–60%; Fig. 3a) is characterized by local increase of peak and mean flow velocities. Peak velocities range above 120 cm/s (4-MHz probe). (b) *Moderate stenosis* (60%–80%; Fig. 3b) shows a distortion of the normal pulsatile flow in addition to a local in-

crease of peak and mean frequencies. Peak systolic flow decelerations are found in the poststenotic segment. The peak velocity ranges from 120–240 cm/s. (c) *Severe stenosis* (more than 80%; Fig. 3c) produces markedly increased peak flow velocities exceeding 240 cm/s and occasionally reaching 500 cm/s. In addition, pre- and poststenotic spectra are dampened compared with the contralateral unaffected carotid artery. Retrograde flow direction of the ophthalmic artery may occur. (d) *Subtotal stenosis* (more than 95%; Fig. 3d) is characterized by a signal of variable, usually low frequencies, which decrease once a stenosis becomes pseudo-occlusive. This condition is difficult to separate from complete occlusion and may be misdiagnosed. *ICA occlusion* is characterized by the absence of any signal in the ICA, damped spectra of the CCA, and sometimes retrograde perfusion of the ophthalmic artery.

Fig. 3a–d. Doppler spectra and CDFI of different ▶ grades of ICA stenosis. **a** Mild stenosis. **b** Moderate stenosis. **c** Severe stenosis. **d** Subtotal stenosis

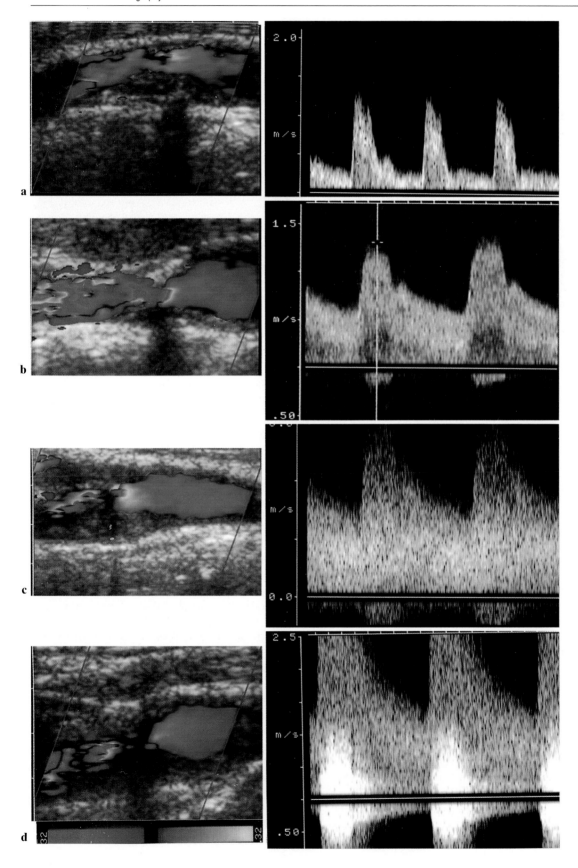

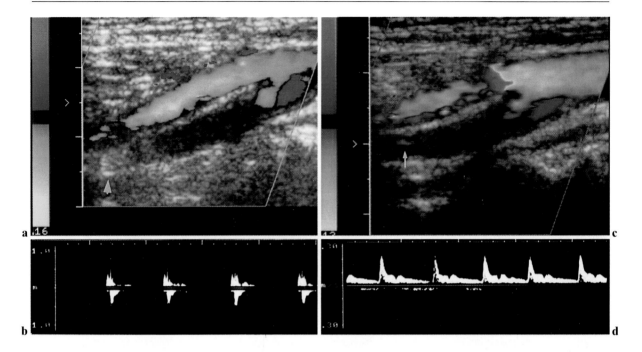

Fig. 4a–d. Internal carotid artery dissection. **a** Absent color-coded Doppler signals in the internal carotid artery with a tapering lumen and a pseudo-occlusion more distally (*arrow*). Flow reversal at the origin of the ICA (*blue*). **b** Typical high-resistance Doppler spectrum of acute ICA dissection with absent diastolic flow and low-flow bidirectional signal components. **c** A few *red* Doppler signals (*arrow*) and the B-mode echotomogram indicate beginning resolution of the pseudoocclusion 2 weeks later. **d** Reappearance of diastolic blood flow in the corresponding Doppler spectrum confirms partial resolution of the dissection

(e) In patients with *carotid dissection* (Fig. 4), a typical bi- or triphasic „to and fro" signal can be recorded, which may be traced from the bifurcation throughout the course of the ICA to the submandibular region. Severe intracranial obstructions within the carotid siphon or the middle cerebral artery (MCA) may lead to dampened spectra in the ipsilateral extracranial carotid artery. In addition, alterations of flow direction and signal frequency may occur in the ophthalmic artery depending on the site and degree of the lesion. (f) Intracranial arteriovenous malformations (AVM) and shunts may lead to increased flow velocities in the ipsilateral proximal vessel segments. Therefore, the presence of an intracranial AVM can sometimes be assumed from extracranial Doppler examinations.

Stenosis in the vertebral artery can be assessed directly if located at the origin or at the atlas loop (Fig. 5). The criteria for classifying the degree of the lesion are the same as those in the carotid system. Severe lesions in distal vessel segments or in intracranial segments and the basilar artery may lead to reduced flow velocities at locations where the vessel can be recorded. Without additional information from B-mode imaging about the vessel lumen size it is not possible to separate obstructive lesions from anatomical variations such as hypoplasia and deep cervical collateral pathways. The same is true for the differentiation between occlusion and aplasia. Since the vertebral artery can regularly be recorded only at two sites with the hand-held Doppler technique, the sensitivity and specificity for detecting vertrebral artery obstructions producing more than 50 % lumen narrowing are lower than those for similar processes in the carotid system [51]. The combination of CW Doppler techniques with high-resolution B-mode imaging and color Doppler flow imaging of the extra- and transcranial Doppler sonography for the intracranial segments of the vertebral and basilar arteries considerably increases the diagnostic accuracy in the vertebrobasilar circulation [31, 137].

In patients with severe lesions of the proximal *subclavian arteries* Doppler methods are excellent noninvasive tools for the detection of associated

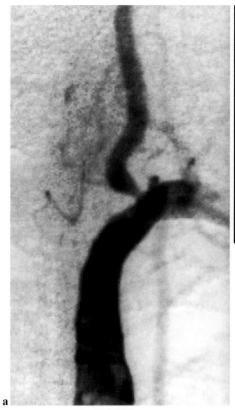
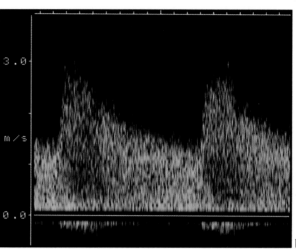

a

b

Fig. 5. Angiography (**a**) and Doppler spectrum (**b**) of a proximal stenosis of the vertebral artery

flow alterations in the vertebral arteries [55, 140]. Various stages of flow abnormalities can be distinguished in the mosly benign condition of the „*subclavian steal phenomenon*" (Fig. 6). Severe obstructions of the innominate artery lead to complex hemodynamic alterations within the ipsilateral carotid and vertebral arteries including reversed flow signals [103].

Advantages and Limitations

Freely hand-held Doppler methods are simple, inexpensive, and noninvasive. In experienced hands they provide reliable data about lesions producing more than 40 % lumen narrowing in the carotid system. Extracranial brain-supplying arteries are accessible, including the vertebral arteries. PW Doppler methods in principle provide similar results in the *intracranial* large arteries provided the Doppler sample volume is adequately positioned. Lesions of less than 40 % lumen narrowing cannot be reliably detected by Doppler sonography alone. These systems provide

no information concerning the morphology and surface of a plaque. The diagnostic accuracy in the vertebrobasilar system is more limited than in the carotid system. In severe stenotic lesions with very high flow velocities CW Doppler is superior to PW Doppler in adequately measuring the maximal frequency. The diagnostic accuracy of CW Doppler is considerably increased when used in combination with duplex methods.

Ultrasound Imaging

Sonographic imaging techniques such as conventional duplex scanning and color Doppler flow imaging (CDFI) have been established as routine methods for the evaluation of carotid and vertebral arterial disease. In some neurovascular laboratories duplex scanning is performed in selected patients after CW Doppler sonography, whereas in other centers duplex system analysis is directly used for the assessment of extracranial obstructive lesions. Doppler sonography provides relevant information about normal and pathological

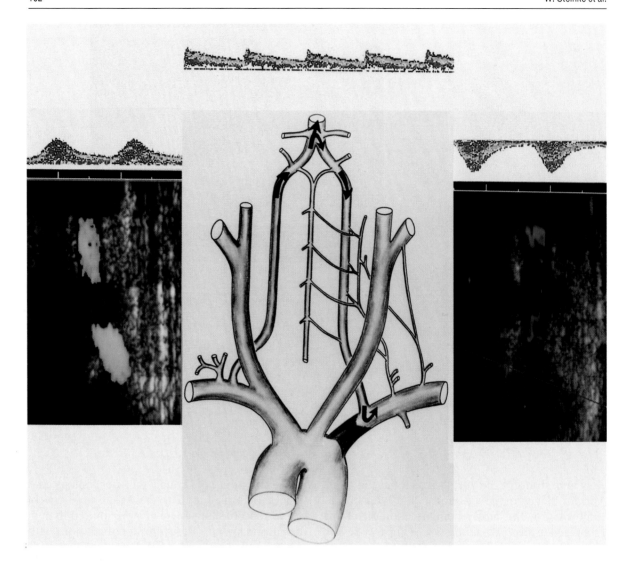

Fig. 6. Schematic drawing, Doppler spectra, and CDFI of a patient with a proximal obstruction of the left subcalvian artery and reversed flow signals (*blue*) in the ipsilateral vertebral artery (subclavian steal phenomenon). Orthograde flow direction is seen in the right vertebral artery (*red*) and in the basilar artery

application, and interpretation of B-mode echotomograms, PW Doppler spectra, and color-flow signals in various cerebrovascular conditions.

Instrumentation and Examination

intravascular hemodynamics [7, 51, 65, 67, 112–114, 146], while high-resolution B-mode imaging displays the morphologic features of arterial lesions in detail [38, 53, 54, 142]. CDFI preserves the advantages of conventional Doppler and duplex sonography and additionally visualizes color-coded blood flow patterns superimposed on a gray-scale echotomogram of the vascular structures [90, 91, 129]. In the following sections we describe the examination procedure, extracranial

The basic sonographic principles for high-resolution gray-scale echotomography, PW Doppler sonography and color-coded real-time display of Doppler signals from intravascular blood flow are discussed in in the standard literature. Since the extracranial carotid and vertebral arteries lie close to the skin surface, linear array transducers of conventional and color duplex instruments are commonly used at an ultrasound frequency of 7.5–10.0 MHz. These systems provide high-

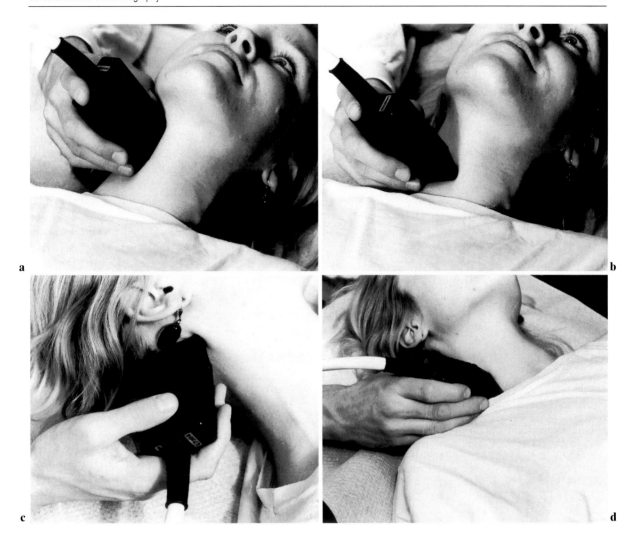

Fig. 7a–d. Transducer position for duplex examination of the extracranial arteries. Anterior-lateral insonation for a longitudinal (**a**) and cross-sectional (**b**) display of the carotid artery. Evaluation of the atlas loop (**c**) and the proximal segment (**d**) of the vertebral artery

resolution B-mode scans and a sufficient spatial and temporal resolution of the color-coded Doppler signals with the disadvantage of a relatively short insonation depth. The emission frequency of the integrated PW Doppler system ranges between 4 and 5 MHz.

The examination should be performed systematically with the patient in a supine position, the neck slightly hyperextended and rotated away from the transducer, which is positioned along the longitudinal axis of the carotid artery (Fig. 7). Alternatively, insonation from posterior-lateral,

behind the sternocleidomastoid muscle, may provide good visualization of the vessel, in particular of the anterior arterial wall.

1. Sequential longitudinal and cross-sectional gray-scale scans are displayed from the most proximal segment of the CCA to the bifurcation and along the ICA to the submandibular region (Fig. 8). Since the bifurcation cannot be visualized simultaneously with both branches in the majority of cases, the CCA is displayed together with either the ICA or the external carotid artery (ECA) in longitudinal sections. Structural vascular abnormalities are characterized according to their echomorphological features.

2. If color flow imaging is available, color-coded Doppler signals are then superimposed for the analysis of the: (a) temporal and spatial extent of

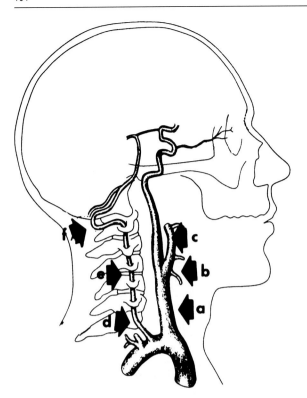

until the cervical vertebrae are displayed to visualize the intertransverse segments of the vertebral artery (Fig. 8, 10). Additional adjustment of the insonation angle is often necessary for adequate display of the vessel lumen and intravascular color-coded flow signals. The Doppler sample volume is positioned in the intertransverse segment to record the Doppler frequency spectrum. The vertebral artery is then followed in a proximal direction, and the pretransverse section below the sixth cervical vertebrum is traced to its ostium in the subclavian artery (Fig. 10), where another PW Doppler spectrum is recorded. Finally, the atlas loop of the vertebral artery is displayed with the probe positioned below the mastoid process and the insonation beam is directed toward the contralateral orbit (Figs. 7, 10).

Clinical Application

Carotid Artery

Normal Carotid Bifurcation

Since atherosclerosis in the carotid system is located predominantly at the bifurcation and the origin of the ICA, local hemodynamic patterns have been analyzed in experimental models and in ultrasound studies using conventional duplex scanning and, more recently, color Doppler flow imaging to identify patterns of hemodynamic and structural interactions relevant in atherogenesis [70, 73, 83, 91, 95, 101, 128, 143, 145]. The complexity of physiological flow separation, which is present in 94%–99% in normal carotid bifurcations, cannot be assessed satisfactorily by means of PW Doppler sonography; however, CDFI displays the distribution of separation zones and their changes during the cardiac cycle in real-time. In recent studies CDFI confirmed the results from in vitro studies that secondary flow occurs at the outer wall of the carotid sinus (Fig. 9). However, the temporal and spatial in vivo distribution of flow separation visualized by blue-coded Doppler signals is highly variable [91, 128]. It frequently occurs at the origin of the ECA as well, and in some cases secondary flow extends from the ICA into the ECA around the flow divider. Flow separation may be absent if smooth plaques fill the carotid sinus, or if there is no common or internal carotid bulb; on the other hand, secondary flow does not exclude small plaques in

Fig. 8. Systematic duplex examination of carotid and vertebral artery segments. Sequential scanning from the proximal common carotid artery (*a*) to the bifurcation (*b*) and the internal/external carotid arteries (*c*) to the submandibular region. Display of the ostium and pretransverse segment (*d*), the intertransverse segments (*e*), and the atlas loop of the vertebral artery (*f*)

physiological flow separation zones in the normal carotid bifurcation, (b) location and pattern of secondary vortices and turbulences adjacent to nonstenotic plaques, and (c) characterization of pre-, intra-, and poststenotic blood flow patterns. The surface structure and geometrical configuration of vascular lesions as well as the relative diameter and area reduction can be assessed from longitudinal and transverse sections.

3. The sample volume of the integrated PW Doppler system is placed in the CCA, ICA, and ECA to confirm vessel indentification according to the Doppler frequency spectrum (Fig. 9). From intrastenotic areas PW Doppler spectra are recorded for the quantitative classification of stenosis.

When the examination of the carotid artery is completed, the probe is shifted laterally from the CCA while maintaining a longitudinal position

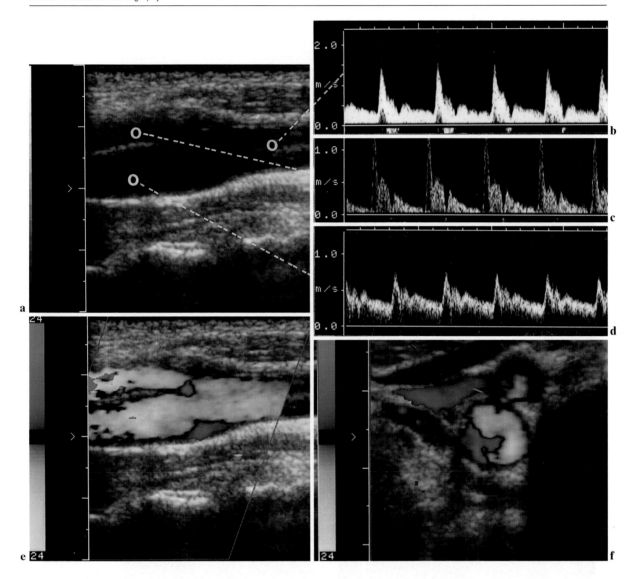

Fig. 9. a High-resolution B-mode echotomogram of a normal carotid bifurcation. **b–d** Doppler spectra of the common carotid artery (**b**), external carotid artery (**c**), and internal carotid artery (**d**). *Circles* indicate position of the PW Doppler sample volume. **e** Color Doppler flow imaging demonstrates small areas of physiological flow separation (*blue*) at the posterior wall of the carotid bulb and the flow divider. **f** Corresponding cross-section displays secondary flow at the outer wall of the ICA extending into the central lumen and a small area of reversed flow in the ECA

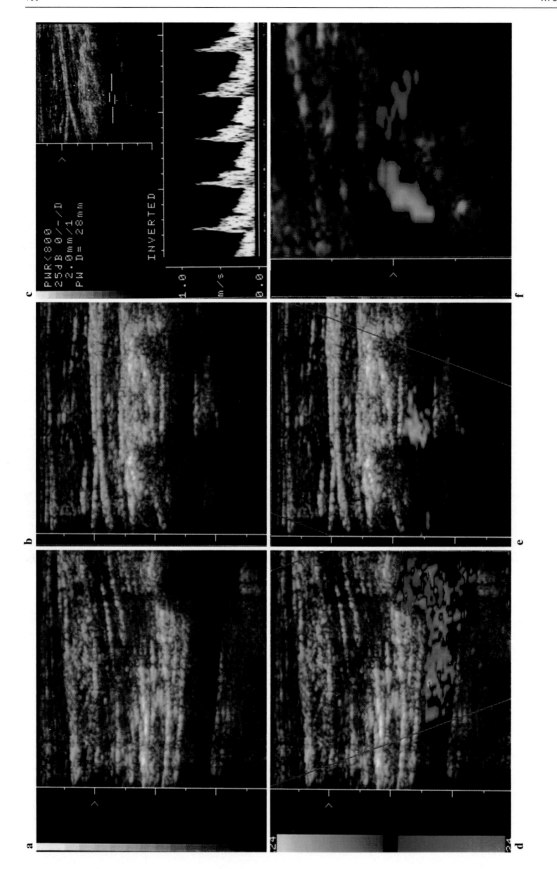

Fig. 10a–f. B-mode echotomograms of the origin of the vertebral artery and proximal pretansverse course (**a**) and the intertransverse segment (**b**). Typical Doppler spectrum (**c**) recorded from an intertransverse segment. Corresponding color Doppler flow imaging of the proximal (**d**), intertransverse segments (**e**), and atlas loop (**f**)

the carotid bifurcation. However, since the assessment of blood flow direction is still limited by CDFI, the three-dimensional complex hemodynamics cannot be analyzed adequately in detail.

Atherosclerotic Plaques

Small atherosclerotic plaques (luminal narrowing <40 %) may be suspected by Doppler sonography if broadening of the frequency spectrum is present, indicating abnormal blood flow components. However, since physiological flow separation and a variety of other hemodynamic variables may confound the interpretation of spectral broadening, ultrasonic imaging techniques are required to detect atherosclerotic lesions and assess plaque morphology. High-resolution B-mode scanning allows characterization of distinct echomorphological features of carotid plaques which correlate with different stages of the disease according to histopathological criteria [27, 38, 40, 54]. In addition, B-mode imaging has been used increasingly to assess changes of the intimal-medial thickness of the carotid artery with regard to vascular risk factors [61]. Using color-coded Doppler signals, which contrast the intravascular lumen, further improves assessment of the plaque surface and configuration [92, 128, 130].

Echogenicity. Plaques with homogeneous gray-scale echoes mainly consist of fibrotic tissue [38, 54]. These lesions are characteristic for the early stages of carotid atherosclerosis; however, they may also be found in hemodynamically relevant stenoses. Ulceration is rare in homogeneous plaques, and no significant correlation exists with the occurrence of focal cerebral ischemia. Heterogeneous lesions represent more advanced disease with deposition of atheromatous matrix, cholesterol accumulation, necrosis, calcification, and intraplaque hemorrhage [38, 54, 142]. Although echolucent areas within the plaque may represent thrombotic material or hemorrhage (Fig. 11), it has been recognized that lipid accumulation may produce similar echogenicity [15]. Many studies report an association between heterogeneous plaques and the occurrence of cerebrovascular events [14, 74, 97, 133]; however, conclusions have often been based on the pathogenetic concept from evaluating the morphology of carotid endarterectomy specimens which suggested a correlation of intraplaque hemorrhage and transient ischemic attacks and stroke [63, 64, 85]. More recent studies have not confirmed this hypothesis [10, 76, 77]. Both homogeneous and heterogenous echogenicity may be associated with acoustic shadowing due to calcification, which represents a major obstacle for adequate visualization of vascular structures in the B-mode echotomogram due to loss of echosignal intensity.

Surface Structure and Plaque Configuration. It is possible to assess smooth, irregular, and ulcerative plaques in the B-mode echotomogram, which has a reasonable sensitivity for the detection of ulcerations in postmortem carotid artery specimens [54]; however, in vivo accuracy in comparison with findings at carotid endarterectomy is markedly lower. In a recent study, both B-mode scanning and angiography had an unsatisfactory diagnostic yield for ulcerative plaques [27]. The quantiative assessment of the plaque size by B-mode imaging alone also had important limitations, as evaluated by Comerota et al. [26] and Zwiebel et al. [147], including a low interobserver reproducibility [108].

Limitations of B-mode echotomography in carotid artery disease may include:
- Assessment of the plaque configuration without sequential transverse and longitudinal cuts
- Detection and classification of stenosis without Doppler spectrum analysis
- Identification of ulcerations and echolucent plaque matrix
- Low inter- and intraobserver reliability
- Limited display of vascular structures due to (a) acoustic shadowing from plaque calcification, (b) high carotid bifurcation, and (c) tortuous vessels.

Color Doppler signals contrast the intravascular lumen, thus improving the visualization of the surface and configuration of vascular lesions. In particular, large echolucent components representing thrombotic material or plaque hemorrhage can be assessed more reliably (Fig. 11). The hemodynamic disturbance at nonstenotic carotid plaques is variable; however, blue-coded Doppler signals indicating turbulent and reversed blood flow are frequently found at surface irregularities surface and within the ulcer crater (Fig. 11). Analysis of the morphologic-hemodynamic interaction at atherosclerotic lesions has suggested that plaque progression is associated with local turbulence [52].

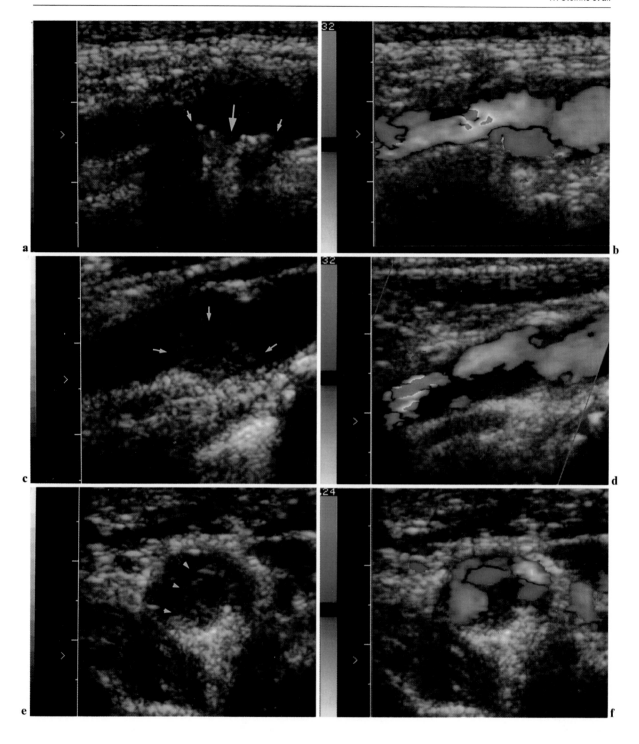

Fig. 11a–f. High-resolution B-mode echotomograms (*left*) and corresponding color Doppler flow imaging (*right*) of carotid plaques (*arrows*). **a** Heterogeneous, partially calcified plaque with a small central niche (*large arrow*). **b** Turbulence (*blue*) fills the ulcer crater. **c, e** Echolucent matrix at the posterior wall of the bifurcation in the longitudinal (**c**) and cross-sectional display at the level of the flow divider (**e**). **d, f** Color Doppler signals improve the assessment of echolucent material due to contrast of the intravascular lumen

Stenosis

The combination of B-mode echotomography and PW Doppler sonography in duplex instruments has considerably improved the accuracy of the noninvasive diagnosis and grading of carotid stenosis. The degree of stenosis is determined from distinct parameters of the Doppler frequency spectrum (Table 1, Fig. 3). Instead of Doppler shift frequencies equivalent flow velocity values can be used after correction of the Doppler insonation angle according to the flow direction in the vessel segment. In CDFI three sources of information are available for the classification of carotid stenosis: (a) the Doppler frequency spectrum, (b) characteristic color flow patterns, and (c) measurement of the residual vessel lumen (Fig. 12).

Doppler Frequency Spectrum. Compared with conventional duplex sonography the time-consuming search for optimal placement of the PW Doppler sample volume is facilitated in CDFI instruments [102]. The assessment of the Doppler spectrum is particularly important since it can be recorded frequently even when plaque calcification obscures adequate visualization of color flow patterns and the residual vessel lumen. Using distinct parameters determined from the Doppler spectrum such as the peak systolic frequency/velocity [113, 135, 146] (Table 1, Fig. 3),

Londrey et al. [84] reported a significantly higher agreement of angiography with CDFI than with standard duplex sonography (86.6 % vs. 79.6 %: p = 0.034).

Color Doppler Flow Patterns. Characteristic patterns of color Doppler signals are found in different categories of stenoses (Fig. 12). Using a prototype DCFI instrument, Hallam et al. [42] reported that a mosaic pattern indicating high blood flow velocity and mixed turbulence was consistently found in high-grade carotid stenosis. Another recent study used color-flow patterns as criteria for the classification of carotid stenosis [128]: (a) Low grade stenosis (40 %–60 %) was characterized by a relatively long segment of decreased color saturation with absent or minimal poststenotic turbulence. (b) In moderate stenosis (61 %–80 %), the decreased color saturation was more circumscribed, and blood flow velocity remained high during diastole. Poststenotic flow was turbulent, and reversal of flow occurred frequently (Fig. 12). (c) High-grade obstructions (81 %–90 %) had a short segment of maximal color fading or aliasing and severe poststenotic turbulence with blue-coded reversal of flow. In addition, pre- and poststenotic flow velocity was reduced compared with the contralateral unaffected carotid artery. For various degrees of stenoses the accuracy of CDFI compared with angiography ranged from 92 %–96 %.

Table 1. Criteria for the classification of ICA stenosis by PW Doppler sonography (4–5 MHz) and CDFI

Diameter stenosis	Color flow pattern	Doppler spectrum			
		Peak systolic		End diastolic	
		Frequency (kHz)	Velocity (cm/s)	Frequency (kHz)	Velocity (cm/s)
Low grade (40 %–60 %)	Color fading only in systole Long segment of color fading Minor turbulence	>4.0	>120	<1.3	<40
Medium grade (61 %–80 %)	Color fading Turbulence and reversed poststenotic flow component Increased flow in diastole	>4.0	>120	>1.3	>40
High grade (81 %–90 %)	Short segment of marked color fading or aliasing Severe poststenotic flow reversal and mixed turbulence (mosaic pattern) Decreased prestenotic flow in the CCA	>8.0	>240	>3.3	>100

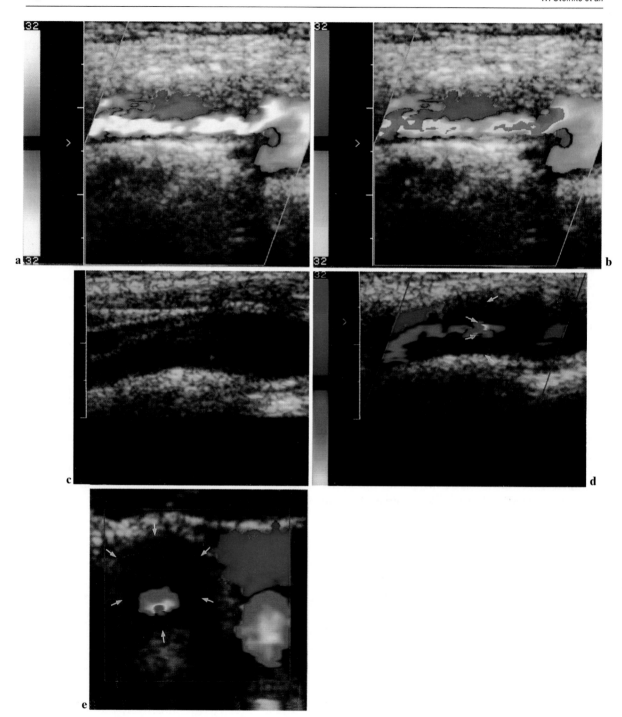

Fig. 12 a–e. Typical color flow pattern of a medium grade carotid stenosis with a segment of intrastenotic markedly increased flow velocity (jet flow), poststenotic turbulence and reversal of flow direction near the vessel wall (*blue*). Different scales of color coding for flow velocity using either varying degrees of saturation of *red* and *blue* (**a**) or a gradual transition from *red* to *yellow* and *blue* to *green*, respectively (**b**). **c** Difficult visualization of a high-grade echolucent carotid stenosis in the B-mode echotomogram. **d** Measurement of the „color flow lumen" in the longitudinal display demonstrates a 75 % diameter reduction. **e** Maximal intrastenotic area reduction in the corresponding cross-section is 88 %. *Arrows*, vessel wall

However, the semiquantitative analysis is limited by a certain variability of color-coded hemodynamic patterns due to variations of the plaque configuration and vessel geometry. Interpretation of blue-coded Doppler signals as turbulence or reversed flow as aliasing phenomenon may be difficult in some cases. In addition, the peak systolic frequency cannot be determined directly from the color-coded Doppler information since each color pixel represents the approximate mean Doppler frequency shift, which is lower than the peak frequency. This is particularly so if turbulence is present, which results in broadening of the Doppler frequency spectrum [22, 93].

Measurement of Residual Vessel Lumen. It has long been recognized that measurements of the residual vessel lumen in B-mode echotomograms have important methodological limitations [26, 108, 147]. The plaque configuration and relative obstruction can be assessed more reliably by CDFI using sequential longitudinal and transverse displays in which the intravascular surface is contrasted by color flow signals [35, 91, 128, 130]. Assuming a concentric stenosis the percentage area reduction in cross-sections is higher than the relative diameter reduction [5]. Erickson et al. [35] assessed the degree of stenosis from the relative reduction in the color flow lumen. They found agreement of CDFI with angiography for the degree of stenosis in 74 % of longitudinal and in 65 % of transverse measurements. In this study angiography underestimated the luminal narrowing in most cases of disagreement. In contrast, recent studies reported a good correlation of transverse lumen reduction on CDFI with diameter reduction on the corresponding angiograms of carotid stenosis [124, 130]. Comparison between CDFI and planimetry of carotid endarterectomy specimens for the assessment of cross-sectional area reduction revealed a high correlation [5].

Occlusion

The diagnosis of carotid occlusion by B-mode echotomography alone without Doppler sonography is not reliable since the residual vascular lumen frequently cannot be visualized adequately in complicated heterogeneous, partially calcified high-grade obstructions. In acute thrombotic occlusion, echolucent material fills the vascular lumen, which can hardly be differentiated on the

gray-scale from blood flow in a patent ICA (Fig. 13). CW Doppler and duplex sonography had a significantly higher accuracy for the diagnosis of ICA occlusion; however, the differentiation from a subtotal stenosis remained difficult. The PW Doppler spectrum and color Doppler signals in ICA occlusion typically demonstrate a marked reduction of the systolic and diastolic blood flow velocity in the CCA and an internalized ECA with high diastolic flow velocity indicating collateral supply via the ophthalmic artery. Color-coded intravascular Doppler signals are absent in the occluded ICA; however, blue-coded flow reversal in the residual stump at the bifurcation (stump flow) may occur (Fig. 13). The capacity of modern CDFI instruments to detect very slow blood flow velocities has markedly improved the sensitivity for the diagnosis of a subtotal ICA stenosis and pseudo-occlusion, which may represent candidates for vascular surgery.

CCA occlusion is a relatively rare condition which can be reliably diagnosed by conventional duplex sonography and color Doppler flow imaging [79, 144]. However, it is more difficult to assess the patency of the ICA distal to the CCA occlusion, the precondition for surgical intervention, and collateral flow from the ECA [11, 29, 110, 132] (Fig. 13). Typically, CDFI displays blue-coded signals in the ECA due to reversed flow direction and orthograde filling of the ICA in the absence of Doppler signals in the CCA.

Dissection

Recent studies have increasingly reported carotid dissection as a cause of transient or permanent ischemic neurological deficits, in particular in young patients [17, 127]. In the majority of cases ICA dissection occurs spontaneously after minor head or neck trauma leading to a typical neurological syndrome, which includes focal cerebral deficits, headache, neck pain, and ipsilateral Horner's syndrome. CW Doppler studies demonstrate a high-resistance Doppler signal with bidirectional signal components (Fig. 4), which can be traced along the course of the ICA in the neck [58]. B-mode scans are either unremarkable at the bifurcation or show a tapering lumen with occasional visualization of a floating intimal flap [30, 127, 134]. Marked blue-coded flow reversal at the origin of the ICA in systole and absent or minimal blood flow in diastole is a typical finding on

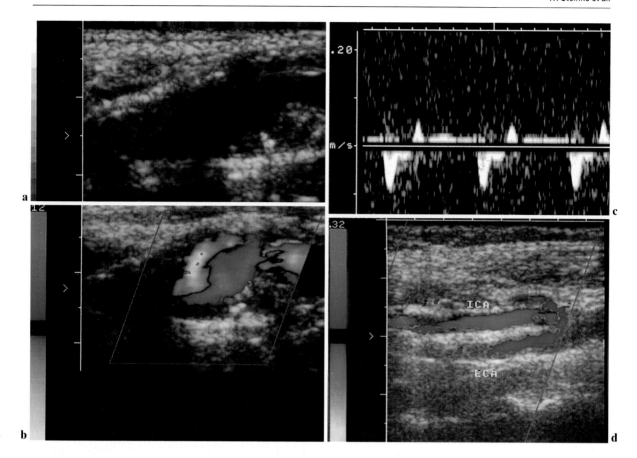

Fig. 13. a–c Internal carotid artery (ICA) occlusion. **a** Difficult visualization of the ICA occlusion due to echolucent thrombotic material; in addition, the B-mode echotomogram demonstrates a large smooth plaque in the carotid bifurcation. **b** Absent color Doppler signals confirm the ICA occlusion. Reversed blood flow is seen in the residual ICA stump (*blue*). **c** Typical biphasic Doppler spectrum with a predominant reversed signal component (stump flow). **d** Common carotid artery occlusion with patent ICA (*red*) supplied from the external carotid artery (ECA) with reversed flow direction (*blue*)

clavian artery, the proximal pretransverse course, and the short intertransverse segments between the third and sixth cervical vertebrae. Although PW Doppler criteria for vertebral artery stenosis have been defined in a few conventional duplex studies, detection and classification of stenosis and occlusion is more difficult than in the carotid system [4, 12, 28]. Intravascular color Doppler signals facilitate identification of the proximal segment and ostium, the predominant location of extracranial vertebral stenosis, as well as the atlas loop (Figs. 8, 10) [9, 137].

CDFI corresponding to the high-resistance bidirectional Doppler signal. Follow-up examinations demonstrate gradual normalization of the Doppler spectrum, indicating recanalization of the ICA within a few weeks to months in more than two-thirds of the patients [58, 127, 131].

Vertebral Artery

Examination of the vertebral artery by standard duplex scanning including analysis of PW Doppler spectra has been limited to the origin of the sub-

Normal Findings

The PW Doppler spectrum recorded routinely from an intertransverse segment of a normal vertebral artery demonstrates a high diastolic flow velocity and low pulsatility, indicating low vascular resistance in the territory of supply (Fig. 10). In a recent study of 42 healthy subjects the mean systolic peak velocity was 56 cm/s (range 19–98 cm/s), the mean diastolic flow velocity 17 cm/s (range

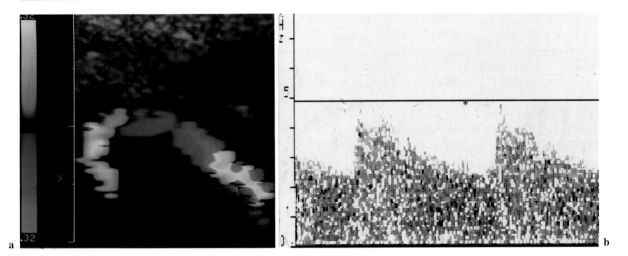

Fig. 14. a Low-grade vertebral artery stenosis proximal to the atlas loop indicated by a segment of marked color aliasing (*yellow*). **b** Systolic peak frequency of 5 KHz in the corresponding Doppler spectrum confirms the vertebral stenosis

6–30 cm/s), and the resistance index [1–(enddiastolic velocity/systolic peak velocity)] ranged from 0.62 to 0.75 [136]. Ackerstaff et al. [4] considered Doppler shift frequencies up to 4 Hz as normal regardless of the presence of spectral broadening.

Pathological Conditions

Hypoplasia. Based on pathoanatomical studies vertebral hypoplasia has been defined as a decrease in vascular lumen to below 2 mm [36]. This finding has been confirmed by results of a recent series using CDFI, which demonstrated a reduction in the systolic and diastolic flow velocities when the lumen of the vertebral artery is smaller than 2 mm [31]. Measurement of the vessel lumen is particularly important since proximal or distal obstructive disease may as well produce abnormal reduction of flow velocity or an intermediate Doppler spectrum, which is characterized by reversal of flow in early systole.

Stenosis and Occlusion. The predominant site of extracranial vertebral artery stenosis is the ostium of the subclavian artery. The atlas loop (Fig. 14) and the intracranial V4 segment are involved less frequently, and stenoses in the intertransverse segments are rare. A peak systolic frequency exceeding 4 kHz assessed by means of the integrated PW Doppler system indicates a relevant vertebral stenosis. Features of color-coded Doppler signals correspond to those of carotid stenosis: with increasing degree of luminal narrowing the segment of decreased color saturation becomes more circumscribed, and turbulence as well as poststenotic reversal of flow are more severe. Hemodynamically significant obstructions of the intracranial vertebral artery produce a high-resistance Doppler waveform with the resistivity index exceeding 0.80 [136]. However, the Doppler spectrum may be normal if flow to the ipsilateral posterior inferior cerebellar artery is preserved. In acute proximal vertebral artery occlusion PW Doppler spectra cannot be recorded, and color Doppler signals are absent in the pre- and intertransverse segments; however, the vascular lumen can frequently be visualized, thus allowing differentiation from vertebral hypoplasia. In some patients with proximal occlusion collaterals to the atlas loop from the ECA and other small cervical arteries may preserve blood flow in the distal vertebral segment, which can be assessed by Doppler sonography and CDFI [137].

Dissection. Dissection of the vertebral artery is one of the most important causes for brainstem strokes in young patients [23, 45]. According to several recent case series the neurological presentation is typically characterized by neck pain, occipital headache, and symptoms of brainstem or cerebellar ischemia in almost 90%, producing a permanent deficit in the majority of patients [41, 68, 94, 120]. Angiography has been the keystone for the diagnosis of vertebral dissection; however, in cases with complete occlusion diagnosis could be confirmed only by demonstrating complete or partial resolution on the follow-up angiogram [41, 120]. Recently, the diagnostic significance of axial magnetic resonance imaging has been emphasized [21]; however, the role of sonographic methods in this condition has not been clearly defined.

Initial Doppler results are more variable than in ICA dissection [130]. In a series of 12 patients with vertebral artery dissection we recorded a high-resistance PW Doppler spectrum in only 33 %, complete occlusion in 25 %, and normal flow velocity in 25 %. Doppler sonography indicated local stenosis in 16 %. In contrast, Hoffmann et al. [60] reported a high-resistance signal in six of ten vertebral dissections. Recanalization occurs in the majority of cases, which can be monitored by Doppler sonography. Structural abnormalities on the B-mode echotomogram are rare, and to date the diagnostic significance of CDFI in this condition has not been established.

Subclavian Steal Phenomenon. Hemodynamically relevant obstructions of the subclavian artery produce abnormal Doppler spectra and color-coded flow patterns in the ipsilateral vertebral artery such as blue-coded retrograde flow. Deflation of a blood pressure cuff on the ipsilateral arm causes an immediately increase in retrograde blood flow velocity in the vertebral artery indicative of a subclavian steal phenomenon. Since both the vertebral artery and vein run side by side within the transverse foramina blue-coded Doppler signals in the vein must be distinguished from reversed arterial blood flow in this situation (Fig. 6). An intermediate flow pattern similar to that seen in hypoplastic vertebral arteries may also be found in normal vertebral arteries distal to a hemodynamically relevant subclavian artery obstruction. Inflation of the blood pressure cuff usually makes the systolic drop disappear, while it is more prominent immediately after deflation.

Advantages and Limitations of CDFI

CDFI has the following advantages for the assessment of extracranial arterial disease compared with standard duplex sonography:
- Preserved capacity of conventional duplex sonography
- Improved orientation and identification of vascular structures
- Faster data acquisition, shorter examination time
- Improved display of: (a) plaque surface, (b) ulcerative lesions, (c) echolucent plaque matrix, and (d) plaque extent
- Analysis of the morphological-hemodynamic interaction in view of: (a) atherogenesis in the normal carotid bifurcation, (b) origin of cerebral embolism, (c) progression of carotid atherosclerosis, and (d) recurrent stenosis after endarterectomy
- Improved diagnosis of: (a) kinking, coiling, and aneurysm of the carotid artery, (b) carotid dissection, (c) carotid body tumor, and (d) vertebral artery hypoplasia, stenosis, and occlusion.

Since the area of maximal blood flow velocity is indicated by color signals, placement of the PW Doppler sample volume is more reliable, which leads to an increased reproducibility of the classification of carotid stenosis [102]. In addition, assessment of the plaque surface morphology and configuration as well as measurement of the residual vascular lumen in transverse and longitudinal sections of stenoses is improved due to the intravascular contrast by color signals.

Some potential limitations of CDFI for the assessment of extracranial arterial disease are evident. These include the following:
- Interpretation of blue-coded Doppler signals as: (a) flow direction towards the insonation plane, (b) reversed flow components, (c) turbulence, and (d) aliasing phenomenon
- Limited spatial and temporal resolution of color signals
- Suboptimal gray-scale resolution
- Coding of mean instead of maximal flow velocity

Plaque calcification, particularly in severe stenosis, may not only obscure the B-mode echotomogram of vascular structures and plaque morphology but also extinguish the color flow signals. Similar to conventional duplex sonography high location of the carotid bifurcation, deep location of the vessels, and the transducer configuration contributed to 11 % technically unsatisfactory examinations in another study [128]. Furthermore, since it is difficult to analyze the spatial and temporal extension of complex flow dynamics form serial two-dimensional tomograms, the display of vascular structures and hemodynamics in three or four dimensions (e.g., time) remains a challenge for the future.

Transcranial Doppler Sonography

High-energy bidirectional pulsed Doppler and duplex sonography for the noninvasive recording of blood flow conditions from intracranial arteries and veins at the base of the skull operate at low frequencies (1–2 MHz) (Fig. 15). Identification of intracranial vessels depends critically on the examination of flow direction, depth control of the Doppler sample volume, and position of the probe in respect to the bone windows (Table 2). Three different approaches may be used: the transtemporal, the transorbital, and the transnuchal.

Normal values of flow velocities of the basal cerebral arteries are given in Table 3. Velocities of intracranial vessels vary with age, hematocrit

[18], end-tidal CO_2 partial pressure, and other parameters. The examiner should be aware of these variables and use a standardized examination procedure [39]. He should also be familiar with the documentation and interpretation of the study. Delegation of the test is not recommended because a correct interpretation of the data usually requires knowledge of the clinical setting and extracranial hemodynamic pecularities. The same applies to decisions regarding the extension or restriction of the basic examination protocol; with increasing complexity of the intracranial hemodynamics it may be necessary to add various functional tests, for example, compression tests. Compression of the CCA may sometimes be used to identify the recorded vessel and to examine the collateral circulation within the circle of Willis.

Table 2. TCD criteria for the identification of basal intracranial vessels using the transtemporal, transorbital, and nuchal approaches

Vessel	Probe	Depth (mm)	Flow direction
Transtemporal approach			
MCA	Medial	30– 65	Towards probe
ACA	Medial	55– 80	Away from probe
ICA	Caudal	55– 75	Towards probe
PCA, P1	Posterior	55– 80	Towards probe
PCA, P2	Posterior	55– 75	Away from probe
Transorbital approach			
Ophthalmic artery		30– 60	Towards probe
ICA, C4, 5		60– 80	Towards probe
ICA, C2, 3		60– 80	Away from probe
Nuchal approach			
Vertebral artery		50–100	Away from probe
Basilar artery		75–120	Away from probe

MCA, middle cerebral artery; ACA, anterior cerebral artery; PCA, posterior cerebral artery; ICA, internal carotoid artery.

Table 3. Normal values of TCD examination: aggregated mean values and standard deviations in normal persons (from [2, 8, 19, 20, 44, 57, 80])

Vessel	Peak velocity (cm/s)	Mean velocity (cm/s)	Enddiastolic velocity (cm/s)
MCA ($n=291$)	89 ± 17.6	60 ± 11.25	42 ± 8.3
ACA ($n=201$)	73 ± 16.7	50 ± 12.4	34 ± 8.5
PCA ($n=201$)	55 ± 12.8	37 ± 9.4	27 ± 6.5
VA/BA ($n=201$)	57 ± 13.8	35 ± 10.25	28 ± 7.5

VA, vertebral artery; BA, basilar artery.

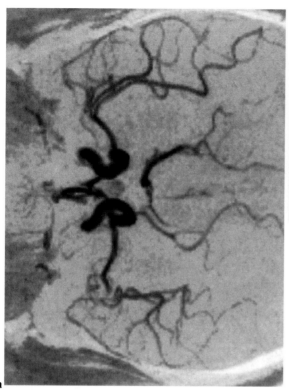

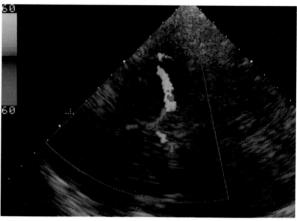

Fig. 15. Magnetic resonance angiography (**a**) and corresponding transcranial CDFI (**b**)

Appropriate safety conditions are to be recognized; a duplex scan of the CCA should be performed prior to compression to exclude plaques or stenosis. Compression should be limited to a few seconds and should be performed in the region of the proximal CCA; the carotid bulb should be avoided. In general, knowledge of the extracranial noninvasive studies is essential to perform the transcrancial Doppler study appropriately and to assure correct interpretation of the results.

Stenosis and Occlusion

As with extracranial arterial disease, the narrowing of intracranial arteries produces flow abnormalities such as local increase in mean and peak flow velocities, the appearance of slow flow signals and reversed flow phenomena in the presence of turbulences, and reduction of pre- or poststenotic flow velocities [56, 81, 125]. The combination of these phenomena depends on the degree of obstruction and allows an estimate of the degree of stenosis in the anterior intracranial circulation (Fig. 16). Whereas stenosis of already

50% lumen narrowing can be reliably detected in arterial segments in line with the ultrasound beam axis such as the M1 segment of the middle cerebral artery (MCA) and the P1 segment of the posterior cerebral artery (PCA; Table 4), stenosis in

Table 4. Detection of intracranial stenoses by TCD in 467 patients investigated prior to selective intra-arterial angiography

	MCA	ICA	PCA	VA	BA
Right positive	24	21	10	19	9
Right negative	438	445	455	442	453
False positive	3	–	–	1	–
False negative	2	1	2	5	5
Sensitivity (%)	92	91	83	79	64
Specificity (%)	99	100	100	99	100
Test accuracy (%)	99	100	100	99	99
Positive predictive value (%)	89	100	100	99	100
Negative predictive value (%)	99	100	99	98	99

ICA, Carotid siphon; VA, vertebral artery; BA, basilar artery.

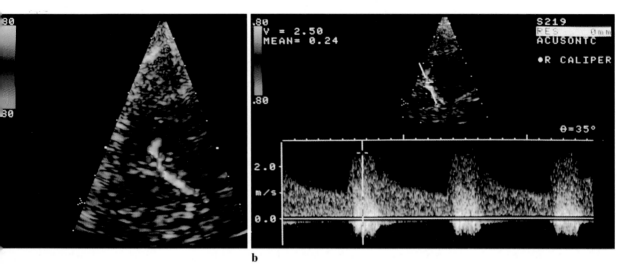

b

Fig. 16. Transcranial CDFI (**a**) and Doppler spectra (**b**) of a patient with a severe stenosis of the M1 segment of the left MCA as documented by intra-arterial digital subtraction angiography and magnetic resonance angiography. Peak flow velocity is 250 cm/s

perpendicular segments such as the distal MCA branches and the communicating arteries are more difficult to evaluate. With increasing obstruction, the delineation of its degree is facilitated with the combination of transcranial Doppler sonography (TCD) and magnetic resonance angiography; this technique seems superior to conventional angiography for the demonstration and quantification of intracranial stenosis [115]. Ongoing research in this area seems to favor TCS and magnetic resonance imaging if standardized parameters are used for validation of obstructive lesions; the difficulty of relating new criteria for stenosis to pathoanatomical specimen is self-evident and represents a major challenge for future investigations [116].

The logical difficulty of reliably documenting occlusion of the M1 segment consists in the absence of any detectable signal – a prerequisite is the differentiation of signals from neighboring vessels [e.g., anterior cerebral artery (ACA) and PCA] to separate conditions of high ultrasound attenuation and poor echo window insonation. In the case of MCA occlusion, dampened spectra in segments proximal to the occlusion are frequently found; reversed flow direction in distal MCA branches and abnormally elevated ipsilateral ACA flow velocities may be present [88].

TCD results in the vertebral-basilar circulation are less reliable than in the anterior circulation due to anatomical variance; the junction of the basilar artery is more difficult to define by TCD criteria alone, and the entire course of the basilar artery can be investigated in 30 % of patients only at great distance from the ultrasound probe resulting in poor signal to noise ratio [96]. Similar to TCD within the anterior circulation, partial obstructions are displayed more easily than total occlusion: stenosis of the distal vertebral and basilar arteries can be diagnosed with a sensitivity of 79 % and 64 % and a specificity of 99 % and 100 %, respectively; however, the sensitivity for the detection of occlusion is 36 % for the basilar artery [59]. This is of major clinical importance in patients suspected of suffering from acute thrombosis of the basilar artery. We believe that the combination of magnetic resonance and TCD techniques represents the highest available standard in noninvasive diagnostics [116].

Vasospasm in Subarachnoid Hemorrhage

TCD has already been used for a decade in the detection, quantification, and follow-up of vasospasms after subarachnoid hemorrhage (SAH) [3, 44, 122]. Initial reports claimed that this method mirrors the degree of obstruction commonly demonstrated in the angiogram of stroke prone patients after SAH. Striking pitfalls however, have questioned, a simple focal arterial lumen narrowing as the cause of Doppler flow pattern alterations similar to that known from atherosclerosis. In subarachnoid vasospasm the pathophysiology is more complex; elevated intracranial pressure may cause an increase in vasomotor resistance of capillary and arteriolar vessels and hence dampen the Doppler flow velocity in proximal major arteries. This may result in a false-negative Doppler result despite angiographically demonstrable vasospasm. On the other hand, local blood flow turbulences may be found despite a normal appearance of the angiogram if peripheral vasomotor dysregulation and large vessel vasoconstriction occur subsequent to SAH. In addition, TCD findings are greatly influenced by changing therapeutic concepts such as the standard calcium channel blocker application in patients with SAH; only 28 % of these patients have a significant increase in flow velocities prior to the onset of delayed ischemic stroke, which could also indicate that an arterial vasospasm distal to the insonated proximal segment is responsible for the final event [75]. Another important limitation of TCD in patients with SAH is the restriction to the territory of the MCA because of the rather poor diagnostic accuracy in the ACA territory, a frequent site of aneurysms [78].

Intracranial Collateralization of Significant Extracranial Lesions

TCD allows noninvasive assessment of the intracranial circulation in the presence of stenosis or occlusion of the extracranial cerebral arteries.

TCD criteria for collateral channels are as follows:

Anterior communicating artery
– Retrograde flow direction in the ipsilateral ACA
– Increased peak and mean velocities in both ACAs
– Increased velocities and low frequency signals in the midline (75–85 mm), anterior communicating artery functional stenosis
– Decrease of MCA velocity during contralateral CCA compression

Posterior communicating artery
– Increased velocities in the ipsilateral PCA (P1)
– Increased velocities in the basilar artery
– Low-frequency signals in the region of the posterior communicating artery (60–70 mm depth)

Leptomeningeal anastomosis
– Increased velocities in proximal and distal vessel segments (e.g., PCA – P1 and P2), partly retrograde flow signals in distal vessel segments (e.g., retrograde flow direction in distal MCA branches)

Ophthalmic collateral
– Retrograde flow direction of the ophthalmic artery.

Flow velocities in the MCA distal to significant stenosis and occlusion vary with regard to the efficacy of the intracranial collateralization. In addition, they sometimes correlate with clinical features: Schneider et al. [118] described reduced MCA velocities and pulsatility index values ipsilateral to a symptomatic carotid occlusion whereas Rautenberg et al. [104] reported normal peak and mean velocities in asymptomatic patients indicating adequate collateralization. Both observations have encouraged further studies to test the hemodynamic reserve capacities within the circle of Willis with regard to the individual prognosis in oligo- and asymptomatic patients with extracranial arterial disease: for example, CO_2 test was used to assess the intracranial reserve capacity [138]. In combination with TCD, this test addresses vasomotor regulation directly. Based on dilation or constriction of small cerebral arterioles – similar but not identical with mechanisms involved in cerebral autoregulation, – the CO_2 test assesses the reactivity of the peripheral arterioles to changing pCO_2 levels. Hypercapnea, artificially induced by administration of CO_2 in the air, leads to vasodilation and reduced vasomotor resistance in the peripheral arteriolar bed with subsequently increased blood flow velocities in the proximal large arteries of the affected vascular territories. If the diameter of these large vessels remains constant at least for some time [62] or is less affected than smaller arteries by changing concentration of CO_2 in blood, the relative changes in blood flow velocities may mirror cerebral tissue perfusion. A major limitation of the diagnostic significance of this test derives from the adaptation of vessel caliber changes to alternating pCO_2 levels [37] and the large variability of compensatory networks and perfusion territories by overlapping microcirculatory systems. In addition, the efficacy of major vessel collateral pathways outside the area of examination may be important (e.g., leptomeningeal anastomosis). Although this method has also been used by several authors to assess the intracranial reserve capacity in patients with significant extracranial disease [13, 111, 141] results of these studies thus far, have been discouraging. At present in patients with extracranial arterial disease, the clinical validity of the CO_2 test for the prediction of the individual prognosis remains obscure.

Whereas extracranial Doppler techniques allow noninvasive diagnosis and follow-up of carotid dissections [58], TCD enables assessment of the intracranial hemodynamics and its changes during follow-up [69]. Sequential TCD recordings are helpful in detecting delayed hemodynamic changes of the intracranial circulation when extracranial reperfusion has already occurred. Recanalization of carotid dissection is a frequent finding during follow-up, however, persisting intracranial collateral pathways and persistence of hemodynamic distal obstructions may indicate the need for further treatment in these patients with increased risk for cerebral ischemia.

Noninvasive assessment of blood flow alterations within the basilar artery in patients with subclavian steal phenomena of the vertebral arteries is another important diagnostic option. In the majority of patients who present with an oligosymptomatic or asymptomatic subclavian steal phenomenon, flow direction of the basilar artery is orthograde, but about one-third of patients have intermediate stages of flow. Retrograde flow direction of the basilar arteries is rare (3%) and usually occurs only in patients with multivessel extracranial arterial disease or severe abnormalities within the circle of Willis [55, 71]. About 40% of patients with subclavian steal phenomenon show minor alterations of flow velocity in the basilar artery during hyperemia of the ipsilateral arm. Whether the findings can be used to sustain the decision between surgical and medical treatment deserves further investigations in an appropriate prospective trial.

In patients with obstructions of the *innominate artery* TCD shows complex intracranial hemodynamic alterations. Abnormal flow patterns in these patients are characterized by a damped signal spectrum during early systole, associated with a soft whispering audio signal, which is due mainly to delayed peak blood flow velocity. Latent steal phenomena can be demonstrated in various intracranial vessels during postischemic hyperemia of the upper extremities. In patients with innominate artery obstructive disease this steal phenomenon seems to be frequently associated with the occurrence of symptoms [103].

Dolichoectatic Arteries

In patients with intracranial dolichoectatic arteries such as the megadolicho-basilar artery significantly reduced peak and mean velocities can be recorded by TCD. This is of clinical importance because in combination with computed tomography or magnetic resonance imaging TCD offers completely noninvasive diagnosis of such an anomaly [106]. A considerable number of patients with intracranial dolichoectatic arteries suffers from transient ischemic attack or stroke [121]. The dramatic reduction in flow velocities which can often be observed in these patients suggests a thromboembolic cause of these ischemic events in slow flow territories.

Arteriovenous Malformations, Fistulas

TCD allows a noninvasive insight into the hemodynamic aspects of intracranial AVMs [82, 119]. Due to the low peripheral resistance proximal segments of feeding vessel show high peak and mean velocities with a low pulsatility index. Feeding vessels can be identified by the lack of CO_2 reactivity. A linear relationship between mean velocity, diameter of feeder, and volume of AVM has been reported [46]. Pulsatile flow can be observed in draining veins. Transcranial color-coded duplex sonography allows selective recordings of small vessel segments within the AVM if the malformation can be investigated directly. TCD is particularly useful in the follow-up of patients with and without treatment (e.g., surgery, radiation) and as a monitoring tool during therapeutic intravascular embolization [99]. TCD provides useful information about the changes of velocity in the feeding vessels during intravascular occlusive procedures to guide the interventional radiologist. In patients with carotid-cavernous sinus fistulas TCD can detect abnormal velocity patterns including high velocities and low frequency signals in the region of the shunt.

Intracranial Pressure

Simultaneous measurements of systemic blood pressure, intracranial pressure as monitored by epidural devices, and Doppler signals of the basal cerebral arteries have shown that a progressive reduction in diastolic and systolic velocities can be found with increasing intracranial pressure. Various patterns of flow alterations have been demonstrated in different regions of the brain, indicating the existence of varying pressure gradients inside the skull [47]. If the intracranial pressure is greater than the diastolic blood pressure, Doppler signals of the basal cerebral arteries are severely altered. Mild or moderate increase in intracranial pressure can be compensated by an increase in the systemic blood pressure; in this situation TCD findings remain normal.

Brain Death

In brain-dead patients three different patterns of flow alterations have been reported [48]: oscillating flow, systolic spikes, and zero flow. Zero flow is difficult to interpret and may be misleading because insufficient echo windows cannot be excluded if sequential examinations are not available. It has been shown that TCD can be used to confirm brain death with a sensitivity of 91.3 % and a specificity of 100 % [100]. Typical TCD signals suggestive of brain death should be detectable in more than one vessel. These results indicate that TCD is a valid bedside noninvasive method to confirm the diagnosis of brain death. Appropriate guidelines for performance and interpretation should be taken into account [139].

Monitoring

The recording of flow velocities in intracranial arteries enables the monitoring of circulatory changes during major surgery, interventional neuroradiological procedures, and in the intensive care unit. Due to its excellent time resolution, TCD is an ideal tool for rapid detection of changes of the intracranial circulation.

TCD has been used in carotid endarterectomy to monitor MCA velocity during ipsilateral ICA clamping [49]. Since the majority of patients show only a minor decrease in MCA velocity during the clamping phase, and few present with postoperative neurological deficits, TCD results should be intrepreted with caution [43, 49, 66, 117, 118]. These findings suggest that shunting during carotid surgery should be performed on a selective basis according to monitoring results. In a large retrospective study severe reduction in MCA velocity during carotid clamping was found in only 7.2 % of patients [43]. The effect of carotid clamping and the need for shunting can also be assessed preoperatively using a carotid compression test during recording of ipsilateral MCA flow velocity.

High-intensity transcranial signals (HITS) suggestive of microembolism have been detected by TCD monitoring during angiography and open heart and carotid surgery [98, 105, 109, 126]. At present the clinical relevance of these TCD findings during surgery or angiography is unclear [49, 66, 87].

TCD monitoring has also been used to detect spontaneous HITS in patients with transient ischemic attack or stroke [123], with heart valve prosthesis and with intracranial arterial disease [32]. Results reported so far concerning the frequency of detection of HITS suggestive of microemboli from the heart or the proximal arteries to the intracranial circulation, however, are controversial [107]. In patients with heart valve prosthesis thousands of clinically silent events can be recorded whereas in patients with symptomatic carotid stenoses HITS are rare events. At present it is unclear whether it will be possible to differentiate between different pathological cerebral embolic materials [86], and whether the appearence of HITS is associated with an increased risk of functional or morphological brain damage.

TCD examination of the basal intracranial vessels during intravenous contrast injection can be used for the detection of right-to-left shunts (e.g., patent foramen ovale) by documentation of microbubbles reaching the brain (Fig. 17, [25, 33]). Monitoring of cerebral hemodynamics during orthostatic maneuvers allows noninvasive assessment of autonomic functions which is useful in patients with autonomic neuropathy, autonomic failure and pandysautonomia. In these patients abnormal decreases in flow velocities within basal cerebral arteries can be detected during orthostatic stress (Fig. 18). Routine measurements of intracranial flow velocities during orthostatic stress may be of value in patients with syncope and ortostatic dysregulation.

Functional Investigations

Assessment of changes of blood velocity during neuronal activation by mental activity or light exposure have been reported [1, 34]. These findings show that TCD is able to detect changes in blood

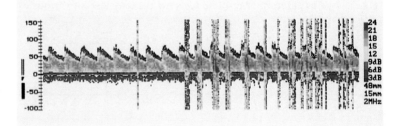

Fig. 17. Multiple micro-bubbles appearing in the right MCA of a patient after intravenous injection of a contrast agent containing air bubbles indicative for a right-left shunt

flow during activation of distinct brain areas. In patients with migraine with or without aura blood flow changes induced by neuronal coupling with variable visual stimuli have been found to be significantly higher than in controls (Ries et al., in preparation). Thus visual stimulation can be used as a diagnostic test.

Transcranial Color Doppler Flow Imaging

Transcranial CDFI may image the basal cerebral arteries [16]. In the case of sufficient echo windows orientation and identification of distinct vessel segments are easier and better than with the nonimaging method. At present no reliable data concerning the failure rate in adults in a large group of patients are available. In our own experience the failure rate is higher, and the examination time is longer than with the nonimaging method. However, particularly in complex situations the visualization of vessel segments is extremely helpful and pathological conditions such as AVMs can easily be imaged. Furthermore, transcranial CDFI allows correction for the angle of insonation when determining blood flow velocities. Whether the diagnostic accuracy for the detection of occlusive intracranial arterial disease of transcranial CDFI is superior to blind TCD remains to be seen in the future.

Advantages and Limitations

TCD is a simple bedside method for recording of flow velocities in basal intracranial arteries. It can be repeated due to excellent time resolution and monitoring of intracranial circulation can easily be performed. In experienced hands intracranial occlusive disease can be diagnosed reliably in the anterior circulation. Assessment of intracranial hemodynamics in patients with severe extracranial arterial disease is possible [6, 24].

Due to insufficient echo windows not all patients can be investigated. In about 5 % of patients predominantly elderly women (20 %) only insufficient signals can be recorded from intracranial vessels due to ossification. Because of numerous anatomical variations the diagnostic value in the posterior circulation is limited. The method depends critically on the skill of the examiner. The combination of TCD and magnetic resonance angiography has shown to increase the diagnostic accuracy, and the use of functional tests provides insight into a variety of diseases such as migraine and syncope. In any case one must keep in mind that not blood flow volume but blood velocity is measured by TCD [72].

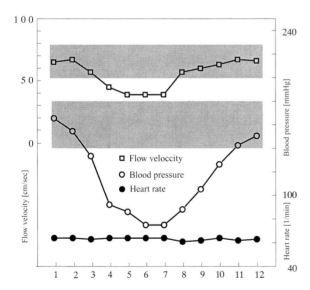

Fig. 18. Polygraphic registration of cerebral blood velocity, mean blood pressure, and heart rate in a patient with syncope. Marked decrease in cerebral blood flow velocity and blood pressure during orthostatic stress

Table 5. Use of different ultrasound tests for the diagnosis of various extra- and intracranial vascular diseases

	Carotid lesions					
	Small plaques	Fresh thrombus, ulcer	Stenosis	Occlusion	Dissection	Dilation
Hand-held						
CW Doppler	–	–	++	++	++	–
PW Doppler	–	–	+	+	+	–
Duplex						
B-Mode	++	+	+	–	–	++
+ PW Mode	++	+	++	+	+	++
+ Color Mode	++	++	++	++	++	++

Diagnostic significance: –, none; (+), limited: +, reasonable; ++, excellent

Table 6. Use of different ultrasound tests for the diagnosis of various extra- and intracranial vascular diseases

	Supra-aortic submandibular lesions	Vertebral lesions			Intracranial processes			
		Stenosis	Occlusion	Steal	Vaso-spasms, collaterals	Raised pressure	HITS	Neuro-vascular dysfunction
Hand-held								
CW Doppler	–	+	(+)	++	–	–	–	–
PW Doppler	+	+	+	++	++	++	++	++
Duplex								
+ PW Mode	(+)	(+)	(+)	(+)	–	–	–	–
+ Color Mode	+	+	+	+	+	–	–	–
Monitoring	–	–	–	–	++	+	++	–
Echocontrast	–	–	–	–	–	–	++	–
Functional	–	–	–	+	–	–	–	++

Diagnostic significanes: –, none; (+), limited; +, reasonable; ++, excellent.

Conclusions

Cerebrovascular ultrasonography has improved continuously since its introduction. Today a variety of different ultrasound techniques are available for noninvasive examination of the brain-supplying extra- and intracranial arteries. The diagnostic value of the different methods for frequent clinical indications is shown in Tables 5 and 6. The highest diagnostic accuracy can be obtained by combining different methods according to the indiviual patient problem.

References

1. Aaslid R (1987) Visually evoked dynamic blood flow response of the human cerebral circulation. Stroke 17: 771–775
2. Aaslid R, Markwalder TM, Nornes H (1982) Non-invasive transcranial Doppler ultrasound recording of flow velocity in basal cerebral arteries. J Neurosurg 57: 769–774
3. Aaslid R, Huber P, Nornes H (1984) Evaluation of cerebrovascular spasm with transcranial Doppler ultrasound. J Neurosurg 60: 37–41
4. Ackerstaff RGA, Hoeneveld H, Slowikowski JM, Moll FL, Eikelboom BC, Ludwig JW (1984) Ultrasonic duplex scanning in atherosclerotic disease of the innominate, subclavian and vertebral arteries. A comparative study with angiography. Ultrasound Med Biol 10: 409–418
5. Alexandrov AV, Bladin CF, Magissano R, Norris JR (1993) Measuring carotid stenosis. Stroke 24: 1292–1296

6. American Academy of Neurology, Therapeutics and Technology Assessment Subcommitee (1990) Assessment: transcranial Doppler. Neurology 40: 680–681

7. Arbeille P, Lapierre F, Patat F, Benhamou AC, Alison D, Dusorbier CH, Pourcelot L (1984) Evaluation du degre des stenoses carotidiennes par l'analyse spectrale du signal Doppler. Arch Mal Coeur 77: 1097–1107

8. Arnolds BJ, von Reutern GM (1987) Transcranial Doppler sonography. Examination technique and normal reference values. Ultrasound Med Biol 12: 115–123

9. Bartels E (1992) Farbkodierte Dopplersonographie der Vertebralarterien. Vergleich mit der konventionellen Duplexsonographie. Ultraschall Med 13: 59–66

10. Bassiouny HS, Davis H, Massawa N, Gewertz BL, Glagov S, Zarins CK (1989) Critical carotid stenoses: morphologic and chemical similarity between symptomatic and asymptomatic plaques. J Vasc Surg 9: 202–212

11. Belkin M, Mackey WC, Pessin MS, Caplan LR, O'Donnell TF (1993) Common carotid artery occlusion with patent internal and external carotid arteries: diagnosis and surgical management. J Vasc Surg 17: 1019–1028

12. Bendick PJ, Jackson VP (1986) Evaluation of the vertebral arteries with duplex sonography. J Vasc Surg 3: 523–530

13. Bishop CCR, Powell S, Insall M, Rutt D, Browse NL (1986) Effect of internal carotid artery occlusion on middle cerebral artery blood flow at rest and in response to hypercapnea. Lancet I: 710–712

14. Bluth EI, Kay D, Merritt CRB, Sullivan M, Farr G, Mills NL et al (1986) Sonographic characterization of carotid plaque: detection of hemorrhage. AJR 146: 1061–1065

15. Bock RW, Lusby RJ (1992) Carotid plaque morphology and interpretation of the echolucent lesion. In: Labs KH, Jäger KA, Fitzgerald DE, Woodcock JP, Neuerburg-Heusler D (eds) Diagnostic vascular imaging. Arnold, London, pp 225–236

16. Bogdahn U, Becker G, Winckler J, Greiner K, Perez J, Meurers B (1990) Transcranial color-coded real-time sonography in adults. Stroke 21: 1680–1688

17. Bogousslavsky J, Regli F (1987) Ischemic stroke in adults younger than 30 years of age. Cause and prognosis. Arch Neurol 44: 479–482

18. Brass LM, Pavlakis SG, De Vivo D, Piomelli S, Mohr JP (1989) Transcranial Doppler measurements of the middle cerebral artery. Effect of hematocrit. Stroke 19: 1466–1469

19. Büdingen HJ, Staudacher T (1987) Die Identifizierung der Arteria basilaris mit der transkraniellen Dopplersonographie. Ultraschall 8: 95–101

20. Büdingen HJ, von Reutern GM (1994) Ultraschalldiagnostik der hirnversorgenden Arterien. Thieme, Stuttgart

21. Bui LN, Brant-Zawadzki M, Verghese P, Gillan G (1993) Magnetic resonance angiography of cervicocranial dissection. Stroke 24: 126–131

22. Cape EG, Sung HW, Yoganathan AP (1991) Basics of color Doppler imaging. In: Lanzer P, Yoganathan AP (eds) Vascular imaging by color Doppler and magnetic resonance. Springer, Berlin Heidelberg New York, pp 73–86

23. Caplan LR, Zarins CK, Hemmatti M (1985) Spontaneous dissection of the extracranial vertebral arteries. Stroke 16: 1030–1038

24. Caplan LR, Brass LM, DeWitt LD, Adams RJ, Gomez C, Otis S, Wechsler LR, von Reutern G-M (1990) Transcranial ultrasound: present status. Neurology 40: 696–700

25. Chimowitz MI, Nemec JJ, Marwick TH, Lorig RJ, Furlan AJ, Salcedo EE (1991) Transcranial Doppler ultrasound identifies patients with right-to-left cardiac or pulmonary shunts. Neurology 41: 1902–1904

26. Comerota AJ, Cranley JJ, Cook SE (1981) Real-time B-mode imaging in diagnosis of cerebrovascular disease. Surgery 89: 718–729

27. Comerota AJ, Katz ML, White JV, Grosh JD (1990) The preoperative diagnosis of the ulcerated carotid atheroma. J Vasc Surg 11: 505–510

28. Davis PC, Nilsen B, Braun IF, Hoffmann JC Jr (1986) A prospective comparison of duplex sonography vs angiography of the vertebral arteries. AJNR 7: 1059–1064

29. Dashefsky SM, Cooperberg PL, Harrison PB, Reid JDS, Araki DN (1991) Total occlusion of the common carotid artery with patent internal carotid artery. J Ultrasound Med 10: 417–421

30. De Bray JM, Dubas F, Joseph PA, Causeret H, Pasquier JP, Emile J (1989) Etude ultrasonique de 22 dissections carotidiennes. Rev Neurol 145: 702–709

31. Delcker A, Diener HC (1992) Die verschiedenen Ultraschallmethoden zur Untersuchung der Arteria vertebralis — eine vergleichende Wertung. Ultraschall Med 13: 213–220

32. Diehl RR, Sliwka U, Rautenberg W, Schwartz A (1993) Evidence for embolization from a posterior cerebral artery thrombus by transcranial Doppler monitoring. Stroke 24: 606–608

33. Di Tullio M, Sacco RL, Venketasubramanian N, Sherman D, Mohr JP, Homma S (1993) Comparison of diagnostic techniques for the detection of a patent foramen ovale in stroke patients. Stroke 24: 1020–1024

34. Droste DW, Harders AG, Rastogi E (1989) A transcranial Doppler study of blood flow velocity in the middle cerebral arteries performed at rest and during mental activites. Stroke 20: 1005–1011

35. Erickson SJ, Mewissen MW, Foley WD, Lawson TL, Middleton WD, Quiroz FA et al (1989) Stenosis of the internal carotid artery: assessment using color Doppler imaging compared with angiography. AJR 152: 1299–1305

36. Fisher CM, Gore I, Okabe N, White PD (1965) Atherosclerosis of the carotid and vertebral arteries — extracranial and intracranial. J Neuropathol Exp Neurol 24: 455–476

37. Fujii K, Heistad D, Faraci FM (1991) Flow mediated dilation of the basilar artery in vivo. Circ Res 69: 697–705

38. Goes E, Janssens W, Maillet B, Freson M, Steyaert L, Osteaux M (1990) Tissue characterization of atheromatous plaques: correlation between ultrasound image and histological findings. J Clin Ultrasound 18: 611–617

39. Gomez CR, Brass LM, Tegeler CH, Babikian VL, Sloan MA, Feldmann E, Wechsler LR (1993) The transcranial Doppler standardization project. J Neuroimag 3: 190–192

40. Gray-Weale AC, Graham JC, Burnett JR, Byrne K, Lusby RJ (1988) Carotid artery atheroma: comparison of preoperative B-mode ultrasound appearance with carotid endarterectomy specimen pathology. J Cardiovasc Surg 29: 676–681

41. Greselle JF, Zenteno M, Kien P, Castel JP, Caille JM (1987) Spontaneous dissection of the vertebrobasilar system. J Neuroradiol 14: 115–123

42. Hallam MJ, Reid JM, Cooperberg PL (1988) Colorflow Doppler and conventional duplex scanning of the carotid bifurcation: prospective, double-blind, correlative study. AJR 152: 1101–1105

43. Halsey JH (1993) Risks and benefits of shunting in carotid endarterectomy. Stroke 23: 1583–1587

44. Harders A (1986) Neurosurgical applications of transcranial Doppler sonography. Springer, Vienna New York

45. Hart RG (1988) Vertebral artery dissection. Neurology 38: 987–989

46. Hassler W (1986) Hemodynamic aspects of cerebral angiomas. Springer, Vienna New York

47. Hassler W, Steinmetz H, Gawlowski J (1988) Transcranial Doppler ultrasonography in raised intracranial pressure and in intracranial circulatory arrest. J Neurosurg 68: 745–751

48. Hassler W, Steinmetz H, Pirschel J (1989) Transcranial Doppler study of intracranial circulatory arrest. J Neurosurg 71: 195–201

49. Hennerici M (1993) Can carotid endarterectomy be improved by neurovascular monitoring? Stroke 24: 637–638

50. Hennerici M, Freund HJ (1984) Efficacy of CW-Doppler and duplex-system examinations for the evaluation of extracranial carotid disease. J Clin Ultrasound 12: 155–161

51. Hennerici M, Neuerburg-Heusler D (1994) Gefäßdiagnostik mit Ultraschall. Thieme, Stuttgart

52. Hennerici M, Steinke W (1989) Untersuchungen zur Entwicklung extrakranieller Karotisplaques mit der farbkodierten Duplexsonographie. In: Kessler C (ed) Plättchenfunktion und Gefäßwand. TM, Hameln, pp 207–215

53. Hennerici M, Steinke W (1991) Carotid plaque developments: aspects of hemodynamic and vessel wall-platelet interaction. Cerebrovasc Dis 1: 142–148

54. Hennerici M, Reifschneider G, Trockel U, Aulich A (1984) Detection of early atherosclerotic lesions by duplex scanning of the carotid artery. J Clin Ultrasound 12: 455–464

55. Hennerici M, Klemm C, Rautenberg W (1988) The subclavian steal phenomenon: a common vascular disorder with rare neurologic deficits. Neurology 38: 669–673

56. Hennerici M, Rautenberg W, Schwartz A (1987) Transcranial Doppler ultrasound for the assessment of intracranial arterial flow velocity. II. Evaluation of intracranial arterial disease. Surg Neurol 27: 523–532

57. Hennerici M, Rautenberg W, Sitzer G, Schwartz A (1987) Transcranial Doppler ultrasound for the assessment of intracranial arterial flow velocity. I. Examination technique and normal values. Surg Neurol 27: 439–448

58. Hennerici M, Steinke W, Rautenberg W (1989) High-resistance Doppler flow pattern in extracranial carotid dissection. Arch Neurol 46: 670–672

59. Hennerici M, Mohr JP, Rautenberg W, Steinke W (1992) Ultrasound imaging and Doppler sonography in the diagnosis of cerebrovascular diseases. In: Barnett HJM, Mohr JP, Stein BM, Yatsu F (eds) Stroke. Churchill Livingstone, New York, pp 241–268

60. Hoffmann M, Sacco RL, Chan S, Mohr JP (1993) Noninvasive detection of vertebral artery dissection. Stroke 24: 815–819

61. Howard G, Sharrett R, Heiss G, Evans GW, Chambless LE, Riley WA, Burke GL (1993) Carotid artery intimal-medial thickness distribution in general populations as evaluated by B-mode ultrasound. Stroke 24: 1297–1304

62. Huber P, Handa J (1967) Effect of contrast material, hypercapnea, hyperventilation, hypotonic glucose and papaverine on the diameter of cerebral arteries. Invest Radiol 2: 17–32

63. Imparato AM, Riles TS, Gostein F (1979) The carotid bifurcation plaque: pathologic findings associated with cerebral ischemia. Stroke 10: 238–245

64. Imparato AM, Riles TS, Mintzer R, Baumann FG (1983) The importance of hemorrhage in the relationship between gross morphologic characteristics and cerebral symptoms in 376 carotid artery plaques. Ann Surg 197: 195–203

65. Jacobs NM, Grant EG, Schellinger D, Byrd MC, Richardson JD, Cohan SL (1985) Duplex carotid sonography: criteria for stenosis, accuracy, and pitfalls. Radiology 154: 385–391

66. Jansen C, Vriens EM, Eickelboom BC, Vermeulen FEE, van Gijn J, Ackerstaff RGA (1993) Carotid endarterectomy with transcranial Doppler and electroencephalographic monitoring: a prospective study in 130 operations. Stroke 24: 665–669

67. Johnston KW, Baker WH, Burnham SJ, Hayes AC, Kupper AC, Poole MA (1986) Quantitative analysis of continuous-wave Doppler spectral broadening for the diagnosis of carotid disease: results of a multicenter study. J Vasc Surg 4: 493–504

68. Josien E (1992) Extracranial vertebral artery dissection: nine cases. J Neurol 239: 327–330

69. Kaps M, Dorndorf W, Damian MS, Agnoli L (1990) Intracranial haemodynamics in patients with spontaneous carotid dissection. Eur Arch Psychiatr Neurol Sci 239: 246–256

70. Kerber CW, Heilman CB (1992) Flow dynamics in the human carotid artery. I. Preliminary observa-

tions using a transparent elastic model. AJNR 13: 173–180

71. Klingelhöfer J, Conrad B, Benecke R, Frank B (1989) Transcranial Doppler ultrasonography of carotid-basilar collateral circulation in subclavian steal. Stroke 19: 1036–1042

72. Kontos HA (1989) Validity of cerebral arterial blood flow calculations from velocity measurements. Stroke 20: 1–3

73. Ku DN, Giddens DP, Phillips DJ, Strandness DE Jr (1985) Hemodynamics of the normal carotid bifurcation: in vitro and in vivo studies. Ultrasound Med Biol 11: 13–26

74. Langsfeld M, Gray-Weale AC, Lusby RJ (1989) The role of plaque morphology and diameter reduction in the development of new symtoms in asymptomatic carotid arteries. J Vasc Surg 9: 548–557

75. Laumer R, Steinmeier R, Gönner F, Vogtmann T, Priem R, Fahlbusch R (1993) Cerebral hemodynamics in subarachnoid hemorrhage evaluated by transcranial Doppler sonography. I. Neurosurgery 31: 1–9

76. Leen EJ, Feeley TM, Colgan MP, O'Malley MK, Moore DJ, Hourihane DOB, Shanik GD (1990) „Haemorhagic" carotid plaque does not contain haemorrhage. Eur J Vasc Surg 4: 123–128

77. Lennihan L, Kupsky WJ, Mohr JP, Hauser A, Correll JW, Quest D (1987) Lack of association between carotid plaque hematoma and ischemic cerebral symptoms. Stroke 18: 879–881

78. Lennihan L, Petty G, Fink E, Solomon R, Mohr JP (1993) Transcranial Doppler detection of anterior cerebral vasospasm. J Neurol Neurosurg Psychiatry 56: 906–909

79. Levine SR, Welch KMA (1989) Common carotid artery occlusion. Neurology 39: 178–186

80. Lindegaard K-F, Bakke SJ, Grolimund P, Aaslid R, Huber P, Nornes H (1985) Assessment of intracranial hemodynamics in carotid artery disease by transcranial Doppler ultrasound. J Neurosurg 63: 890–898

81. Lindegaard K-F, Bakke SJ, Aaslid R, Nornes H (1986a) Doppler diagnosis of intracranial arterial occlusive disorders. J Neurol Neurosurg Psychiatr 49: 510–518

82. Lindegaard KF, Grolimund P, Aaslid R, Nornes H (1986b) Evaluation of cerebral AVM's using transcranial Doppler ultrasound. J Neurosurg 65: 335–344

83. LoGerfo FW, Nowak MD, Quist WC (1985) Structural details of boundary layer separation in a model human carotid bifurcation under steady and pulsatile flow conditions. J Vasc Surg 2: 263–269

84. Londrey GL, Spadone DP, Hodgson KJ, Ramsey DE, Barkmeier LD, Sumner DS (1991) Does color-flow imaging improve the accuracy of duplex carotid evaluation? J Vasc Surg 13: 659–662

85. Lusby RJ, Ferrell LD, Ehrenfeld WK, Stoney RJ, Wylie EJ (1982) Carotid plaque hemorrhage. Its role in production of cerebral ischemia. Arch Surg 117: 1479–1488

86. Markus HS, Brown MM (1993) Differentation between different pathological cerebral embolic ma-

terials using transcranial Doppler in an in vitro model. Stroke 24: 1–5

87. Markus H, Loh A, Israel D, Buckenham T, Clifton A, Brown MM (1993) Microscopic air embolism during cerebral angiography and strategies for avoidance. Lancet 341: 784–787

88. Mattle H, Grolimund P, Huber P, Sturzenegger M, Zurbrügg HR (1988) Transcranial Doppler sonographic findings in middle cerebral artery disease. Arch Neurol 45: 289–295

89. Melis-Kisman E, Mol JMF (1970) L'application de l'effet Doppler à l'exploration cérébrovasculaire—Rapport préliminaire. Rev Neurol 122: 470–472

90. Merritt CRB (1987) Doppler color flow imaging. J Clin Ultrasound 15: 591–597

91. Middleton WD, Foley WD, Lawson TL (1988a) Flow reversal in the normal carotid bifurcation: color Doppler flow imaging analysis. Radiology 167: 207–209

92. Middleton WD, Foley WD, Lawson TL (1988b) Color-flow Doppler imaging of carotid artery abnormalities. AJR 150: 419–425

93. Mitchell DG (1990) Color Doppler imaging: principles, limitations, and artifacts. Radiology 177: 1–10

94. Mokri B, Houser OW, Sandok BA, Piepgras DG (1988) Spontaneous dissections of the vertebral arteries. Neurology 38: 880–885

95. Motomiya M, Karino T (1984) Flow patterns in the human carotid artery bifurcation. Stroke 15: 50–56

96. Mull M, Aulich A, Hennerici M (1990) Transcranial Doppler ultrasonography versus arteriography for assessment of the vertebrosbasilar circulation. J Clin Ultrasound 18: 539–549

97. O'Donnell TF, Erdoes L, Mackey WC, McCullough J, Shepard A, Heggerick P et al (1985) Correlation of B-mode ultrasound imaging and arteriography with pathologic findings a carotid endarterectomy. Arch Surg 120: 443–449

98. Padayachee TS, Gosling RG, Bishop CC, Beurnand K, Browse NL (1986) Monitoring MCA blood velocity during carotid endarterectomy. Br J Surg 73: 98–100

99. Petty GW, Massaro AR, Tatemichi TK, Mohr JP, Hilal SK, Stein BM, Salomon RA, Duterte DI, Sacco RL (1990a) Transcranial Doppler ultrasonographic changes after treatment for arteriovenous malformations. Stroke 21: 260–266

100. Petty GW, Mohr D, Pedley TA, Tatemichi TK, Lennihan L, Duterte DI, Sacco RL (1990b) The role of transcranial Doppler in confirming brain death: sensitivity, specificity and suggestions for performance and interpretation. Neurology 40: 300–303

101. Phillipps DJ, Greene FM, Langlois Y Jr, Roederer O, Strandness DE Jr (1983) Flow velocity patterns in the carotid bifurcations of young, presumend normal subjects. Ultrasound Med Biol 9: 39–49

102. Polak JF, Dobkin GR, O'Leary DH, Wang AM, Cutler SS (1989) Internal carotid artery stenosis: accuracy and reproducibility of color-Doppler-assisted duplex imaging. Radiology 73: 793–798

103. Rautenberg W, Hennerici M (1988) Pulsed Doppler assessment of innominate artery obstructive disease. Stroke 19: 1514–1520

104. Rautenberg W, Hennerici M (1991) Intracranial hemodynamic measurements in patients with severe asymptomatic extracranial carotid disease. Cerebrovasc Dis 1: 216–222

105. Rautenberg W, Schwartz A, Hennerici M (1987) Transkranielle Dopplersonographie während der zerebralen Angiographie. In: Widder B (ed) Transkranielle Dopplersonographie bei zerebrovaskulären Erkrankungen. Springer, Berlin Heidelberg New York, pp 144–148

106. Rautenberg W, Aulich A, Röther J, Wentz KU, Hennerici M (1992) Stroke and dolichoectatic intracranial arteries. Neurol Res 14: S 201–203

107. Rautenberg W, Ries S, Bäzner H, Hennerici M (1993) Emboli detection by TCD monitoring. Can J Neurol Sci 20 (S4): 138 (abstract)

108. Ricotta JJ, Bryan FA, Bond MG, Kurtz A, O'Leary DH, Raines JK et al (1987) Multicenter validation study of real-time (B-mode) ultrasound, arteriography, and pathologic examination. J Vasc Surg 6: 512–520

109. Ries F, Eicke M (1987) Auswirkungen der extrakorporalen Zirkulation auf die intrazerebrale Hämodynmik — Erklärung postoperativer neuropsychiatrischer Komplikationen. In: Widder B (ed) Transkranielle Doppler-Sonographie bei zerebrovaskulären Erkrankungen. Springer, Berlin Heidelberg New York, pp 100–103

110. Riles TS, Imparato AM, Posner MP, Eikelboom BC (1984) Common carotid occlusion. Ann Surg 199: 363–366

111. Ringelstein EB, Sievers C, Ecker S, Schneider PA, Otis SM (1988) Noninvasive assessment of CO_2 induced cerebral vasomotor response in normal individuals and patients with internal carotid artery occlusions. Stroke 19: 963–969

112. Rittgers SE, Thornhill BM, Barnes RW (1983) Quantitative analysis of carotid artery Doppler spectral waveforms: diagnostic value of parameters. Ultrasound Med Biol 9: 255–264

113. Robinson ML, Sacks D, Perlmutter GS, Marinelli DL (1988) Diagnostic criteria for carotid duplex sonography. AJR 151: 1045–1049

114. Roederer GO, Langlois YE, Jager KA, Primozich JF, Beach KW, Phillips DJ, Strandness DE Jr (1984) The natural history of carotid arterial disease in asymptomatic patients with cervical bruits. Stroke 15: 605–613

115. Röther J, Wentz KU, Rautenberg W, Schwartz A, Hennerici M (1993a) Magnetic resonance angiography in vertebrobasilar ischemia. Stroke 24: 1310–1315

116. Röther J, Schwartz A, Rautenberg W, Wentz KU, Hennerici M (1993b) Middle cerebral artery assessment by magnetic resonance angiography and transcranial Doppler. Neurology 45: A414–415

117. Sandmann W, Kolvenbach R, Willeke F (1993) Risks and benefits of shunting in carotid endarterectomy. Stroke 24: 1098 (letter)

118. Schneider PA, Rossman ME, Torem S, Otis SM, Dilley RB, Bernstein EF (1988) Transcranial Doppler in the management of extracranial cerebrovascular disease: implications in diagnosis and monitoring. J Vasc Surg 7: 223–231

119. Schwartz A, Hennerici M (1986) Non-invasive transcranial Doppler ultrasound in intracranial angiomas. Neurology 36: 626–635

120. Schwartz A, Mull M, Aulich A (1991) Vertebral artery dissection proved by follow-up. Neuroradiology 33 [Suppl]: 440–442

121. Schwartz A, Rautenberg W, Hennerici M (1993) Dolichoectatic intracranial arteries: review of selected aspects. Cerebrovasc Dis 3: 273–279

122. Seiler RW, Grolimund P, Aaslid R, Huber P, Nornes H (1986) Cerebral vasospasm evaluated by transcranial ultrasound correlated with clinical grade and CT-visualized subarachnoid hemmorrhage. J Neurosurg 64: 594–600

123. Siebler M, Sitzer M, Steinmetz H (1992) Detection of intracranial emboli in patients with symptomatic extracranial carotid artery disease. Stroke 23: 1652–1654

124. Sitzer M, Fürst G, Fischer H, Siebler M, Fehlings T, Kleinschmidt A, Kahn T, Steinmetz H (1993) Between-method correlations in quantifying internal carotid stenosis. Stroke 24: 1513–1518

125. Spencer M, Whisler D (1986) Transorbital Doppler diagnosis of intracranial arterial stenosis. Stroke 17: 916–921

126. Spencer MP, Thomas GI, Nicholls SC, Sauvage LR (1990) Detection of middle cerebral artery emboli during carotid endarterectomy using transcranial Doppler ultrasonography. Stroke 21: 415–423

127. Steinke W, Aulich A, Hennerici M (1989) Diagnose und Verlauf von Carotisdissektionen. DMW 114: 1869–1875

128. Steinke W, Kloetzsch C, Hennerici M (1990a) Variability of flow patterns in the normal carotid bifurcation. Atherosclerosis 84: 121–127

129. Steinke W, Kloetzsch C, Hennerici M (1990b) Carotid artery disease assessed by color Doppler flow imaging. AJNR 11: 259–266

130. Steinke W, Hennerici M, Rautenberg W, Mohr JP (1992a) Symptomatic and asymptomatic high-grade carotid stenoses in Doppler color flow imaging. Neurology 42: 131–137

131. Steinke W, Rautenberg W, Schwartz A, Sliwka U, Hennerici M (1992b) Ultrasonographic diagnosis and monitoring of cervicocephalic arterial dissection. Cerebrovasc Dis 2: 195 (abstract)

132. Steinke W, Rautenberg W, Sliwka U, Hennerici M (1993) Common carotid artery occlusion: clinical significance of a patent internal carotid artery. J Neurol Sci 20: s4: 140 (abstract)

133. Sterpetti AV, Schultz RD, Feldhaus RJ, Davenport KL, Richardson M, Farina C, Hunter WJ (1988) Ultrasonographic features of carotid plaque and the risk of subsequent neurologic deficits. Surgery 104: 652–660

134. Sturzenegger M (1991) Ultrasound findings in spontaneous carotid artery dissection. Arch Neurol 41: 1057–1063

135. Taylor DC, Strandness DE Jr (1987) Carotid artery duplex scanning. J Clin Ultrasound 15: 635–644

136. Trattnig S, Hübsch P, Schuster H, Pölzleitner D (1990) Color-coded Doppler imaging of normal vertebral arteries. Stroke 21: 1222–1225

137. Trattnig S, Schwaighofer B, Hübsch P, Schwarz M, Kainberger F (1991) Color-coded sonography of vertebral arteries. J Ultrasound Med 10: 221–226

138. Tuteur P, Reivich M, Goldberg HI, Cooper ES, West JW, McHenry LC, Chernik N (1976) Transient responses of cerebral blood flow and ventilation to changes in PaCo2 in normal subjects and patients with cerebrovascular disease. Stroke 7: 584–590

139. von Reutern GM (1991) Zerebraler Zirkulationsstillstand. Dtsch Arztebl 88: B2844–B2848

140. von Reutern G-M, Pourcelot L (1978) Cardiac-cycle dependant alternating flow in vertebral arteries with subclavian artery stenosis. Stroke 9: 229–236

141. Widder B, Paulat K, Hackspacher J, Mayr E (1986) Transcranial Doppler CO2-test for the detection of hemodynamically critical carotid artery stenoses and occlusions. Eur Arch Psychiatr Neurol Sci 236: 162–168

142. Wolverson MK, Bashiti HM, Peterson GJ (1983) Ultrasonic tissue characterisation of atheromatous plaques using high resolution real time scanner. Ultrasound Med Biol 9: 599–609

143. Zarins CK, Giddens DP, Bharadvaj BK, Sottiurai VS, Mabon RF, Glagov S (1983) Carotid bifurcation atherosclerosis. Circ Res 53: 502–514

144. Zbornikova V, Lassvik C (1991) Common carotid artery occlusion: haemodynamic features. Cerebrovasc Dis 1: 136–141

145. Zierler RE, Phillips DJ, Beach KW, Primozich JF, Strandness DE Jr (1987) Noninvasive assessment of normal carotid bifurcation hemodynamics with color-flow ultrasound imaging. Ultrasound Med Biol 13: 471–476

146. Zwiebel WJ, Knighton R (1990) Duplex examination of the carotid arteries. Semin Ultrasound CT MRI 11: 97–135

147. Zwiebel WJ, Austin CW, Sackett JF, Strother CM (1983) Correlation of high-resolution, B-mode and continuous-wave Doppler sonography with arteriography in the diagnosis of carotid stenosis. Radiology 149: 523–532

Quantitative Ultrasonography of Carotid and Femoral Arteries

J. Wikstrand and I. Wendelhag

Introduction

The aim of the present chapter is to provide an overview on how to measure early atherosclerosis in humans with ultrasound. Atherosclerosis is a disease affecting the intima leading to intimal thickening, but there is no method available at present which can measure only intima thickness in vivo (Fig. 1). However, intima-media thickness may be measured with ultrasound and an increase in intima-media thickness in atherosclerotic prone areas is used as an indicator of intimal thickening. There is a long latent period (often many decades) until the atherosclerotic disease manifests itself as a changed lumen configuration [1] (Fig. 2), and our focus is mainly on the early phases of atherosclerosis before flow disturbances occur.

The present development of noninvasive methods capable of quantitating atherosclerosis in carotid and femoral arteries in a valid way will very likely be of great importance for the clinical assessment of these arteries; and also for clinical research relating to the pathophysiology of atherosclerosis and for the evaluation of preventive measures in randomized clinical trials [2–7]. With an ever-increasing number of studies underway, however, it is important to reach a consensus on standardized investigational routines and on the use of well-defined, generally accepted end points. This will simplify comparisons between different groups, and also aid uniform interpretation of results.

Pignoli and coworkers published their important observations on ultrasound measurement of intima plus media thickness in 1986 [8]. They concluded that B-mode imaging represented a useful approach for measurement of the intima-media complex of human arteries in vivo. However, their experiments were performed only on the far walls only, because the typical double-line pattern on which measurements were made could only be consistently and repeatably visualized on far walls, and not on near walls. Therefore they concluded that the results of their experiments could only be applied to far wall measurements.

With the technique available at present, however, the typical double-line pattern can often also be recorded from the near wall of the carotid artery and the question arises whether near wall intima-media thickness can be measured accurately from these images (Fig. 3). The aim of the present chapter is to discuss some of the fundamental principles of the ultrasound method that indicate that measurements should be made on the so-called leading edges of echoes, which permit accurate quantitation of the lumen diameter and the far wall intima-media thickness in carotid and femoral arteries [2, 10, 11]. A further aim is to comment briefly on some other aspects of ultrasound investigation of these arteries.

Results from In Vitro Experiments: Definition of Near and Far Wall Intima-Lumen and Lumen-Intima Interfaces

In the ultrasound image the arterial wall nearest the transducer is called the "near wall" and the farthest wall is called the "far wall," independent of the angle of the transducer. The upper demarcation line of an echo is defined as the "leading edge" and the lower demarcation line as the "far edge." The thickness of an anatomical structure, e.g., intima-media complex, is measured as

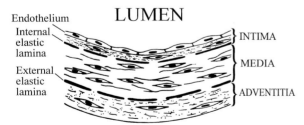

Fig. 1. Anatomy of the arterial wall with its different layers

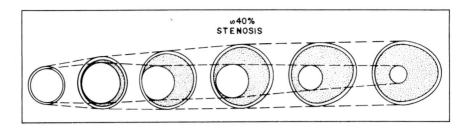

Fig. 2. Diagrammatic representation of a possible sequence of changes in atherosclerotic arteries, leading eventually to lumen narrowing. The artery initially enlarges *(left to right)* in response to plaque accumulation to maintain an adequate, if not normal, lumen area. Early stages of lesion development may be associated with overcompensation. At more than 40% stenosis, however, the plaque area continues to increase to involve the entire circumference of the vessel, and the artery no longer enlarges at a rate sufficient to prevent narrowing of the lumen [l]. (Reprinted by permission of The New England Journal of Medicine, 316: 1371, 1987)

which are not possible to standardize or control for, such as gain-setting and individual composition of adventitia tissue. It is too early, however, to conclude that near wall estimates of intima-media thickness achieved by measurements performed on far edges are redundant. Future studies will have to be done to define the relevance of near wall measurements.

It should be noted that the leading edge of the near wall adventitia echo in most cases is well the distance between the leading edges of two different echoes.

Figures 4 and 5 illustrate two in vitro experiments. The results from these experiments contribute to the understanding of how the inner, thin echoes are created (the echoes nearest the lumen). The figures also nicely illustrate that the thickness of an echo (as that created by the transition between blood and the vessel wall) has no biological significance, and measurements should therefore be performed on the leading edge of an echo (see legends to Figs. 4 and 5 for further comments).

Near Wall Measurements

The adventitia, in contrast to the media, is normally quite echogenic, with bright echoes produced also by the adventitia tissue adjacent to the adventitia-media interface. This means that the echoes produced by the inner part of the adventitia are overlapping echoes produced by the adventitia-media interface in the near wall as illustrated in Fig. 6. This explains why accurate measurements of near wall intima-media thickness cannot be made. This problem cannot be easily overcome by making the reading on the far edge of the adventitia echo since, by definition, the location of this is always clearly below the true location of the adventitia-media transition. Furthermore, the location of the far edge of the adventitia echo is dependent on several factors

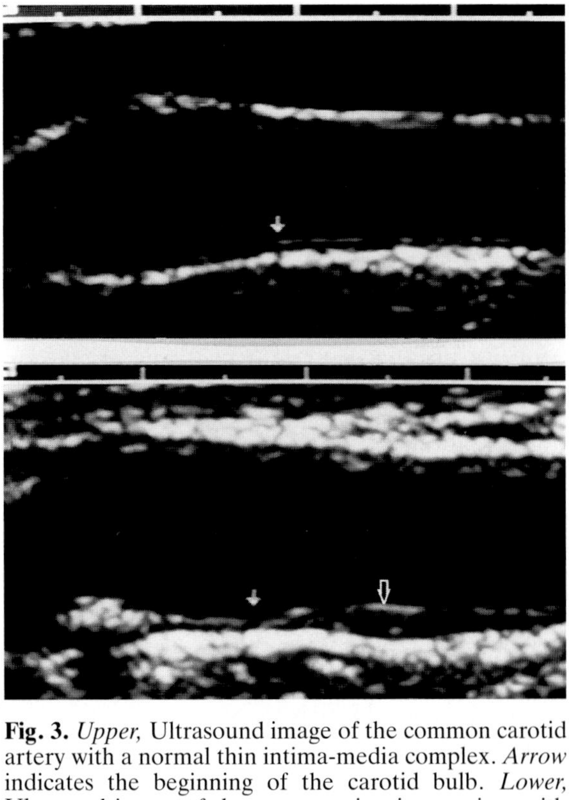

Fig. 3. *Upper,* Ultrasound image of the common carotid artery with a normal thin intima-media complex. *Arrow* indicates the beginning of the carotid bulb. *Lower,* Ultrasond image of the same section in a patient with familial hypercholesterolemia and with an increase in intima-media thickness indicated by the *right unfilled arrow.* The *filled arrow* indicates the beginning of the carotid bulb. Notice the plaque in the carotid bulb *to the left of the filled arrow* and how calcification within the plaque causes an echo shadow below the plaque. (From [9], by permission)

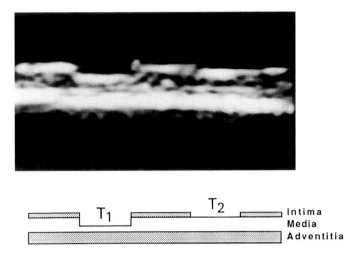

Fig. 4. In vitro experiment with a piece of arterial wall mounted in a solution bath. The intima and part of the media were removed at various depths using a corneal trepanation instrument (T_1 and T_2). For a detailed description see [10]. The ultrasound image shows that the upper echo created by the transition between solution and the vessel wall was very similar whether created by the intact intima or by other vessel wall structures after trepanation into the media. (From [10], by permission)

defined as is near wall intima-lumen interface (except in echogenic plaques, see below), and therefore total wall thickness of the near wall may be measured in an accurate way. However, including adventitia thickness in wall thickness measurements does not appear ideal when the interest is in assessing atherosclerosis.

Near Wall Intima-Lumen Interface

The near wall intima-lumen interface is defined by the leading edge of the second echo from the near wall as discussed above (see A in Fig. 6). This echo is well defined since normally the media has a low echogenic structure and therefore produces no echoes disturbing the mostly highly echogenic intima-lumen interface.

Lumen Diameter

Measurement of lumen diameter ought to be done from the leading edge of the echo from the near wall intima-lumen interface to the leading

Fig. 5. In vitro experiment with an intact carotid artery mounted in a solution bath. For a detailed description see [10]. The artery was ligated at one end, while the other end was connected to a syringe filled with buffer solution and some air, which was introduced into the vessel so that an air bubble was slowly created along the intima-buffer solution interface in the near wall. High-contrast resolution is created by the intima-air interface. The ultrasound image shows how the leading edge of the inner, thin echo in the near wall coincides with the leading edge of the echo from the air bubble, when the air bubble extends to the right. Thus the leading edge of this echo defines the intima-lumen interface. Also observe the echo shadow below the air bubble. The echo shadow *(S)* in the lower part of the image indicates how far the air bubble has reached. (From [10], by permission)

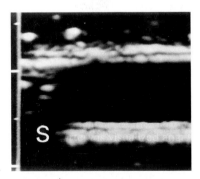
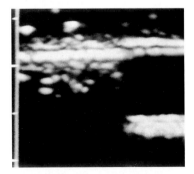
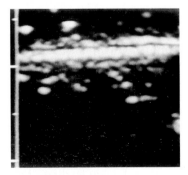

Time

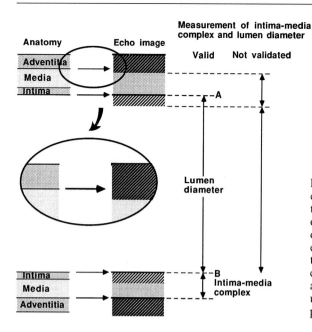

Fig. 6. Illustration of the anatomical correlates to echoes that may be recorded from an artery. Observe that all measurements are performed on leading edges of the different echoes, that any thickness of an echo is of no interest, and that the thickness of an anatomical entity (e.g., the intima-media complex) is defined by the distance between the leading edges of two different echoes. The figure also illustrates that the near wall adventitia-media interface cannot be identified in the ultrasound image *(encircled)*. (Adopted from [10], by permission)

edge of the echo from the far wall lumen-intima interface (distance between A and B in Fig. 6). Thus, the two leading edges defining lumen diameter of the common carotid artery can be easily recorded in most cases. However, the intima-lumen interface of the near wall of the femoral artery is difficult to visualize in many cases, probably due to the curved nature of the common femoral artery. Thus, in some cases, and with present technique, a true measurement of lumen diameter cannot be performed in the femoral artery [12].

Far Wall Intima-Media Thickness

The leading edge echo from the lumen-intima interface from the far wall can be recorded in the majority of cases.

Until recently it has been generally accepted that the leading edge of the second bright echo from the far wall is created by the media-adventitia interface, thus enabling valid measurements of far wall intima-media thickness to be made. In a recent report from a study comparing ultrasound measurements with histological measurements, however, the authors concluded that the distance between the two leading edges in the far wall corresponded best with total wall thickness (including adventitia) and not with the extent of the intima-media complex alone as has been previously proposed [13]. The results from this study

contrast with the observations made by Pignoli et al. [8] and also with the results from another recently published ultrasound-pathological comparison, however [14]. The authors of the latter study concluded that the intima-media thickness of the carotid artery can be accurately measured in the far wall projection. Further studies are needed to resolve the controversy. Until more data are available, we will continue to use the expression "intima-media complex" for the variable defined by the distance between the two leading edges in the far wall.

Discussion

The Leading Edge Principle

The anatomical location of a biological structure is always defined by a leading edge of an echo, and the thickness of a structure as the distance between the leading edges of two different echoes. In spite of the similarity of the near and far wall images the thickness of the intima-media complex can only be measured accurately in the far wall position [11, 14]. This is because it is only in the far wall that the intima-media complex is defined by leading edges from echoes of interest. Recent data reevaluating in vitro measurements of arterial wall segment thicknesses obtained by histology and by current vascular sonography also indicate that only far wall intima-media thickness, in

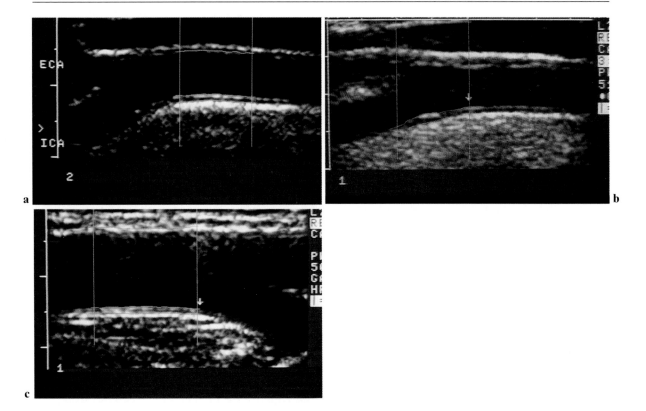

Fig. 7. a Ultrasound image of the common carotid artery. Measurement of intima-media thickness is made along a 10-mm-long section just proximal to the carotid bulb. The measurement area is defined by two vertical reference lines in the analyzing program. **b** Ultrasound image of the common carotid artery with the carotid bulb. Measurement of intima-media thickness is made along a 10-mm-long section distal to the beginning of the bulb. **c** Ultrasound image of the femoral artery. Measurement of intima-media thickness is made along a 15-mm-long section of the common femoral artery proximal to the bifurcation into the superficial and the profound femoral arteries. The distal of the two vertical reference lines defining the measurement area is set where the far wall of the common femoral artery starts to bend and form the profound femoral artery. This transition is used as an internal marker, as the femoral artery does not have a bulb like the carotid artery

contrast to near wall intima-media thickness, may be accurately measured [14].

It may therefore be concluded that until more experience is gathered main outcome variables in ultrasound studies of atherosclerosis should preferably be from the far wall. If analyses of the near wall are performed they ought to be separately presented. Future studies will have to be per-

formed to define any usefulness of near wall measurements.

If lumen diameter is measured, this measurement should be read from the leading edge of the intima-lumen interface of the near wall as illustrated in Fig. 6. Present experience indicates that it is more difficult to visualize the intima-lumen interface of the near wall of the femoral artery than of the carotid artery, probably due to the curved nature of the femoral artery [12].

Common Carotid, Carotid Bulb, and Internal Carotid Artery

Our own, and also the experience of others, indicates that good-quality multiple scans of the far wall of the straight part of the common carotid artery may be achieved in nearly every case [6]. But, in accordance with other groups [6], we have found that the percentage of missing images is so high from the internal carotid artery that it is questionable if it is meaningful to try to routinely perform quantitative measurements of intima-media thickness in the internal carotid artery in all subjects. If measurements are routinely performed in the carotid bulb, which we would recommend, it should be noted that the bulb of the internal carotid artery is not always located in the far wall position. It might be advisable to note the topographical location of the arteries in the far wall position and also analyze if there are any differences between different topographical situations. The development of atherosclerosis typically begins with an increased intima-media thickness in the bifurcation area, i.e., in the proximal part of the internal carotid artery and the carotid bulb, and the intima-media complex is often thicker here than in the straight part of the common carotid artery. To be able to make a correct comparison of the results from different laboratories, it is therefore very important to report where the measurements were performed.

Quantifications of Plaques

A thorough scanning is performed to record the occurrence of plaques in all investigated subjects in our laboratory. Independent of the location in the carotid arteries, i.e., internal, external, and common carotid artery and carotid bulb, all plaques in both the near and the far wall are identified and recorded. A semiquantitative visual scoring of plaque size is performed (see Table 1) [12]. Further studies are needed to define the usefulness of any quantification of plaques (area, base, height, composition, etc.), especially in prospective studies. One important question to be addressed is how blindness should be preserved if one wants to return to the same plaque in prospective studies.

Not all atherosclerotic plaques are the same even if they are similar in size and location. Some plaques may stabilize, like an inactive volcano. For others, plaque formation may continue with complications such as hemorrhage, necrosis, in-

flammation, sclerosis, or calcification that can alter the vulnerability of plaques to disruption. It would be highly desirable to develop methods with the possibility of identifying plaques with different qualitative characteristics. Calcification gives intense echoes and often also an echo shadow (see Fig. 3). However, although work is ongoing the possibility of identifying in vivo plaques with different qualitative tissue characteristics seems to be limited at present.

Differences in Recording and Analysis Techniques

We have commented on certain aspects of measuring intima-media thickness and lumen diameter in the carotid and femoral arteries. We recognize at the present time several differences in the recording and analysis routines between different laboratories. Some investigate only the common carotid artery, others the common carotid, the carotid bulb, and the internal carotid artery, and still others both the carotid and femoral arteries. Some perform measurements of just single maximal intima-media thickness, sometimes from several locations in the carotid artery region, and present scores from these measurements (see below), while others perform measurements along a predefined section of the artery of interest and from these measurements calculate means and maximum values. In our own laboratory we have chosen the latter way of analysis [12].

These measurements give values for intima-media thickness and lumen diameter along a predefined 10-mm-long section of the common carotid artery and the carotid bulb, respectively, and from a 15-mm-long section of the common femoral artery (Fig. 7a–c). We believe that these measurements may give more valuable information than just measurements of single maximum values that

Table 1. Grading of the occurrence and size of plaques in the carotid and femoral arteries by visual scoring (from [11])

Grade 0: No plaque

Grade 1: One or more small plaques
          Arteria carotis: each less than approximately $10 \, mm^2$
          Arteria femoralis: each less than approximately $20 \, mm^2$

Grade 2: Moderate to large plaques

Grade 3: Plaque leading to disturbances in blood flow defined by the pulsed Doppler curve
          Arteria carotis: peak systolic flow velocity $>1.2 \, m/s$
          Arteria femoralis: 100 % increase in peak systolic flow velocity and loss of reverse flow

may not be from the same location in prospective studies. Furthermore, it is recommended that analyses are performed on images frozen via ECG-triggering (top of R wave) to minimize variability depending on changes in intima-media thickness and lumen diameter occurring during the cardiac cycle [3, 5, 11, 15]. Real-time images are always recorded to complement the frozen images in order to simplify a valid judgement of what the frozen images show. Since we believe that the best quality on both registration and analyses is achieved if the responsible technologist fully masters both registration and analyses, we have organized the work in the laboratory so that each technologist is involved in and masters both.

If the sum from several measurements from different sections of the carotid artery is used in a describing score, it is also important to report in addition to the score the separate means or maximum values from each section of the artery. Otherwise, it will be almost impossible to compare study results from different research groups, as these types of scores are often individually created. There is at present no consensus regarding whether and how these scores should be formed and used.

Fig. 8. Common carotid artery presented as an image intensity plot

Automated Reading

To measure the thickness of intima-media complex most research laboratories utilize some kind of computerized analyzing system. The thickness is measured by manually tracing the different interfaces of interest. One research group has reported an automated method for tracing the different interfaces [16]. In collaboration with Chalmers University of Technology we are currently developing a new reading system for automated detection of echo interfaces, including optional interactive corrections by the human operator. The new analyzing program will also make it possible to display the ultrasound image as a landscape representing image intensity by vertical height thus complementing the standard grayscale image. We will also evaluate whether this kind of presentation will allow a more reliable interpretation of the ultrasound image (Fig. 8).

Carotid Vs. Femoral Arteries

Instead of investigating carotid arteries bilaterally we have chosen to investigate the right carotid artery and the right femoral artery in order to be able to follow the development in two different

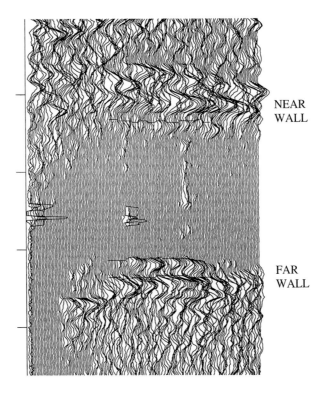

NEAR
WALL

FAR
WALL

arterial regions. Each recording session takes approximately 45 min to perform (including ECG recording and blood pressure measurements) and because of limited time we have elected not to investigate both arterial regions bilaterally in all studies.

Clinical Relevance

We see an increasing use of the quantitative ultrasound method primarily in the evaluation of preventive measures in randomized clinical trials. In the interpretation of results from these trials several important issues should be addressed: (a) How should changes in intima-media thickness depending on changes in lumen diameter be handled? (b) How should missing data be handled? (c) Is intima-media thickness measured by ultrasound in carotid and femoral arteries an appropriate surrogate variable for coronary atherosclerosis?

Changes in Lumen Diameter

One way of normalizing for drug-induced effects of changes in lumen diameter on intima-media thickness is to calculate cross-sectional area of the intima-media complex and use that as the primary surrogate end point [11, 17]. Suppose a randomized trial compares two agents where one drug dilates the vessel while the other reduces the lumen diameter. Since vessel wall mass must be unchanged in the short-term perspective a decrease in wall thickness occurs after the former drug but an increase after the latter. Cross-sectional area will, however, be unchanged (Fig. 9). In the recently presented large-scale MIDAS study [6, 18] comparing a thiazide diuretic with a calcium antagonist (isradipine) in hypertensives, a difference in intima-media thickness was recorded after 6 months, with a thicker intima-media thickness in those randomized to the diuretic. Unfortunately, lumen diameter was not investigated in this study. However, theoretical calculations show that the results regardig the thicker intima-media complex in the diuretic group could be explained by just a 3 % decrease in lumen diameter. After 3 years of follow-up there was a trend towards significantly more cardiovascular complications in those randomized to isradipine than in those randomized to diuretic (see further comments below) [18].

Subjects Lost to Follow-up

Subjects get lost to follow-up in long-term, prospective, randomized trials for many reasons. Often it cannot be excluded that treatment may have negatively affected the disease process in those lost to follow-up, which may introduce a bias when interpreting the results. One way of handling this problem is to compare treatment groups using a nonparametric scoring test in which the highest score is given to all patients lost to follow-up. This way of analysis should preferably be stated prospectively in the study protocol [2].

Value of Surrogate End Points

Is it possible to use the intima-media thickness in the carotid artery as a surrogate variable for coronary atherosclerosis? As yet, there is no clear answer to this question and the answer may also partly depend on which surrogate variable is used. We cannot take for granted that measurements performed in the common carotid artery bring the same information as measurements performed in the carotid bulb or in the internal carotid artery (or scores from these measurements). At present we cannot even with certainty claim that an increased thickness of the intima-media complex in the carotid artery without doubt indicates atherosclerosis at the location where the measurement was performed. The proof is yet to come that simple surrogate ultrasound end points from the carotid or femoral artery can substitute for measurements of coronary atherosclerosis and for hard end points such as myocardial infarction, stroke, and cardiovascular death (Fig. 10) [2, 4].

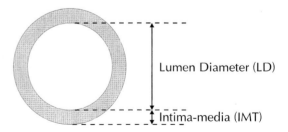

Cross-sectional intima-media area (A)

$$A = \pi(\frac{LD}{2} + IMT)^2 - \pi(\frac{LD}{2})^2$$

Fig. 9. Illustration with the formula for calculation of mean cross-sectional area of the intima-media complex

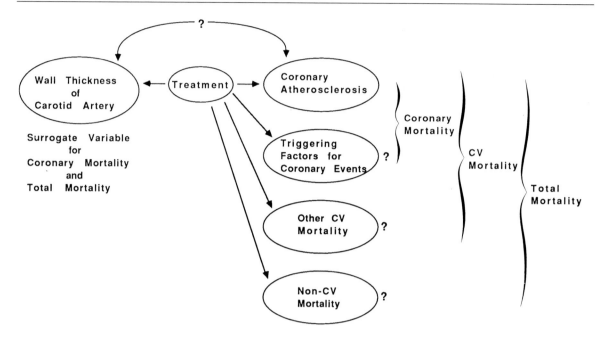

Fig. 10. Diagrammatic representation of relationship between a surrogate end point (intima-media thickness) and coronary atherosclerosis, and "hard" end points like coronary and total mortality. (From [2], by permission)

There are many examples in the literature where results from surrogate variables have been misleading [2], e.g., results from the CAST study [19], the INTACT study [20], and recently results from the MIDAS study [18]. Nevertheless, ultrasound evaluation of vascular disease looks increasingly promising as a noninvasive, cost-effective method for the future [4].

Conclusion

Methods capable of quantitatively evaluating early atherosclerotic manifestations in a safe, valid, and reproducible way in prospective studies of humans would be of great importance for epidemiological and clinical research relating to the pathophysiology of atherosclerosis and also for the evaluation of preventive measures particularly in randomized clinical trials.

The ultrasound method is a promising technique, with a great potential for refined, computerized, quantitative analyzing techniques. However, atherosclerotic manifestations are complex struc-

tures and, therefore, difficult to measure. Thus, there is a need for improved interaction between pathologists and researchers, who use different methods to measure atherosclerosis in vivo, to increase our understanding of what the recordings show. In addition, agreement about standardized measurement routines and end points should be reached. This will simplify comparisons between different studies and will also aid uniform interpretation of results. Furthermore, more studies are needed to clarify the relationship between the thickness of the intima-media complex in large arteries (surrogate end points) and coronary atherosclerosis and coronary heart disease.

Hard end points like myocardial infarction and sudden death are usually due to a combination of an underlying atherosclerotic disease and triggering or precipitation factors such as left ventricular electric instability, plaque instability, or a disturbed thrombogenesis-fibrinolysis balance. It might be advisable, therefore, to combine different surrogate variables (for both the underlying atherosclerotic disease and triggering or precipitation mechanisms) to obtain a broader perspective of the disease process.

An intervention may or may not be effective in treating the condition of interest but could be harmful in other respects. Therefore, total mortality should be considered, as well as cause-specific fatal and nonfatal events, in addition to the primary surrogate variables whenever possible.

References

1. Glagov S, Weisenberg E, Zarins CK, Stankunavicius R, Kolettis GJ (1987) Compensatory enlargement of human atherosclerotic coronary arteries. N Eng J Med 316: 1371–1375
2. Wikstrand J, Wiklund O (1992) Frontiers in cardiovascular science: quantitative measurements of atherosclerotic manifestations in human. Arterioscler Thromb 12: 114–119
3. Salonen JT, Salonen R (1993) Ultrasound B-mode imaging in observational studies of atherosclerotic progression. Circulation 87 [Suppl II]: 56–65
4. Lees RS (1993) Non-invasive detection of vascular function and dysfunction. Curr Opinion Lipidol 4: 325–329
5. Bots ML, Hofman A, de Bruyn AM, de Jong PTVM, Grobbee DE (1993) Isolated systolic hypertension and vessel wall thickness of the carotid artery. The Rotterdam Elderly Study. Arterioscler Thromb 13: 64–69
6. Furberg CD, Borhani NO, Byington RP, Gibbons ME, Sowers JR (1993) Calcium antagonists and atherosclerosis. The multicenter isradipine/diuretic atherosclerosis study. Am J Hypertens 6: 24S–29S
7. Blankenhorn DH, Selzer RH, Crawford DW, Barth JD, Liu C-r, Liu C-h, Mack WJ, Alaupovic P (1993) Beneficial effects of colestipol-niacin therapy on the common carotid artery. Two- and four-year reduction of intima-media thickness measured by ultrasound. Circulation 88: 20–28
8. Pignoli P, Tremoli E, Poli A, Oreste P, Paoletti R (1986) Intimal plus medial thickness of the arterial wall: a direct measurement with ultrasound imaging. Circulation 74: 1399–1406
9. Wendelhag I, Wiklund O, Wikstrand J (1992) Arterial wall thickness in familial hypercholesterolemia: ultrasound measurement of intima-media thickness in the common carotid artery. Arterioscler Thromb 12: 70–77
10. Wendelhag I, Gustavsson T, Suurküla M, Berglund G. Wikstrand J (1991) Ultrasound measurement of wall thickness in the carotid artery: fundamental principles and description of a computerized analysing system. Clin Physiol 11: 565–577
11. Wikstrand J, Wendelhag I (1994) Methodological considerations of ultrasound investigation of intima-media thickness and lumen diameter. J Int Med 236: 565–570
12. Wendelhag I, Wiklund O, Wikstrand J (1993) Atherosclerotic changes in the femoral and carotid arteries in familial hypercholesterolemia. Ultrasonographic assessment of intima-media thickness and plaque occurrence. Arterioscler Thromb 13: 1404–1411
13. Gamble G, Beaumont B, Smith H, Zorn J, Sanders G, Merrilees M, MacMahon S, Sharpe N (1993) B-mode ultrasound images of the carotid artery wall: correlation of ultrasound with histological measurements. Atherosclerosis 102: 163–173
14. Wong M, Edelstein J, Wollman J, Bond MG (1993) Ultrasonic-pathological comparison of the human arterial wall. Verification of intima-media thickness. Arterioscler Thromb 13: 482–486
15. Persson J, Stavenow L, Wikstrand J, Israelsson B, Formgren J, Berglund G (1992) Noninvasive quantification of atherosclerotic lesions. Reproducibility of ultrasonographic measurement of arterial wall thickness and plaque size. Arterioscler Thromb 12: 261–266
16. Gariepy J, Massonneau M, Levenson J, Heudes D, Simon A (1993) Evidence for in vivo carotid and femoral wall thickening in human hypertension. Hypertension 22: 111–118
17. Furberg CD, Byington RP, Craven TE (1994) Lessons learned from clinical trials with ultrasound endpoints. J Int Med 236: 585–590
18. McClellan K (1994) Views & Reviews: Unexpected results from MIDAS in atherosclerosis. Weekly Inpharma 932: 4
19. The Cardiac Arrhythmia Suppression Trial (CAST) Investigators (1989) Preliminary report: effect of encainide and flecainide on mortality in a randomized trial of arrhythmia suppression after myocardial infarction. N Eng J Med 321: 406–412
20. Lichtlen PR, Hugenholtz PG, Rafflenbeul W, Hecker H, Jost S, Decker JW (1990) Retardation of angiographic progression of coronary artery disease by nifedipine. Lancet 335: 1109–1113

Abdominal and Pelvic Vascular Ultrasonography

K. Haag and P. Lanzer

Introduction

Indications for abdominal color flow mapping (CFM) include nearly all suspected vascular abnormalities in the abdomen, i.e., the vessels of the portal circulation, upper abdominal arteries, renal vessels, abdominal aorta, vena cava inferior, and blood vessels of the pelvis [1]. However, the quality of CFM data depends greatly on the anatomical site of the vessel, the patient's condition (bowel gas, obesity, compliance, ascites, postoperative dressings), operator's skill and experience. The sonographer performing abdominal CFM should be thoroughly familiar with normal B-mode sonography, standard Duplex techniques, and the anatomy of the abdominal organs and their vasculature. Correct data interpretation also requires an understanding of vascular pathology and hemodynamic principles. An operational understanding of color (Doppler) imaging, instrumentation, and technology is also needed to avoid misinterpretation of artifacts.

Establishing a routine abdominal CFM protocol aids in producing consistent and reproducible results. To avoid respiratory effects on venous hemodynamics it is preferable to acquire all quantitative data during breath holding. Fasting also facilitates the examination and is necessary for the validity of quantitative data of portal flow measurements. Gentle pressure on the transducer avoids interference with venous hemodynamics. It is essential that examinations begin with conventional B-mode sonography to define the topography and morphology of the abdominal organs. The operator notes the position, size, and texture of the parenchymal organs and documents any structural abnormality [2]. CFM is then used to identify the vessels of interest and to determine their flow characteristics. Whenever possible the vessels are examined in both longitudinal and transverse along the standard imaging planes [3]. To minimize errors the vessels should be examined along their complete course. Basic imaging planes and transducer orientations for an abdominal CFM examination have recently been outlined. Quantitative flow is measured at present using the standard Doppler methods [4]. To perform reliable Doppler and gray-scale imaging related measurements the examiner should be familiar with the potential sources of errors [5, 6] and with the essentials of splanchnic hemodynamics [7]. Quantitative assessments of flow directly from the CFM data will become increasingly available in the future [8].

In this chapter flow velocity is given as the maximum flow velocity (corrected for Doppler angle and time averaged in veins) because this does not depend critically on the electronic equipment or geometry of the ultrasound beam, both responsible for systematic errors (overestimation of mean flow velocity). In vessels with laminar flow conditions, for example, the portal circulation in patients with portal hypertension, mean flow velocity (averaged over the cross-section) can be approximated using the relation: mean flow velocity = $0.5 \times$ maximum flow velocity. Flow rates are estimated by multiplying mean flow velocity with the cross-section area of the vessel.

Portal System

Potential indications for a CFM examination of the portal system include:

- Liver cirrhosis
- Portal hypertension, ascites of unknown etiology, esophageal varices
- Thrombosis of the portal vein, superior mesenteric vein, splenic vein
- Venoocclusive disease, Budd-Chiari syndrome
- Splenomegaly
- Monitoring of portosystemic shunts
- Space-occupying lesions in the liver
- Abdominal trauma

– Gastrointestinal bleeding without endoscopically confirmed cause
– Liver transplantation

Examination Technique

A complete examination of the portal circulation should include evaluation of (a) portal vein, (b) intrahepatic branches of the portal vein in both the right and left liver lobe, (c) hepatic veins, (d) hepatic arteries (see below), (e) splenic vein, (f) superior mesenteric vein, (g) collateral vessels and (h) a check of the celiac trunk and the superior and inferior mesenteric arteries (see below). The topographic anatomy and hemodynamics [9, 10] of the portal venous system should be reviewed and well understood.

The examination begins by locating the portal vein. The ultrasonic beam is directed obliquely in the right upper quadrant between the umbilicus and the costophrenic angle. In this orientation the portal vein can be visualized in its long axis from the venous confluence to its division into the right and left branches (Fig. 1). For quantitative analysis a large anatomic angle between the course of the vein and the ultrasonic beam makes a more caudal approach necessary. In patients with ascites, bowel gas, or abdominal dressings the vein can be imaged laterally from the right side using an oblique transducer orientation. The left main portal branch is imaged from ventral epigastric with a transverse transducer orientation. Higher order portal vein branches are identified within the liver parenchyma.

The hepatic veins are imaged from the right upper quadrant with a transverse transducer orientation at the midclavicular line. The imaging of the left veins is often facilitated from a more left lateral orientation while the patient holds his breath in deep inspiration. The veins of the right liver lobe are frequently better visualized from a more right lateral oblique position (Fig. 2).

The splenic vein is typically examined from the epigastrium longitudinally in a coronal plane or transversally in a left parasagittal plane. This approach allows visualization of the vessel from the end at the portal vein to the tail of the pancreas (Fig. 3). The hilar segment can be visualized from the left lateral using the spleen as an echogenic window. Blood flow should be also assessed in several parenchymal branches if splenic infarction is suspected.

The superior mesenteric vein can be imaged following its oblique course by orienting the transducer from left caudal to right lateral in the right upper quadrant. Frequently large angles of insonation require moving the transducer more cranially or caudally from its original position to obtain Doppler flow measurements.

The inferior mesenteric vein displays a more variable anatomic course and is frequently identified at the confluence with the splenic vein or the superior mesenteric vein.

The right and left gastric veins can be identified close to the venous confluence where they empty into the portal vein or into the splenic vein, respectively. The recognition of a retrograde gastric venous flow is important in diagnosis of portal hypertension (Fig. 4). Infrequently, downstream filling of a thrombosed portal vein via the right gastric vein is observed.

The umbilical vein joins the left branch of the portal vein where it is easily identified (Fig. 5). Varicose veins of the gastric cardia and the esophagus are recognized as tortuous vascular structures at the level of the epigastrium and the left upper quadrant. When there is splenic obstruction, the short gastric veins can be visualized as short stumps originating from the splenic vein close to the hilus and moving upward toward the greater curvature of the stomach. Other small vessels providing collateral circulation in the presence of a portal hypertension move from the hilar segment of the splenic vein downward and into the retroperitoneum. Other portacaval collateral pathways occasionally documented by CFM are the veins of the gallbladder walls emptying into the veins of the liver capsula. Small veins originating in the territory of the inferior mesenteric vein and joining the hemorrhoidal plexus of the inferior and middle rectal vein are also occasionally seen with CFM.

In addition to the evaluation of the native portal vasculature, CFM is becoming an important method to assess the functional status of surgically constructed portosystemic shunts [11]. Proximal and distal splenorenal shunts are best seen in a cross-sectional view with the transducer in the left lateral or anterior position. Portocaval shunts are visualized using techniques described for portal vein imaging in short- and long-axis views along the hepatoduodenal ligament (Fig. 6). Mesocaval shunts are visualized along the superior mesenteric vein (Fig. 7). If the shunt is functioning, flow reversal is seen at the level of its

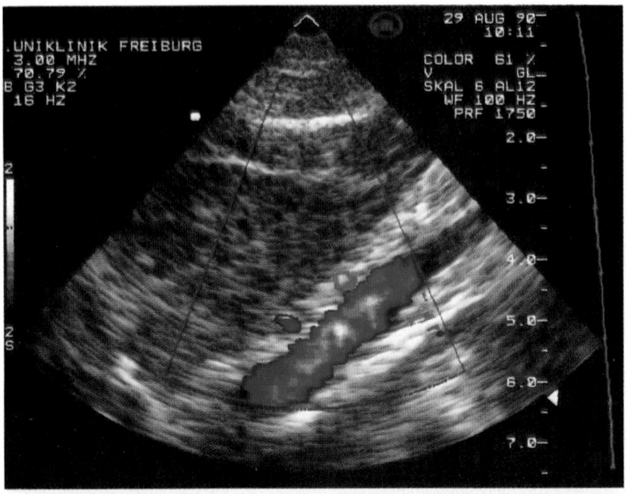

Fig. 1. Normal portal vein. *Blue,* hepatopetal flow from the venous confluence to the hepatic portal; *white (within the vessel),* higher flow velocity in the central portions of the vessel; *red spot (ventral to the portal vein),* proper hepatic artery. Several figures in this section have been published in [20]; all CFM images were produced by Ultramark 9, ATL, Solingen, Germany)

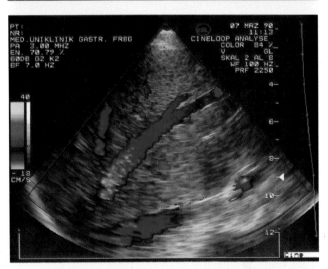

Fig. 2. Right lateral view of the hepatic veins of the right liver lobe

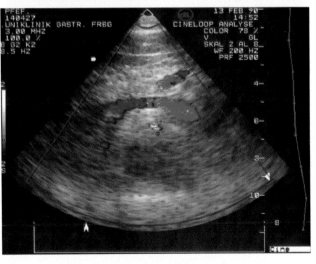

Fig. 3. Splenic vein in its long axis (transverse transducer orientation). *Red,* blood flow towards the transducer; *blue,* blood flow away from the transducer; *colored spots (ventral and dorsal to the splenic vein),* splenic artery and superior mesenteric artery

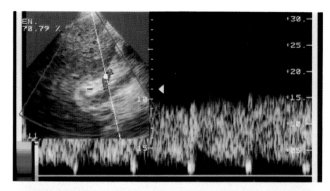

Fig. 4. Right gastric vein in a patient with liver cirrhosis and a portal hypertension (view along the hepatoduodenal ligament). *Red*, hepatofugal retrograde blood flow. The frequency spectrum shows a time-constant (monophasic) flow pattern

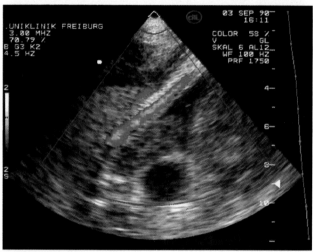

Fig. 5. Collateral umbilical circulation in a patient with liver cirrhosis, portal hypertension, and ascites

proximal anastomosis. Transjugular intrahepatic portosystemic stent-shunts [12] are visualized from ventral epigastric or from a right lateral oblique position (Fig. 8).

To allow correct interpretations of the CFM quantitative data in the portal system it is important to perform all examinations consistently in fasting patients during breath holding in midexpiraton or during a quiet respiration.

Pathologic Findings

Normal Doppler waveforms and the flow directions within the veins of the portal system must be recognized to allow correct assessment of pathology [13]. Recognition of abnormal flow patterns using CFM greatly facilitates and shortens the examination by quickly determining the optimal sampling site for Doppler related measurements.

Liver Cirrhosis and Portal Hypertension

The CFM findings should be interpeted within the context of the entire diagnostic picture. Individual findings are often nonspecific and misleading. The effect of liver cirrhosis on portal circulation is variable. The flow pattern is relatively monophasic, as in a healthy state. However, reduced maximum flow velocity (MFV) in the portal vein is a nearly obligate feature, maximum flow velocity being lesser than 30 cm/s. In patients with intact splanchnic vessels a decrease in portal maximum flow velocity to 20 cm/s or lower clearly indicates portal hypertension [14] independently of its origin. Increased portal vein diameter (greater than 13 mm) is frequent but not obligate [15]. Especially in patients with large spontaneous portosystemic shunts portal vein diameter is often in the normal range. Decreased as well as normal flow rates [16–23] of the portal vein have been reported. In our own experience the flow rates (normal values: 600–1 000 ml/min) in patients with cirrhosis can be normal, decreased, or even elevated

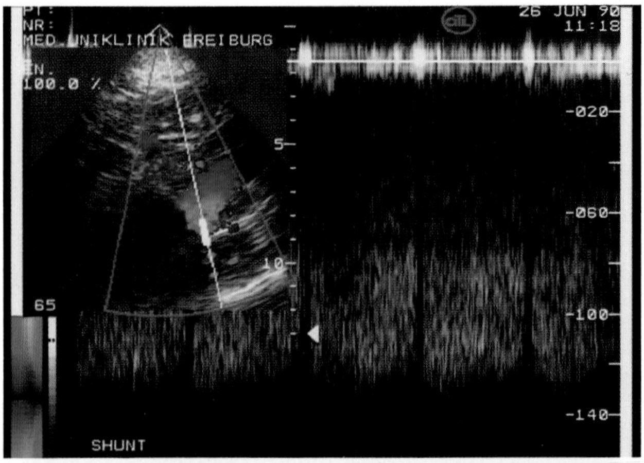

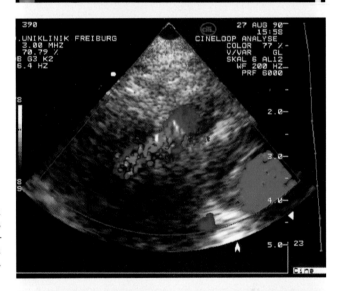

Fig. 6. Portocaval shunt. The patency of the shunt and a high flow velocity are demonstrated ($V_{max}=130$ cm/s)

Fig. 7. Mesocaval shunt. A mesocaval shunt in a transverse section caudally to the renal arteries is demonstrated. The patency of the shunt is documented by the turbulent flow (*mosaic color*) from the superior mesenteric vein to the cava inferior. *Right bottom* (*red*), aorta

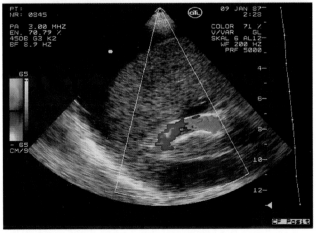

Fig. 8. Transjugular intrahepatic portosystemic stent-shunt from a right lateral view. The metallic stent is easily recognized in the normal B-mode image, and the good shunt function is characterized by an constant high flow velocity without significant turbulences along the shunt tract

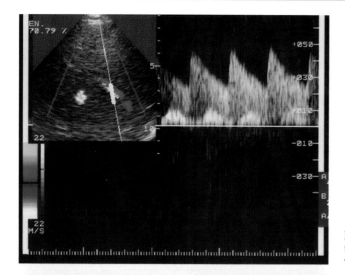

Fig. 9. Predominance of arterial blood flow over the portal venous blood flow in a patient with liver cirrhosis

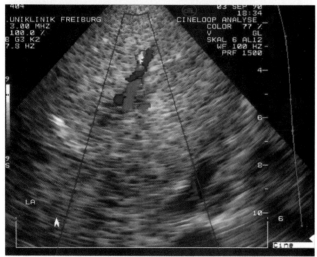

Fig. 10. Liver cirrhosis-portal flow reversal. The blood in the branches of the hepatic artery and portal vein flows in opposite directions. *Red*, hepatopetal arterial flow; *blue*, hepatofugal venous flow

[24]. We observe high flow rates most frequently in patients with early stages of cirrhosis, splenomegaly, or patent umbilical vein. Only in patients with advanced cirrhosis do the flow rates tend to decline reaching subnormal levels.

In the great majority of patients with advanced liver cirrhosis the arterial Doppler flow signal „dominates" over the portal venous Doppler flow signal whereas in healthy subjects the portal flow signal „dominates" (Fig. 9). The „dominance" is assessed using a wider-range gate spanning both the vein and the accompanying artery. The „dominant" flow is qualitatively assigned to the vessel based on the relative intensities of the respective frequency spectra. This criterion corresponds to the increasing importance of arterial blood flow („arterialization") in liver cirrhosis [25]. In the presence of the „dominance" of the arterial flow signal the direction of the arterial and the portal flow should be noted. In the majority of patients flow is unidirectional, as in normal subjects. In patients with advanced cirrhosis a reversal of the intrahepatic portal flow direction can be seen in some segments of the liver. Only in a few patients (5 %) can flow reversal in nearly all liver segments and in the portal vein be documented by CFM (Fig. 10).

CFM greatly facilitates identification of collateral vessels with hepatofugal flow in the coronary veins of the stomach (Fig. 4), umbilical and parumbilical vein (Fig. 5), dilated short veins of the stomach walls, perisplenic and retroperitoneal vessels, superficial abdominal and gallbladder varicose veins (Fig. 11) [25].

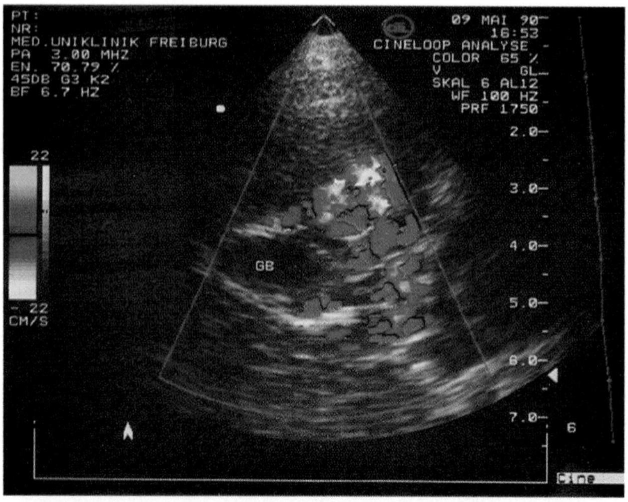

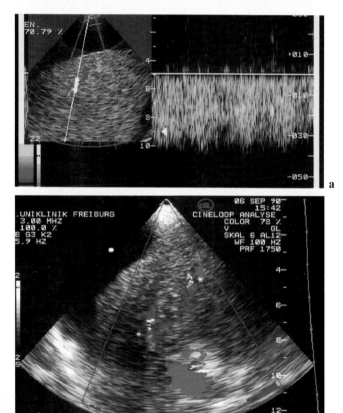

Fig. 11. Gallbladder varicose veins in a patient with chronic pancreatitis and portal vein thrombosis but without liver cirrhosis. The blood replenishes the intrahepatic portal branches and provides for considerable portal perfusion of the liver

Fig. 12 a, b. Regional compression of a peripheral hepatic vein in liver cirrhosis. **a** $V_{max} > 30$ cm/s is demonstrated in the Doppler velocity tracing, **b** Flow velocity normalization down stream to the stenosis (*)

In our experience some patients with liver cirrhosis complicated by splenomegaly the splenic vein flow increases four- to fivefold the normal (normal in our laboratory: 200–300 ml/min), contributing to the severity of the portal hypertension by about 50 %.

The flow in the hepatic venous circulation in patients with cirrhosis can also vary. Wave form analysis (e.g., loss of pulsation) may give a hint to the diagnosis of cirrhosis. However, in our experience more characteristic is a *regional* flow acceleration, which can be easily demonstrated by CFM. As a rule flow velocity increases along the hepatic vein by more than threefold, exceeding 30 cm/s (Fig. 12) and declines after the regional acceleration to the previous level. These changes may be less prominent in patients with reduced portal flow. Flow acceleration is thought to be due to regional vein compressions secondary to regenerative nodules. However, flow accelerations in the central parenchymal branches of large hepatic veins are also occasionally observed in healthy subjects secondary to diaphragmatic hepatic compression during inspiration. To ascertain pathology flow accelerations should therefore also be documented in the peripheral branches of the hepatic veins. Due to the frequency of regional hepatic flow differences multiple segments of liver parenchyma should be evaluated. Regional flow acceleration can also be observed in the presence of space occupying lesions in the liver. Therefore liver metastases should be considered even when they cannot be seen on B-mode images. It should be noted that despite severe portal hypertension sometimes observed in the case of liver fibrosis (e.g., schistosomiasis, early stages of primary biliary cirrhosis) or hepatic venoocclusive disease regional flow acceleration in the hepatic veins is absent. The diagnostic CFM criteria for liver cirrhosis and portal hypertension are also as follows:

– Maximum flow velocity in the portal vein less than 20 cm/s; maximum flow velocity greater than 30 cm/s excluding liver cirrhosis except the case of portal vein stenosis
– Regional flow acceleration in the peripheral hepatic veins to more than 30 cm/s
– Hepatofugal flow in collaterals (umbilical vein, coronary vein, short gastric veins) or in the portal, splenic, or mesenteric vein
– „Arterialization" of the liver
– Absence of diameter and velocity changes in the splenic and superior mesenteric vein at increased pressure on the transducer

Portal Vein Thrombosis

A complete or incomplete portal vein thrombosis of various etiologies based on the absence of color-coded and Doppler signal is reliably detected on the CFM examination [25]. An acute portal vein thrombosis should always be excluded by Duplex or CFM because the hypoechoic fresh thrombus can easily be overlooked on the B-mode image. After a few days portal vein thrombosis is now often documented on the B-mode image by direct visualization of the echogenic organized thrombus within the vessel lumen [2]. Old thrombosis (older than 3 months) is characterized by the change to an echogenic fibrotic cord. In about one-third of patients the thrombosed vessel can be observed to be surrounded by numerous small collaterals (Fig. 13), the appearance of which is termed in Duplex imaging „cavernous transformation" [26]. Occasionally, reconstitution of the portal vein or its branches with a partially patent lumen, residual flow, and regional acceleration can be documented. The isolated thrombosis of intrahepatic branches of the portal vein is often induced by a hepatocellular carcinoma (see below).

Splenic Vein Thrombosis

Splenic vein thrombosis (SVT) may occur in a variety of pathologic conditions either in isolation or in conjunction with thrombosis involving other splanchnic veins [27]. The patency of the splenic vein should routinely be established in patients with suspected pathology of the pancreas and gastric vein varicosis [28]. Based on our experience the CFM is useful in SVT detection. SVT is documented by the absence of the color-coded flow at the level of the body of the pancreas and by visualization of collaterals in the proximity of the hilum of the spleen. In patients with incomplete obliteration of the splenic vein the upstream blood flow velocity in the proximity of the splenic hilus is in our experience often reduced, usually to less than 15 cm/s. In contrast to patients with portal hypertension, in whom splenomegaly is a common finding, it appears to be less frequent in patients with isolated, incomplete SVT.

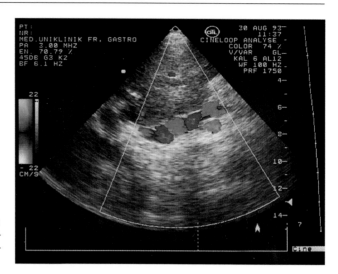

Fig. 13. Portal vein thrombosis. The changes from red to blue and vice versa are typical for the tortuous course of the collateral vessel corresponding to the so-called cavernous transformation

Thrombosis of the Superior Mesenteric Vein

Superior mesenteric vein thrombosis occurs in isolation or in conjunction with thrombosis of other splanchnic veins. It is often found in patients with identifiable coagulopathy and in those with a previous history of thrombosis [20]. The association between thrombosis of the superior mesenteric vein and pathology of the head of the pancreas mandates further diagnostic evaluations of this region when superior mesenterie vein thrombosis is detected. Experience in our laboratory shows that CFM is useful in the diagnosis of superior mesenteric vein thrombosis. Acute or subacute thrombosis of the SMV usually appears as an anechoic or hypoechoic cord on the B-mode image with absent Doppler and color-coded flow on the CFM. The consequences of superior mesenteric vein thrombosis are more serious than those of splenic vein thormbosis, and it often results in intestinal ischemia, necrotizing enterocolitis, and peritonitis. Only if collateral flow mitigates mesenteric congestion and prevents intestinal necrosis can larger collaterals be observed in the chronic stage mimicking the superior mesenteric vein. However, the normally smooth curvilinear course of these vessels is often interrupted to follow a tortuous trajectory toward the hepatic porta.

Budd-Chiari Syndrome, Hepatic Veno-occlusive Disease

The etiology of Budd-Chiari syndrome and of hepatic veno-oclusive disease and the associated duplex findings have been reviewed [30–32]. As portal hypertension is present in these patients, the portal circulation must be checked according to the criteria presented above. In the case of an acute *complete* Budd-Chiarj syndrome no flow is detectable in the hepatic veins, and the flow direction in the portal branches is reversed. After a few days the thrombosis is recognized in the B-mode ultrasound as an echogenic material filling the enlarged hepatic veins. However, it should be noted that an incomplete and chronic Budd-Chiari syndrome is much more frequent than the complete obstruction of the hepatovenous outflow. Slow blood flow in the portal vein [33], unusual tortuosity of the hepatic veins, intrahepatic hepatovenous shunts from right to left or vice versa, and a markedly increased flow velocity in the remaining still patent hepatic veins near the confluence with the inferior vena cava can often be recognized (Fig. 14). Hepatovenous outflow obstruction located directly at the confluence with inferior vena and caused by a membrane („web") is characterized by intrahepatic dilatation of the hepatic veins, absence of pulsatile flow pattern, and highly turbulent flow at the stenosis, with maximum flow velocity exceeding at least 150 cm/s. Especially in this case is CFM the method of choice for diagnosis and follow-up after catheter dilatation (Fig. 15).

In patients with veno-oclusive disease the hemodynamics of the large hepatic veins may be regular. In these cases diagnosis by CFM is difficult and requires concomitant examination of the hepatic arteries [34]. Only in severe cases are the findings prominent, corresponding to those in liver fibrosis (see above). The examination shows

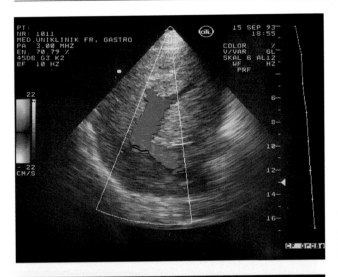

Fig. 14. Chronic Budd-Chiari syndrome. From a right lateral view the dilated right hepatic vein changes its direction and drains to the caudate lobe

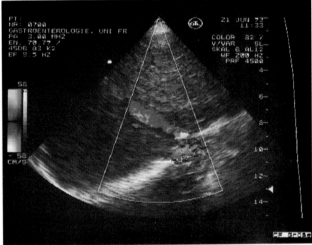

Fig. 15. Chronic Budd-Chiari syndrome. The highly turbulent flow at the junction to the inferior vena cava corresponds to the membranous stenosis caused by a „web," which was confirmed by angiography. After dilation using a 12 mm balloon catheter portal pressure gradient decreased by 50%

the signs of portal hypertension with a reversed or bidirectional flow pattern and/or decrease in the volumetric flow rates in the portal vein [30], but regional flow acceleration in the hepatic veins typical for liver cirrhosis is absent. Only the sudden onset of symptoms and patient's history (e.g., chemotherapy with dacarbazine for malignant melanoma, history of bone marrow transplantation) lead to the diagnosis, which must be confirmed by biopsy and histologic examination. However, hepatic graft-versus-host disease after bone marrow transplantation may result in similar changes of hepatic perfusion, and cannot be reliably differentiated from veno-occlusive disease despite of some differences in arterial blood flow, for example, an elevated Pourcelot index (resistive index, RI) in patients with veno-occlusive disease [34]. Hepatic storage diseases and amyloidosis can mimic veno-occlusive disease and liver fibrosis. Occasionally, high blood flow velocity (> 30 cm/s) along the whole course of the hepatic veins and loss of pulsatility are observed.

Tricuspid Insufficiency and Congestive Heart Failure

In patients with tricuspid incompetence or congestive heart failure the intrahepatic veins are typically dilated. The blood flow pattern in the portal vein suggestive of congestive heart faillure includes monophasic pulsatile forward flow with maximum flow velocity during ventricular diastole, rarely reversed flow during systole, biphasic pancyclic forward flow [35], and increased pulsatility [36]. Increased flow pulsatility in the portal vein [37] and markedly decreased maximum forward

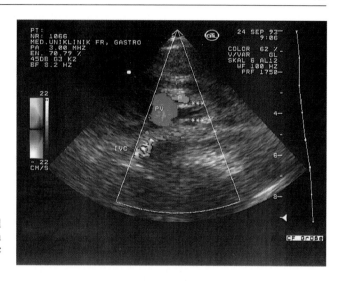

Fig. 16. Thrombosis of a proximal splenorenal shunt (***). Color signals are detected only from the portal vein (*PV, blue*), superior mesenteric artery (*A, red*), and inferior vena cava (*IVC*)

systolic flow velocity or systolic flow reversal in the hepatic vein [28] appear to be associated with tricuspid incompetence. In a few patients systolic backflow results in a pulsatile flow profile in the superior mesenteric and splenic veins. However, in contrast to patients with arterioportal shunts due to large hemangiomas or hepatocelluar carcinoma the flow direction remains in most cases hepatopetal throughout the entire length of the cardiac cycle.

Portosystemic Shunts

Compared to simple duplex imaging CFM allows a faster and more reliable determination of patency of the portosystemic shunts (Fig. 16). In addition, CFM appears superior in assessing the patency of the distal splenorenal shunts and in evaluations of shunt anastomoses [11]. Based on our experience a partial shunt obstruction should be suspected when the maximum flow velocity within the shunt lumen exceeds 200 cm/s (normal range established in our laboratory: 50–150 cm/s). However, quantitative Doppler measurements within the shunt lumen can be difficult at times due to the presence of local hematomas, deep and tortuous shunt position, or echogenicity of the walls of the synthetic grafts. In these patients it is preferable to measure shunt flow upstream in the afferent vessel. Here, the blood flow pattern typically fluctuates and undulates with respiration: based on standards in our laboratory the expected minimum volumetric flow rate exceeds 500 ml/min in distal splenorenal

shunts and 1 000 ml/min in the other portosystemic shunt types.

In our patients following a succesful shunt implantation reducing portal hypertension is reflected by disappearance of preoperatively documented flow in the paraumbilical vein. The exception to this observation appears to be the splenorenal shunt. Here, adequate shunt function appears to be consistent with flow reduction of 50 % in the umbilical vein. Figures 6 and 7 represent some of the typical CFM findings in patients with portosystemic shunts. Recently, a nonoperative technique for the treatment of portal hypertension has been developed (for review see [12]), the so-called transjugular intrahepatic portosystemic stent-shunt. Portal hemodynamics associated with these stent-shunts (diameter about 1 cm) are characterized by high flow in the portal vein (maximum flow velocity: > 30 cm/s; flow: 1.5–2 l/min) and maximum flow velocities up to 150 cm/s within the stent (Fig. 8). Shunt insufficiency due to intima hyperplasia in the draining hepatic vein is accompanied by a decrease in portal and shunt flow below 1 l/min. In some cases where the whole shunt body is continuously visualized by CFM the portosystemic pressure gradient can be estimated from the shunt maximum flow velocity according to Bernoulli's formula ($4 \times V^2$). Thus, maximum flow velocity exceeding 200 cm/s corresponds to a gradient of more than 15 mmHg and indicates significant shunt stenosis.

Liver Transplantation

In the case of poor liver function after liver transplantation (low bile production, high bilirubin, high serum transaminases) not only the arterial but also the portal blood supply should be checked. As a rule the maximum flow velocity in the portal vein should be greater than 30 cm/s, as in a normal genuine organ. The CFM has become the method of choice to exclude portal vein thrombosis or high-grade stenosis at the anastomosis. The signs of Budd-Chiari syndrome can be observed if the cranial anastomosis with the vena cava inferior is too narrow or thrombosed. Graft rejection may be accompanied by a decrease in portal perfusion and by loss of pulsatility in the hepatic veins while changes in arterial blood flow are inconstant.

Portal Venous Gas

A very rare but characteristic phenomenon can be observed by CFM when gas bubbles are transported along the portal vessels. This phenomenon, termed portal venous gas, occurs in anaerobic necrotizing enterocolitis, toxic megacolon in ulcerative colitis, after the use of a Sengtaken balloon to stop bleeding from esophageal varices, and after excessive bowel dilatation by gas. The CFM examination shows bright spots moving together with the bloodstream, and the frequency spectrum appears coarser than normal (Fig. 17). This corresponds to the acoustic impression of short metallic-clear tones similar to that coming from gas bubbles within the bowel. In severe cases the gas bubbles can be observed directly in the B-mode image together with gas accumulation at the venous confluence and in the periphery of the liver.

Arteriovenous Fistulas

Arteriovenous fistulas and shunts are due to congenital abnormalities, for example, Osler-Rendu-Weber disease, to stub injuries with penetration of the liver (Fig. 18), rarely to laparoscopic liver biopsy (Fig. 19), but in most cases to hepatocellular carcinoma (see below). In only a few cases does arterioportal shunting contribute significantly to portal hypertension.

Upper Abdominal Arteries

The indications for a CFM examination of the celiac trunk and its branches and the superior and inferior mesenteric arteries include those presented above ("Portal System"). Stenoses near the origin from the aorta can be confirmed or excluded if abdominal angina is suspected. CFM examination of the upper abdominal arteries before a transjugular intrahepatic portosystemic stent-shunt (see "Portal System") to exclude significant stenosis of the hepatic arteries or the celiac trunk makes angiography unnecessary. In the first days after liver transplantation the arterial blood supply of the graft should be checked by CFM.

Examination Technique

The examination begins by locating the celiac trunk at its origin from the abdominal aorta. The longitudinal transducer orientation facilitates separation from the superior mesenteric artery. In a transverse transducer orientation the proximal segments of the common hepatic artery and the splenic artery can be visualized. The hepatic artery and the superior mesenteric artery can be imaged in their long axis left parallel to the portal vein and the superior mesenteric vein, respectively (see "Portal System: Examination Technique").

The ultrasonographer should be familiar with the common arterial variations of the upper abdominal arteries [39]. In particular, the common origin of the celiac trunk and the superior mesenteric artery in the celiacomesenterial trunk should be recognized. In this anomaly high blood flow with accompanying flow disturbance are frequently demonstrated on CFM. Also the anomalous origin of the right or common hepatic artery from the superior mesenteric artery may pose a differential diagnostic puzzle to an unsuspecting examiner. Knowledge of normal Doppler flow patters is important to assess pathology [26].

Pathologic Findings

Celiac Trunk and Superior Mesenteric Artery

Stenoses of the celiac trunk and those up to approximately 5 cm from the origin in the superior mesenteric artery can, in our experience be reli-

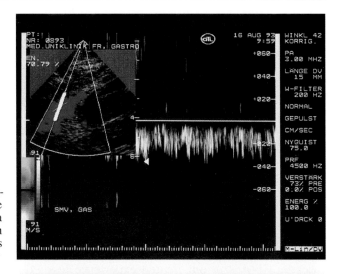

Fig. 17. Portal venous gas in the superior mesenteric vein after esophageal balloon tamponade and mesenteric emphysema. In this patient with a minor content of gas bubbles, detected neither in B-mode nor in CFM, the frequency spectrum is coarser than normal, indicating its high sensitivity

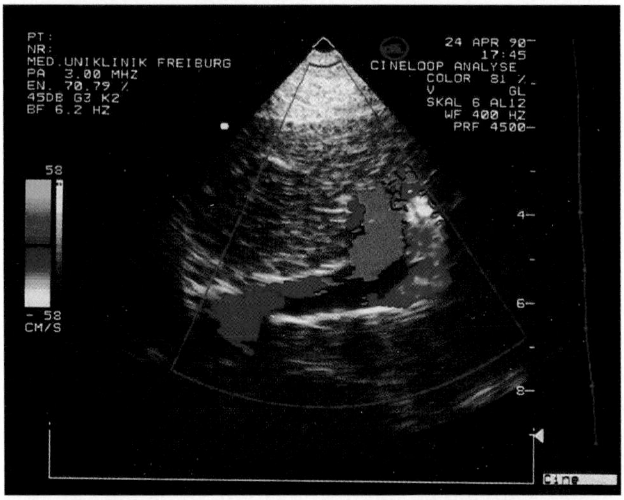

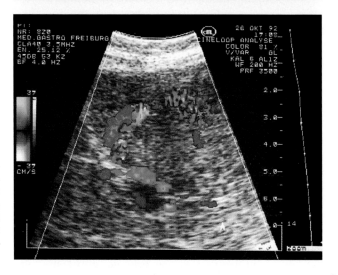

Fig. 18. Arterioportal fistula (*white*) from the left hepatic artery to the left main portal vein due to a stub injury with penetration of the left liver lobe near the falciform ligament (transverse transducer orientation). The slight hepatofugal blood flow in the left main branch oft the portal vein indicates that the fistula has some hemodynamic significance

Fig. 19. Arterioportal fistula after multiple laparoscopic liver biopsies in the left liver lobe (transverse section). As indicated by the different color the blood flow in the afferent artery (*red*) has the opposite derection compared to that in the portal branch (*blue*). Hepatofugal portal blood flow is observed down to the left main branch of the portal vein

ably confirmed or excluded by CFM examination. A hallmark of hemodynamically significant stenosis that has been advocated is a V_{max} greater than 300 cm/s [40]. The increase in V_{max} can be less in long, complex lesions. In these patients CFM typically reveals a highly turbulent flow pattern. Less pronounced turbulent color-coded flow pattern at the origin of the upper abdominal arteries often represents complex flow at branch points and should not be confused with a poststenotic flow field. Although proximal stenoses are usually atherosclerotic, obstructions resulting from mechanical compression from carcinoma of the body of the pancreas or enlarged lymph nodes should also be considered.

Detection of distal superior mesenteric artery stenoses by CFM is in our limited experience less consistent. A pronounced downstream decrease in the RI can raise suspicion of an upstream stenosis. However, the sensitivity of this sign, when present, has not been established.

In an occlusion of the celiac trunk the arterial blood is supplied to the liver via the arcades of the pancreatic arteries and the gastroduodenal artery. Blood flow in the common hepatic artery may be reversed under these circumstances. Proximal occlusions of the superior mesenteric artery are documented by the absence of the color-coded signal on the CFM. A concomitant increase in compensatory flow with a prominent diastolic flow component in the inferior mesenteric artery and the celiac trunk has been observed in our laboratory in several patients with this rare pathology.

Based on examinations in our laboratory the normal values for V_{max}, RI, and volumetric flow rates (VFR) in the celiac trunk and superior mesenteric artery are: V_{max}=100–200 cm/s and 70–180 cm/s; RI=0.6–0.75 and above 0.80 (fasting); VFR= 600 ± 100 ml/min and 500 ± 100 ml/min (fasting). However, the blood flow to the intestine is subject to a great number of intrinsic factors, including metabolic, myogenic and extrinsic (e.g. nervous system), hormone, and drug-regulatory variables [7, 41], thus making meaningful and reproducible measurements difficult. The ability to increase the blood flow in response to a meal has been considered a means to determine the reactivity of the splanchnic arterial circulation [42, 43]. However, due to complexity of postprandial hemodynamics the clinical utility of this test remains uncertain [44]. An increase in diastolic blood flow in the mesenteric arteries is observed in inflammatory bowel disease independently of its origin, in peri-

tonitis, in graft-versus-host disease after bone marrow transplantation, and in patients with subtotal stenosis or occlusion of the distal aorta.

Hepatic and Splenic Arteries

Duplex [26, 45] and more recently CFM [46] have been advocated primarily to establish patency of the hepatic artery in liver transplant recipients. Hepatic artery thrombosis represents the most common vascular complication after liver transplantation and requires prompt retransplantation [46]. The occlusion is characterized by the absence of arterial blood flow in the liver and the hepatic artery. Sometimes a biphasic oscillating flow profile proximal to the anastomosis is observed. Relevant stenosis of the anastomosis may be accompanied downstream by low systolic and relatively high diastolic flow velocity (RI <0.5). As mentioned above, the CFM examination should also be extended to the portal, hepatovenous, and caval circulation. At very high perfusion due to excessive splenomegaly (> 2 l/min) arterial blood flow in the graft may be very low and difficult to detect, especially in the right liver lobe.

CFM checks after liver transplantation include:

– Hepatic artery and its intrahepatic branches
– Portal vein (V_{max} >30 cm/s), intrahepatic branches
– Hepatic veins (pulsatile flow, no dilatation)
– Inferior vena cava (no congestion, no stenosis)
– Iliac veins (no congestion)

Pathologic arterial flow pattern with high flow velocities and low RI values arise if intrahepatic arteriovenous shunts are present. Occasionally these shunts arise after a stub injury penetrating the liver or after biopsy, and rarely may be responsible for portal hypertension.

Splenic artery stenoses are of less clinical importance with the exception of when they are detected in patients with pancreas transplantation [47]. In these patients an increased RI (higher than 0.7) is highly correlated with episodes of rejection.

An extremely tortuous course of the splenic artery occasionally mimics the CFM findings associated with splenic artery aneurysm. In contrast, aneurysms, pseudoaneurysms, and mesenteric fistulas may simulate B-mode findings of a

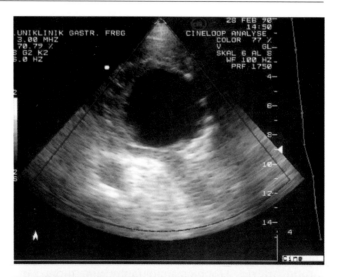

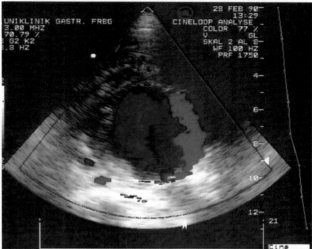

Fig. 20 a,b. Pseudoaneurysm of the splenic artery. **a** In a patient with chronic pancreatitis a pseudocyst was diagnosed by B-mode sonography. After an episode of gastrointestinal bleeding no bleeding source was identified endoscopically. **b** Color Doppler flow mapping examination revealed a circular pulsatile blood flow and confirmed the diagnosis of pseudoaneurysm

pseudocyst of the pancreas. Distinction is easily made, however, by CFM, where a circular blood flow in the presumed pseudocyst is documented (Fig. 20).

Renal Arteries

The indications for a CFM study of the renal vasculature are: renal artery stenosis, renal artery occlusion, renal vein thrombosis, arteriovenous fistula, acute renal failure, and monitoring of renal transplant.

Examination Technique

The entire course of both renal arteries should be examined. In the majority of patients it is not feasible to examine their entire length from an anterior approach. To aid in the examination of the hilar segments of the renal arteries its intrarenal posterior and anterior branches, and the segmental, interlobar, and arcuate arteries, the lateral approach with the patient in the contralateral decubitus positon via the renal parenchyma is recommended [47]. To document pathology the proximal, central, and caudal segmental arteries along with the interlobar arteries which ascend perpendicularly to the renal capsule should be examined.

Examination of the renal veins begins laterally. First, the parallel course of the interlobar and segmental veins to the corresponding is evaluated. Subsequently the course of renal veins is followed medially. The examiner should be familiar with common anatomic variants and typical Doppler flow findings [48, 49].

Pathologic Findings

Renal Artery Stenosis

Renal artery stenosis (RAS) is an important and treatable cause of systemic hypertension [50, 51]. Due its ability reliably to detect stenoses in the carotid arteries Doppler sonography and more recently CFM have been proposed as means to exclude hemodynamically significant RAS in patients with systemic hypertension. A significant RAS has been reported to be present based on the decrease in volumetric flow rates, changes in spectral Doppler flow characteristics, increase in maximum flow velocity, and the ratio of peak renal artery to aortic velocities (for review see [49], as well as changes in acceleration characteristics of the flow pulse, when the translumbar approach is used [52]. A simple differentiation of the degree of stenosis is presented in Table 1. Despite high rates for both sensitivity and specifity, between 83% and 97% [53–58], routine screening for renovascular systemic hypertension by Doppler sonographic methods seems to be questionable due to the low (3%) prevalence of renal vascular hypertension [59, 60]. Even at a presumed sensitivity and specifity of 95% a false-positive diagnosis would be expected in more than 50% of patients [61]. Therefore, the CFM examination should be used in selected patients with medical history, clinical examination (stenotic sound in 50% [53]), and suboptimal response to medical treatment, all suggestive of RAS. The reliability of RAS detection also appears to be determined by the experience and skill of the operator as well as the pathologic substrate, i.e., location of the stenosis and the presence of accessory renal arteries. Therefore, unequivocal recommendations regrading the utility in suspected vasculogenic renal hypertension depend on the individual experience and preferences of the examiner at this stage [62–64].

Based on our experience proximal stenoses of the renal artery located close to the origin from the abdominal aorta can be reliably detected by the CFM based on peak velocity (in our laboratory $V_{max} > 200$ cm/s), loss of the systolic window, and/or color-coded flow turbulence criteria (Fig. 21). However, the increase in V_{max} and in the intensity of the turbulence is highly dependent not only on the severity but also on the geometry of the lesions. For example, in our experience the increase in V_{max} is often less and the intensity of turbulence higher in long complex lesions. The detection of more distal lesions depends on the operator's ability to interrogate the distal course of the vessel. In some patients in whom continuous visualization of the renal arteries is not feasible a marked peripheral decrease in the RI may be indicative of an upstream, hemodynamically significant stenosis. The stenosis in an accessory renal artery is often detected only by segmental differences in the RI. As the ratio between systolic and end-diastolic flow velocity depends on aortic systolic and diastolic blood pressure, extrarenal factors such as heart rate, total peripheral resistance, and aortic compliance affect the RI. Therefore, changes in the RI in comparison to the contralateral kindney, to segments of the same side, or along the course of the vessel are more reliable than its absolute value. An RI smaller than 0.5 („normal range": 0.6–0.7), however, is highly suspect for an upstream RAS.

Table 1. CFM criteria for renal artery stenosis (RAS)

	normal	Ineffective RAS	Effective RAS
Maximum flow velocity (cm/s)	<150	<200	>200
Turbulence	No	Little	Loss of systolic window
Peripheral decrease in RI	<10%	<10%	>10% (not obligate)

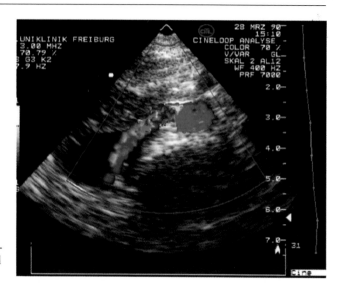

Fig. 21. Renal artery stenosis. Turbulent flow is visualized (*green*) at the origin of the right renal artery from the aorta (*red*) in a transverse view

Renal Artery Occlusion

Absence of renal blood flow may be secondary to thromboembolic or traumatic occlusion. Depending on the site of the embolization or thrombosis the renal blood flow ceases completely or segmentally. Acutely the B-mode image may appear normal. Absence of flow should therefore be confirmed by lack of color filling of the renal artery and/or its branches. In some patients with collaterals to the renal capsula retrograde poorly pulsatile flow within the interlobular arteries is observed. In patients with chronic renal failure and small fibrotic kidneys the renal artery blood flow may be very low, making a distinction to an occlusion difficult.

Renal Vein Occlusion

Ten years ago Doppler techniques were proposed to assess patients with renal vein thrombosis (RVT) [65]. Reduction in blood flow velocity in the central segments of the renal veins resulted in a moderate sensitivity (85%) and specificity (56%). Using CFM the diagnosis of renal vein thrombosis has become more reliable. The CMF findings depend on the site, extent, and age of the thrombosis. Complete acute thrombosis near the renal hilum is characterized by the absence of venous flow signals in the context of a bidirectional arterial flow. Thereby the time course of the retrograde flow velocity during the diastole exhibits a sigmoid pattern (Fig. 22). The B-mode image shows findings similar to those accompanying urinary tract obstruction with dilated renal veins. Based on our experience in patients with chronic renal vein thrombosis a low, predominantly systolic flow in the ipsilateral renal artery and a residual perfusion of the renal parenchyma are usually present. Depending on whether the segmental veins are involved the thrombotic process or not, irregular segmental veins may be observed which are not accompanied by segmental arteries. The flow in the renal vein compared to the flow in the inferior vena cava lacks pulsatility and respiratory variation. CFM often also reveals collaterals originating at the renal hilum, the left testicular and ovarian veins. In some patients it is difficult to distinguish between compression of the (left) renal vein, for example, by enlarged paracaval lymphatic nodules, and central thrombosis as flow velocity is decreased and collaterals can develop under both conditions.

Arteriovenous Fistulas

Arteriovenous renal parenchymal fistulas, for example, as a result of biopsy, can be recognized on the CFM based on localized flow turbulence at the site of the fistula. Rarely, a marked decrease in the RI and increased flow velocities in the supplying artery and arterialization of the venous efferent limb indicate significant arteriovenous shunting [48].

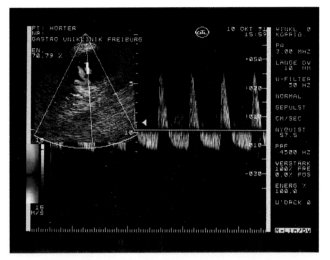

Fig. 22. Acute vein thrombosis in a renal transplant. Systolic antegrade flow is followed by an retrograde flow during the diastole as shown in the frequency spectrum

Renal Transplant

Vascular causes of a posttransplant renal failure include renal artery or vein occlusion and stenosis, and renal vascular acute allograft rejection [49]. CFM has some advantages over scintigraphic procedures and is now the method of choice to monitor transplant perfusion. The examination technique and normal Doppler flow signals in the transplant's vasculature have been described [49]. The sonographer should attempt to visualize the entire course of both the artery and the vein in its long axis. Several sonographic criteria have been used successfully to identify the transplant's renal artery stenoses, including a direct visualization of the stenotic lumen, perivascular artifacts around the stenotic lumen, spectral broadening, increase in peak flow velocity, and auditory impression of turbulence [67, 68]. It should be noted that an increase in flow velocity to more than 200 cm/s due to sharp bending does not necessarily indicate hemodynamically significant stenosis in contrast to atherosclerotic lesions in the native renal arteries (Table 1). Detection of arterial and venous thrombotic occlusions based on the absence of Doppler and/or color-coded flow signals (for review see [49, 68]) or on the presence of a retrograde arterial flow during diastole [69], as described above (complete acute renal vein thrombosis), have proven highly reliable.

The ability of duplex and CFM imaging to detect acute vascular rejection based mainly on an increase in the RI due to the presumably high impedance circulation in immunologically induced acute proliferative vasculitis has been proposed by some investigators [70, 71] but refuted by others [72]. Based on a large number of examinations it appears that an increased RI indeed frequently accompanies episodes of acute vascular rejections; however, it can also be associated with other vascular and nonvascular graft complications [73]. In the absence of venous congestion a sharp increase in RI within a few days from below 0.7 to above 0.9 can be considered as specific for vascular rejection.

Abdominal Aorta, Vena Cava Inferior, and Blood Vessels of the Pelvis

Only a limited experience has been accumulated in CFM diagnosis of abdominal aortic, inferior vena cava, and pelvic vascular pathology. Therefore predictions of the clinical utility of CFM in this vascular territory would be premature and speculative.

Based on our preliminary experience CFM is able to visualize both abdominal aortic aneurysms and dissections. In the former a clear distinction between the patent lumen with a disturbed flow pattern and hypoechoic intraluminal thrombus is possible (Fig. 23). In the latter the patent or thrombosed true and false lumen have also been successfully identified. In these patients blood flow in the true and the false lumen can be documented to be out of phase. Similarly, our early experience suggests that CFM might become useful in the identification of abdominal aortic stenoses and occlusions based on an stenotic increase in flow velocity (normal values in our laboratory:

60–140 cm/s), the loss of the systolic window and turbulent color-coded flow pattern. In patients with a high-grade subtotal stenosis and occlusions the upstream flow velocity is low and the flow pattern bidirectional, whereas downstream typically no flow signal can be recorded. In the presence of distal aortic occlusion CFM frequently identifies the presence of dilated collaterals with a prominent diastolic flow, for example, the superior mesenteric artery.

Based on initial experience stenoses, occlusions, and aneurysms (Fig. 24) of the pelvic arteries can also be documented by CFM similarly to those in other vascular territories. A consistent and accurate quantitation of the grades of the stenoses, however, appears more difficult due to the often suboptimal incidence angle of the Doppler beam. The value of CFM in diagnosis of patients with a suspected vasculogenic impotence [74, 75] is currently under evaluation.

Thromboses of the inferior vena cava and those of the common, external, and internal iliac veins have been successfully visualized by CFM in several patients with this disorder studied in our laboratory (Fig. 25). Thrombosis of the inferior vena cava is visualized as a hypoechoic cord with an absent color-coded intraluminal flow. Upstream to the thromboses the blood flow is slow; downstream it shows reduced respiratory variation and loss of the normal pulsatile pattern. In patients with invasive malignant processes such as hypernephroma and leiomyosarcoma it is not possible to distinguish clearly between tumor and thrombus. The examination of patients with thrombosis of the inferior vena cava should include the search for the presence of collateral circulation. It is often possible to document epigastric inferior and the ascending lumbar veins with the cranially directed blood flow and the testicular or ovarian veins with the caudally directed blood flow. The large lumbar veins are occasionally confused with the persistent left inferior vena cava which drains the left lower extremity. In patients with a suspected thrombosis of the internal iliac veins a comparison of the findings with the contralateral vessel often aids the diagnosis. Stenoses of the inferior vena cava have been recognized in a few patients based on a increased flow velocity (V_{max}=150 cm/s) and the presence of turbulence in the color-coded flow map. However, an undue pressure of the transducer can simulate stenosis and must be avoided. In patients after liver transplantation significant stenosis at the caval anasto-

moses is suspected if there is congestion of the inferior vena cava and renal and iliac veins. Stenosis of the proximal anastomosis can be differentiated from the caudal one by CFM considering the concomitant effects on portal and arterial liver perfusion. CMF findings characteristic of a Budd-Chiari syndrome (see above) lead to the diagnosis of a problem with the proximal anastomosis. For therapeutic consequences the diagnosis should be confirmed or excluded immediately by radiologic evaluation (transfemoral cavography).

Tumor Vessels

An increase in flow velocities due to arteriovenous anastomoses in patients with hepatocellular carcinoma [76, 77] and hypernephroma [49] has been documented by duplex sonography. More recently, several vascular patterns on CFM have been proposed to indicate the presence of hepatocellular carcinoma [78]. Based on our experience presently available CFM technology does not allow a systematic evaluation of vessels smaller than 1 mm in diameter. However, it is these arteries which are felt to be pathologic arteries detected indirectly on CFM images based on regional flow accelerations in parenchymal veins. However, these findings are nonspecific, and liver cirrhosis must also be excluded. Arteries are either of low resistance and low RI (Fig. 26) or high resistance and high RI (Fig. 27) [76]. Probably the most specific sign of hepatocellular carcinoma not visible in the B-mode image is the gross regional difference in arterial blood flow. High diastolic flow in an afferent artery (low resistance) and retrograde, fequently pulsatile flow in the branch of the portal vein can be interpreted as indirect signs of multiple parenchymal arterioportal shunts. However, absence of pathologic arteries detectable by CFM does not exclude the presence of a hepatocullular carcinoma [79]. In patients with liver hemangiomas the flow within the arteriovenous shunts is usually slow and frequently evade Doppler sonographic detection, with the exception of giant hemangiomas associated with a prominent diastolic flow in the supplying artery. Blood supply of benign tumors of the liver such as hepatic adenoma and focal nodular hyperplasia is of arterial origin: however, these lesions cannot be reliably differentiated from hepatocellular carcinoma by CFM despite typical

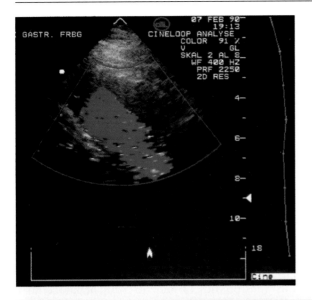

Fig. 23. Thrombosed abdominal aortic aneurysm. The patent lumen is visualized (*blue*) whereas the thrombosed lumen is hypoechoic, and there is no flow signal

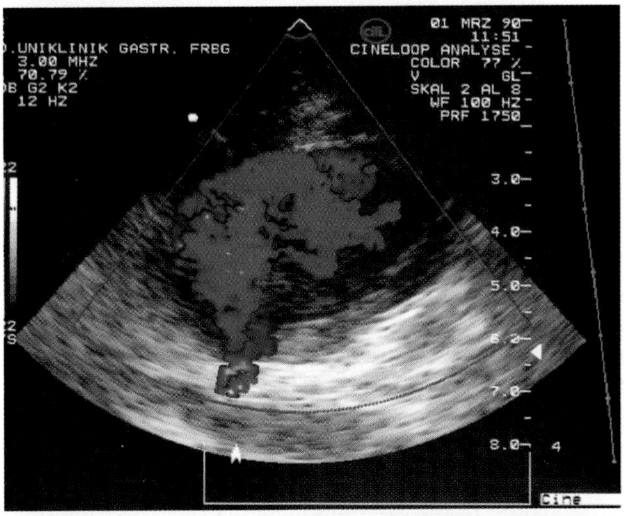

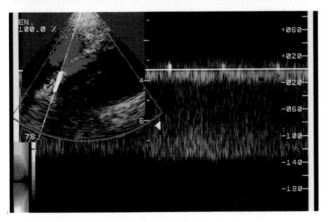

Fig. 24. False aneurysm of the right external illiac artery at end-systole. Following a routine coronary angiography in this patient a pulsatile tumor in the right groin was shown by color Doppler flow mapping to be a pseudeoaneurysm. An arteriovenous fistula was excluded because the blood left the pseudoaneurysm during diastole by the same path as it entered during systole

Fig. 25. Distal thrombosis of the inferior vena cava. The blood of the left renal is drained via the partially thrombosed cranial portion of the inferior vena cava

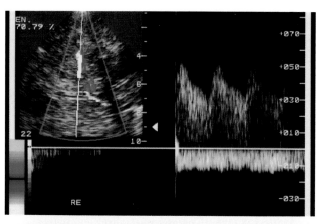

Fig. 26. Intrahepatic artery with a high diastolic blood flow. In a patient with hepatocellular carcinoma retrograde hepatofugal flow in the accompanying branch of the portal vein was observed, thus indicating an arterioportal shunting as demonstrated by Doppler

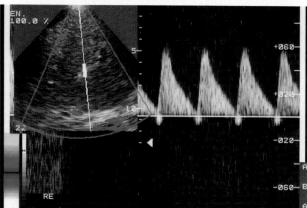

Fig. 27. Intrahepatic artery with a diminished diastolic blood flow. In a patient with hepatocellular carcinoma the end-diastolic flow velocity normally accounting for approximately 30 % of the systolic flow velocity was absent due to increased peripheral resistance

findings due to arterioportal shunting in patients with this carcinoma [79–81]. Perfusion of metastases is usually low and cannot be analyzed sufficiently by CFM at present [76, 78].

Summary

CFM is a novel ultrasonic method for assessing the intra-abdominal and pelvic vascular pathology. The method represents an extension of the well-established principles of duplex sonography to a planar color-coded flow mapping. Although new and presently subject to extensive ongoing clinical evaluations, the CFM technology holds great promise in the noninvasive diagnosis of diseases involving the intra-abdominal vasculature. Compared to duplex imaging, identification of the intra-abdominal and pelvic vessels is faster and more complete: visualization of both large tortuous and small parenchymal vessels is facilitated and greatly enhanced. Initial clinical results indicate that CFM will likely become the leading sonographic modality in the noninvasive diagnosis of a variety of gastrointestinal, renal, and pelvic vascular disorders. However, determination of its ultimate diagnostic value in each of the individual fields awaits the results of more extensive clinical experience in a greater number of medical centers. Improved flow sensitivity and quantitative flow mapping should further enhance the relevance of CFM in the abdominal and pelvic vascular diagnostics in the future. Transpulmonary ultrasound contrast agents may improve the sensitivity of flow mapping preferentially in smaller vessels [82].

References

1. Evens RG (1991) Doppler sonographic imaging of the vascular system. JAMA 265: 2382–2387
2. Goldberg BB (ed) (1984) Abdominal ultrasonography. J. Wiley & Sons, New York
3. Foley WD, Erickson SJ (1991) Color Doppler flow imaging. Amer J Roentgenol 156: 3–13

4. Taylor KJW, Burns PN, Wells PNT (eds.) (1988) Clinical applications of Doppler ultrasound. Raven Press, New York
5. Gill RW (1985) Measurement of blood flow by ultrasound: accuaracy and sources of error. Ultrasound Med Biol 11: 625–641
6. Wilson LS, Dadd MJ, Gill RW (1990) Automatic vessel tracking and measurement for Doppler studies. Ultrasound Med Biol 16: 645–652
7. Kvietys PR, Barrowman JA, Granger DN (eds) (1987) Pathophysiology of splanchnic circulation. CRC Press, Boca Raton
8. Landwehr P, Schindler R, Heinrich U, Doelken W, Krahe T, Lackner K (1991) Quantification of vascular stenosis with color Doppler flow imaging: in vitro investigations. Radiology 178: 701–704
9. Sherlock S (1989) Diseases of the liver and biliary system. Blackwell Scientific Publications, Oxford, Chapter 10
10. Grant EG, Schiller VL, Millener P, Tessler FN, Perrella RR, Ragavendra N, Busuttil R (1992) Color imaging of the hepatic vasculature. AJR 159: 943–950
11. Grant EG, Tessler FN, Gomes AS, Holmes CL, Perrella RR, Duerinckx AJ, Busuttill RW (1990) Color Doppler imaging of portosystemic shunts. Amer J Roentgenol 154: 393–397
12. Haag K, Ochs A (1993) Transjugular intrahepatic portosystemic stent-shunt (TIPS) in the treatment of portal hypertension. Current Opinion in Gastroenterology 9: 435–440
13. Taylor KJW, Burns PN (1985) Duplex Doppler scanning in the pelvis and abdomen. Ultrasound Med Biol 11: 643–658
14. Zironi G, Gaiani S, Fenyves D, Rigamonti A, Bolondi L, Barbara L (1992) Value of measrement of mean portal flow velocity by Doppler flowmetry in the diagnosis of portal hypertension. J Hepatol 16: 298–303
15. Lafortune M, Marleau D, Breton G, Viallet A, Lavoie P, Huet P.-M (1984) Portal venous system measurements in portal hypertension. Radiology 151: 27–30
16. Ohnishi K, Saito M, Nakayama T, Iida S, Nomura F, Koen H, Oduda K (1985) Portal venous hemodynamics in chronic liver disease: effects of posture change and excercise. Radiology 155: 757–761
17. Moriyasu F, Nishida O, Ban N, Nakamura T, Sakai M, Miyake T, Uchido H (1986) „Congestion index"of the portal vein. Amer J Roentgenol 146: 735–739
18. Bolondi L, Gandolfi L, Arienti V, Caletti GC, Corcioni E, Gasbarrini. G, Labo G (1982) Ultrasonography in the diagnosis of portal hypertension: diminished response of portal vessels to respiration. Radiology 142: 167–171
19. Carlisle KM, Halliwell M, Read AE, Wells PNT (1992) Estimation of total hepatic blood flow by duplex ultrasound. Gut 33: 92–97
20. Haag K, Lanzer P (1991) Color Doppler Imaging of Abdominal Vessels. In: Lanzer P, Yoganathan A (eds) Vascular imaging by color doppler and magnetic resonance. 241–265 Springer Verlag Berlin, Heidelberg, New York
21. De Vries PJ, Van Hattum J, Hoekstra JBL, De Hooge P. Duplex Doppler measurements of portal flow in normal subjects. J Hepatol 1991; 13: 358–363
22. Kinoshita H, Sakai K, Kubo S, Yamazaki O (1989) Measurement of human portal blood flow by continuous thermodilution. J Surgical Res 46: 235–240
23. Zoli M, Marchesini G, Cordiani MR, Pisi P, Brunori A, Trono A, Pisi E (1986) Echo-Doopler measurement of splanchnic blood flow in control and cirrhotic subjects. J. Clin. Ultrasound 14: 429–435
24. Haag K, Weimann A, Zeller A, Spamer C, Sellinger M, Rössle M (1992) Milzgröße und duplexsonographisch bestimmter Blutfuß in der V. lienalis und der V. portae bei Lebercirrhose. Bildgebung (Imaging) 59: 80–83
25. Ralls PW (1990) Color Doppler sonography of the hepatic artery and portal venous system. Amer J Roetgenol 155: 517–525
26. Taylor KJW (1988) Gastrointestinal Doppler ultrasound. In: Taylor KJW, Burns PN, Wells PNT (eds) Clinical applications of Doppler ultrasound. Raven Press, New York p. 162–200
27. Vogelzang RL, Gore RM, Anschuetz SL, Blei AT (1988) Thrombosis of the splanchnic veins: CT diagnosis. Amer J Roetgenol 150: 93–96
28. Marn CS, Glazer GM, Williams DM, Francis IR (1990) CT-angiographic correlation of collateral venous pathways in isolated splenic vein occlusion: new observations. Radiology 175: 375–380
29. Harward TRS, Green D, Bergan JJ, (1989) Mesenteric vein thrombosis. J Vasc Surg 9: 328–333
30. Brown BP, Abu-Yousef M, Farmer R, LaBrecque D, Gingrich R (1990) Doppler sonography: a noninvasive method for evaluation of hepatic venooclusive disease. Amer J Roentgenol 154: 721–724
31. Stanley P (1989) Budd-Chiari syndrome. Radiology 170: 625–627
32. Grant EG, Perrella R, Tessler FN, Lois J, Busuttil R (1989) Budd-Chiari syndrome: the results of duplex and color Doppler imaging. Amer J Roentgenol 152: 377–381
33. Hosoki T, Kuroda C, Tokunoga K, Marukawa T, Masuike M, Kozuka T (1989) Hepatic venous outflow obstruction: evaluation with pulsed Duplex sonography. Radiology 170: 733–737
34. Herbetko J, Gripp AP, Buckley AR, Phillips GL (1992) Venoocclusive liver disease after bone marrow transplantation. Findigs at duplex sonography. AJR 158: 1001–1005
35. Duerinckx AJ, Grant EG, Perella RR, Szeto A, Tessler FN (1990) The pulsatile portal vein in cases of congestive heart failure: correlation of duplex Doppler findings with right atrial pressure. Radiology: 176: 655–658
36. Hosoki T, Arisawa J, Marukawa T, Tokunaga K, Kuroda C, Kozuka T, Nakano S (1990) Portal blood flow in congestive heart failure: pulsed duplex sonographic findings. Radiology 174: 733–736
37. Abu-Yousef MM, Milam SG, Farmer RM (1990) Pulsatile portal vein flow: a sign of tricuspid regurgitation on duplex Doppler sonography. Amer J Roentenol 155: 785–788

38. Abu-Yousef MM (1991) Duplex Doppler sonography of the hepatic vein in tricuspid regurgitation. Amer J Roentgenol 156: 79–83

39. Wenz W (1972) Abdominale Aniographie. Springer Verlag, Berlin

40. Seitz K, Kubale R (1988) Duplexsonographie der abdominalen und retroperitonealen Gefaesse. VCH, Weinheim

41. Granger DN, Richardson PDI, Kvietys PR, Mortillaro NA (1980) Intestinal blood flow. Gastroenterology 78: 837–863

42. Qamar MI, Read AE, Skidmore R, Evans JM, Wells PNT (1984) Transcutaneous Doppler ultrasound measurement of the superior mesenteric artery blood flow in man. Gut 27: 100–105

43. Moneta GL, Taylor DC, Helton WS, Mulholland MW, Strandness DE Jr (1988) Duplex ultrasound measurements of postprandial intestinal blood flow: effect of meal composition. Gastroenterology 95: 1294–1301

44. Taylor GA (1990) Blood flow in the superior mesenteric artery: estimation with Doppler US. Radiology 174: 15–16

45. Flint EW, Sumkin JH, Zajko AB, Bowen A (1988) Duplex sonography of hepatic artery thrombosis after liver transplantation. Amer J Roentgenol 151: 481–483

46. Hall TR, Diarmid S, Grant EG, Boechat M, Busuttil RW (1990) False-negative duplex Doppler studies in children with hepatic artery thrombosis after liver transplantation. Amer J Roentgenol 154: 573–575

47. Isikoff MB, Hill MC (1980) Sonography of the renal arteries: left lateral decubitus position. Amer J Roentgenol 134: 1177–1179

48. Lusza G (1963) X-ray anatomy of the vascular system. J.B. Lippincott Co. Philadelphia and Toronto

49. Rigsby CM, Burns PN, Taylor KJW (1988) Renal duplex sonography. In: Taylor KJW, Burns PN, Wells PNT (eds) Clinical applications of Doppler ultrasound. Raven Press, New York p. 201–245

50. Tegtmeyer CJ, Sos TA (1986) Techniques of renal angioplasty. Radiology 161: 577–586

51. McNeil BJ, Varady PD, Burrows BA, Adelstein SJ (1975) Measures of clinical efficacy: cost-effectiveness calculations in the diagnosis and treatment of hypertensive renovascular disease. N Engl J Med 293: 216–221

52. Handa N, Fukunaga R, Etani H, Yoneda S, Kimura K, Kamada T (1988) Efficacy of echo-Doppler examination for the evaluation of renovascular disease. Ultrasound Med Biol 14: 1–5

53. Distler A, Spies KP, Fobbe F (1992) Diagnostik der renovaskulären Hypertonie. Dt Ärzteblatt 89: Heft 11 A₁ 923–931

54. Haag K, Blum U, Gries P, Baumann S, Sellinger M, Spamer C (1992) Überlegenheit der Farbdopplersonographie bei der nicht-invasiven Diagnostik von Nierenarterienstenosen In: Anderegg A, Despland P, Henner H, Otto R (eds) Ultraschalldiagnostik '91, Springer Verlag Berlin Heidelberg New York, pp 131–134

55. Norris CS, Pfeiffer JS, Rittgers SE, Barnes RW (1984) Noninvasive evaluation of renal artery stenosis and renovascular resistance. J Vasc Surg 1: 192–201

56. Stavors AT, Parker SH, Yakes WF et al (1992) Segmental stenosis of the renal artery: pattern recognition of tardus and parvus abnormalities with duplex sonography. Radiology 184: 487–492

57. Taylor DC, Kettler MD, Moneta GL, Kohler TR, Kazmers A, Beach KW, Strandness DE (1988) Duplex ultrasound scanning in the diagnosis of renal artery stenosis: prospective evaluation. J Vasc Surg 7: 363–369

58. Zoller WG, Hermans H, Bogner JR, Hahn D, Middeke M (1990) Duplex sonography in the diagnosis of renovascular hypertension Klin. Wochenschr. 68: 830–334

59. Anderson G H, Blakeman N, Streeten DHP (1988) Prediction of renovascular hypertension: comparison of clinical diagnostic indices. Am. J. Hypertens 1: 301–304

60. Distler A, Köhler H. (1982) Angiopathien der Niere. In: Losse H, Renner E (eds) In: Klinische Nephrologie, vol II. Georg Thieme Verlag Stuttgart New York, 215–240

61. Pickerin TG (1991) Diagnosis and evaluation of renovascular hypertension. Indications for therapy. Circulation 83 (Suppl. 1): 147–154

62. Hansen KJ, Tribble RW, Reavis SW, Canzanello VJ, Craven TE, Plonk GW, Dean RH (1990) Renal duplex sonography: evaluation of clinical utility. J Vasc Surg 12: 227–236

63. Berland LL, Koslin B, Routh WD, Keller FS (1990) Renal artery stenosis: prospective evaluation of diagnosis with color duplex US compared with angiography. Radiology 174: 421–423

64. Dresberg AL, Pauschter DM, Lammert GK, Hale JC, Troy RB, Novick AC, Nally JV Jr, Weltevreden AM (1990) Renal artery stenosis: evaluation with color Doppler flow imaging. Radiology 177: 749–753

65. Avashi PS, Grenne ER, Scholler C, Fowler CR (1983) Noninvasive daignosis of renal vein thrombosis by ultrasonic echo-Doppler flowmetry. Kidney Int 23: 882–887

66. Middleton WD, Kellman GM, Melson GL, Madrazo BL (1989) Postbiopsy renal transplant arteriovenous fistulas: color doppler US characteristics. Radiology 171: 253–257

67. Taylor KJW, Morse SS, Rigsby CM, Bia M, Schiff M (1987) Vascular complications in renal allografts: detection with duplex Doppler US. Radiology 162: 31–38

68. Grenier N, Douws C, Morel D, Ferriere J-M, Guillou ML, Potaux L, Broussin J (1991) Detection of vascular comlications in renal allografts with color Doppler flow imaging. Radiology 178: 217–223

69. Kaveggia LP, Perella RR, Grant EG, Tessler FN, Rosenthal JT, Wilkinson A, Danovitch GM (1990) Duplex Doppler sonography in renal allografts: the significance of reversed flow in diastole. Amer J Roentgenol 155: 295–298

70. Rifkin MD, Nedleman L, Pasto ME, Kurtz AB, Foy PM, McGlynn E, Canico C, Baltarovich OH, Pennell RG, Goldberg BB (1987) Evaluatin of renal transplant rejection by duplex Doppler exami-

nation: value of the resistive index. Amer J Roentgenol 148: 759–762

71. Rigsby CM, Burns PN, Weltin GG, Chen B, Bia M, Taylor KJW (1987) Doppler signal quantitation in renal allografts: comparison in normal and rejecting transplants, with pathologic correlation. Radiology 162: 39–42

72. Drake DG, Day DL, Letourneau JG, Alford BA, Sibley RK, Mauer SM, Bunchman TE (1990) Doppler evaluation of renal transplants in children: a prospective study with histopathologic correlation. Amer J Roentgenol 154: 785–787

73. Warshauer DM, Taylor KJW, Bia MJ, Marks WH, Weltin GG, Rigsby CM, True LD, Lorber MI (1988) Unusual causes of increased vascular impedance in renal transplants: duplex Doppler evaluation. Radiology 169: 367–370

74. Paushter DM (1989) Role of duplex sonography in the evaluation of sexual impotence. Amer J Roentgenol 153: 1161–1163

75. Schwartz AN, Wang KY, Mack LA, Lowe M, Berger RE, Cyr DR, Feldman M (1989) Evaluation of normal erectile function with color flow Doppler sonography. Amer J Roentgenol 153: 1155–1160

76. Taylor KJW, Ramos I, Morse SS, Fortune KL, Hammers L, Taylor CR (1987) Focal liver masses: differential diagnosis with pulsed Doppler US. Radiology 164: 643–647

77. Taylor KJW, Ramos I, Carter D, Morse SS, Snower D, Fortune KL (1988) Correlation of Doppler US tumor signals with neovascular morphologic features. Radiology 166: 57–62

78. Tanaka S, Kitamura T, Fujita M, Nakanishi K, Okuda S (1990) Color Doppler flow imaging of liver tumors. Amer J Roentgenol 154: 509–514

79. Ohnishi K, Nomura F (1989) Ultrasonic Doppler studies of hepatocellular carcinoma and comparison with other hepatic focal lesions. Gastroenterology 97: 1489–1497

80. Tanaka S, Kitamra T, Fujita M, Kasugai H, Inoue A, Ishiguro S (1992) Small hepatocellular carcinoma: differentiation from adenomatous hyperplastic nodule with color Doppler flow imaging. Radiology 182: 161–165

81. Börner N, Brennecke R, Schild H, Meyer J (1988) Farbcodierte Dopplersonographie bei fokal nodulärer Hyperplasie. Ultraschall in Klinik und Praxis (Suppl 1): 16

82. Feinstein SB, Cheirif J, Ten Cate FJ, Silverman PR, Heidenreich PA, Dich C, Desir RM, Armstrong WF, Quinones MA, Shah PM (1990) Safety and efficacy of a new transpulmonary ultrasound contrast agent: initial multicenter clinical results. J Am Col Cardiol 16, 2: 316–324

Peripheral Vascular Ultrasonography

G. L. Moneta and J. M. Porter

Peripheral vascular ultrasonography as currently practiced involves the use of both continuous wave and duplex techniques. Both methods may be applied to the diagnosis of arterial and venous disorders and have achieved widespread clinical acceptance.

Arterial Applications

Continuous Wave Doppler

Vascular ultrasound began with application of the continuous wave Doppler to the diagnosis of arterial disease. Continuous wave based techniques are still the most frequently employed testing methods for extremity arterial occlusive disease in most noninvasive vascular laboratories.

Ankle Brachial Index

The use of the continuous wave Doppler in the determination of ankle brachial systolic blood pressure ratios (ABI) remains the single most useful noninvasive diagnostic test in the evaluation of peripheral artery occlusive disease. The ABI for each leg is determined with the patient supine. The highest brachial artery systolic pressure (left or right arm, whichever is greater) determined with a continuous wave Doppler is used as the reference pressure (denominator) in the ABI calculation. This is compared to the highest pressure measured at the ankle from the dorsalis pedis, posterior tibial, or peroneal positions in each leg. It is assumed that the brachial artery pressure is an accurate reflection of central aortic pressure, and that the arteries collapse appropriately in response to inflation of a blood pressure cuff. The ABI may be falsely elevated in patients with pressure reducing brachiocephalic occlusive disease (decreased denominator) or significant tibial artery calcification (increased numerator). A change in ABI between examinations of more than 0.15 is considered significant. While determination of an ABI cannot localize the site of a pressure reducing stenosis, the test has gained widespread acceptance as a simple, accurate and reproducible method of defining overall severity of arterial occlusive disease in a particular extremity (Table 1).

Exercise Testing

Doppler-determined pressures can be combined with treadmill exercise testing in the evaluation of patients with possible intermittent claudication. After determining a resting supine ABI the patient walks on a treadmill at a standardized incline and rate. The test lasts for 5 min or until claudication symptoms force the patient to stop. Time to onset and location of symptoms are recorded. At test completion the patient is immediately placed supine, and ABIs are calculated every 30 s until they have returned to baseline. A drop of 20% from the baseline level combined with appropriate ischemic symptoms is usually required to confirm a diagnosis of intermittent claudication [1]. The greater the drop in exercise-induced ABI and the longer the time required to return to baseline, the greater is the extent of the patients lower extremity arterial occlusive disease [2] (Fig. 1).

Table 1. Correlation of ankle brachial index (ABI) with clinical severity of arterial occlusive disease

ABI	Clinical correlation
1.1 ± 0.2	normal
0.6 ± 0.2	intermittent claudication
0.3 ± 0.1	Ischemic rest pain
0.1 ± 0.1	Impending tissue necrosis

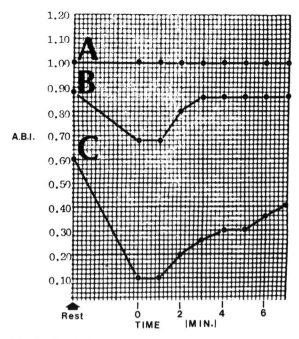

Fig. 1. Treadmill exercise test curves. *A,* Normal response to treadmill walking. *B,* Typical of a patient with mild to moderate intermittent claudication; the ankle brachial index *(ABI)* drops with exercise but returns rapidly to baseline after exercise. *C,* More severe disease. The resting ABI is lower and falls dramatically with exercise *(time O),* and recovery of pedal pressures is delayed. (From [1])

Segmental Pressures

Multiple pneumatic cuffs placed on the leg can be combined with Doppler-determined pressures and ABIs to determine arterial pressure in different segments of the limb in an effort to localize occlusive lesions. Usually four cuffs are used on each leg: (a) as proximal on the thigh as possible, (b) just above the knee, (c) immediately below the knee, and (d) just proximal to the malleoli [3]. Often the test is combined with qualitative analysis of Doppler analog waveforms.

The examination begins by placing a continuous wave Doppler probe over the most prominent Doppler signal at the ankle. The high-thigh cuff is inflated until the Doppler signal disapears. The cuff is slowly deflated, and the pressure at which there is return of an audible arterial signal is the high thigh pressure. Above-knee, below-knee, and ankle pressures are determined in a similar fashion and waveforms recorded from each site as well (Fig. 2).

While theoretically attractive, there are a number of potential problems and limitations in the interpretation of segmental limb pressures and/or waveforms. In practice waveform interpretation is almost always qualitative and provides little quantitative information. Pressures may be artifactually elevated by using too narrow cuffs (cuffs should be 20 % greater in width than the diameter of the limb at the point where they are applied) [4], or in the presence of calcific vessels. A 20 mmHg gradient between cuffs is indicative of significant intervening stenosis [5]. In patients with multilevel disease, however, diminished proximal pressures may mask more distal gradients. While a diminished high-thigh pressure ideally reflects impaired iliac artery inflow, similar findings may be produced by common femoral artery disease or by stenoses involving both the profunda femoris and the proximal superficial femoral artery. Additionally, it is not possible to distinguish between long- and short-segment occlusions or between vessels that are occluded from those that remain patent but highly stenotic. These limitations combined with the need in both atherosclerosis research and interventional radiology to precisely characterize lesions has led to the current intense interest in the application of duplex scanning to peripheral arteries.

Color Flow Duplex Scanning

Equipment/Personnel

Color flow duplex scanning (CFDS) facilitates duplex examination of the extremity vessels, particularly the iliac, tibial, pedal, and forearm arteries (Fig. 3). CFDS can be used to measure the length of arterial occlusions and identify the site of reconstitution of an occluded vessel (Fig. 4). While the color flow image is useful in identifying points of turbulence associated with arterial stenosis, it does not permit optimal quantification of degrees of stenosis [6]. Subocclusive levels of stenosis are best determined by velocity waveform analysis. The optimum use of CFDS applied to the extremity arteries is to identify the vessels and areas suspicious for stenosis with the color flow image and then quantify the stenosis into broad categories with spectral analysis.

Extremity CFDS requires a selection of transducers. For iliac vessels 2- or 3-MHz probes are usually best. Infrainguinal vessels can be exa-

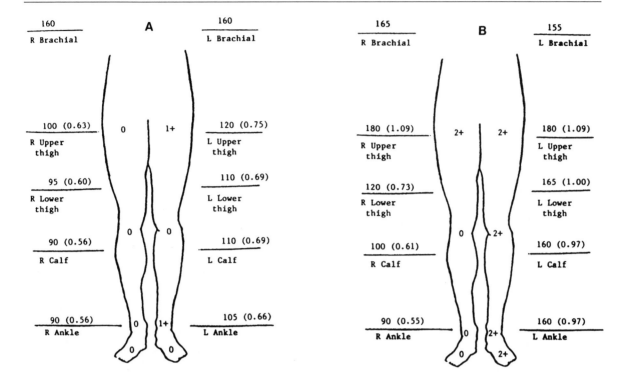

Fig. 2. Segmental limb pressures in patients with iso-lated aortoiliac disease (**A**) and right leg femoropopli-teal disease (**B**). Note that there is little subsequent drop in segmental pressure beyond the areas of hemo-dynamically significant disease. (From [1])

mined in all but the largest legs using a 5-MHz probe. Distal tibial vessels occasionally are best examined with 7.5- or 10-MHz transducers [7]. Angle correction is a practical necessity in ex-tremity arterial CFDS. Not all vessels can be in-sonated at the ideal 60° angle. Angles between 30° and 70° can, however, almost always be obtained and provide information sufficiently accurate for clinical usefulness.

Technique

Lower extremity arterial CFDS includes examina-tion of the aorta, iliac, common and superficial fe-moral, and popliteal arteries and, when indicated, tibial arteries as well. To reduce intra-abdominal gas the examination is best carried out in the morning after an overnight fast [8]. The examina-tion is performed with the patient supine. The only exception is the popliteal artery which is best examined with the patient prone. (Large genicu-late collateral vessels secondary to a popliteal artery occlusion or stenosis are easily interpreted as the popliteal artery when this area is examined from a medial approach). Often tibial artery exa-minations are facilitated by identifying the vessel near the ankle and following it proximally [7].

A point-to-point examination technique of each individual arterial segment should be used. Peak systolic velocities (PSV) are recorded from multi-ple sites, usually the proximal, middle, and distal portion of each arterial segment. Areas of high PSV, indicating a significant stenosis (Fig. 5) and points within the vessel without filling by color flow and without an associated Doppler signal di-agnostic of occlusion are also recorded.

When used clinically, extremity CFDS is made more efficient by prior physical examination and selected use of segmental pressures. Abnormal-ities on physical and continuous wave Doppler ex-aminations can direct the technologist to examine with special care selected locations with CFDS and hopefully shorten the overal time of the ex-amination. Currently a straightforward complete CFDS examination of both legs from the aorta to the ankles takes about 1 h. Complex examinations may require considerably longer.

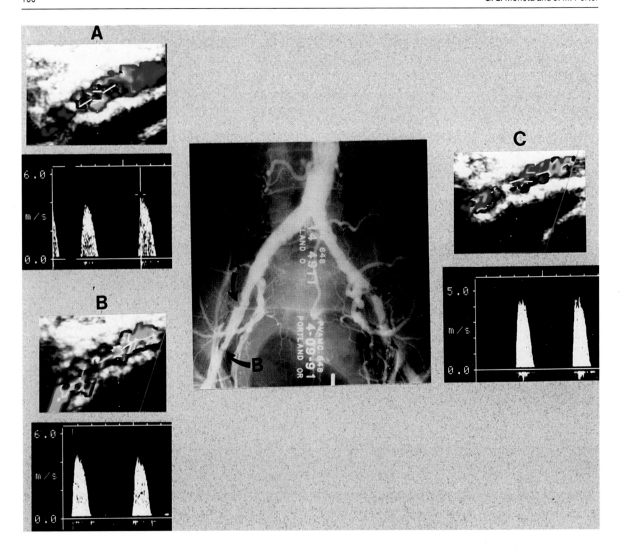

Fig. 3 A–C. High peak systolic velocities indicate multiple areas of stenosis in a patient with bilateral thigh and buttock claudication. (From [12])

Velocity Waveforms/Classification of Stenosis

Velocity waveforms obtained from normal peripheral arteries are triphasic. There is a short reverse flow component at end-systole and end-diastolic flow is near zero in these high-resistance vessels. The triphasic waveform is maintained throughout the length of the extremity as long as there is no significant occlusive lesion [9] (Fig. 6). PSVs in the suprageniculate vessels steadily decrease from proximal to distal (Table 2) while velocities in continuously patent tibial arteries remain relatively constant from proximal to distal [7,10].

Markedly depressed PSVs and absence of the reverse flow component indicate a pressure reducing lesion proximal to the site of examination. Although criteria exist for subclassifying lesions of less than 50% [9] (Table 3), for clinical purposes a stenotic lesion identified with CFDS is usually classified as under 50%, 50%–99%, and occlu-

Table 2. Peak systolic velocities in normal arteries above the knee

Artery	Peak systolic velocity (cm/s)
External iliac	119.3±21.7
Common femoral	114.1±21.9
Superficial femoral	
Proximal	90.8±13.6
Distal	93.6±14.1
Popliteal	68.8±13.5

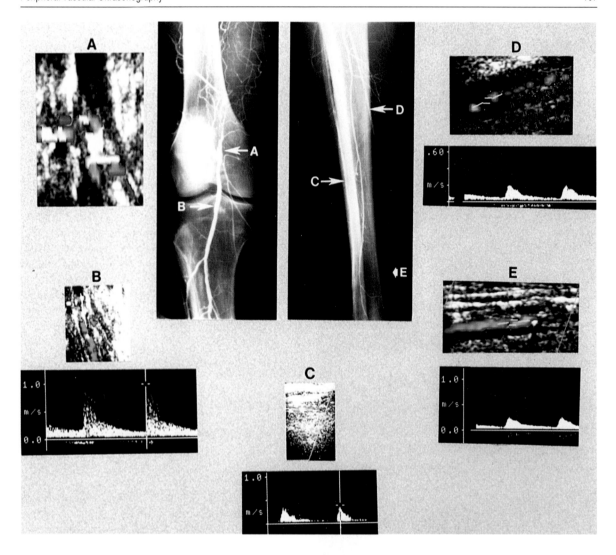

Fig. 4A–E. CFDS delineates reconstitution of the popliteal artery (**A, B**) and establishes patency of the tibial runoff vessels (**C–E**) in a patient with superficial femoral artery occlusion. (From [12])

Table 3. University of Washington spectral criteria for CDFS-detected stenosis in lower extremity arteries

Stenosis	Criteria
0%	Normal waveforms and velocities
1%–19%	Normal waveforms and velocities; spectral broadening is present primarily on the downslope of the systolic portion of the curve
20%–49%	Normal waveform with marked spectral broadening: there is a 30% or more increase in peak systolic velocity
50%–99%	Reverse flow component is lost from the waveforms; peak systolic velocity is increased 100% or more
Occluded	No flow can be detected at multiple sites in adequate visualized arterial segment

sion. Velocity waveforms vary somewhat with cardiac output, arterial inflow, and outflow resistance; thus patients undergoing CFDS must be considered individually. Waveforms must be analyzed proximal and distal to sites suspicious for significant stenosis. Elevated PSVs (greater than 100% of the immediate proximal arterial segment) suggest a stenosis of at least 50% at the examination site [10]. A velocity greater than 200 cm/s in an above-knee artery is also a reliable predictor of a greater than 50% stenosis [11] (Fig. 3, 5). We have applied the criteria noted above and in Table 3 in a blinded, prospective

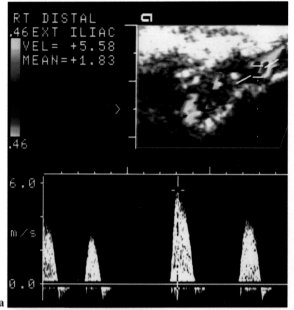

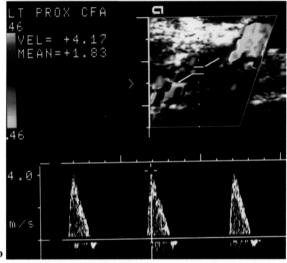

Fig. 5a,b. PSV of 558 cm/s in the right distal external iliac artery (**a**) and PSV of 417 cm/s in the proximal portion of the left common femoral artery (**b**) mark specific sites of flow limiting stenoses in a patient bilateral lower extremity claudication

study to 150 consecutive preoperative vascular surgical patients (286 extremities) undergoing both angiography and CFDS [12]. Each limb was classified based on segmental pressures and clinical examination as normal, isolated aortoiliac disease, infrainguinal disease only, or as multilevel aortoiliac and infrainguinal disease. Of 2036 arterial segments from the popliteal artery cephalad, 99 % were successfully visualized with CFDS; 95 % of anterior and posterior tibial

artery segments and 80 % of peroneal artery segments were also successfully imaged. In vessels proximal to the tibials, CFDS was evaluated for its ability to detect a greater than 50 % angiographic stenosis and distinguish stenosis from occlusion. In the tibial arteries CFDS was assessed for its ability to predict continuous patency from the level of the popliteal trifurcation to the ankle. Results are summarized in Table 4. Of note is the observation that the patient's arterial involvement did not significantly affect the accuracy of CFDS. While we found accuracy of CFDS in patients with multilevel disease was not significantly different from those with hemodynamically significant disease limited to above or below the groin, others have found the detection of distal stenoses more difficult in the presence of proximal disease [13]. We also found CFDS was able to distinguish stenosis from occlusion in 97 % of ileo-femoral-popliteal arteries [12].

Clinical Applications

Current clinical applications of CFDS includes both the evaluation of preprocedure or nonoperative patients, as well as patients who have had surgical or endovascular arterial reconstruction.

Nonoperative or Preoperative Patients. CFDS can serve as a screening test for angiography. Patients with an absolute indication for arterial reconstruction such as severe ischemic pain or pedal gangrene obviously require a complete evaluation,

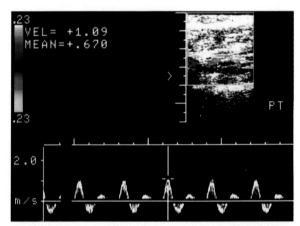

Fig. 6. Velocity recording from the distal posterior tibial *(PT)* artery from a normal volunteer. The arterial waveform in the absence of occlusive disease is triphasic throughout the length of the leg

Table 4. Accuracy of arterial CDFS in comparison to angiography in 150 preoperative patients (286 limbs) with lower extremity arteriosclerosis (from [13])

Clinical			Location			
Classification[a] (no. limbs)	Iliac[b]	SFA[b]	Popliteal[b]	AT[c]	PT[c]	Per[c]
Aortoiliac (n=44)	94/100	77/99	No lesions	100/100	100/100	90/73
Femoral-popliteal-tibial (n=117)	71/99	92/98	67/99	96/73	100/75	80/76
Multilevel (n=45)	92/98	78/97	69/98	81/85	89/71	79/57
All (n=286)[d]	89/99	87/98	67/99	93/75	97/74	

SFA, Superficial femoral artery; AT, anterior tibial artery; PT, posterior tibial artery; Per, peroneal artery.
[a] Clinical classification based on physical examination and segmental Doppler pressures.
[b] Sensitivity/specificity for detecting >50 % stenosis and/or occlusion.
[c] Sensitivity/specificity for detecting continuous patency from popliteal trifurcation to the ankle.
[d] Includes limbs clinically felt to be normal.

evaluation, usually including arteriography, to guide therapy to avoid amputation. However, patients with only intermittent claudication do not require arterial reconstruction to avoid limb loss. Occasional claudicating patients who do not respond to medical or exercise therapy and do not want to undergo the discomfort and more prolonged recovery period of a surgical reconstruction may be candidates for an endovascular procedure. Patients such as this who thouroughly understand the limited durability and small but real risk of most endovascular reconstructions are ideal for screening with CFDS. If an appropriate lesion is found, the patient can be scheduled for an interventional procedure. If an appropriate lesion is not found ateriography can be avoided. The utility of CFDS to screen patients for possible endovascular reconstructions has now been reported from a number of centers. Jäger initially reported a series of patients who were selected for transluminal angioplasty based on symptoms, physical examination, and lower extremity CFDS [14]. Cossman has also documented the accuracy of CFDS in selecting patients for treatment with the excimer laser. Although it is now clear that laser angioplasty offers no clear advantage over conventional balloon dilatation, Cossman's study made the important point that CFDS can very accurately determine the length of extremity arterial occlusions and thus their potential suitability for an endovascular procedure [11]. Edwards et al. reported 110 patients with lower extremity angiography preceded by CFDS [15]. Based on the duplex study 50 patients were scheduled for percutaneous angioplasty prior to actu-

ally obtaining the arteriogram. In 47 of the 50 patients (94 %) the anticipated endovascular procedure was performed. Similary, van der Heijden et al. from University Hospital Utrecht reported 51 arterial lesions in 31 patients that were determined by CFDS to be suitable for transluminal angioplasty. In 48 of the 51 lesions CFDS accurately predicted the location and character of the lesion as confirmed by arteriography at the time of angioplasty. The authors noted that CFDS was also useful in determining puncture sites and catheter routes for percutaneous transluminal angioplasty [16].

At the Portland, Oregon Veteran's Affairs Hospital we have performed a small number of lower extremity surgical arterial reconstructions based on physical examination and CFDS alone. To date we have noted no complications and are currently systematically evaluating the clinical settings in which CFDS may be appropriate without angiography prior to surgical arterial reconstruction. That such an approach may be possible in vascular surgical patients has been suggested by Kohler et al. [17]. In that study individual vascular surgeons were found to make similar clinical decisions without consideration of whether information on a patient's arterial anatomy was obtained with CFDS or arteriography.

Intra-arterial Pressure Gradients. The ability of CFDS to predict pressure gradients across individual stenoses has not been established. Such information would obviously be useful in planning certain arterial reconstructions. Cardiologists frequently use velocity measurements to estimate

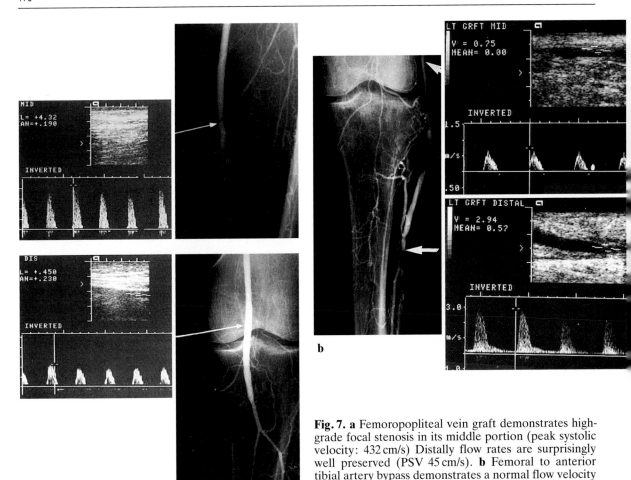

Fig. 7. a Femoropopliteal vein graft demonstrates high-grade focal stenosis in its middle portion (peak systolic velocity: 432 cm/s) Distally flow rates are surprisingly well preserved (PSV 45 cm/s). **b** Femoral to anterior tibial artery bypass demonstrates a normal flow velocity of 75 cm/s about the knee despite a nearly occlusive stenosis at the distal anastomosis (PSV 294 cm/s)

pressure gradients across heart valves using the simplified Bernoulli equation. With some basic assumptions the Bernoulli equation can be simplified to: $P=4(V_{max})^2$ where P is the pressure gradient (mmHG) across a stenosis and V_{max} is the maximal intrastenosis blood flow velocity [18].

The simplified Bernoulli equation for predicting pressure gradients with CFDS has produced conflicting results in peripheral arteries. Some investigators have reported excellent correlation in animal models between measured and calculated pressure gradients [19], while others have reported little correlation [20]. As clinical studies comparing duplex determined iliac artery pressure gradients and angiographic pull-back catheter measurements have also reported variable results. In one study of 18 patients correlation was poor ($R=0.54$) [20] while in another study of 11 patients it was excellent ($R=0.90$) [22]. A larger prospective evaluation of 60 patients produced in-termediate results ($R=0.62$) [23]. It will be interesting to see under what circumstance, if any, CFDS velocities will prove consistently accurate in estimating iliac artery pressure gradients.

Postoperative Patients. CFDS is ideal for monitoring the results of extremity arterial reconstructions. It is currently the method of choice for postoperative monitoring of lower extremity vein grafts. Clinical follow-up alone is clearly inadequate for identifying vein grafts at risk for near term thrombosis. Many vein grafts fail without premonitory changes in pulse status, symptoms, or ankle pressure. Vein grafts fail as often in limbs with stable serially obtained ABIs as in limbs with deteriorating ABIs [24].

Nearly 80% of vein graft failures result from stenosis in the graft itself or its inflow and outflow arteries [25, 26]. It is now clear that postoperative surveillance of vein grafts using CFDS can reliably identify such stenoses prior to graft thrombosis. Vein grafts monitored for stenosis using CFDS and revised appropriately have better overall patency than grafts revised only for recurrent symptoms, worsening physical exam, or falling ABI [27, 28]. Grafts revised prior to thrombosis appear to have late patency rates as good as vein grafts that do not develop detectable stenosis and never require revision [29].

For in situ vein grafts a PSV below 45 cm/s in the distal portion of a 3- to 4-mm graft is a good marker for short-term graft failure [30]. This velocity value is, however, not absolute as many vein grafts, both in-situ and reversed, can have a over 50 % stenosis despite an isolated PSV of 45 cm/s or higher [27, 31]. (Fig. 7) In addition, many reversed vein grafts may have less than 45 cm/s velocity in the larger distal portion of the graft with no detectable stenosis [31].

Because stenosis is associated with subsequent vein graft failure, screening for stenosis is becoming the standard for CFDS surveillance of lower extremity vein grafts. A PSV greater than two times the PSV in the immediately preceding portion of the graft or a PSV of at least 200 cm/s indicates the presence of a more than 50 % stenosis at the site of the high velocity. (Fig. 7) Use of the color flow image alone does not discriminate as well for high-grade vein graft stenosis as do PSV criteria [32].

Most vascular surgeons now recommend repair of high-grade vein graft stenoses when identified in patients who are suitable candiates for operative or percutaneous intervention. Given the propensity for vein grafts to fail early following implantation, a program of CFDS graft surveillance every 3 months in the first 1–2 years postoperatively appears prudent. If the graft remains patent without the need for revision during this time, surveillance examinations can probably be carried out on a yearly basis.

CFDS can be used to monitor sites of endovascular arterial reconstructions and may be predictive of the durability of these procedures. Kinney et al. found that when the immediate postprocedure duplex evaluation suggested a residual stenosis of more than 50 %, even if associated with a technically satisfactory angiographic result, the incidence of clinical and/or hemodynamic failure at 3 months and 1 year was 45 % and 88 %, respectively. If, however, the postprocedure duplex examination showed less than 50 % stenosis, failure rates at 3 and 18 months were only 7 % and 20 % [33] (Fig. 8).

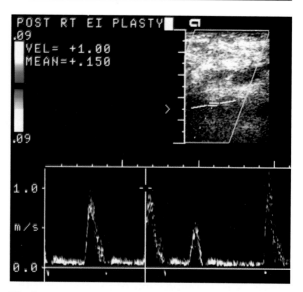

Fig. 8. A normal peak systolic velocity (100 cm/s) at the angioplasty site of a right external iliac artery suggests short term failure of the procedure is unlikely (see text)

Venous Applications

Acute Deep Venous Thrombosis

The diagnosis of acute deep venous thrombosis (DVT) requires objective confirmation. History and physical examination alone lead to the correct diagnosis in no more than 50 % of patients [34]. In the hands of an experienced and skilled observer a continuous wave Doppler examination of the deep veins is reasonably accurate. Sensitivities and specificities for the detection of acute lower extremity DVT average 92 % and 81 %, respectively [35]. The disadvantages of using the continuous wave Doppler to detect acute DVT are obviously lack of hard-copy documentation of findings, the inability to distinguish between normal venous channels and collateral vessels, and the extreme technician dependence of the procedure. It is therefore not surprising that CFDS is now by far the preferred noninvasive examination for the detection of acute DVT in both the lower and upper extremities.

Technique/Diagnostic Criteria

Iliac/Superficial Femoral and Popliteal Veins. With the exception of the popliteal vein, which is examined in the lateral positon, venous CFDS of the lower extremity veins is performed with the patient supine and the legs mildly externally rotated and lowered 10°–20°. Low-megahertz probes are required for examination of the abdominal veins. These are visualized longitudinally and assessed with the Doppler for spontaneous flow, variation of flow with respiration, and response to a Valsalva maneuver. The CFDS criteria for diagnosis of DVT are: (a) noncompressible vein, (b) no spontaneuous flow, (c) no color filling of the lumen, (d) no flow variation with respiration, (e) visible distension, and (f) prominent collateral vessels. While compression of the vein with the ultrasound probe is an important feature of examination of the deep veins below the inguinal ligament (see below), it is usually not an important part of the examination of the abdomonal veins.

Infrainguinal deep veins are examined in longitudinal and cross-section. Usually a 5-MHz transducer is used. Distal tibial veins may be best examined with a 7.5- or 10-MHz transducer. As with the iliac veins, infrainguinal veins are assessed for spontaneous flow, variation of flow with respiration, and response to Valsalva maneuver. Lack of detectable flow implicates thrombus at the examination site. Failure of lower extremity venous flow to increase with expiration or decrease with inspiration implies the presence of a thrombus proximal to the examination site. Sustained increased flow in response to a Valsalva maneuver suggests valvular incompetence proximally (see „Chronic Venous Insufficiency").

Infrainguinal veins are also examined by applying gentle pressure to the vein walls with the ultrasound transducer in an attempt to coapt their walls. Failure of the vein walls to coapt with gentle probe pressure generally indicates an intraluminal thrombus. Although easy to understand conceptually, this portion of the test can be difficult to interpret. Confusing echos produced by overlapping fascial plans at the level of the adductor canal can make confirmation of compression of the superficial femoral vein difficult at this level. In addition, failure to observe tibial vein compression with probe pressure does not always indicate the presence of an intraluminal thrombus [36]. Detection of coaption of tibial vein walls is presumably difficult because of the small size of

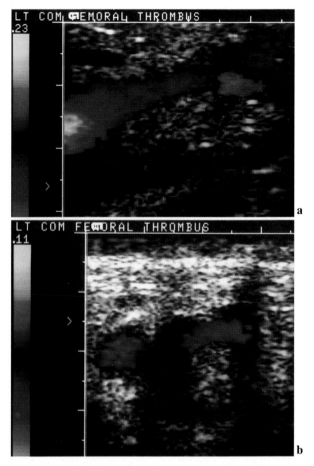

Fig. 9. Longitudinal (**a**) and across-sectional (**b**) views of a large but nonocclusive common femoral vein thrombus in a patient with acute deep venous thrombosis

the vessels and, at least in the upper calf, their deep anatomic location. It is recommended always to confirm the presence or absence of flow with the Doppler and color flow components of the examination.

Often the thrombus can be visualized either directly using the gray scale image or indirectly as lack of filling of the lumen with color during color flow examination. The latter can be of particular importance in the detection of a subocclusive thrombus (Fig. 9). When thrombi are visible, their echo characteristics may help to determine their age and distinguish acute from chronic venous occlusion [37]. A smooth homogeneous thrombus, perhaps with a free-floating component, suggests an acute process. An irregular, adherent thrombus with a heterogeneous echo pattern implies a more chronic process. Chronic thrombi are also more frequently associated with venous dilatation and visible collateral vessels usually not seen with acute DVT.

Accuracy

CFDS is highly accurate in the detection and exclusion of venous thrombosis in the popliteal, superficial femoral, and common femoral vein. Compared to venography, sensitivities and specificities exceed 90 % [35]. Errors in the diagnosis of acute DVT in the thigh using CFDS relate primarily to difficulty in compressing the superficial femoral vein at the abductor canal and misidentification of chronic thrombi as acute. Errors can be minimized by using color flow and Doppler to confirm that an incompressible vessel is in fact truly not patent and by closely studying the echo characteristics of a visualized thrombus and noting the presence of significant venous collateral vessels.

The accuracy of CFDS for the detection of calf vein thrombosis is less accepted than that for the more proximal veins. Older studies suggest duplex scanning does not reliably visualize all tibial veins [38, 39]. A more recent study, however, claims success with CFDS in visualization of all the axial tibial veins from the ankle to the popliteal fossa [40]. Duplex appears poor in the detection of isolated tibial vein thrombosis when examinations are performed primarily for surveillance in patients at risk for DVT. Barnes et al. examined the lower extremity deep veins in 78 patients undergoing total hip or knee arthroplasty. In 52 % of the 25 patients with venographically confirmed postoperative DVT, thrombi were isolated to the calf veins but were not detected by duplex scanning [41]. Conversely, when there is proximal DVT, CFDS detects concurrent tibial vein thrombosis quite well, with reported sensitivities and specificities of up to 95 % when compared to phlebography [42].

There is not sufficient data to justify the use of CFDS to rule out the presence of calf vein thrombosis in patients who are not found to have a proximal venous thrombosis. If symptomatic isolated calf vein thrombosis is suspected clinically, and it is the decision of the attending physician to treat with anticoagulation, we recommend either obtaining a phlebogram or repeating the CFDS every 2–3 days to document possible progression of a suspected thrombosis into the popliteal vein

and then treating with anticoagulation based on the presence of a proximal venous thrombus.

Chronic Venous Insufficiency

Proper function of venous valves in the axial deep and superficial veins is critical to avoid the sequela of chronic venous insufficiency (CVI). CFDS in patients with possible CVI is used to locate sites of reflux in the axial veins and to quantify venous reflux with respect to volume flow of reflux and reflux duration.

Technique of Examination

Vascular laboratory testing of valvular reflux using CFDS requires the creation of a transvalvular

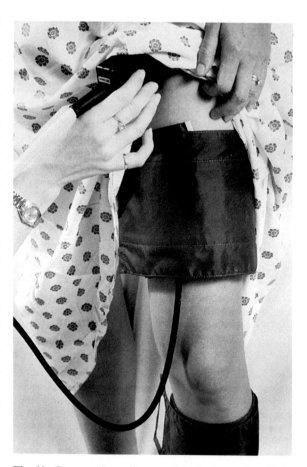

Fig. 10. Pneumatic cuffs are placed about the thigh, calf, and forefoot to quantify venous reflux using the technique of distal cuff deflation (see text for details)

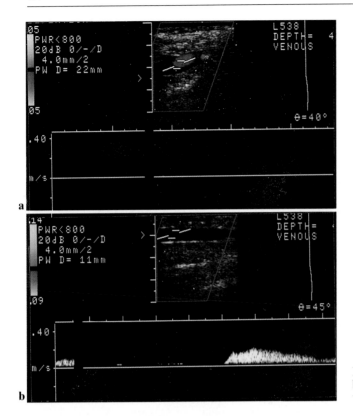

Fig. 11. Normal (<0.5 s; **a**) and abnormal (>0.5 s; **b**) reflux as determined by duplex scanning using the distal cuff deflation technique

pressure gradient that is of both physiologic magnitude and sufficient duration to exceed normal valve closure time. The preferred method of using CFDS to locate and quantify venous reflux involves examining the patient upright and employs distal deflation of pneumatic cuffs to induce valvular reflux and simulate conditions occurring with with calf muscle contraction and relaxation [43].

With the patient upright and without weight bearing on the extremity to be examined, pneumatic cuffs connected to an automatic inflation and deflation device are placed around the thigh, calf, and forefoot. (Fig. 10, Table 5) Each level is examined separately. The transducer is placed over the vein to be examined, proximal to and less

than 5 cm from the pneumatic cuff. The cuff is inflated to a standard pressure (Table 5) for 3 s and then deflated in less than 0.3 seconds. Some reflux with cuff deflation is normal. However, 95 % of normal valves close within 0.5 s. Valvular reflux that exceeds 0.5 s is therefore considered to be abnormal [43] (Fig. 11). With an experienced technician, examination of the common femoral, superficial femoral, popliteal, posterior tibial, and greater and lesser saphenous veins in each leg requires about 30 min.

Clinical Application

In addition to identifying sites of abnormal valvular reflux CFDS may be able to provide a measure of total reflux that is predictive of the risk of ulceration. Time to valve closure, venous diameter (D), peak reflux velocities (PRV), and calculated volume flow at peak reflux (VFPR) can be determined in individual venous segments: $VFPR = (D/2)^2 \times PRV$. It has been suggested the total of the measured VFPRs obtained from single sites in the mid-greater saphenous, lesser saphenous, and popliteal veins may be predictive of lipo-

Table 5. Cuff inflation pressures and widths for quantifying venous reflux using the distal cuff deflation technique

Anatomic site	Cuff pressure	Cuff width
Thigh	80 mmHg	24 cm
Calf	100 mmHg	12 cm
Foot	120 mmHg	7 cm

dermatosclerosis or venous ulceration. In a series of 47 patients with symptomatic CVI, total VFPR summed from the above sites that exceeded 10 ml/s was associated with a 66% incidence of lipodermatosclerosis. Limbs with total reflux of under 10 ml/s did not have lipodermatosclerosis [44]. These data suggest that reconstructive and/or ablative procedures for CVI may be individualized based on site and severity of valvular reflux. As examples, a patient with a venous ulcer and a cumulative VFPR of 14 ml/s, 9 ml/s of which originates in the superficial system, may be best treated with superficial venous ablation (sclerotherapy or surgery). In contrast, a patient with a VFPR of 18 ml/s within the popliteal segment and normal superficial veins may be best treated with some form of deep venous reconstruction.

Conclusion

Ultrasound-based techniques have been of great importance in the noninvasive evaluation of arterial and venous disease. These physiological based studies serve to elevate vascular diagnosis from subjective impressions to hard data based on physiologic principles. They result directly in improved patient care and are important in numerous research studies relevant to vascular disease. Despite the emergence of additional imaging methods ultrasound will remain the primary noninvasive vascular diagnostic technique for the forseeable future.

References

1. Moneta GL, Porter JM. (1991) Diagnosis of chronic lower extremity ischemia. In: Wells SA (ed) Current problems in Surgery. Volume XVIII. Mosby Year Book, St. Louis, MO, p. 29.
2. Feinberg RL, Gregory RT, Wheeler JR, et al. (1992) The ischemic window: a method for the objective quantitation of the training effect in exercise therapy for intermittent claudication J Vasc Surg 16: 244–50.
3. Heintz SE, Bowe GE, Slaymaker EE, et al. (1978) Value of arterial pressure measurements in the proximal and distal part of the thigh in arterial occlusive disease. Surg Gynecol Obstet 146: 337–343.
4. Kirkendall WM, Burton AC, Epstein FH, et al. (1967) Recommendations for human blood pressure determination by sphygmomanometers: report of a subcommittee of the Post-Graduate Education Commitee. American Heart Association. Circulation 36: 980–988.
5. Bridges RA, Barnes RW. (1987) Segmental limb pressures. In: Kempczinski RF, Yao JSTC (eds). Practical noninvasive vascular diagnosis. 2nd ed. Year Book, Chicago, p. 112–26.
6. Hatsukami TS, Primozich JF, Zierler RE, et al. (1992) Color Doppler imaging of infrainguinal arterial occlusive disease. J Vasc Surg 16: 527–33.
7. Caster JD, Cummings CA, Moneta GL, et al. (1992) Accuracy of tibial artery duplex mapping (TADM). J Vasc Tech 16: 63–8.
8. Moneta GL, Caster JD, Cummings CA, et al. (1990) Duplex scanning of peripheral arteries: technique, accuracy, current and future applications. Dynamic Cardiovasc Imag. 3: 124–33.
9. Jäger KA, Phillips DJ, Martin RL, et al. (1985) Noninvasive mapping of lower arterial lesions. Ultrasound Med Biol 11: 515–21.
10. Jäger KA, Ricketts HJ, Strandness DE Jr. (1985) Duplex scanning for evaluation of lower limb arterial disease. In: Bernstein EF (ed). Noninvasive diagnostic techniques in vascular disease. CV Mosby, St Louis, MO, p. 619–31.
11. Cossman DV, Ellison JE, Wagner WH, et al (1989) Comparison of contrast arteriography to arterial mapping with color-flow duplex imaging in the lower extremities. J Vasc Surg 10: 522–9.
12. Moneta G:, Yeager RA, Antonovic R, et al. (1992) Accuracy of lower extremity arterial duplex mapping. J Vasc Surg 15: 257–83.
13. Allard L, Cloutier G, Durand L-G. (1993) Limitations of ultrasonic duplex scanning for diagnosing lower limb arterial stenoses in the pressure of adjacent segment disease. J Vasc Surg 9: 650–57.
14. Jager KA, Johl H, Seifer H, et al. (1986) Perkutane transluminale angioplastic (PTA) ohue vorausgehude diangosische arteriographic (abstract) VASA Suppl 15: 24.
15. Edwards JM, Coldwell DM, Goldman ML, et al. (1991) The role of duplex scanning in the selection of patients for transluminal angioplasty. J Vasc Surg 13: 69–74.
16. Van Der Heijden FHWM, Legemate A, van Leeuwen MS, et al. (1993) Value of duplex scanning in the selection of patients for percutaneous transluminal angioplasty. Eur J Vasc Surg 7: 71–76.
17. Kohler TR, Andros G, Porter JM et al. (1990) Can duplex scanning replace arteriography for lower extremity arterial disease? Ann Vasc Surg 4: 280–278.
18. Hatle L, Angelsen B, (1985) Physics of blood flow. In: Harte L, Angelsen B. (eds). Doppler ultrasound in cardiology. Lea and Fegiber, Philadelphia, p. 8–31.
19. Faccenda F, Usu Y, Spencer MP. (1985) Doppler measurement of the pressure drop caused by arterial stenosis: an experimental study; a case report. Angiology 36: 899–905.
20. Kohler TR, Nicholls SC, Zierler RE, et al. (1987) Assessment of pressure gradient by Doppler ultrasound: experimental and clinical observations. J Vasc Surg 6: 460–469.
21. Langsfeld M, Nepute J, Hershey FB, et al. (1988) The use of deep duplex scanning to predict hemodynamically significant aortoiliac stenoses. J Vasc Surg 7: 395–399.

22. Legemate DA, Teenwen C, Hoeneveld H, et al. (1993) How can the assessment of the hemodynamic significance of aortoiliac stenosis by duplex scanning be improved? A comparative study with intraarterial pressure measurement. J Vasc Surg 17: 676–684.

23. Barnes RW, Thompson BW, MacDonald CM, et al. (1989) Serial noninvasive studies do not herald postoperative failure of femoropopliteal or femorotibial bypass grafts. Ann Surg 210: 486–494.

24. Donaldson MC, Mannick JA, Whittemore AD. (1992) Causes of primary graft failure after in situ saphenous vein bypass grafting. J Vasc Surg 15: 113–120.

25. Mills JL, Fujitani RM, Taylor SM. (1993) The characteristics and anatomic distribution of lesions that cause reversed vein graft failure: a five-year prospective study. J Vasc Surg 17: 195–206.

26. Idu MM, Blankenstein JD, de Gier P, et al. (1993) Inpact of a color-flow duplex surveillance program on infrainguinal vein graft patency: a five year experience. J Vasc Surg 17: 42–53.

27. Mattos MA, van Bemmelen PS, Hodgsdon KJ, et al. (1993) Does correction of stenoses identified with color duplex scanning improve infrainguinal graft patency? J Vasc Surg 17: 54–66.

28. Bandyk DF, Schmitt DD, Seabrook GR, et al. (1989) Monitoring functional patency of in situ saphenous vein bypass: the impact of a surveillance protocol and elective revision. J Vasc Surg 9: 286–296.

29. Bandyk DF, Cato RF, Towne JB. (1985) A low blood flow velocity predicts failure of femoropopliteal and femorotibial bypass grafts. Surgery 98: 799–809.

30. Chang BB, Leather RP, Kaufmann JL, et al. (1990) Hemodynamic characteristics of failing infrainguinal in situ vein bypass. J Vasc Surg 12: 596–600.

31. Luscombe J, Moneta GL, Cummings CA, et al. (1993) Post operative surveillance of infrainguinal reverse vein grafts: an hypothesis for improving examination efficiency. J Vasc Tech 17: 291–294.

32. Buth J, Disselhoff B, Sommeling C, et al. (1991) Color flow duplex criteria for grading stenosis in infrainguinal vein grafts. J Vasc Surg 14: 716–728.

33. Kinney E, Bandyk DF, McWissen M, et al. (1991) Monitoring functional patency of percutaneous transluminal angioplasty. Arch Surg:

34. Cranley JJ, Canes AJ, Sull WJ (1976) The diagnosis of deep venous thrombosis: fallibility of clinical signs and symptoms, Arch Surg III: 34–36.

35. Moneta GL, Strandness DE Jr (1989) Basic data concerning noninvasive vascular testing. Ann Vas Surg 3: 190–193.

36. Polak JR, Culrer SS, O'Leary DH (1989) Deep veins of the calf: assessment with color Doppler flow imaging. Radiology 171: 481–485.

37. Hobson RW, Mintz BL, Jamil Z, et al. (1991) Current status of duplex ultrasoundography in the diagnosis of acute deep venous thrombosis. In: Bergan JJ, Yao JST (eds) Venous disorders. Saunders, Philadelphia, pp 55–62.

38. Vogel P. Laing FC, Jeffery RBJr et al. (1987) Deep venous thrombosis: of the lower extremity: US evaluation. Radiology 163: 747–751

39. Cronan JJ, Dorfamn GS, Scola FH, et al (1987) Deep venous thrombosis: US assessment using vein compression. Radiology 162: 191–194.

40. van Bemmelen PS, Bedford G, Strandness DE Jr. (1990) Visualization of calf views by color flow imaging. Ultrasound Med Biol: 15–17.

41. Barnes RW, Nix ML, Branes CL, et al (1989) Perioperative asymptomatic venous thrombosis; role of duplex scanning versus venography. J Vas Surg 9: 251–260.

42. Sumner DS, Londrey GL, Spadone DP, et al, (1991) Study of deep venous thrombosis in high risk patients using color flow Doppler. In: Bergan JJ, Yao JST (eds) Venous disorders. Saunders, Philadelphia, pp. 63–76.

43. van Bemmelen PS, Bedford G, Beack K, et al. (1989) Quantitative segmental evaluation of venous valvular reflux with duplex ultrasound scanning. J Vasc Surg 10: 425–431.

44. Vasdelois SN, Clarke GM, Nicolaides AN (1989) Quantification of venous reflux by means of duplex scanning. J Vasc Surg 10: 670–677.

Part II
Invasive Techniques in Periinterventional Evaluations

Section I
Radiographic Angiography

Imaging Technology

J. Niepel

Introduction

Conventional catheterization laboratories with film-changer technology allow only diagnostic evaluations. Nowadays, however, for example, in the United States, more than 80 % of laboratories perform interventional procedures routinely. The number of strictly diagnostic laboratories continues to decrease, and we expect that by 1995 all angiographic laboratories will be converted to allow diagnostic as well as interventional procedures. Special angiographic equipment is required to perform neurovascular interventions. The rapid development of vascular interventional procedures has been greatly facilitated by advances in modern imaging technology and such techniques as digital fluoroscopy, on-line digital substraction angiography (DSA), roadmapping, and viewing of digital reference images.

Vascular interventions require simple and safe manipulation of the equipment, convenient handling, fast recall of images, looping of runs from the entire study, easy display of the pre- and postprocedure images, and simplified quantification of stenoses and other lesions. State-of-the-art angiographic imaging technology is further aided by such modalities as computed tomography, magnetic resonance angiography, and ultrasound, which allow the simultaneous display of all relevant data on one viewing station.

General Requirements for Angiographic Laboratories

Monoplane laboratories are standard for general angiography and are often used as combination laboratories for general and cardiac applications. Figure 1 shows a typical room layout for a state-of-the-art monoplane laboratory, with a movable gantry for general angiography and interventions and a floor-mounted table. Biplane laboratories, used mainly for cardiac and neurovascular diagnoses and interventions, have an additional second gantry, generally mounted in rails on the ceiling, and physiological monitoring devices, included in the monitor system. Figure 2 shows a typical room layout for a state-of-the-art biplane laboratory for angiocardiography, with a ceiling-supported table. Figure 3 presents the Bicor installation for angiocardiography.

Gantry

The gantry consists of the stand and a C or U arm system. Most stands in the market can be turned into a parking position to provide unimpeded access to the patient. In the case of biplane systems the second system is usually ceiling supported to provide more space on the floor. When not in use, this system can be parked away to allow undisturbed monoplane examinations.

For angiographic studies a wide choice of projections is necessary. Therefore, typically the C or U arm systems are used which allow complete three-dimensional positioning over a wide range of angles. Isocentric positioning (positioning of the object of interest in the center point of the C or U arm rotation) must be easy. It is often aided by light indicators, to allow angulation without having to reposition the patient. For cardiac (especially pediatric) cases a biplane rather than a monoplane system may be advantageous (Table 1). A biplane system enables simultaneous acquisition of two projections of the same vessel segment with each injection, thus reducing the amount of contrast medium that is required. Biplane systems are often preferred for neuroradiology because switching from one projection to the other is much faster than angulating the system to the different projections. To reduce the radiation exposure the image intensifier should always be used in overtable position (Fig. 2).

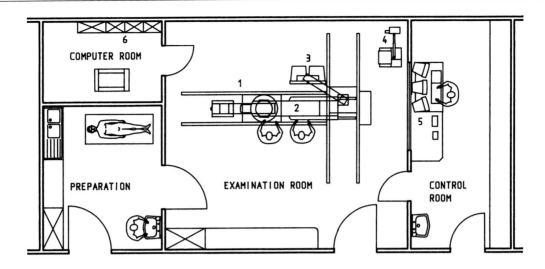

Fig. 1. Room layout of a monoplane laboratory for general angiography and interventions (Multistar). *1* Angiography system, *2* examination table, *3* monitor support, *4* injector, *5* control console, *6* cabinets for generator and imaging system

Several years ago stationary gantries were used exclusively and they remain the most frequently used systems in interventional cardioloy and neuroradiology. However, in general interventional radiology, particularly in peripheral angiographic studies, a movable gantry is preferable (Table 2). Peripheral run-offs are often performed with a stepping gantry in DSA or in conventional continuous scanning. If the table is moved, stepwise or continuously, the physician must follow the patient. Keeping the patient stationary during the study reduces motion artifacts and improves image quality. Motion artifacts are further reduced by stabilization and immobilization of the knees and feet.

Table

The table and mattress should allow comfortable positioning of the patient; this is particularly important in long interventional procedures. The width of the table is limited to allow the system free angulation, with the image intensifier positioned as close as possible to the patient. Narrow tables require an arm rest. The table should be "shadow-free" for all projections over the full length of the patient. It must be possible to perform fluoroscopy from head to toe without restrictions. A motorized table facilitates control of speed. Stepwise movement of the table is an alternative to gantry stepping. A table with head-up or down-tilt is required in some neurovascular studies.

Floor-mounted tables are frequently used, but ceiling-suspended tables provide more space on the floor. Some studies, such as the four-chamber view in pediatric cardiac examinations, are made possible by using a swiveling table. Swiveling, however, is not necessary if the gantry can be rotated around the head end (Table 3). Free and easy

Table 1. Applications for monoplane and biplane systems

Application	Monoplane	Biplane
Cardiac	Sufficient, but an extra injection for each projection is necessary	Saves dose and contrast medium; faster for interventions
Peripheral vascular	Sufficient	Not necessary; higher price
Neurovascular	Sufficient for diagnostic purposes	Preferred for interventions; quick switching between different projections

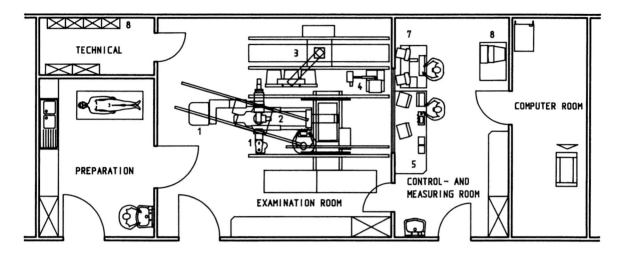

Fig. 2. Room layout of a biplane laboratory for angio-cardiography and interventions (Bicor T.O.P.). *1* Angiography system, *2* examination table, *3* monitor support, *4* injector, *5* control console, *6* cabinets for generator und imaging system, *7* physiological monitoring, *8* workstation

access to the patient is important, particularly in emergencies. In this case the table can be moved footward or turned, or the gantry can be pivoted in a free position. The table height should allow comfortable working for any person's height, thus requiring adjustability over a wide range.

System Geometry

Setting the isocenter requires special light indicators, which are projected onto the patient. To allow quantification a readout for the geometric factors such as source-to-image distance and image intensifier size is required. Display of gantry angulations is necessary to find and reproduce the required projections. A preprogramming device for system angulation often permits faster operation.

Fig. 3. Biplane installation for angiocardiography (Bicor)

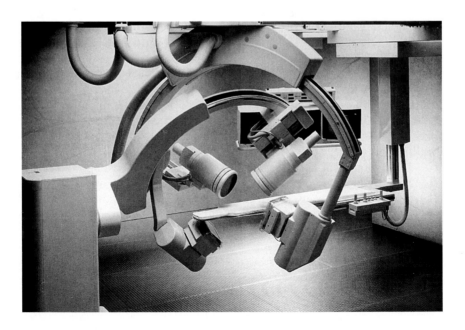

Table 2. Applications for stationary and movable stands

Application	Stationary	Movable
Cardiac	Sufficient	Not necessary; higher price
Peripheral vascular	Not recommended; physician must follow the table; better quality with resting patient	Preferred system
Neurovascular	Sufficient	Not necessary; higher price

Table 3. Applications and additional table features

Application	Step movement	Tilting table	Swiveling table
Cardiac	Not necessary; higher price	Not necessary; higher price	Four-chamber view; alternative: gantry angulation
Peripheral vascular	Necessary if stationary gantry	Not necessary; higher price	Advantageous for arm angiography
Neurovascular	Not necessary; higher price	Some studies	Not necessary; higher price

Imaging System

Generator, X-Ray Tube

Modern angiographic studies require powerful generators and X-ray tubes with high loadability. Loadability depends on the heat-storage capacity of the tube anode. The reason for this requirement is not to increase the dose of the exposure but, depending on the kind of study, the necessity to perform fluoroscopy and acquisition within a range of about 63–76 kV, to conform to the iodine X-ray absorption characteristics and to keep the exposure time as short as possible.

The selection of an optimum generator and X-ray tube depends on the overall requirements of the imaging system and the type of study to be performed. For fluoroscopy and acquisition of small to medium-sized objects the X-ray tubes should have a small focus of 0.4–0.6. For studies using digital imaging with magnification up to factor 2 a 0.3 focus is adequate. Geometrical magnification is of interest almost only in neuroradiology. The microfocus of 0.1 or 0.2 which was used for extreme magnification on film changers is no longer necessary. This technique has been almost completely replaced by DSA, which often gives better results with less magnification because of its high signal to noise ratio and its high contrast performance. The standard focus for angiograms, except for neuroangiograms, is 1.0. Under normal conditions a geometric magnification of 1.2–1.4 provides sufficient resolution to investigate lesions in vessels with a lumen less than 1 mm in diameter.

Collimation, Filtering

The best possible collimation is required to assure optimal radiation protection and image quality. Square and circular (iris) collimation are offered for general angiography. The high absorption differences between heart and lung fields require a compensation which is very often achieved with straight or heart-shaped filters. Special semitransparent filters are used for the head and neck and between the legs. These filters are sometimes integrated into the collimator. Such collimators allow one to cone in and to adjust the filters by remote control. In some collimators these settings can be preprogrammed. These filters are wedge shaped so that their edges do not appear in DSA images. Additional copper filters can be selected automatically for fluoroscopy to harden the beam and minimize skin dose without adversely affecting the image quality.

Image Intensifiers

Image itensifiers are electronic devices employed to transform the X-ray profile into a visible image by conversion of X-ray photons within the cesium iodide input screen. This image is transformed in the photocathode, a thin semiconductor layer on the inner side of the phosphor layer of the input screen, into an electron "image." The electron optics of the tube, which is normally formed by the input screen itself, the cathode, two or more cylindrical electrodes, and in some tubes a disc-shaped electrode and anode, focuses the electrons onto the output screen where they, again, produce a visible image. The electronic image is thereby enhanced by minification. The small output image of an image intensifier is transferred by an optical system to the television and/or cine camera. This optical system consists of the high-speed collimating lens, the light distributor containing a mirror system to simply reflect or split the light beam, and the television or cine camera optics. In the light distributor a light-measuring system is also integrated which controls the fluoroscopic dose rates and exposure dose.

The size of the image intensifier is chosen according to the kind of examination to be performed. For cardiac applications a 23-cm (9-in.) image intensifier is optimal. The diameter of the input field must allow a sufficient field of view for cardiac applications. The outer dimensions must be small enough to bring the image intensifier close to the patient in all projections, guaranteeing the best possible image quality. For laboratories performing both cardiac and general angiography a 33-cm (13-in.) image intensifier is ideal; this allows peripheral studies of both legs simultaneously in about 80% of all patients. For pediatric and neuroradiologic vascular examinations the 33-cm (13-in.) image itensifier is preferable. Although this size may not be ideal for extreme projections in adult cardiology, standard diagnostic and interventions can be performed without

limitation. With the three or four selectable input field sizes this image intensifier can be very well adapted to all practical needs. The standard image itensifier for general angiographic applications should have 40-cm (16-in.) input field diameter (Table 4). All peripheral vascular studies can be performed with this size. Peripheral run-offs with both legs simultaneously are covered with six or seven steps regardless how tall the patient is.

All types of image intensifiers offer a selection of different input sizes, the so-called "zoom modes" in addition to the full size. The image intensifier types for vascular diagnoses usually offer three or four different entrance sizes. The advantages of smaller input sizes are better spatial resolution and larger display of small areas. This makes them very useful for small vessels and improves visualization during interventional procedures. The signal to noise ratio is not affected because the dose rate is automatically adapted to the field size.

Radiation Protection

Long fluoroscopic times and a high number of exposures require the use of very effective radiation protection for the examiner. In general angiography with interventions the highest exposures for the physician are measured at his hands because the operating field is relatively close to the central beam. Also critical are the thyroid and eyes. In cardiology the physician's eyes are exposed to higher exposure than the hands. The maximum allowed exposure, however, has been known to be exceeded in only very few cases. This depends very much on the workload and the kind of study performed. In general angiography the exposure in an average DSA run of 10 s with 1.5 frames/s and a dose of 2 μGy/frame is equivalent to that of about 1.5 min of conventional fluoroscopy. Simple angioplasty with 10 min fluoroscopic time and four DSA runs exposes the physician to one-fifth of that of more complex revascularization with

Table 4. Recommeded image intensifizer sizes for angiographic laboratories

Image intensifier	Application
23 cm (9 in.)	Angiocardiography laboratories
33 cm (13 in.)	Laboratories for neuroradiology and combined application of general angiography and angiocardiography
40 cm (16 in.)	General angiography

60-min fluoroscopic time and ten DSA runs. In complicated neurologic interventions the exposure could even be higher.

In cardiac angiography with conventional cine exposures the exposure in a single cine run with 30 frames/s and 6-s duration is equivalent to that of 45 s of fluoroscopy. For diagnostic cases a fluoroscopic time of 5 min and eight cine runs are very common. In the case of digital cine exposure and pulsed fluoroscopy, both with 15 frames/s, the radiation exposure to the physician is cut in half.

The specific exposure in the various procedures cannot be given. In the literature this varies by a factor of 10. It depends very much on the kind of work, the selected dose values, and the patient's condition. It may be mentioned that the use of the zoom modes of the image intensifiers means an increase in dose, usually by a factor of 2 for each step.

A large window made of absorbing acrylic glass (0.5 mm lead equivalent) with a special body-shaped contour (in neurology and cardiac angio-

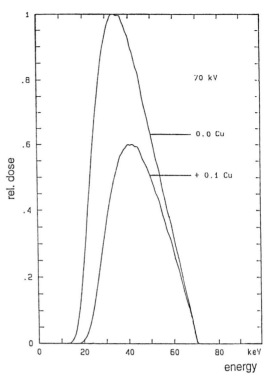

Fig. 5. X-ray spectra with and without 0.1 mm Cu additional filtration

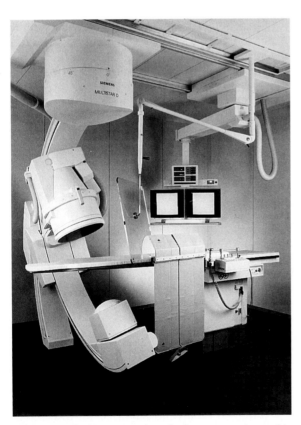

Fig. 4. Radiation protection devices on angiographic systems (Multistar)

graphy) or rectangular profile (in general angiography) can be placed close to the patient. The lower body can be protected by a lead curtain without hindering angulation (Fig. 4). In addition, all means should be used to reduce the dose in fluoroscopy. There are fluoroscopic modes available which allow digital fluoroscopy to be performed with half the normal dose by reducing the frame rate; these modes include Supervision (Siemens) and digital pulsed fluoroscopy. Advanced image processing keeps the image quality and signal to noise ratio at the same level as in standard continuous fluoroscopy. The use of adaptive dose filters hardens the X-ray beam and reduces skin dose. These filters (0.1 mm copper) do not degrade the image quality and are activated automatically during fluoroscopy. The dose reduction is about 40 % in the 70-kV range. The respective spectra are shown in Fig. 5.

In addition to the technical features of an installation, which allow reduction of radiation exposure to the personnel in the examination room, there are also application-related measures which must be observed. Increased distance to source is the best radiation protection; doubling the distance results in one-fourth of the exposure. The best possible collimation not only reduces the amount of radiation but also improves image quality. In addition to the radiation protection devices of the installation mentioned above, lead aprons, thyroid protection, and lead eyeglasses should be worn. Of equal importance is the extensive use of such dose-reducing features as last image hold (LIH), variable frame rate, and dose-reducing fluoroscopy modes. Also, the lowest possible number of frame and dose/frame and frame rates should be chosen.

Image Processing

Acquisition Mode

The output image of an image intensifier (see above) is converted in the television camera pickup tube into an electric image pattern, which is scanned in different modes by an electron beam and produces an analog television signal. The video signal is processed in the video amplifier with a linear or logarithmic characteristic or a special contrast gradient, adapted to specific needs. The signal processing depends on the selected mode in fluoroscopy or exposure. This analog signal is digitized by the analog to digital converter to produce the digital image. The image can be stored in digital form or processed further (see below). For display this digital image must again be converted into an analog image by the built-in digital to analog converter.

High-resolution television systems are used in modern imaging systems. The best image display available today is accomplished by upscanning a 1024-line image to 2048 lines and displaying this image flicker-free with 120 Hz on a large (54-cm) monitor with an antireflex coating (Display 2000, Siemens). Some of the postprocessing modalities, such as filtering and windowing, can already be implemented in the acquisition mode and, if necessary, can be modified later. Automatic maximum peak opacification or manual selection at the time of best filling provides a desired static image display at the end of the acquisition.

Image Postprocessing

Digital images can be stored, summarized, edge enhanced, filtered with different kernels, or inverted and subtracted. Motion artifacts can be eliminated by pixel shift, i.e. shifting the filling image against the mask image in all directions by whole pixels or portions of them down to 0.1 pixels. The brightness and contrast of the image can be changed by "windowing." The "window" is a limited number of gray steps within the overall range. The position within this window can be shifted to higher or lower densities, thus influencing the brightness. The processed image can be stored and/or transferred to a second monitor and used for comparisons of before and after a procedure or as a reference image for manipulation of the guidewire or catheter during interventions. "Roadmapping" produces a substracted image under fluoroscopy with a pilot injection. The roadmap image shows a section of a vessel overlayed on the current fluoroscopic image. This facilitates correct positioning of the interventional devices. Another very important postprocessing feature is quantification. The lumen of a stenosed vessel, length of a stenotic artifact, ventricular volume, ejection fraction, and wall motion can be measured and documented on the diagnostic images or printed out separately. Different methods of calibration may be used. "Annotation" allows the marking of findings and the writing of additional text onto the images.

Imaging Technology

General

Angiographic imaging is performed today in pulsed mode. About 10 years ago the continuous mode was standard; the exposure dose during continuous radiation was about twice as high. With the pulse mode technique the radiation exposure is far below the dangerous level for tissue irradiation even in long studies (e.g., those necessary for diagnosis of cerebral aneurysms). About 60% of all general angiographic procedures are peripheral run-offs. With modern techniques such as on-line DSA the radiation exposure is low in comparison to the conventional film-changer technique. The diagnostic quality is better, and the number of necessary repeats is much lower with on-line DSA because the examiner can monitor the bolus directly.

In the early years of DSA most neuroradiologic and peripheral vascular studies were performed with intravenous injections. However, in the past ten years intravenous injections have been used less frequently. Intra-arterial injections are the most commonly used today. The high fluoroscopic image quality today allows highly selective studies. The main advantage of intra-arterial injection is the high image quality gained with a small amount of contrast medium. In addition, fewer images are acquired due to easier timing. On the other hand, the advantages of intravenous injection are less invasiveness and the less reaction of the patient to the contrast medium due to the lower intravascular concentration. The most significant practical advantage is that intravenous DSA can be easily applied on a outpatient basis. Nevertheless, due to the often suboptimal image quality intravenous DSA studies today remain reserved to a small number of specific cases, such as screening for grafts.

Cardiac Angiographic Imaging Technology

Equipment

Heart and coronary catheterization is most commonly performed via the femoral approach (Judkins). The approach via the brachial artery (Sones) is less frequent. For the arm approach, an additional stable arm rest is required.

To obtain complete diagnostic information the right and left coronary systems are typically studied in at least eight different projections. The left ventricle is usually visualized in two projections, i.e., 30° right anterior oblique (RAO) and 60° left anterior oblique (LAO). If a biplane system is used, both projections for the left ventricle can be carried out simultaneously, thus reducing the necessary amount of contrast medium and saving time. While ventriculograms normally do not need caudal or cranial angulations, these angles are needed for the coronaries. Therefore the C arm must allow RAO, LAO, cranial and caudal projections. These are usually carried out with a C arm plus an L arm or two C arms in one gantry system. The gantry is in most cases a floor-mounted unit and is used as a monoplane installation. It is advantageous for the isocenter of the C arm system to permit upward and downward movement to adapt to the height of the person manipulating the catheter.

In biplane systems the second plane is very often a ceiling-suspended C arm system for RAO and LAO projections. This system can usually be pivoted to allow cranial or caudal projections.

It can also be moved out completely to provide unimpeded working space for the floor stand when used as a monoplane system. Biplane installations are very important for pediatric cardiology to reduce the amount of contrast medium and radiation (less positioning, lower fluoroscopic time).

The table in cardiac examination rooms may be suspended from the ceiling or mounted on the floor. The lowest position must still allow easy access to the patient as well as his transfer. Furthermore, it must be possible to move the table footwards and to move the gantry out to provide free access to the patient in the case of an emergency. Isocentric positioning for cardiac studies is very important. This enables the examiner to achieve all projections by simply angulating the C arm only. Some units permit preprogramming of standard projections. To allow repeated image acquisition in given projections some units store all spatial angulations together with the images, thus allowing a proper repositioning of the gantry.

Fluoroscopy

Digital pulsed fluoroscopy is typically used to allow proper positioning of catheters and interventional devices. Short radiation pulses reduce motion artifacts and guarantee sharp images. On-line filtering and special computing provide better spatial resolution, simultaneously reducing the noise. The total fluoroscopic dose can be reduced by decreasing pulse repetition rates. Decreasing the frame rate to 15 frames reduces the standard dose rate by 50 %. For routine applications, such as positioning the patient, advancing the guide wire or catheter or checking the balloon position during a dilatation 15 frames/s is fully adequate. With rapidly moving targets, such as the right coronary artery, the stroboscopic effect may be disturbing. In these situations 30 frames/s is preferable.

Continuous fluoroscopy, digitized, corresponding to 30 frames/s, is also possible and offers all image-manipulating techniques that are possible with digital image acquisition. Conventional non-digital fluoroscopy cannot be manipulated. For interventional procedures, which require the highest image quality, many systems offer the so-called high-contrast fluoroscopy mode. This mode provides continuous fluorscopy with a much higher milliampere value than in standard fluoroscopy, thus keeping the tube voltage virtually independent of the patient's absorption. Thus the contrast medium or the catheters are imaged at a kilovolt level that provides the best possible contrast, ranging between 63 and 70 kV.

Cine Imaging

In conventional cardiac catheter laboratories the diagnostic images are recorded on 35-mm cine film at 15–60 frames/s. The images are simultaneously stored on magnetic tape (e. g., S-VHS) for instant review. Modern digital cardiac catheter laboratories are equipped with two modes of acquisition. With the standard acquisition technique images are generated in a way similar to that in cine film imaging, using the same dose/frame rate but without exposing a film; the images are stored digitally. The image quality is excellent and fulfills all clinical requirements. The second diagnostic acquisition mode provides a low-dose alternative, called digital cine mode. Although the exposure dose is only 40 % of the standard cine dose, the image quality is still high and fully adequate for routine diagnostics.

Quantitative evaluation in nondigital laboratories can be carried out only from single frames. All methods for cine frame evaluation are very time consuming. In digital laboratories with or without cine film cameras the images are usually stored in digital format. This allows optimizing of image quality by postprocessing features such as filtering and windowing. Image manipulation such as zooming, roaming, and inverting are also possible.

Quantification

On-line quantification is available only with digital imaging. Measuring of stenosis by geometric edge detection and densitometry, ventricular volume, or ejection fraction are performed automatically after defining the area of interest.

Calibration

Calibration is necessary for all quantitative measurements and can be performed by several methods. "Dot" calibration is very common; this uses four radiopaque dots arranged in a square on the input of the image intensifier. The distance between the dots on the image intensifier entrance is known, and their distance in the image is measured. The specific geometric conditions such as focus to image intensifier, object to image intensifier distance, and zoom mode must be taken into account. A calibration factor is derived from this information and is used to calculate the correct size of the target of interest. "Cath" calibration uses the known size of the catheter within the vessel of interest. This therefore automatically includes the geometry in the calibration process. Another possibility is "Grid" calibration. Here a radiopaque grid is recorded in a separate acquisition run. Provided the grid was recorded under the same geometric conditions as the vascular region of interest in the diagnostic scene, the calculated results will be correct. If quantification for more than one scene is necessary, the first calibration factor can be preserved as long as the geometric conditions (source-intensifier distance and object-intensifier distance) are not changed.

Storing Images

The memory of digital units is sufficient to store all acquired images from at least one patient. Often the memory size of the imaging device is sufficient to store all data acquired on a given day.

Digital Cardiac Imaging, Features

State-of-the-art digital imaging offers more than the above features. The Hicor system from Siemens, for instance, includes the following features that are very useful for cardiac and coronary imaging, particularly when coronary interventions are performed:

Automap either selects the reference images or scenes automatically according to the C arm position or angulates the C arm to the stored position of a recalled reference image. It is possible to split the screen horizontally or vertically.

Corner reduced display displays a live fluoroscopic and roadmap image on the same monitor, with the roadmap image in a freely selectable corner of the monitor.

Dynamic reference images (Dynamp) is an additional orientation aid during coronary interventions. The reference scenes are ECG synchronized automatically to the live fluoroscope. Sequences of an ECG-related R-R interval are displayed in an endless loop.

Landmark option allows addition of a certain percentage of a mask image (anatomic background) to a subtracted image. This enables one to see the relationship of an opacified vessel to the surrounding anatomy.

Multimap displays up to 16 reference images simultaneously on the monitor for selection of a reference image or scene.

Before/after comparisons display the respective images side by side for evaluation of the intervention.

Static roadmap is a single image that can be selected from a cine scene for the purpose of catheter guidance or device placement.

Integrated systems in a heart catheter laboratory allows the transfer of hemodynamic data from the measuring system computer to the digital imaging device and their recording with the acquired diagnostic images. The ECG, for instance, can be used to synchronize the acquired images with the Dynamap modality of the Hicor system.

Peripheral Imaging Technology

Methods of Peripheral Imaging

Approximately 60% of studies in general angiography are performed to visualize the vasculature of the lower extremities. The majority of interventions are also performed here. For peripheral studies the femoral artery is punctured, and the catheter tip is placed in the abdominal aorta. The renal arteries are often visualized in separate runs. Imaging is therefore necessary from the pelvis down to the feet. Most studies are performed in postero-anterior projection. Angulations of up to 30% RAO/LAO are generally used for the renal and iliac arteries. Lateral views are employed to visualize abdominal aortic aneurysm. Cranial or caudal projections are rarely used.

Conventional Methods. The conventional method for performing peripheral examinations is the cut-

film changer, with table stepping. Test exposures are made to determine the correct exposure values; blood flow is measured for programming of the proper stepping and determining the appropriate number of exposures. Nevertheless, important vessel segments may be missed, and repeats are often necessary. Long cassettes, used in a changer, lessen the number of repeat examinations required, but the handling is more cumbersome.

Digital Methods. DSA represents an important advance in peripheral angiography. Its use in conjunction with large-image intensifiers enables the extremities to be imaged segmentally in six or seven separate runs with excellent image quality. The bolus is followed on screen. The images can be manipulated and evaluated with all possibilities offered by digital imaging. A useful feature particularly in balloon sizing is the on-line quantification of lesions. Printing of the diagnostically relevant images reduces total film consumption and simplifies archiving.

The use of digital imaging in angiography makes digital fluoroscopy possible and thus further improves fluoroscopic image quality via digital image enhancement. The roadmap feature further enables interventions such as balloon dilatation and embolization. These features are especially helpful in difficult procedures requiring tiny guide wires or very thin catheters. Documenting the situation before and after the intervention is accomplished simply by pressing a button on the foot switch.

A combination of peripheral stepping technology and DSA, called Perivision, has recently been developed by Siemens. This allows on-line DSA of peripheral run-off examinations. With this technique it is advantageous to step the gantry and to fix the patient's knees and feet to avoid movement during the procedure. Pixel shift can be used to compensate for minor motions such as those caused by the unavoidable reaction to the contrast medium. The greatest advantage is on-line display of subtracted images which enables the operator to control the stepping and thus to follow the course of the bolus.

The necessary number of images and, correspondingly, the radiation dose are lower than in conventional segmental DSA. The amount of contrast medium required is about the same as in conventional run-offs. The resulting image quality is high, and interventions can be performed immediately following the diagnostic image acquisition.

Another method for performing digital peripheral run-offs is the so-called "Bolus chasing" which is offered by several manufacturers. This is carried out by moving the table or gantry manually during acquisition, providing a nonsubtracted image display. The number of images is normally higher than with Perivision. Subtraction is possible only in the first and last steps. The necessary mask images can be obtained if the procedure is performed in the same way in which these step images were acquired before the contrast medium filled the vessel or in the last step after the bolus disappears. Substracted images show better quality especially in the lower leg.

Image Display

For documentation the peripheral study is usually recorded on multiformat film using a laser printer. Two hardcopies with six images each generally suffice. One hardcopy contains representative images of each segment of the leg, and the other shows the images from the renal arteries and angulated projections of the iliac arteries. More extensive documentation may be necessary only in complex cases. Improved image presentation is provided by the so-called "long-leg display" that is currently being developed; this combines the images of each segment into a single image showing the complete vasculature of the legs (Fig. 6).

Neuroradiologic Imaging Technology

Equipment

For diagnostic neuroradiology and interventions a stationary gantry permitting a wide range of angulation is sufficient. Biplane installation allows a reduction in examination time. The skull should always be positioned isocentrically to be able to change the projections rapidly. Unimpeded access to the patient's head is necessary. A rotating gantry with park position or a wide range of table movement is necessary to allow full access to the patient. The table must be narrow at the head end

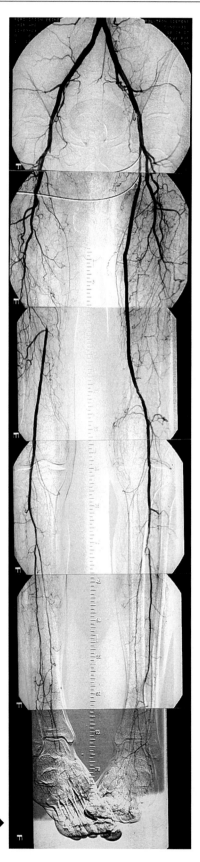

Fig. 6. Long-leg display of a peripheral run-off study in ▶ DSA (Perivision)

to allow straight lateral projections without excessive magnification. The head should be fixed in an appropriate radiopaque holder. For some types of examination, such as myelograms, a tilting table is required. As the examination may last up to several hours, especially in neurologic interventions, a comfortable mattress and arm rests are obligatory.

If no geometric magnification is needed, a standard angiographic X-ray tube with a 0.6 and 1.0 focus is sufficient. If magnification with a factor of more than 1.5 is planned, the X-ray tube should provide an additional 0.3 focus. The entrace field of the image intensifier should have a diameter of 12- or 13-in. to allow some magnification for the survey exposure. The zoom modes of the image intensifier are very important. A smaller input field offers higher resolution. High definition is needed especially for selective studies and the sometimes very complicated interventions within small vessels. Further requirements for the image intensifier include high detection quantum efficiency ($>60\%$), high contrast ratio ($>20:1$), and high resolution)>4 mm^{-1}; spatial frequency) for the full entrance field. The television system should have high resolution with more than 20 MHz bandwidth. The digital system must offer a 1024×1024 matrix throughout the entire imaging chain, from acquisition to processing to display.

Cutfilm Changer Versus Digital Acquisition

The relative merits of images from a cutfilm changer and those from digital hardcopy images are a subject of on-going debate. Resolution in a film-changer image may be higher than that in a digital image, but the higher contrast with digital imaging – especially in DSA – compensates for the lower resolution. On the other hand, the digital system offers so many possibilities to improve the image quality that digital imaging should be the system of choice. Interventions cannot be performed as easily without digital imaging.

Rotational Angiography

In rotational angiography the imaging system is rotated around the patient during the acquistion. This technique, which is possible only with a digital imaging system, provides more projections of the vascular region of interest with a single injection. This is of great help in orientation and offers the best way in which to detect and to define aneurysms.

Archiving

Cardiac Angiography

The cine camera is still the medium of choice for dynamic studies of the heart. The 35-mm cine film is internationally standardized and can be shipped anywhere for evaluation. The medium offers very high quality long-term storage and high definition. The contrast (gradient curve) can be easily adapted to individual needs. It can be evaluated with special projectors or projected onto the wall even in large auditoriums. Negative aspects include the high price, the need for relatively expensive darkroom equipment, handling of chemicals, time-consuming quality control, a relatively high storage volume requirement, and the necessity of viewing the films in a darkened room.

The "cineless" catheter laboratory is therefore finding increasingly use. Super-VHS videotape is a less expensive alternative for storage of dynamic studies. The image quality is lower than cine standards and also about $20\%-30\%$ below the quality offered by a digital image but in general it is sufficient for archiving of dynamic studies. The videotape is inexpensive, easy to archive and to handle. The diagnostically relevant images should be stored on a hardcopy or videoprinter. Another possibility is digital archiving on streamer tape (one patient per tape, similarly as with cine). Evaluation does not require a digital imaging system. The tape can be reviewed on an external workstation. Furthermore, a laser disc can be used for digital or analog archiving.

Peripheral, Neurovascular Angiography

For long-term archiving the standard today is documentation of images using a laser printer. Digital archiving of the selected images or the complete study on an optical disc or magnetic tape is also possible. Optical discs are available in two types: the write-once/read-many-times disc (WORM) and the magneto-optical disc (MOD; erasable). Several types of digital magnetic tape recording devices are offered on the market, with varying standard and recording speed. The recording speed depends on the matrix and the compression factor.

Multimodalities

Angiography remains the definite diagnostic modality for a large proportion of vascular diseases. For comprehensive vascular diagnostics it is of great interest to display on a single monitor the images from various modalities, such as ultrasound, computed tomography, and magnetic resonance angiography, and to compare them with the angiographic digital images. This is already possible on some workstations. The next step, of special interest in neuroradiology, is to merge these images. The initial steps in this direction are now being taken.

Glossary

- *Biplane system:* an X-ray system containing two C or U arms to produce two simultaneous projections acquired with a single injection
- *Catheter calibration:* use of the known dimension of a catheter to obtain a calibration factor for quantitative measurements
- *Continuous mode:* continuous radiation (fluoroscopy)
- *Contrast gradient:* the function of signal processing which influences the resulting image contrast
- *Digital cine mode:* a pulsed acquisition similar to cine but without a cine camera, images being digitally processed and stored
- *Dot calibration:* the use of four radiopaque dots in a defined distance on the image intensifier entrance to obtain a calibration factor for quantitative measurements
- *Exposure:* (a) image acquisition; (b) the amount of direct or scattered radiation to which a person is exposed

- *Geometric conditions:* the focus to image intensifier distance and the object to image intensifier distance, defining the magnification factor
- *Grid calibration:* the use of a radiopaque grid to replace the object under the same geometrical conditions to obtain a calibration factor for quantitative measurements
- *Image intensifier system:* the image intensifier, including an antiscatter grid, light distributor, television camera, and for conventional cardiac applications a cine camera
- *Isocenter:* the center point around which the C or U arm system is angulated
- *Isocentric positioning:* positioning of the area of interest in the isocenter (for any system angulation the target remains in the center of the image)
- *Kernel:* a neighborhood of pixels whose values are used to filter the pixel in the center of the neighborhood
- *Loadability:* the heat-storage capacity of the anode that limits the power that can be applied to an X-ray tube over a given period (measured in kilowatt-seconds)
- *Monoplane system:* an X-ray system with a single C or U arm equipped with the X-ray tube and image intensifier system which can be angulated around the patient
- *Movable gantry:* an X-ray system (C or U arm) that can be moved horizontally from the head to the foot end, or vice versa, continuously or stepwise (resting patient in peripheral studies)
- *Pixel shift:* in DSA, moving the mask or filling image by whole pixels or portions of a pixel either up/down (Y) or left/right (X) to compensate for movement of the target between mask and filling during acquisition
- *Pulsed fluoroscopy:* radiation in short pulses with selectable repetition rate for fluoroscopy
- *Pulsed mode:* (see pulsed fluoroscopy)
- *Stationary gantry:* a fixed floor- or/and ceiling-mounted X-ray system (for peripheral studies the table must be moved)
- *Stroboscopic effect:* imaging of rapidly moving targets with a pulsed mode of low frequencies stepwise from image to image

Angiographic Contrast Agents

W. Krause

Introduction

Contrast enhancement of the vessel lumen is required to visualize blood vessels using X-ray technology, due to similar radiodensity of blood and the surrounding tissues. Research on contrast agents began shortly after the discovery of X-rays by W. C. Röntgen in 1895 [1]. Sodium and lithium iodide and strontium bromide were the first water-soluble contrast media introduced into clinical practice, in 1923 [2]. Iodine was identified as an atom with a sufficiently high atomic weight difference to organic tissue and has therefore been used exclusively as the X-ray absorbing atom in contrast agents until the present. The blood concentration of iodine must be greater than 1 mg/ml for adequate contrast enhancement. The first contrast agent, sodium iodide, however, was rather toxic. Subsequent research was therefore directed to safe packaging of iodine in molecules with reduced toxicity. The noniodine remainder of the contrast molecule has three purposes: to increase solubility to 370 mg iodine/ml, to stabilize the iodine atom, and to mask the iodine to make it "biologically invisible" to the body thereby reducing the inherent toxicity of the halogen atom. The first urographic contrast medium with organically bound iodine was Uroselectan, which became available in 1929 [6]. The introduction of a second iodine atom into this molecule led to Uroselectan-B, the first angiographic contrast agent [7]. The first of the modern substances based exclusively on the triiodobenzene ring system was introduced between 1953 and 1956 [7–9].

An ideal contrast agent exclusively absorbs X-rays without interacting with the organism. The optimum contrast agent is therefore characterized by: (a) high density difference (positive or negative) relative to surrounding tissue, (b) biological inertness/no interaction with the organism, (c) easy handling (low viscosity), (d) rapid and complete excretion, and (e) low price. Presently available contrast agents carry at least three iodine atoms per molecule and provide an adequate tissue/vessel lumen density difference. The present chapter deals with physicochemical properties and pharmacokinetics of modern contrast media. The price of the contrast media has received substantial attention following the introduction of nonionic substances which are five to ten times more expensive than the conventional ionic agents, particularly in the context of the cost containment policies in health care. Thus far, however, the synthesis of low-price contrast agents has not been successful. The alternative approach to visualize vessels by reverting the tissue/vessel lumen X-ray contrast for example, by injecting CO_2 [3–5] has not been widely accepted in clinical settings.

Chemistry

Stable binding of iodine and chemical masking have been achieved by coupling of the iodine atoms to a benzene ring. This moiety allows the symmetrical introduction of three iodine atoms and the concomitant "hydrophilic shielding" necessary to improve solubility and tolerance. All modern contrast agents are derivatives of triiodobenzene. The coupling of hydrophilic groups is performed either via a carboxyl or an amine group. Among the three possible basic structures – triiododiaminobenzoic acid, triiodoisophthalamic acid, and triiodotrimesic acid – only derivatives of the first two have reached the market; no trimesic acid derivative is presently available. The first widely used ionic contrast agent was diatrizoate, which was introduced in 1953 and is still an important compound either as pure sodium, meglumine salts, or mixtures thereof. Other ionic compounds include iothalamate (Conray), ioxithalamate (Telebrix), iodamide (Uromiro), ioglicate (Rayvist), and metrizoate (Isopaque).

The first nonionic compound, metrizamide (Amipaque), was introduced in 1969 [10]. The draw-

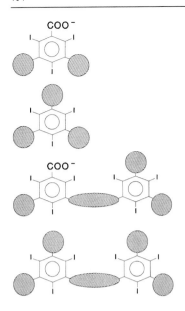

Ionic Monomer

Ionic
High osmolality
High chemotoxicity

Nonionic Monomer

Low osmolality
Good tolerance
Low viscosity

Ionic Dimer

Ionic
High chemotoxicity
Low osmolality

Nonionic Dimer

Isotonic
Good tolerance
High viscosity

Fig. 1. Types of contrast media according to chemical structures

back of this substance is its chemical instability, and therefore it had to be distributed in a freeze-dried form and reconstituted before use. The first ready-to-use nonionic contrast medium was iopamidol (Isovue, Niopam, Solutrast) followed by iohexol (Omnipaque), iopromide (Ultravist), and ioversol (Optiray).

At present there are four chemically different types of contrast agents available: ionic and nonionic monomers and ionic and nonionic dimers (Figs. 1, 2).

Sufficient chemical stability of the compounds to achieve shelf-lives of up to 5 years has been reached by additives to the preparation. These include buffering systems to maintain a definite pH value and chelating agents to mask trace levels of metals such as iron which would initiate deiodination processes. Monitoring of stability is performed by measuring pH, free iodide, and amine groups. Another possibility of degradation includes intramolecular rearrangement which is observed in some contrast agents.

Physicochemical Parameters

Contrast agents can be classified according to the physicochemical characteristics of water solubility, electrical charge, osmolality, viscosity, and hydrophilicity.

Sufficient *water solubility* is the basic requirement for any angiographic contrast agent. Considering the highest available concentration is 370 mg iodine per milliliter, which is equivalent to approximately 800 mg substance; this means that in a 100-ml bottle ca. 80 g or about 55 % is the contrast agent and only 45 % water. No other class of compounds used in medicine have concentrations this high.

Electrical charge, which is an exclusive characteristic of ionic contrast agents (generally negative charge of a carboxyl group), has been identified as one of the major factors contributing to undesired biological activity ("chemotoxicity") of the ionic X-ray contrast agents. Ionic contrast agents are salts of iodine-containing, negatively charged ions (anions) and of positively charged counterions (cations, most commonly Na^+ or meglumine$^+$). The latter do not contribute to the absorption of X-rays. However, they do influence the interaction with biological systems such as proteins or enzymes. The iodine-containing anions bind circulating ions such as Ca^{2+} [11], thereby interfering with membranes and their electrical charges. As a result, bradycardia, alterations in T wave configuration, and, rarely, ventricular fibrillation may occur [31, 32]. To avoid these side effects the modern compounds are electrically neutral.

Osmolality describes the number of molecules in solution in terms of milliosmoles per kilogram. It is influenced by the concentration of contrast agent, association/dissociation effects, and hydration. Since for ionic compounds only the negatively charged ion (anion) is the carrier of iodine,

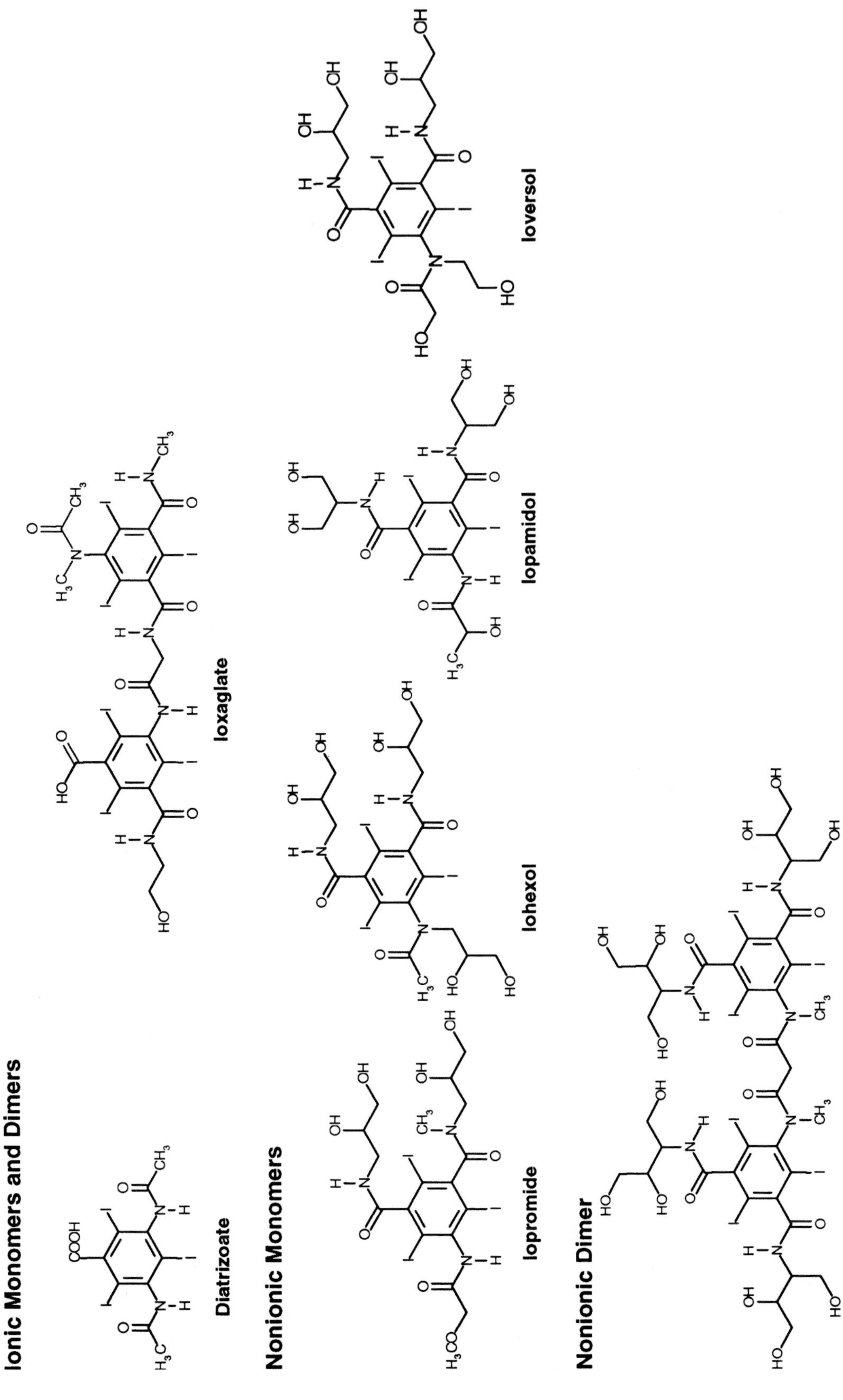

Fig. 2. Structural formulas of the most commonly used contrast agents

the positively charged ion (cation) which is needed as counterion, unnecessarily increases the number of molecules in solution by a factor of 2 and therefore contributes considerably to osmotic effects. High-osmolar, ionic contrast media (HOCM) are characterized by osmolalities in the range of 1500 mosm/kg and low-osmolar nonionic monomeric substances (LOCM) of 600–800 mosm/kg [12]. This is still approx. twice the value of blood (300 mosmol/kg). Isotonicity at clinically relevant concentrations (300 mg iodine/ml) has been achieved for the dimers iotrolan and iodixanol. The importance of lowering osmolality cannot be overestimated. It is known that next to the electrical charge most effects of HOCM are related to their high osmotic pressure. Osmolality-related adverse effects include hemodynamic effects such as depression in myocardial contractile performance and a subsequent decrease in blood pressure and in dP/dt followed by an increase in left ventricular end-diastolic pressure [13–17]. Bradycardia [18] and an increase of blood pressure in the lung circulation, pain, endothelial damage, blood-brain barrier disturbance, thrombosis, and thrombophlebitis have also been reported. Osmolatities of selected presently available contrast media are illustrated in Fig. 3.

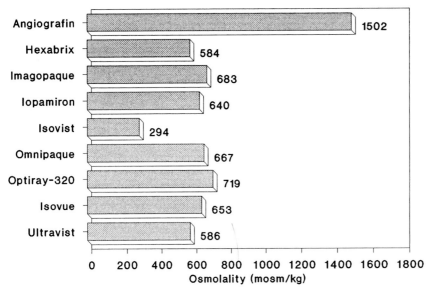

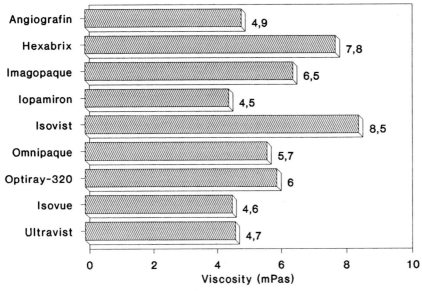

Fig. 3. Comparison of osmolalities and viscosities of different contrast media at a concentration of 300 mg iodine/ml (except for Optiray, 320 with 320 mg iodine/ml) and 37 °C. Date are mean values of four batches and two bottles each

The *viscosity* of a solution is a measure of its fluidity and is given in millipascals. It is influenced by the size of the molecule (larger molecules have higher viscosities), the shape of the molecule, and the possibility of intermolecular interactions (formation of aggregates), which increases this parameter. There is an inverse relationship with temperature; increasing the temperature of the solution sharply decreases viscosity. Contrast media are therefore often warmed to 37 °C before injection. For ionic compounds there is a clear dependence of viscosity on the counterions used. Sodium salts have lower values than meglumine salts. Viscosity has a direct impact on the handling of the solution, limiting the injection rate at higher viscosities. Lower viscosity is generally preferable in angiography, where narrow catheters and high injection rates are used, but there are some indications for high-viscosity compounds, for example, when rapid dilution should be prevented. The viscosities of commercially available contrast media are illustrated in Fig. 3.

The *hydrophilicity* of a molecule is determined by measuring its partition between a lipophilic organic phase such as *n*-butanol or *n*-octanol and an aqueous buffer. On a gross scale hydrophilicity is responsible for the biological tolerance to the compound; lower hydrophilicity results in higher protein binding and better permeability of cell membranes. Therefore it is desirable to increase the hydrophilicity to increase tolerance. Among the currently used nonionic monomeric contrast agents, however, hydrophilicity is already at such a level that any further increase results in no additional improvements; on the contrary, it would increase osmolality and viscosity and therefore be counterproductive.

Pharmacokinetics

The pharmacokinetics of all iodinated contrast agents (ionic and nonionic, monomer and dimer) used for angiography are practically identical [19, 20]. Following rapid intravenous injection there is a biphasic decline in blood levels characterized by half-lives of 3–10 min for the first phase and 1.5–2 h for the second. The first phase can be attributed to distribution within the vascular system and diffusion from the intravascular space into the extracellular tissue, and the second phase corresponds to renal elimination from the intravascular compartment (Fig. 4).

The *distribution* of contrast agents within the body is determined by their extremely high hydrophilicity. As a consequence protein binding is low (<5 %), and cell membranes are not crossed to any significant extent. These compounds are therefore not able to pass the blood-brain barrier, are not excreted in breast milk, and are not absorbed after oral administration in significant amounts. Their volume of distribution is practically identical to that of the extracellular space volume (0.25 l/kg).

Due to their highly hydrophilic character *biotransformation* is not necessary and, indeed, has never been described for any angiographic contrast agent. Deiodination is normally not observed in the organism. The amount of free iodide

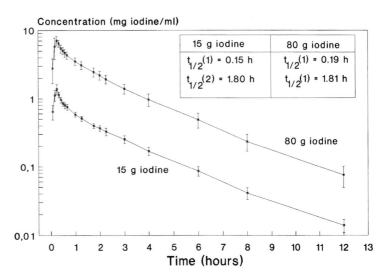

Fig. 4. Plasma levels of iopromide in 12 healthy male volunteers (mean ± SD) after an intravenous 15-min infusion of 15 g iodine or 80 g iodine

is probably due to degredation of the contrast agent within the preparation [21]. Iodide levels in formulations are typically below 10 µg/ml. At a total dose of 100 ml contrast medium, less than 1 mg free iodide is administered. This amount does not compromise the function of an intact thyroid gland. In patients with hyperthyrosis the use of contrast agents should be avoided whenever possible. Whenever indicated, a prophylactic treatment with perchlorate and thiamazol is mandatory (see below).

Elimination of contrast agents proceeds rapidly and mainly via the kidneys (>95 % of dose), and here glomerular filtration is the predominant mechanism. Active tubular excretion has been observed for ionic monomeric contrast agents and tubular reabsorption for nonionic compounds or ionic dimers [22]. These processes, however, comprise only very small proportions of the injected dose. As a consequence the total clearance of the contrast agents is practically identical to the individual glomerular filtration rate. The elimination of iodine or the decline in enhancement on computed tomography has therefore been used to determine the glomular filtration rate in patients [23, 24]. Impaired renal function prolongs the half-life of contrast agents up to 10 h or more. Extrarenal (biliary) excretion is increased in these patients up to 20 % of the dose as compared to less than 5 % in normal subjects. Due to the excellent tolerance of nonionic contrast agents their application might even be considered in dialysis patients [25, 26]. Doses in renal risk patients must be minimized (<2 ml/kg) and the following measures taken: discontinuation or dose reduction of potentially nephrotoxic comedication (nonsteroidal antirheumatics, aminoglycosides, hydroxyethyl starch infusions), premedication by sufficient hydration (500–1500 ml physiological saline) and diuretics (furosemide, 20 mg i.v.) and continuous dopamine infusion (3–4 µg/kg/min). If renal function deteriorates, mannitol infusion (up to 25 g/ 3 h), then dopamine and furosemide as given above, and, if necessary, hemodialysis [27] are administered. It has been shown that contrast agents are easily dialyzable (55 ml/min at a blood flow of 200 ml/min), and that they can be effectively removed from the body by hemodialysis. Half-lives, total clearance, and routes of elimination are independent of the injected dose in the clinically relevant dose range.

In summary, the pharmacokinetic properties of iodinated contrast agents are (a) low protein binding (<5 %); (b) no passage of membranes: minimal intracellular uptake, negligible blood-brain barrier passage, and minimal excretion into breast milk; (c) rapid extravasation and distribution in the extracellular space with a half-life of 0.1–0.2 h; (d) rapid renal excretion by glomerular filtration with a half-life of 1–2 h; (e) no biotransformation; and (f) minimal absorption/enterohepatic recirculation.

Biological Interactions of Contrast Media

Contrast agents are among the best tolerated compounds used in medicine. Extremely high doses are administered in man, up to 1.5 g iodine per kilogram of body weight, which means more than 100 g iodine, and which is in some cases injected at a high rate; despite this, however, the incidence of side effects is extraordinarily low (Fig. 5). Adverse events may be classified according to severity (mild, moderate, severe, fatal; Table 1), target organ (kidneys, heart, skin), dependence on dose (dose dependent, dose independent), or time of appearance (early, late reactions). The side effects reported for HOCM and LOCM are the following: minor: nausea, vomiting, urticaria, pruritis, pain at injection site, transient arrhythmia; moderate: severe vomiting, extensive urticaria, headache, bronchospasm, edema (face or larynx); severe: nausea + vomiting + diarrhea, syncope, convulsion, shock + hypotension, cardiac arrest, pulmonary edema. Their possible mechanisms are summarized in Table 1.

Effects on electrophysiology are observed mainly after intracoronary or intracardiac injection of contrast media. These include a reduction in the rate of depolarization and a prolongation of the PR interval and may result in transient bradycardia, heart block, or sinus arrest [13–18, 28, 29]. Transient alterations in T wave configuration are osmolality related and are therefore reported for HOCM. The ionic character of HOCM results in the binding of calcium. As a consequence ventricular fibrillation can occur in up to 1 out of 200 cardiac angiographic procedures [30]. Additives to the preparation or the use of LOCM reduces this risk. There is evidence that nonionic LOCM lead to less bradycardia and ventricular fibrillation and fewer T wave alterations than HOCM [31, 32].

The *hemodynamic effects* of contrast media include a depression in myocardial contractility fol-

Table 1. Interaction of HOCM and LOCM with various systems of the organism

System	HOCM	LOCM	Cause/Remarks
Endothelium			
Vascular	Shrinkage of cell volume, opening of junctions, vesicle proliferation	Minor effect	Related to osmolality and chemotoxicity
Blood-brain barrier	Disruption, opening of tight junctions	Smaller effect	Related to osmolality and chemotoxicity
pH			Electrical charge
Blood	Decrease	No effect	
Intracellular	Increase	No effect	
Vascular tone	Decrease	Smaller effect	Osmolality
Blood volume	Marked increase	Less increase	Osmolality-related hemodilution
Hematocrit	Strong decrease	Weak decrease	Osmolality-related hemodilution
Plasma electrolytes	Transient decrease/strong decrease (Ca^{2+})	Little effect	Osmolality-related hemodilution/electric charge
Erythrocytes	Echinocyte formation, crenation, increased aggregability	Little or no effect	Osmolality and chemotoxicity; dose-related
Leukocytes	Histamine release	Minor histamine release	No direct correlation with adverse reactions, higher in "reactor" patients; osmolality related?
Lymphocytes	Rare immediate allergylike reactions	Extremely rare immediate allergylike reactions	Antibody formation controversial; no dose dependence
Platelets	Inhibition of aggregation	No effect	Dose-proportional; lipophilicity related? Ca^{2+} binding?
Arachidonic acid metabolism	Stimulation of metabolism, decreased inactivation of PGE $_2$	Stimulation of metabolism	Reactive process of irritation
Blood coagulation	Increase in coagulation time	No effect	Dose-related inhibition of thrombin
Fibrinolysis	Slight activation?	Slight activation?	tPA activation?
Complement system	Decrease in complement hemolytic activity	Minor decrease in complement hemolytic activity	Unknown mechanism; no direct correlation with clinical adverse reactions
Enzyme systems			Electrical charge, lipophilicity
Acetyl-cholinesterase,	Inhibition	Minor effect	
Alcohol-dehydrogenase	Inhibition	Minor effect	
β-Glucuronidase,	Inhibition	Minor effect	
Hexokinase	Inhibition	Minor effect	

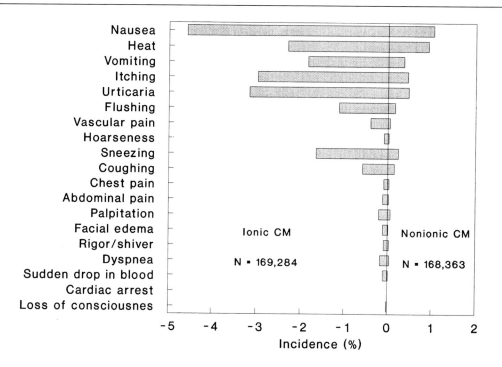

Fig. 5. Side effects of contrast media (*CM*). (From [71])

lowed by a decrease in blood pressure and in d*P*/d*t* and an increase in left ventricular enddiastolic pressure [15, 33–36]. This may provoke or exacerbate myocardial ischemia especially in patients with preexisting hemodynamically relevant coronary stenosis or heart failure. Nonionic LOCM have been shown less likely to produce ischemia [14–16]. Another, dose-dependent characteristic of HOCM is vasodilatation, which is experienced by the patient as a sensation of warmth or even pain. With LOCM or isotonic agents this effect is reduced or not observed [37].

The *blood coagulation system* is more influenced by ionic contrast media (HOCM and LOCM) which show anticoagulant and antiplatelet activities [38–45]. These agents act similarly to antithrombotic agents. Nonionic compounds interact to a lesser extent with this system. Prolonged contact of blood and contrast medium should therefore be avoided. Alternatively, the addition of heparin to the preparation (5 IU/ml) or its coadministration may be advisable.

Acute renal insufficiency is provoked in rare cases by the injection of contrast media. Risk factors for this side effect include diabetes mellitus, multiple myeloma, and dehydration [46]. The se-

verity of such reactions ranges from a transient change in laboratory parameters to the need for dialysis or even – in very rare cases – to permanent injury. LOCM are reported to exhibit a lower incidence for this side effect [47, 48].

In addition to the above side effects, there is the general class of „allergy-like" reactions, with an incidence of 1 %–2 %. These can be divided into two groups: the mild and dose-dependent release of mediators, which cannot be inhibited by corticosteroids, and the second stage, which seems to be dependent on preexisting allergy or priming factors, and which can be controlled by corticosteroids. Allergylike symptoms include nausea, vomiting, urticaria, bronchospasm and laryngospasm, edema and – in very rare cases – vascular collapse. The incidence of severe reactions is approximately 0.1 % and that of mortality below 1 in 10 000 patients. None of the many factors proposed to explain the cause of these reactions, such as histamine release, antibody formation, complement activation, and changes in leukotriene formation, can be made unequivocally responsible for these effects. Psychological factors such as stress and anxiety of the patient may play a considerable role. Since a clearly defined cause of allergylike reactions cannot be found, pretesting and pretreatment of the patients remains controversial [49, 50]. A careful history of known allergies or previous allergylike effects is mandatory.

The known risk factors include renal and cardiac insufficiency, diabetes, and advanced age. General prophylaxis of allergylike side effects includes administration of corticosteroids (32 mg methylprednisolon, Urbason, p.o. 12 and 2 h before contrast medium) against direct toxic reactions and atropine (0.75 mg i.v.) against vasovagal effects [75]. Concomitant treatment with antihistaminics ($H_1 + H_2$; 0.1 mg/kg demetindenmaleate, Fenistil, i.v. plus cimetidine, Tagamet, 5 mg/kg i.v.), and corticosteroids has proven useful in high-risk patients [51, 52]. Other prophylactic measures include high water load and discontinuation of potentially interacting comedication such as biguanides and drugs affecting renal clearance. LOCM are reported to have a lower incidence in anaphylactoid reactions than HOCM [53, 54]. Details on the treatment of minor and major allergylike reactions are summarized below ("Prevention/Premedication and Treatment of Side Effects", Table 4).

The debate about the superiority of nonionic contrast media over ionic agents has long been the subject of much controversy. A substantial number of clinical results have by now, however, clearly shown the incidence of side effects to be decreased by a factor of 3–10 with nonionic versus ionic contrast media (Table 2). The nature of adverse reactions seems to be identical for ionic and nonionic compounds. With HOCM side effects are observed in 0.5%–24% of cases, depending on the investigator, as opposed to 0.7%–3% with nonionic contrast media [49, 50, 55–71]. The incidence of fatal reactions is probably also decreased, but this cannot be confirmed unequivocally since with ionic compounds this event is only seen in 1 out of 10000–100000 cases. To assist the physician in the decision as to whether and when to use nonionic LOCM several authorities have issued guidelines. The American College of Cardiology (ACC) recommends using nonionic contrast agents in "selected patients at

Table 2. Comparison of side effects of HOCM and LOCM in a number of clinical studies

Reference	Contrast medium	Total (%)	Severe side effects (%)	Deaths
Ansell [62]	HOCM	–	0.02	1:41000
Coleman [56]	HOCM	8.5	0.08	0:10000
Davies [60]	HOCM	9.7	0.11	0:4000
Fischer [49]	HOCM	–	0.05	1:52000
Leonello [50]	HOCM	1.3	0.03	1:10000
Hartman [66]	HOCM	–	–	1:75000
Hobbs [63]	HOCM	–	0.05	1:93000
Katayama [71]	HOCM	12.7	0.22	1:170000
	LOCM	3.1	0.04	1:170000
Lasser [68]	LOCM	8.3	0.4	0:6000
Michel [65]	HOCM	0.5	0.01	1:59000
Palmer [69]	HOCM	3.8	0.09	1:40000
	LOCM	1.2	0.02	0:30000
Pinet [64]	HOCM	6.0	0.04	1:91000
Schrott [67]	LOCM	2.1	0.01	0:50000
Shehadi [61]	HOCM	4.7	0.07	1:17000
Toniolo [57]	HOCM	–	–	1:85000
Witten [59]	HOCM	6.8	0.1	1:33000
Wolf [70]	HOCM	4.1	0.4	0:6000
	LOCM	0.7	0.0	0:7000
Wolfromm [58]	HOCM	–	0.04	1:61000

high risk for hemodynamic complications (including congestive heart failure, severe aortic stenosis, cardiogenic shock and left main coronary artery disease) during cardiac catheterization and in patients with a history of allergic reaction to contrast medium" [72]. In general, the ACC recommends that the physician in consultation with the patient should determine the choice of contrast agent. The American Society of Cardiovascular and Interventional Radiology proposes the use of LOCM compounds [73] for painful examinations and in patients with marked anxiety, hemodynamic instability or limited cardiac reserve, or an inability to tolerate a marked osmotic load. Various other conditions for which there is contradictory or incomplete evidence include age (low versus high), hyperosmolar states (dehydration), renal failure, prior reactions and strong allergic diathesis or asthma. The Australian guidelines recommend [74] that high-risk patients, asthmatic subjects, and patients aged over 50 years should receive only nonionic contrast media, and that low-risk patients should receive corticosteroid pretreatment (methylprednisolone, 32 mg 12 and 2 h before injection) prior to injection of the contrast agent. If pretreatment cannot be arranged, or if the study is urgent, the use of nonionic contrast agents is recommended. In Central Europe, Scandinavia, and Japan the use of HOCM has been practically discontinued, and only LOCM are used.

In summary, HOCM and LOCM seem to exhibit the same quality of side effects whereas the quantity is clearly different. Ionic HOCM elicit a three to ten times higher risk of provoking adverse reactions than nonionic LOCM.

Indications for Contrast Media Use

Ionic contrast media have been in use for angiographic indications for more than 30 years. In cardioangiography the mixed sodium/meglumine salt of diatrizoate (Urografin) has been shown to be better tolerated than pure sodium or meglumine salts. Increasingly high doses and rapid injection rates in multiple-disease patients may, however, result in undesirable side effects. To reduce the adverse reactions associated with the use of ionic contrast agents, nonionic substances are recommended. In terms of the above characteristics, nonionic LOCM are well tolerated and safe to administer. Guidelines for the use of LOCM have been issued by several authorities (see above).

Recommended concentrations and volumes for angiographic indications are summarized in Table 3 and general handling and storage advice is presented in Table 4.

Table 3. Concentration and dose recommendations for various techniques of contrast media administration

Technique	Concentration (mg iodine/ml)	Dose (ml)
Angiopraphy		
Abdominal	300	5–50
Aorta	300–370	10–50
Cardiac	370	40–60
Cerebral	300	4–12
Coronary	370	4–8
DSA i.a.	75–300	6–60
DSA i.v.	300–370	50–150[a]
Extremities	300	10–70
Phlebography	150–300	20–50

DSA, Digital subtraction angiography.
[a] Multiple injections of 20–50 ml.

Table 4. Recommendations for the handling of contrast media

	Recommendation
Storage	At room temperature in the dark Not in the refrigerator
Shelf-life	2–5 years See expiration date
Handling before use	Take from the dark immediately before use Use only clear solutions Crystals may be solubilized by warming up to 80 °C If solution does not become clear, discard Viscous preparation may be injected at 37 °C
Handling after opening	Use within 4 h; under no circumstances use after 12 h Do not pour out of container Do not resterilize

Prevention/Premedication and Treatment of Side Effects

The incidence of adverse reactions is markedly decreased when nonionic LOCM instead of ionic HOCM (diatrizoate) or LOCM (ioxaglate) are used. However, side effects can also occur with nonionic compounds.

Patients with *allergic history* must be pretreated with corticosteroids (32 mg methylprednisolone, Urbason p. o. 12 and 2 h before contrast medium) or antihistaminics (0.1 mg/kg demetindenmaleate, Fenistil, i. v. plus cimetidine, Tagamet, 5 mg/kg i. v.). In patients with *hyperthyroidism* the use of iodinated contrast media should be avoided. If used, prophylaxis with perchlorate (2–3 mg Irenat) and thiamazol (2 × 20 mg) or carbimazol (3 × 10 mg) from 4 days before until 3 weeks after contrast medium is mandatory. *Phaeochromocytoma* patients should be pretreated for approximately 2 weeks with individual doses of α-blocking agents to avoid hypertensive crisis or sudden decrease in blood pressure. In *sickle-cell anemia* the deformation of erythrocytes due to osmotic overload is less marked with LOCM than with HOCM. Deformed and rigid erythrocytes are unable to pass narrow capillaries, resulting in stasis and possibly tissue damage. Intra-arterial injections must be performed with special caution [76] for both groups of contrast media (blood exchange to decrease hemoglobin S to less than 20 % prior to arteriography) since even LOCM, unless they are isotonic to blood, elicit erythrocyte deformation and ensuing complications. In patients with *impaired renal function* (renal insufficiency, diabetes, cardiac insufficiency, myeloma, advanced age) the use of contrast medium is to be restricted. Serum creatinine values should be measured, the doses minimized (<2 ml/kg), and nephrotoxic medication (nonsteroidal antirheumatics, aminoglycosides, hydroxyethyl starch) discontinued. Prophylactic measures also include high water load (500–1000 ml physiological saline), the administration of diuretics (furosemide, 20 mg i. v.) and dopamine (continuous infusion, 3–4 µg/kg per minute), and the avoidance of re-

Table 5. Treatment of contrast media adverse reactions. (From [75])

Adverse reaction	Mild reaction	Severe reaction
Heat, nausea, vomiting	Fresh air, oxygen (2–6 l/min)	Valium (5–10 mg i. v.)
Urticaria	None	Diphenhydramine (50 mg p. o. or i. m.) or hydroxyzine (25 mg p. o. or i. m.) Cimetidine (300 mg p. o. or i. v.) Epinephrine (1:1000; 0.3 ml s. c.)
Angiodema	Local cooling; epinephrine (1:1000; 0.3 ml s. c.); oxygen (2–6 l/min) Diphenhydramine (50 mg i. m.); Cimetidine (300 mg p. o. or i. v.)	
Bronchospasm	Epinephrine (1:1000; 0.3 ml s. c.) Oxygen (2–6 l/min) Albuterol or metaproterenol (two breaths)	Add aminophylline (250 mg i. v.) Intubation If prolonged, add: Hydrocortisone (250 mg i. v.) Diphenhydramine (50 mg i. m.) Cimetidine (300 mg i. v.) If necessary, add: Morphine (5 mg i. v.)
Hypotension with bradycardia	Trendelenberg position Intravenous fluids	Atropine (0.75 mg i. v.) If ineffective: Dopamine (5–10 µg/kg per minute i. v.)
Hypotension with tachycardia	Trendelenberg position Intravenous fluids If no response but remaining mild, epinephrine (1:1000; 0.3 ml s. c.)	Intravenous fluids Epinephrine (1:10 000; 3 ml i. v.) Oxygen (2–6 l/min) Intubation If persistent: Dopamine (5–10 µg/kg per minute i. v.)
Pulmonary edema	Oxygen (2–6 l/min) Raise head and body Furosemide (40 mg i. v.)	If unconscious: Intubation If agitated: Morphine (10–15 mg i. v.) Epinephrine (1:1000; 0.3 ml s. c.)

peated contrast medium injections within a short period of time. If renal function deteriorates, the injection of mannitol (25 g/3 h) is recommended and then dopamine/furosemide as given above. In the case of further deterioration of renal function, hemodialysis must ultimately be instituted. Risk evaluation is also mandatory for *pregnant women,* and X-ray diagnosis should be performed only if it is vital and unavoidable. *Breast feeding* of newborns has not been generally considered as a problem since contrast media are not excreted in the milk and are not absorbed in the gastrointestinal tract of the infant to any significant amounts. Although contrast media induced side effect are very rare, especially with nonionic LOCM, the physician and personnel must be aware of potential side effects and must know how to treat them. The availability of well-trained personnel and therapies for the treatment of side effects is mandatory. Table 5 summarizes the effective treatment of side effects [75].

Future Developments

The past 20 years have shown the development of safe and well-tolerated contrast media for angiographic purposes. Modern nonionic monomeric substances exhibit relatively low osmolalities and low viscosities. The nonionic dimers to appear soon for angiographic indications will be even isotonic to blood. Is there still any need for further research and development? For cardiac/coronary applications higher concentrations, for example, 400 mg iodine/ml, would be of benefit. Additionally, the combination of isotonicity and low viscosity would represent further progress. Monomeric compounds with these characteristics are presently under development. However, these will not be available before 1998.

Other possible developments in the future require new technological improvements on the part of the medical equipment industry. Monochromatic X-rays, for example, would be useful to operate at the K edge of iodine. This could considerably increase both patient safety by reducing radiation intensity and imaging efficiency by increasing specificity.

A further line of research involves compounds that do not extravasate. These substances are thought to have molecular weights greater than 40 000. For this purpose polymers on the basis of dextrane or other backbones have been synthetized. These molecules are too large to pass through the endothelial gaps into the extravascular space. The problem still to be solved, however, is improving tolerance and retention in the body of considerable proportions of the injected dose. Compounds which do not leave the vessel lumen would have the advantage of clear delineation of vascular fine structures and of prolonging the imaging time for hyper- or hypovascularized tumors in, for example, the liver. The future will show whether these desirable compounds can be synthetized and can become clinically available.

References

1. Haschek E, Lindenthal TO (1896) Ein Beitrag zur praktischen Verwertung der Photographie nach Röntgen. Wien Klin Wochenschr 9: 63–64.
2. Osborne ED, Sutherland CG, Scholl AF, Rowntree LG (1923) Roentgenography of urinary tract during excretion of sodium iodide. JAMA 80: 368–373.
3. Shifrin EG, Plich MB, Verstandig AG, Gomori M (1990) Cerebral angiography with gaseous carbon dioxide CO_2. J Cardiovasc Surg (Torino) 31: 603–606.
4. Strunk H, Schild H, Mortasawi MA (1992) Arterial interventional measures using carbon dioxide CO_2 as a contrast medium. RöFo 157: 599–600.
5. Mladinich CRJ, Akins WW, Weingarten KE, Hawkins IF (1991) Carbon dioxide as angiographic medium. Comparison to various methods of saline delivery. Invest Radiol 26: 874–878.
6. Binz A, Rath A, von Lichtenberg A (1931) The chemistry of uroselectan. Z Urol 25: 297–301.
7. Wallingford VH (1953) The development of organic iodide compounds as X-ray contrast media. J Am Pharmacol Assoc (Sci Ed) 42: 721–728.
8. Langecker H, Harwart A, Junkmann K (1954) 3,5-Diacetylamino-2,4,6-trijodbenzoesäure als Röntgenkontrastmittel. Naunyn-Schmiedebergs Arch Exp Pathol 222: 584–590.
9. Hoppe JO, Larsen HA, Coulston FJ (1956) Observation on the toxicity of a new urographic contrast medium, sodium 3,5-diacetamido-2,4,6-triiodobenzoate (Hypaque sodium). J Pharmacol Exp Ther 116: 394–403.
10. Almén T (1969) Contrast agent design. Some aspects on the synthesis of water-soluble agents of low osmolality. J Theor Biol 24: 216–226.
11. Morris TW, Sahler LG, Fischer HW (1982) Calcium binding by radiopaque media. Invest Radiol 17: 501–505.
12. Krause W, Miklautz H, Kollenkirchen U, Heimann G (1994) Physiocochemical parameters of X-ray contrast media. Invest Radiol, 29: 72–80.
13. Higgins CB (1985) Cardiotolerance of iohexol, a survey of experimental evidence. Invest Radiol 20: 565–569.

14. Bettmann MA, Bourdillon PD, Bary WH, Brush KA, Levin DC (1984) Contrast agents for cardiac angiography: effects of a nonionic agent vs. a standard agent. Radiology 153: 583–587.
15. Gertz EW, Wisneski JA, Chiu D, Akin JR, Hu C (1985) Clinical superiority of a new nonionic contrast agent (iopamidol) for cardiac angiography. J Am Coll Cardiol 5: 250–258.
16. Gerber KH, Higgins CB, Yuh YS, Koziol JA (1982) Regional myocardial hemodynamic and metabolic effects of ionic and nonionic contrast media in normal and ischemic states. Circulation 65: 1307–1314.
17. Bashore TM, Davidson CJ, Mark DB (1988) Iopamidol use in the cardiac catheterization laboratory: a retrospective analysis of 3313 patients. CARDIO 5: 4–10.
18. Thomson KR, Evill CA, Fritzsche J, Benness GT (1980) Comparison of iopamidol, ioxaglate and diatrizoate during coronary arteriography in dogs. Invest Radiol 15: 234–241.
19. Hartwig P, Mützel W, Taenzer V (1989) Pharmacokinetics of iohexol, iopamidol, iopromide, and iosimide compared with meglumine diatrizoate. In Taenzer V, Wende S (eds.) Recent developments in nonionic contrast media. Thieme Verlag, Stuttgart, p. 220–223.
20. Feldman S, Hayman A, Hulse M (1984) Pharmacokinetics of low- and high-dose intravenous diatrizoate contrast media administration. Invest Radiol 19: 54.
21. Wang YCJ (1980) Deiodination kinetics of water-soluble radiopaques. J Pharm Sci 69: 671–675.
22. Zurth C (1984) Mechanism of renal excretion of various X-ray contrast materials in rabbits. Invest Radiol 19: 110–115.
23. Almén T, Bergquist D, Frennby B, Hellsten S, Lilja B, Nyman U, Sterner G, Tornquist C (1991) Use of urographic contrast media to determine glomerular filtration rate of each kidney with computed tomography and scintigraphy. Invest Radiol 26: S72–74.
24. Effersoe H, Rosenkilde R, Groth S (1990) Measurement of renal function with iohexol or a comparison of iohexol, ^{99m}Tc-DTPA, and ^{51}Cr-EDTA clearance. Invest Radiol 25: 778–782.
25. Corradi A, Menta R, Cambi V (1990) Pharmacokinetics of iopamidol in adults with renal failure. Arzneim Forsch 40: 830–832.
26. Waaler A, Svaland M, Fauchald P (1990) Elimination of iohexol, a low osmolar nonionic contrast medium, by hemodialysis in patients with chronic renal failure. Nephron 56: 81–85.
27. Scherbach JE, Kollath J, Riemann HE (1991) Unerwünschte Kontrastmittelwirkungen an der Niere, in Peters PE, Zeitler E (eds.) Röntgenkontrastmittel – Nebenwirkungen, Prophylaxe, Therapie. Springer-Verlag, Berlin, p. 65–69.
28. Hirshfeld JW Jr, Laskey W, Martin JL, Groh WC, Untereker W, Wolf GL (1983) Hemodynamic changes induced by cardiac angiography with ioxaglate: comparison with diatrizoate. (1983) Am J Cardiol 2: 954–957.
29. Feldman RL, Jalowiec DA, Hill JA, Lambert CR (1988) Contrast-media related complications during cardiac catheterization using Hexabrix or Renografin in high risk patients. Am J Cardiol 61: 1334–1337.
30. Johnson LW, Lozner EC, Johnson S (1989) Coronary arteriography 1984–1987: a report of the Registry of the Society for Cardiac Angiography and Intervention. I. Results and complications. Cathet Cardiovasc Diagn 17: 5–10.
31. Piao ZE, Murdock DK, Hwang MH, Raymond RM, Scanlon PJ (1988) Contrast media induced ventricular fibrillation: a comparison of Hypaque-76, Hexabrix and Omnipaque. Invest Radiol 23: 466–470.
32. Missri J, Jeresaty RM (1990) Ventricular fibrillation during coronary angiography: reduced incidence with nonionic contrast media. Cathet Cardiovasc Diagn 19: 4–7.
33. Friesinger GC, Schaffer J, Criley JM, Gaertner RA, Ross RS (1965) Hemodynamic consequences of the injection of radiopaque material. Circulation 31: 730–740.
34. Vine DL, Hegg TD, Dodge HT, Stewart DK, Frimer M (1977) Immediate effect of contrast medium injection on left ventricular volumes and ejection fraction. Circulation 56: 379–384.
35. Bettmann MA (1982) Angiographic contrast agents: conventional and new media compared. Am J Roentgenol 139: 787–794.
36. Cohan RH, Dunnick NR (1987) Intravascular contrast media: adverse reactions. AJR 149: 665–670.
37. Hagen B, Klink G (1983) Contrast media and pain: hypotheses on the genesis of pain occurring on intra-arterial administration of contrast media. In Taenzer V, Zeitler E (eds.) Contrast media in urography, angiography and computerized tomography, Thieme Verlag, Stuttgart, p. 50–56.
38. Stormorken H, Skalpe IO, Testart MC (1986) Effect of various contrast media on coagulation, fibrinolysis, and platelet function: an in vitro and in vivo study. Invest Radiol 21: 348–354.
39. Robertson HJF (1987) Blood clot formation in angiographic syringes containing nonionic contrast media. Radiology 163: 621–622.
40. Gabriel DA, Jones MR, Reece NS (1991) Platelet and fibrin modification by radiographic contrast media. Circ Res 68: 881–887.
41. Dawson P, Hewitt P, Mackie IJ (1986) Contrast, coagulation, and fibrinolysis. Invest Radiol 21: 248–252.
42. Grollman JH Jr, Liu CK, Astone RA, Lurie MD (1988) Thromboembolic complications in coronary angiography associated with the use of nonionic contrast medium. Cathet Cardiovasc Diagn 14: 159–164.
43. Au PK (1991) Nonionic contrast media and intracatheter clot formation during use of a perfusion balloon catheter. Cathet Cardiovasc Diagn 22: 235–236.
44. Davidson CJ, Mark DB, Pieper KS (1990) Thrombotic and cardiovascular complications related to nonionic contrast media during cardiac catheterization: analysis of 8,517 patients. Am J Cardiol 65: 1481–1484.
45. Hwang MH, En Piano A, Murdock DK (1989) The potential risk of thrombosis during coronary angio-

graphy using nonionic contrast media. Cathet Cardiovasc Diagn 16: 209–213.

46. Rich MW, Crecelius CA (1990) Incidence, risk factors, and clinical course of acute renal insufficiency after cardiac catheterization in patients 70 years of age or older: a prospective study. Arch Intern Med 150: 1237–1242.

47. Taliercio CP, Vlietstra RE, Ilstrup DM (1991) A randomized comparison of the nephrotoxicity of iopamidol and diatrizoate in high risk patients undergoing cardiac angiography. J Am Coll Cardiol 17: 384–390.

48. Hill JA, Winniford M, Van Fossen DB (1991) Nephrotoxicity following cardiac angiography: a randomized double-blind multicenter trial of ionic and nonionic contrast media in 1194 patients. Circulation 84 (suppl II) 333.

49. Fischer HW, Doust VL (1971) An evaluation of pretesting in the problem of serious and fatal reactions to excretory urography. Radiology 103: 497.

50. Leonello PP, Frewin DB, Russell WJ, Gilligan JE, Jolley PT (1980) Adverse reactions to radiographic contrast media administered by the intravascular route. Aust Radiol 24: 311.

51. Lasser EC, Lang J, Sovak M, Kolb W, Lyon S, Hamlin E (1977) Steroids: theoretical and experimental basis for utilizationin in prevention of contrast media reactions. Radiology 125: 1.

52. Greenberger PA (1987) Clinical studies on the pretreatment of high risk patients submitted to contrast media procedures. Parvez Z (ed) Contrast media. CRC Press, Boca Raton, p. 165.

53. Barrett BJ, Parfrey PS, Vavasour HM (1992) A comparison of nonionic, low-osmolality radiocontrast agents with ionic, high-osmolality agents during cardiac catheterization. N Engl J Med 326: 431–436.

54. Gertz EW, Wisneski JA, Miller R (1992) Adverse reactions of low osmolality contrast media during cardiac angiography: a prospective randomized multicenter study. J Am Coll Cardiol 19: 899–906.

55. Pendergrass HP, Tondreau RL, Pendergrass EP, Ritchie DJ, Hildreth EA, Askovitz SI (1958) Reactions associated with intravenous urography. Historical and statistical review. Radiology 71: 1.

56. Coleman WP, Ochsner SF, Watson BE (1964) Allergic reactions in 10,000 consecutive intravenous urographies. Southern Medical Journal 57: 1401.

57. Toniolo G, Buia L (1966) Risultati di una inchiesta nazionale sugli incidenti mortali da iniizione di mezzi di contrasto organo-iodati. Rad Med II: 625.

58. Wolfromm R, Dehouve A, Degand F, Wattez E, Lange R, Crehalet A (1966) Les accidents graves par injection intraveineuse de substances iodées pour urographie. J Radiol Electr 47: 346.

59. Witten DM, Hirsch FD, Hartman GW (1973) Acute reactions to urographic contrast medium. AJR 119: 832.

60. Davies P, Roberts MB, Roylance J (1975) Acute reactions to urographic contrast media. Br Med J (Clin Res) 2: 434.

61. Shehadi WH, Toniolo G (1980) Adverse reactions to contrast media. Radiology 137: 299.

62. Ansell G, Tweedie MCK, West CR, Evans P, Couch L (1980) The current studies of reactions to intravenous contrast media. Invest Radiol 15: S32.

63. Hobbs BB (1991) Adverse reactions to intravenous contrast agents in Ontario 1975–1989. J Can Assoc Radiol 32: 8.

64. Pinet A, Lyonnet D, Maillet P, Groleau JM (1982) Adverse reactions to intravenous contrast media in urography – results of national survey. In: Contrast media in radiology. Amiel (ed.), Springer-Verlag, Basel, p. 14.

65. Michel JR (1982) Prevention of shocks induced by intravenous urography. In: Contrast media in radiology. Amiel (ed.), Springer-Verlag, Basel, p. 11.

66. Hartman GW, Hattery R, Witten DM (1982) Mortality during excretory urography: Mayo Clinic experience. AJR 139: 919.

67. Schrott KM, Behrends B, Clauß W, Kaufmann M, Lehnert J (1986) Iohexol in der Ausscheidungsurographie. Fortschr Med 104: 153.

68. Lasser EC, Berry CC, Talner LB (1987) Pretreatment with corticosteroids to alleviate reactions to intravenous contrast material: a randomized multiinstitutional study. New England J Med 317: 845.

69. Palmer FJ (1988) The RACR survey of intravenous contrast media reactions – final report. Australia Radiol 32: 426.

70. Wolf GL, Arenson RL, Cross AP (1989) A prospective trial of ionic vs nonionic contrast agents in routine clinical practice: comparison of adverse effects. AJR 152: 939.

71. Katayama H, Yamaguchi K, Kozuka T, Takashima T, Seez P, Matsuura K (1990) Adverse reactions to ionic and nonionic contrast media: a report from the Japanese Committee on the Safety of Contrast Media. Radiology 175: 621.

72. Ritchie JL, Nissen SE, Douglas SR et al. (1993) Use of nonionic or low osmolar contrast agents in cardiovascular procedures. JACC 21: 269–273.

73. Bettmann MA (1989) Guidelines for use of low-osmolality contrast agents. Radiology 172: 901–903.

74. Benness GT (1988) Guidelines revisited. Australas Radiol 32: 424–425.

75. Siegle RL (1992) Contrast reactions, treatment and risk management. Refresher Course # 317, RSNA '92.

76. O'Livieri Russell M, Goldberg HI, Reiss L (1976) Transfusion therapy for cerebrovascular abnormalities in sickle cell disease. J Pediatr 88: 382–387.

Cerebrovascular Angiography

G. P. Teitelbaum and R. T. Higashida

Introduction

A new array of low-profile highly trackable catheters, steerable guidewires, and versatile embolic agents have made possible the rapid expansion of the field of interventional neuroradiology. The treatment of many cranial and spinal vascular malformations, aneurysms, and tumors has been made possible by these newer developments.

Although diagnostic carotid, cerebral, and spinal angiography has become somewhat less frequent due to Doppler sonography, computed tomography, and magnetic resonance imaging, high-quality cranial and spinal angiography are now even more essential in the planning stages of interventional procedures. The individual performing such angiographic procedures must work as a team with the neuro- and vascular surgeons ultimately responsible for the care of such patients and be thoroughly familiar with the indications (see "Appendix") and potential complications associated with such angiographic studies.

Potential Risks of Neurovascular Angiography and Neurointerventional Procedures

Besides the risks of vessel damage, contrast reaction, renal failure, and groin hematoma and pseudoaneurysm common to other transfemoral angiographic procedures, neurovascular procedures carry with them an array of potential neurologic complications.

The risk of permanent neurologic complications from diagnostic neuroangiography should be in experienced hands, less than 1 %. Transient ischemic attacks and other temporary neurologic deficits should occur less than 3 % of the time. Because of these special concerns it is vital to perform a neurologic examination prior to and following the completion of any neurovascular procedure to assess the occurrence of any of complications.

Care must be taken to avoid spasm and dissection of the great vessels during catheterizations since these complications may result in cerebral embolization. Spasm around a catheter tip in either the vertebral or internal carotid arteries may result in a wedge injection and transmission of the entire pressure head of a power injection into the vascular tree examined. Such pressure transmission distally may be sufficient to rupture an intracranial aneurysm. Therefore it is always essential to test the catheter position and the flow rate of the cannulated vessel with a small hand injection of contrast prior to any power contrast injection.

In patients with a high blood pressure, the risk of vasospasm can be reduced by the application of an inch of nitropaste and/or administration of sublingual nifedipine. At times, intra-arterial papavarine (30–60 mg) may be slowly injected to help treat severe, catheter-induced vasospasm.

Major complications occur in 5 %–10 % of neurointerventional cases, including perforation of an intracranial blood vessel (estimated to occur in approximately 1 % of cases) nontarget embolization, stroke, intracranial hemorrhage, cranial nerve injuries, and neurologic injuries due to mass effect (due to thrombosis of a vascular structure).

Neurointerventionalists need to be keenly aware of communications between the external carotid artery (ECA) and intracranial circulation as well as the vascular supply to the cranial nerves and ocular structures in order to lessen the risk of nontarget embolization (see below).

Treatment of mass effect due to thrombosis following neuroembolizations may involve the use of parenteral steroids. Care must be taken to minimize the course of these agents and to taper their dosage during discontinuation. Delayed side effects of steroid use include femoral head necrosis.

Stenoses of the vertebral and carotid arteries may in large part be composed of thrombus. Balloon angioplasty of such lesions without a prior conservative course of anticoagulation may result in cerebral embolization. Balloon angioplasty within the vertebral and basilar arteries resulting in acute arterial dissections with significant flow restriction may precipitate confusion, dysarthria, coma, and respiratory arrest. The standard of care during such angioplasties therefore includes anesthesiology stand-by assistance within the angiography laboratory should emergent endotracheal intubation become necessary.

Angioplasty of basilar artery stenoses carries with it the risk of occluding sufficient paramedian perforating vessels to cause the "locked-in" syndrome. In this condition the patient is unable to speak and is paralyzed although spinothalamic sensation is retained, and some facial and eye movements may be perserved. For this reason basilar artery dilatations are to be approached with extreme caution and should be limited to stenoses of less than 5 mm in length.

A not infrequent complication of transfemoral catheterizations in children under the age of 12 months is common femoral artery occlusion and ipsilateral loss of lower extremity pulses for this complication. In this age group, as long as there is pink coloration and good capillary refill in the toes of the affected side, no immediate intervention, surgical or otherwise, is required or indicated.

Basic Equipment and Catheterization Techniques

The vast majority of adult neurocatheterizations may be accomplished using either a 5.5-F Norman (Cook, Bloomington, IN) or 7-F Berenstein catheter (USCI, Billerica, MA), with the smaller size catheter being useful for patients under the age of 40 years. For patients with highly tortuous great vessel anatomy and for common carotid arteriography, a Simmons II or III 7-F catheter (USCI) may be useful. The Simmons catheters have also been referred to as sidewinder and reverse-curve catheters. Additional useful catheters for cannulating the great vessels would include Hincks and "head hunter" varieties (Cook and other manufacturers).

A high-flow 6-F pigtail flush catheter (Cook) may be used for aortic arch arteriography. Extreme care must be exercised with the use of such multisidehole catheters: They should be vigorously hand-flushed every 2 min and never placed on a pressurized saline drip in order to avoid the risk of catheter-related cerebral thromboembolism. Flush catheters should also be withdrawn from the aortic arch as soon as possible following the performance of a contrast injection.

The most useful guidewires for neurovascular work would include 0.035-in. Bentson (Cook) and angled Glidewire (Medi-tech, Watertown, MA) varieties as well as 0.035-in. exchange wires (260 cm length) of the Newton (Cook), Bentson (Cook), and Glidewire (Medi-tech) varieties. The Bentson wire, the most commonly employed in our practice, is a floppy-tipped straight wire that is distally shapable. The Newton wire, also straight, is somewhat stiffer. The steerable, hydrophylic Glidewire is much stiffer than the Bentson wire but is well suited to navigate particularly tortuous vessels. It is, however, a poor choice for an initial access wire when puncturing the femoral artery.

If multiple catheter exchanges are anticipated during a diagnostic angiogram or during neurointerventional cases, we employ a femoral access sheath. Generally, 4-F sheaths are used in infants and small children whereas 5.5–8.0-F sheaths are utilized in adults, depending upon the type of procedure being performed.

For aortic arch studies a pigtail catheter is positioned 2–3 cm proximal to the origin of the inominate artery. We generally perform adult arch arteriography with the injection of contrast at 30 ml/s with a total volume of 45 ml. Filming is performed in the left anterior oblique plane (with the patient's head turned toward the right) with the acquisition of four or five images/s for 5 s followed by one image/s for 6 s.

For catheterizations of the common carotid arteries a Norman or Berenstein catheter is positioned within the proximal aortic arch, with a Bentson or Glidewire inserted to the distal tip of the catheter, and is rotated so as to direct the tip in a cephalad direction. The catheter is then slowly withdrawn until its tip springs into the ostium of the innominate or left common carotid artery (CCA). Sometimes one first intentionally enters the innominate artery with the catheter tip to catheterize the left CCA. As above, the catheter is slowly withdrawn with the application of slight counterclockwise torque to make the catheter tip spring into the left CCA.

Once the catheter tip is located in either the innominate or left CCA, the guidewire is gently advanced cephalad to the level of the angle of the mandible. In younger patients with fairly straight vascular anatomy, the catheter can then be advanced over the immobilized wire. However, with more tortuous anatomy, other maneuvers are necessary to advance the catheter. As a unit, the catheter and guidewire are advanced forward slighty (<1 cm). Next, mild counterclockwise torque is placed upon the catheter while simultaneously applying traction on the guidewire. These two steps are repeated several times to make the catheter spring forward. One must not allow bucking of the catheter into the aortic arch during these maneuvers. Caution must be exercised to prevent the catheter from advancing beyond the distal guidewire tip (thus avoiding the risks of vasospasm and dissection).

Once in place, the endhole catheter must be immediately double-flushed (one syringe to aspirate blood and a second clean saline syringe to forward flush). A small gentle contrast injection should then immediately be made through the catheter to determine the presence of dissection or vasospasm (evident with contrast stasis or slow flow at the catheter tip). In such cases the catheter should be withdrawn sufficiently to relieve the flow restriction. A small test injection to rule out catheter wedging (due to vasospasm) is also vital if an intracranial aneurysm is suspected. Power injection of contrast through a wedged catheter in such a situation could cause aneurysm rupture. One should never leave a standing column of blood with a catheter with the stopcock closed. Either an endhole catheter should be double-flushed by hand every 2 min or immediately placed to a pressurized and heparinized saline flush.

A 7-F Simmons II or III catheter is usually preferred to catheterize the CCA for the evaluation of carotid bifurcation disease (since only a short length of leading guidewire is necessary to position a reverse curve catheter; wire passage through a suspected stenosis can be avoided). Contrast injection should be at a rate of 6 ml/s for a total volume of 6 ml at an injector pressure setting of no greater than 450 psi. Full-strength nonionic contrast should be used for cut-film technique, whereas more dilute contrast can be used in digital subtraction angiography (with the dilution factor depending upon the type of angiography unit used). We employ only nonionic contrast for all of our neurovascular procedures. We generally film at a rate of four images/s for 4 s followed by one image/s for 8–10 s. Stenoses of the proximal ICA must be accurately assessed in at least two angiographic planes with complete splaying of the carotid bifurcation in one view. If any intraluminal thrombus is visualized within the proximal internal carotid artery (ICA), further ipsilateral CCA injections risk cerebral thromboembolism, and therefore the study is terminated.

In cases of seemingly complete cervical ICA occlusion, careful delayed imaging is essential to assess for any faint opacification of the cervical ICA (usually termed the "string sign" due to a thin layering of contrast along the posterior wall of the ICA) since this denotes a critical proximal ICA stenosis rather than a complete occlusion. One pitfall is the assumption that the faint opacification of the carotid siphon (the sinusoidally shaped distal intracranial segment of the ICA; see below) always represents a string sign. However, this is sometimes merely due to collateral flow to the carotid siphon from branches of the ipsilateral ECA. In general, high-quality digital or cut-film arteriography is necessary to evaluate the carotid bifurcation, especially with regard to the string sign. Cineangiography should not be used for this purpose.

Selective catheterization of the ICA and ECA is accomplished using fluoroscopy with or without digital roadmap imaging, depending on the amount of vessel tortuosity that is present. Catheter position within the ECA must permit adequate filling of all ECA branches, including the proximally located occipital artery. One usually injects 2–3 ml contrast/s for a total volume of 6 ml. Filming is performed in the frontal and lateral planes at a rate of three images/s for 4 s followed by one imgage/s for 7–8 s.

Generally, ICA contrast injections are made with the catheter no higher than the C2 level. The petrous portion of the ICA (see below) is more prone to dissections with catheter manipulations and forceful contrast injections. For cerebral angiography a contrast injection rate of 6 ml/s for a total volume of 8 ml is used in adult patients. If a CCA injection is utilized, the injection rate is increased to 7 ml/s for a total volume of 9 ml. Filming is performed in the frontal (with petrous ridges superimposed over the orbital roofs) and lateral planes at three or four images/s for 4–5 s followed by one image/s for 7 s. A Schullers view (lateral positioning with caudad angulation of image intensifier on the side ipsilateral to carotid injection) is helpful in splaying out the vessels of the M1 bifurcation (see below). Ipsilateral anterior oblique imaging (viewing through the orbit on the side of injection) is useful for demonstrating the ICA bifurcation.

We usually perform vertebral artery catheterizations with either 7-F Berenstein or 5.5-F Norman catheters. The catheter should be advanced only several centimeters into the vessel. The vertebral arteries are smaller and more spasm prone than the carotids. The contrast injection rate for adult vertebral arteriography is usually 5 ml/s for a total volume of 7 ml. Filming of the skull is performed in the Towne's (with the image intensifier angled toward the head) and lateral planes with the acquisition of three images/s for 4 s followed by one image/s for 7–8 s. If there is marked tortuosity or atherosclerotic plaquing of the proximal vertebral arteries, the intracranial distribution of these vessels can be studied using the same skull imaging planes and image acquisition rates but using contrast injection into the proximal subclavian artery with an inflated blood pressure cuff on the ipsilateral upper arm. A contrast injection rate in this situation of 8 ml/s for a total volume of 16 ml would be satisfactory.

To evelute the course of the cervical portion of the vertebral artery the total contrast injection volume can be reduced to 5 ml with filming performed in the ipsilateral oblique plane. For evaluation of the origin of a vertebral artery, contrast can be injected through a selective catheter within the proximal subclavian artery at a rate of 8 ml/s for a total volume of 10–12 ml. Filming of the supraclavicular area is performed in the contralateral oblique plane (with mild Towne's angulation) with the acquisition of four images/s for 4 s followed by one image/s for 5 s.

The above brief catheterization, contrast injection rate, and imaging guidelines are for adult transfemoral procedures. An alternative transbrachial route, using 4-F reverse curve catheters, can be used for outpatient neurovascular procedures. Also, pediatric neurovascular studies require lower profile catheters and smaller injection volumes. However, these more specialized procedures should only be performed by highly experienced neuroangiographers.

Branches of the Aortic Arch

The usual branching order of the great vessels from the aortic arch is the innominate, left CCA and left subclavian arteries (Fig. 1a). The most common anatomic variants and anomalies of the arch include common origin of the innominate and left CCAs (25 %; Fig. 1b), origin of the left CCA from the proximal innominate artery (bovine left CCA; 5 %–10 %; Fig. 1c), separate origin of left vertebral artery (VA) from the arch (5 %), and aberrant right subclavian artery origin from the arch (0.5 %).

Stenoses and irregularities of the great vessels are most commonly caused by atherosclerosis (Fig. 1d, e). Less commonly, stenoses are caused by fibromuscular dysplasia (FMD), dissections, arteritis (especially Takayasu's arteritis), or neurofibromatosis. Long-standing hypertension may result in marked tortuosity of the proximal great vessels.

Extracranial Carotid Arteries

Usually the right CCA arises from the bifurcation of the innominate artery. The left CCA typically arises separately from the aortic arch just distal to

Fig. 1. a Thoracic aortic (arch) digital arteriogram ▶ obtained in the left anterior oblique (LAO) plane demonstrating normal anatomy of the great vessels originating from the aortic arch: innominate (*1*), right internal mammary artery (*2*), right vertebral artery (*3*), right common carotid artery (*4*), right subclavian artery (*5*), left common carotid artery (*6*), left vertebral artery (*7*), left thyrocervical trunk (*8*), left costocervical trunk (*9*), left subclavian artery (*10*), left internal mammary artery (*11*), and left supreme intercostal artery (*12*). **b** LAO digital arch arteriogram revealing annomalous origin of the right subclavian artery (*open arrow*) distal to the left subclavian arterial origin (*curved arrow*). Note the more distal course of the right subclavian artery (*arrows*), as well as the right (*curved open arrow*) and left (*thin arrow*) common carotid arteries. **c** LAO digital arch arteriogram demonstrating the left common carotid artery originating from the innominate artery (*open arrow*). Note the tortuous course of the proximal left common carotid artery (*arrows*). **d** High-grade atherosclerotic stenosis of the proximal innominate artery in a middle-aged man with transient ischemic attacks. **e** Following balloon angioplasty of lesion in **d**, there is now excellent flow through a widely patent innominate artery and resolution of the patient's cerebral ischemic symptoms

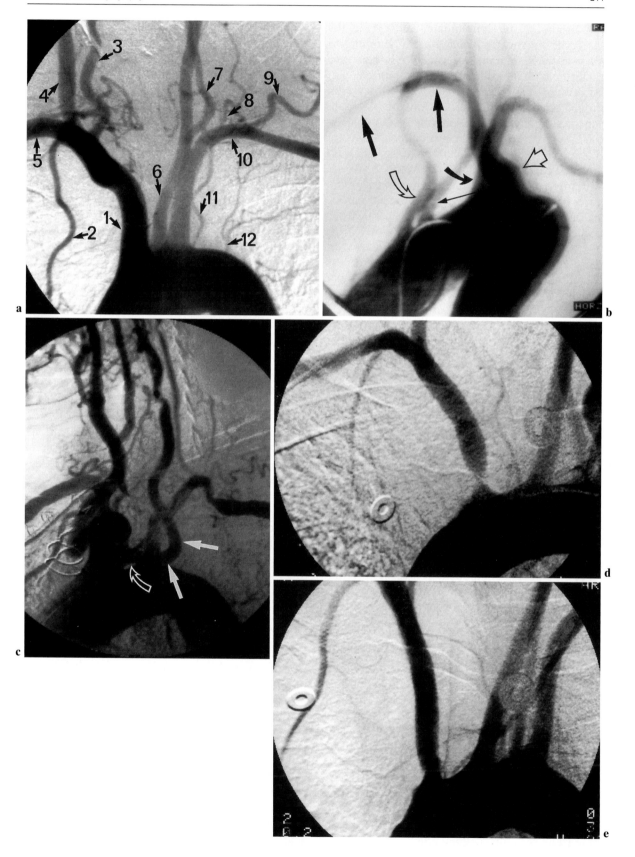

the origin of the innominate artery (Fig. 1a). However, the left CCA may have a common origin with the innominate artery. The common carotid bifurcation into the internal and external carotid arteries is usually located at the C4 level, although this is variable. The proximal ICA usually runs posterolateral to the proximal ECA (Fig. 2a, b). The relatively dilated proximal portion of the ICA is referred to as the carotid sinus. There are no significant cervical ICA branches.

Atherosclerosis is the most common cause of stenoses and occlusions of the extracranial carotid arteries (Fig. 2c). Less common causes of carotid occlusive disease include dissection (either acute or healed; Fig. 2d), arteritis, FMD (Fig. 2e), tumor encasement, and trauma. In cases of suspected complete cervical ICA occlusion delayed imaging is essential to assess for a string sign (see above; Fig. 2f, g) denoting a critical proximal ICA stenosis rather than a complete occlusion (the latter excludes the possibility of carotid endarterectomy). Results of a recent cooperative study suggest that the risk of stroke outweigh the risks of carotid endarterectomy when the degree of symptomatic proximal ICA stenosis is at least 70 %.

Surgical carotid endarterectomy is still the treatment of choice for significant symptomatic proximal ICA stenoses. Balloon angioplasty should be reserved for intrathoracic CCA and high cervical/petrous ICA stenoses associated with cerebral ischemic symptoms since lesions at these locations are more hazardous to access surgically. Extreme caution should be exercised when considering such carotid stenoses for balloon angioplasty since a significant component of these lesions may be due to mural thrombus. Balloon dilatation in these cases without a prior conservative trial of anticoagulation therapy may result in disastrous embolic complications.

Carotid dissections (Fig. 2d) may cause complete occlusion or true lumen restriction and/or irregularity. Carotid dissections may occur spontaneously or may be the result of an underlying disorder such as hypertension or FMD. These lesions may present with ipsilateral neck pain and Horner's syndrome. Partially occluding dissections may require anticoagulation therapy to counter the risk of cerebral embolization.

The most common branching order of the ECA is: superior thyroidal (most proximal), ascending pharyngeal (which sometimes arises from a common trunk with the occipital artery), lingual, occi-pital, facial, posterior auricular, superficial temporal, middle meningeal, accessory meningeal, and internal maxillary arteries (Fig. 2a, c, 3a, b). The middle meningeal artery may occasionally arise from the ophthalmic artery, a branch of the ICA.

The superior thyroidal artery supplies the thyroid and larynx. The ascending pharyngeal supplies mainly the naso- and oropharynx and the tympanic cavity, but it may also provide blood supply to the lower cranial nerves (see below), meninges, and tentorium via its neuromeningeal division. The lingual artery supplies the tongue, floor of the mouth, and submandibular gland. The occipital artery supplies the scalp, and upper cervical musculature. A number of facial artery branches anastomose with other ECA vessels to provide vascular supply to the palate, pharynx, orbit, and face. The superficial temporal and posterior auricular arteries primarily supply scalp, buccal region, and ear structures. The internal maxillary artery gives vascular supply to the temporalis muscle, the meninges via (middle and accessory meningeal arteries), palatine and deep facial structures, turbinates and paranasal sinuses, mandible, and the alveolar ridges.

One needs to be keenly aware of communications between the ECA and intracranial circulation as well as the cranial nerves and ocular structures receiving vascular supply from ECA branches. Muscular branches from the distal occipital artery can communicate with the ipsilateral VA (Fig. 3c, d). The posterior auricular artery may communicate with the ICA via the stylomastoid artery. Facial nerve palsy is a concern during embolization of the occipital and posterior auricular arteries due to potential branches to the stylomastoid foramen. The odontoid arcade and neuromeningeal division of the ascending pharyngeal artery (entering the skull base through the jugular foramen) may communicate with the VA (Fig. 3e). The neuromeningeal division also provides vascular supply to cranial nerves IX–XII and sometimes the gasserian ganglion of the trigeminal nerve. The angular branch of the facial artery communicates with the ophthalmic artery via orbital anastomoses.

From the anterior division of the middle meningeal artery a meningolacrimal branch giving retinal supply may arise (denoted by a curvilinear choroidal blush on a lateral middle meningeal arteriogram; Fig. 3f, h). Thus, middle meningeal arterial embolization proximal to the meningolac-

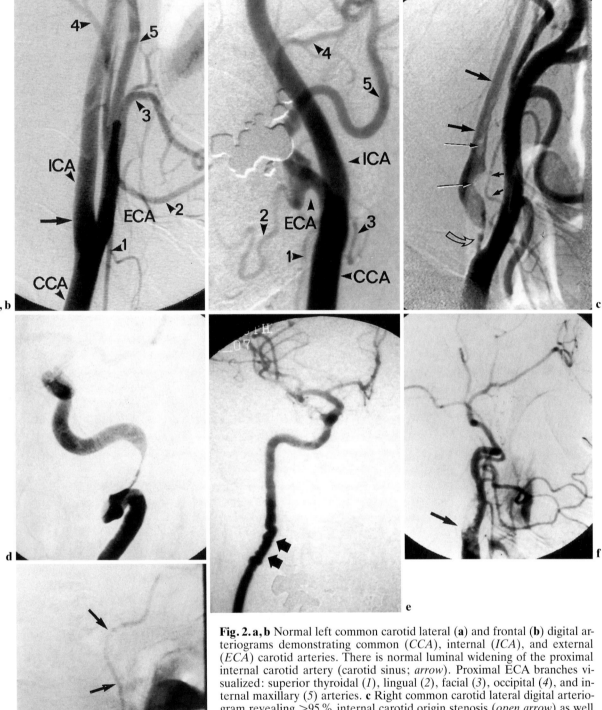

Fig. 2. a, b Normal left common carotid lateral (**a**) and frontal (**b**) digital arteriograms demonstrating common (*CCA*), internal (*ICA*), and external (*ECA*) carotid arteries. There is normal luminal widening of the proximal internal carotid artery (carotid sinus; *arrow*). Proximal ECA branches visualized: superior thyroidal (*1*), lingual (*2*), facial (*3*), occipital (*4*), and internal maxillary (*5*) arteries. **c** Right common carotid lateral digital arteriogram revealing >95 % internal carotid origin stenosis (*open arrow*) as well as diminished distal internal carotid opacification (*arrow*) and intraluminal filling defects due to thrombus (*thin arrows*). Also note course of proximal right ascending pharyngeal artery (*small arrows*). **d** Left common carotid frontal digital arteriogram demonstrating high-grade tapered stenosis of distal cervical portion of the left internal carotid artery caused by dissection. **e** Frontal digital arteriogram showing "beading" of short segment of cervical right internal carotid artery (*arrows*) due to fibromuscular dysplasia. **f** There appears to be complete occlusion of the cervical internal carotid artery at its origin (*arrow*) during the early phase of a left common carotid lateral digital arteriogram. **g** However, delayed images reveal faint opacification of the internal carotid artery ("string sign"; *arrows*) signifying a critical stenosis, rather than complete occlusion, of the internal carotid origin

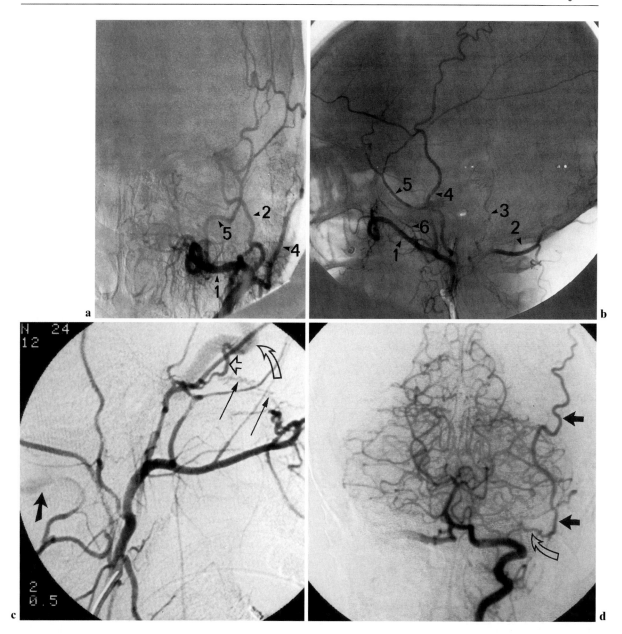

Fig. 3. a, b Frontal (**a**) and lateral (**b**) external carotid artery (ECA) subtraction angiograms demonstrating the following branch vessels: internal maxillary (*1*), occipital (*2*), posterior auricular (*3*), superficial temporal (*4*), middle meningeal (*5*), and anterior deep temporal (*6*) arteries. **c** External carotid lateral digital arteriogram revealing collateral flow from the internal maxillary artery to carotid siphon (*curved open arrow*) via the artery of the foramen rotundum (*thin arrows*) to the infrolateral trunk (lateral mainstem artery; *open arrow-*

head). Also note opacification of the ipsilateral vertebral artery (*arrow*) due to muscular collaterals from the occipital artery. **d** Towne's projection left vertebral digital arteriogram demonstrating filling of the occipital artery (an external carotid branch; *arrows*) via extracranial muscular collaterals (*open arrow*). **e** Left ascending pharyngeal lateral digital arteriogram (anterior, *to the right*) in a 4-year-old girl showing the main vessel (*arrow*) along with its neuromeningeal division (*open arrow*) and odontoid arcade (*smaller arrows*). These

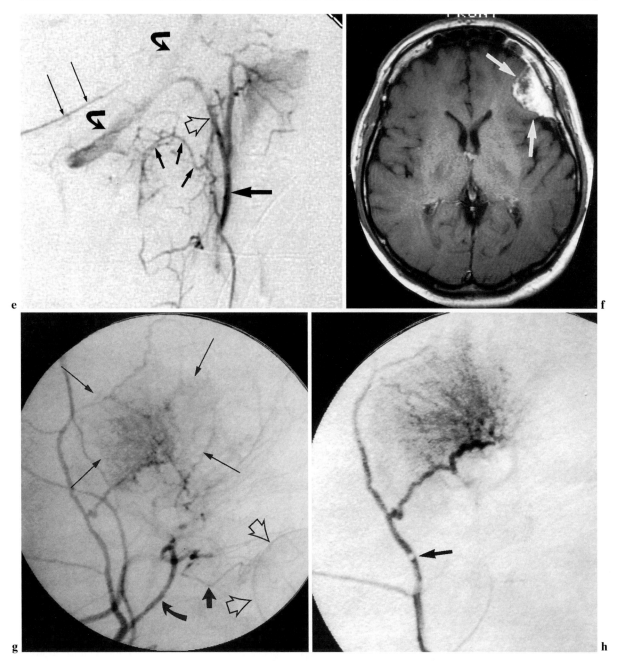

branches possess collateral communications with the ipsilateral vertebral (*curved arrows*) and posterior meningeal (*thin arrows*) arteries. **f** Axial T1-weighted spin
echo magnetic resonance brain image with gadolinium
enhancement revealing a homogenously enhancing left
frontal meningioma (*arrows*). **g** Left external carotid digital arteriogram in same patient as **f** demonstrating meningolacrimal branch (*curved arrow*) arising from the
middle meningeal artery and providing collateral flow
to the ipsilateral ophthalmic artery (*arrow*). Note the

curvilinear choroidal blush (*open arrows*) of the retina
as well as the contrast blush of the meningioma from
middle meningeal artery vascular supply (*thin arrows*).
h Prior to surgical excision of the tumor in **g**, a microcatheter was advanced distally within the middle meningeal artery (*arrow*), beyond the origin of the meningolacrimal artery, to embolize the meningioma with polyvinyl alcohol particles

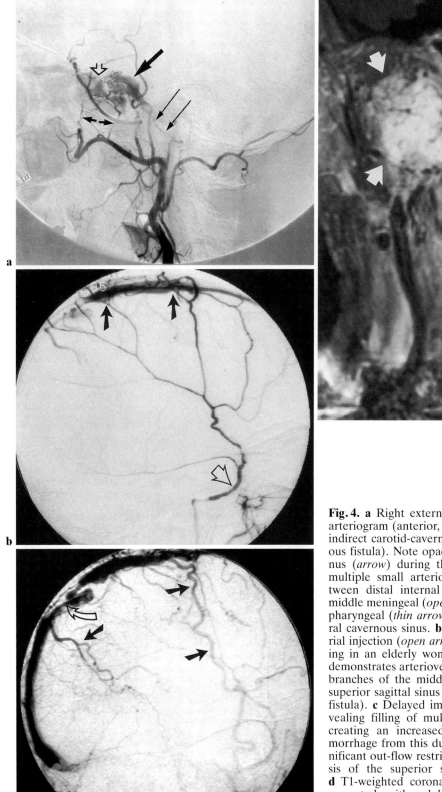

Fig. 4. a Right external carotid lateral subtraction arteriogram (anterior, *to the left*) in patient with an indirect carotid-cavernous fistula (dural arteriovenous fistula). Note opacification of the cavernous sinus (*arrow*) during the arterial phase as well as multiple small arteriovenous communications between distal internal maxillary (*smaller arrows*), middle meningeal (*open arrowhead*), and ascending pharyngeal (*thin arrows*) branches and the ipsilateral cavernous sinus. **b** Left middle meningeal arterial injection (*open arrow*) with lateral digital imaging in an elderly woman with aphasia. The study demonstrates arteriovenous shunting between distal branches of the middle meningeal artery and the superior sagittal sinus (*arrows*; dural arteriovenous fistula). **c** Delayed image from angiogram in **b** revealing filling of multiple cortical veins (*arrows*) creating an increased risk for subarachnoid hemorrhage from this dural fistula. Also note the significant out-flow restriction caused by a tight stenosis of the superior sagittal sinus (*open arrow*). **d** T1-weighted coronal spin-echo magnetic resonance study with gadolinium enhancement demonstrating a large right-sided cervical paraganglioma (*arrows*) displacing the trachea in a 55-year-old woman.

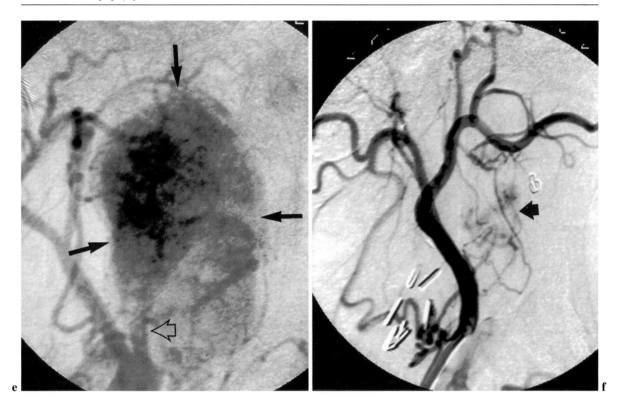

e   f

Fig. 4. e Right external carotid frontal digital arteriogram in same patient showing the highly vascular mass (*arrows*) fed primarily by an enlarged ascending pharyngeal artery (*open arrow*). **f** Following polyvinyl alcohol particle embolization of this artery, pretumor excision, repeat angiogram demonstrates little residual vascular blush within the tumor (*arrow*)

The most common neurointerventional procedures involving branches of the ECA include: treatment of dural arteriovenous fistulas (Fig. 4a–c), preoperative tumor embolization (mainly meningiomas, paragangliomas, and juvenile angiofibromas; Fig. 3f,g, 4d–f), treatment of congenital arteriovenous malformations (AVMs) and fistulas (AVFs), control of intractible epistaxis, and occlusion of posttraumatic pseudoaneurysms and arteriovenous fistulas.

rimal branch risks ipsilateral blindness. While traversing the foramen spinosum, the middle meningeal artery may supply a branch, through the petrous bone, to the facial nerve.

ECA-to-ICA connections arising from the internal maxillary artery include the vidian artery (communicating with the petrous ICA through vidian canal of the sphenoid bone), artery of the foramen rotundum (communicating with the infrolateral trunk/lateral mainstem artery of the cavernous ICA), and the infraorbital artery and orbital branches of the anterior deep temporal artery (communicating with the intracranial circulation via the ophthalmic artery). The artery of the foramen rotundum may supply the V_2 division of the trigeminal nerve passing through the same foramen. The vidian artery may also collateralize with the ascending pharyngeal and accessory meningeal arteries.

Petrous, Cavernous, and Supraclinoid Portions of the Internal Carotid Artery

There are relatively few branches arising from the petrous portion of the ICA traversing the carotid canal (anterior to the jugular foramen). These include the vidian artery (seen in 25% of angiograms), described above, as well as a persistent trigeminal artery (seen on <1% of angiograms), connecting the petrous ICA with the basilar artery (BA) (Fig. 5). The trigeminal artery is an embryonic vessel and is the most common type of carotid-vertebral anastomosis caudad to the circle of Willis. The petrous ICA may take an aberrant course through the middle ear where it may cause pulsa-

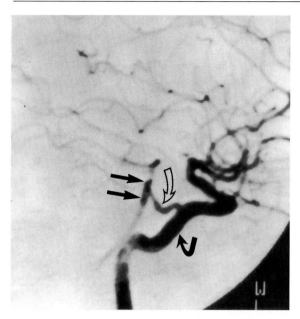

Fig. 5. Lateral right internal carotid digital arteriogram demonstrating a trigeminal artery (*open arrow*) connecting the internal carotid artery (*curved arrow*) with the basilar artery (*solid arrows*)

Fig. 6. a Left ICA frontal digital arteriogram in a 49-year-old woman who sustained blunt head trauma during an assault demonstrating a direct carotid-cavernous fistula (*CCF*) with rapid opacification of the cavernous sinuses (*CS*) as well as superior (*SPS*) and inferior (*IPS*) petrosal sinuses, sphenoparietal sinus (*SphPS*), sigmoid sinus (*SS*), superior (*SOV*) and inferior (*IOV*) ophthalmic veins, and internal jugular vein (*JV*). Note the poor filling of the middle cerebral arterial branches (*small arrows*). **b** Same patient as in **a**. Following transarterial left cavernous sinus detachable balloon embolization (*arrow*) (via the rent in the left ICA), left internal carotid arteriography reveals obliteration of the arteriovenous fistula

Fig. 7. a Lateral internal carotid digital arteriogram displaying the ophthalmic (*1*), posterior communicating (*2*), anterior choroidal (*3*), anterior cerebral (*4*) and middle cerebral (*5*) arteries. The carotid siphon (*S's*), consisting of the cavernous and supraclinoid portions of the internal carotid artery, follows a sinusoidal course. Note plexal point (*open arrow*). **b** Right internal carotid lateral subtraction arteriogram demonstrating the meningohypophyseal trunk (*curved arrow*; emanating from the proximal cavernous internal carotid artery) and artery of Bernasconi and Cassinari (*straight arrows*). Also note the appearance of a normal angiographic sylvian triangle (*solid white lines*), roughly defining the insula. **c** Right common carotid lateral digital arteriogram performed in a middle-aged woman showing a large supraclinoid (within the subarachnoid space) fusiform internal carotid artery aneurysm (*open arrows*) distal to the ophthalmic artery (*solid arrow*). **d** Same patient as in **c**. A lateral skull film, obtained after transcatheter occlusion of the parent internal carotid artery, shows two contrast-filled silicone balloons deposited within the carotid siphon (*open arrows*) and several platinum embolization coils within the aneurysm cavity itself (*solid arrow*). **e** Same patient as in **d**. A postembolization left vertebral lateral digital arteriogram demonstrates filling of the right middle (*solid arrows*) and anterior (*open arrow*) cerebral arteries via collateral flow through the right posterior communicating artery (*thin arrow*). Also note the basilar artery (*curved arrow*)

tile tinnitus and a blue tympanic membrane. Obviously, biopsy of the tympanic membrane in this situation circumstances would be disastrous.

Aneurysms of the petrous ICA are uncommon and are usually congential or posttraumatic. They may cause intracanial embolization and thus warrant detachable balloon ICA occlusion. Deceleration or penetrating injuries may result in arteriovenous fistulas between the ICA and internal jugular vein.

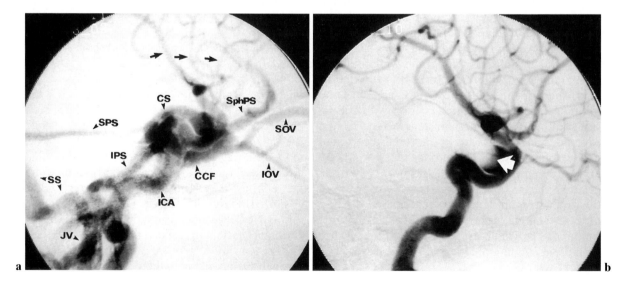

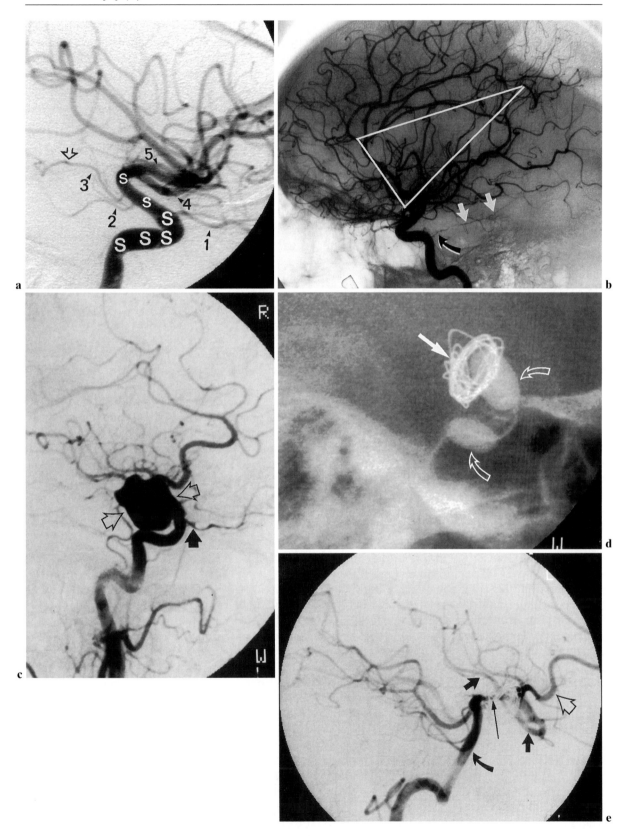

As the ICA exits the petrous bone, it enters the cavernous sinus, a confluence of venous drainage channels within the dura at the base of the brain (Fig. 6a). The paired cavernous sinuses, flanking the pituitary gland, are typically interconnected by circular sinuses. Other important structures traversing the cavernous sinus include cranial nerves III, IV, V_1, V_2, and VI. Within the cavernous sinus, the ICA assumes a sinusoidal shape. This portion plus the terminal ICA cephalad to the cavernous sinus (the supraclinoid portion) make up the carotid siphon (Fig. 7a).

The typical branching order of angiographically visible vessels arising from the carotid siphon is: meningohypophyseal trunk (most proximal), inferolateral trunk (lateral mainstem artery), ophthalmic artery, posterior communicating artery (PCOM), anterior choroidal artery, and anterior and middle cerebral arteries (terminal branches). In approximately 90% of patients the ophthalmic artery is the first branch of the supraclinoid portion of the ICA and thus serves as a demarcation between the intracavernous and subarachnoid segments of the ICA (Fig. 7a).

The meningohypophyseal trunk (Fig. 7b) supplies the tentorium (via the artery of Bernasconi and Cassinari), cavernous sinus dura, posterior pituitary, and at times cranial nerves III–VI. The infrolateral trunk (Fig. 3C) provides vascular supply to the cavernous sinus dura as well as cranial nerves III–VII, and anastomoses with multiple ECA branches including the artery of the foramen of rotundum (Fig. 3C). The ophthalmic artery supplies the globe, orbit and its contents (in conjuction with ECA branches), dura (via the anterior falx artery; rarely, the middle meningeal artery originates from the ophthalmic artery), and may serve as an important collateral pathway with flow received from orbital branches of the facial and internal maxillary arteries.

Aneurysms of the cavernous ICA present a lower risk than those present in the supraclinoid region (subarachnoid space) since rupture of the intracavernous lesions results in a direct carotid-cavernous fistula (Fig. 6), which is far less devastating than intracranial hemorrhage. Very large aneurysms may cause mass effects on adjacent cranial nerves. Symptomatic inoperable fusiform aneurysms of the cavernous and supraclinoid ICA may be treated by occlusion of the parent ICA using detachable balloons (Fig. 7c–e).

The PCOM (Figs. 7e, 8a) serves as a collateral pathway in the circle of Willis (see below), connecting the internal carotid and vertebrobasilar circulations. It runs between the supraclinoid portion of the ICA and the Pl segment of the ipsilateral posterior cerebral artery (PCA). The PCOM supplies important minute perforating branches to the thalamus, hypothalamus, and optic chiasm. Some 30%–35% of intracranial aneurysms occur within the ICA at the origin of the PCOM. A cone- or nipplelike dilatation (<3 mm in greatest diameter), termed an infundibulum, normally occurs at the origin of the PCO from the supraclinoid ICA. This must not be mistaken for an aneurysm.

The anterior choroidal artery (Fig. 7a) usually originates from the ICA just distal to the PCOM and travels posteriorly in the crural cistern subjacent to the optic tract and medial to the uncus of the temporal lobe. It then enters the choroidal fissure of the temporal horn of the lateral ventricle where there is a slight kink in its contour called the plexal point. Distal to the plexal point the anterior choroidal artery supplies the choroid plexus of the lateral ventricle and anastomoses with the lateral posterior choroidal artery. The anterior choroidal artery is quite strategic. Its occlusion may cause the devastating consequences of hemiplegia, hemiparesis, and/or homonymous quadrant- or hemianopsia due to thrombosis of minute perforators arising proximal to the plexal point serving the internal capsule, optic tract, thalamus, basal ganglia, a portion of the cerebral peduncle, and substantia nigra.

Circle of Willis

The circle of Willis (Fig. 8a) is an important vascular collateral ring at the base of the brain surrounding the optic chiasm and pituitary stalk. It is composed of (from posterior to anterior) the basilar artery bifurcation (basilar tip), paired proximal P1 segments of the PCAs (PCA proximal to its junction with the PCOM), paired PCOMs, paired distal ICAs, paired proximal A1 segments of the anterior cerebral arteries (ACAs) and the anterior communicating artery (ACOM; linking both ACAs). This vascular ring is actually present in its complete form, i.e., no hypoplastic or absent segments, in only approximately 25% of persons. In about 20% the PCA arises directly from the supraclinoid ICA (fetal origin; Fig. 8b, c). The PCOM is hypoplastic in more than 30% of the population. Hypoplasia or absence may be seen

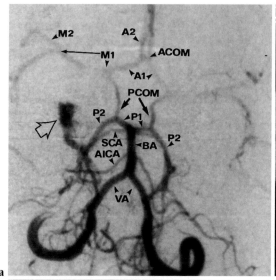

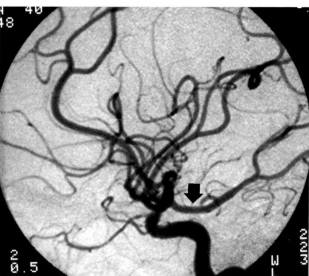

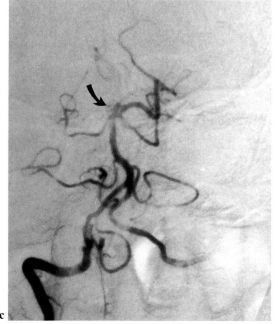

Fig. 8. a Submentovertex view (extreme neck extension with caudal angulation of the image intensifier) left vertebral digital arteriogram with excellent opacification of the circle of Willis in this patient with a right temporal lobe arteriovenous malformation (*open arrow*) fed primarily by an anterior temporal branch of the right posterior cerebral artery. Note the components of the circle of Willis: basilar artery (*BA*), P1 segments (*P1*), posterior communicating arteries (*PCOM*), A1 segements (*A1*), and anterior communicating artery (*ACOM*). Also note the vertebral arteries (*VA*), anterior inferior cerebellar arteries (*AICA*), superior cerebellar arteries (*SCA*), P2 segment of the posterior cerebral arteries (*P2*), M1 and M2 segments of the middle cerebral arteries (*M1, M2*), and the A2 segment of the anterior cerebral arteries (*A2*). **b** Right internal carotid lateral digital arteriogram (anterior, *to the left*) demonstrating fetal origin of the right posterior cerebral artery (*arrow*). **c** Same patient as in **b**. Right vertebral frontal digital arteriogram demonstrating absence of opacification of the right posterior cerebral artery (*arrow*) due to its fetal origin from the right internal carotid artery

in the A1 segment of the ACA. The ACOM is multiple in up to 40 % of cases.

Vital perforating vessels arising from the circle of Willis include branches to the thalamus, limbic system, reticular activating system, cerebral peduncles, posterior limb of the internal capsule, and occulomotor nerve nucleus from the basilar tip, P1 (most proximal PCA) segments, and the PCOMs. Branches to the optic chiasm and pituitary stalk may arise from the PCOMs and terminal ICA segments. Medial lenticulostriate arteries arise from the A1 segments and supply the internal capsule,

hypothalamus, and basal ganglia. Approximately 14 % of the time, the recurrent artery of Heubner originates from the A1 segment (more commonly it arises from the ACA distal to the ACOM) to supply the anterior limb of the internal capsule, a portion of the globus pallidus, and the head of the caudate nucleus. Small perforators originate from the ACOM supplying the limbic system and optic chiasm. Occlusion of these perforators risks akinetic mutism and bitemporal hemianopsia.

The circle of Willis is the most frequent site for intracranial aneurysm, with 30 %–35 % of these lesions occurring within the ACOM and ICA (at the PCOM origin), each. Approximately 5 % of intracranial aneurysms are located at the basilar tip. The circle of Willis is also subject to atherosclerotic, thromboembolic, and other forms of vascular occlusive disease including vasospasm following subarachnoid hemorrhage.

Anterior Cerebral Artery

The initial portion of the ACA, between the terminal ICA and the ACOM is termed the A1 segment (Fig. 9a). This segment passes anteromedially to enter the interhemispheric fissure where it follows a generally cephalad curvilinear course around the genu and body of the corpus callosum (Fig. 9b). The A2 segment begins distal to the ACOM and extends to the distal ACA. The A2 segment supplies the head of caudate nucleus, portions of the globus pallidus and internal capsule (via the recurrent artery of Heubner), and the anterior two-thirds of the medial cerebral cortex.

The first two branches of the A2 segment are the orbitofrontal and frontopolar arteries which provide vascular supply to the inferomedial frontal lobe cortex as well as the olfactory bulb and tract (Fig. 9b). Next, the ACA bifurcates into the pericallosal and callosal marginal arteries (Fig. 9b). A well-defined callosal marginal artery is present in about 50 % of cerebral arteriograms. This vessel roughly follows the course of the cingulate sulcus as it extends posterosuperiorly. Its three major branches are the anterior, middle, and posterior internal frontal arteries. When the callosal marginal artery is diminutive or absent, these three branches usually arise directly from the pericallosal artery.

The pericallosal artery runs between the corpus callosum and the cingulate gyrus (Fig. 9b). Its branches include the paracentral, superior internal parietal (precuneal), and inferior internal parietal arteries. Distally, the pericallosal artery courses around the splenium of the corpus callosum where it anastomoses with the splenial artery of the PCA.

There is significant variability in the normal ACA, including varying degrees of A1 segment hypoplasia. The A1 segment may have a markedly attenuated caliber and terminate in the orbitofrontal or frontopolar artery. It is not unusual to observe lack of opacification of the ACA during an ICA contrast injection (Fig. 9c) and visualization of both ACAs during injection of the contralateral ICA. There may be one or more communicating vessels between the A2 segments distal to the ACOM. A single or azygous ACA supplying both cerebral hemispheres may occur uncommonly, arising in the midline from the confluence of the right and left A1 segments (Fig. 9d). A higher incidence of pericallosal artery aneurysms may be associated with this anomaly.

ACA occlusion would affect cortical territories for motor and sensory functions of the contralateral lower extremity. Frontal lobe infarctions caused by deficient ACA blood flow may result in cognitive disorders, altered personality/initiative, disinhibited behavior and speech, incontinence, and akinetic mutism (in cases of bilateral frontal lobe infarctions).

The course of the ACA (as well as other intracranial vessels) can be altered and distorted as a result of intracranial masses, cerebral edema, and focal blood collections. However, as computed tomography and magnetic resonance imaging have largely replaced angiography in the diagnosis of intracranial masses, the angiographic localization of intracranial masses will not be broached in this chapter.

Middle Cerebral Artery

The middle cerebral artery (MCA) follows a complex course and provides vascular supply to a wide expanse of both deep and cortical structures within the frontal, parietal, temporal, and, sometimes, lateral occipital lobes. Great variability exists in MCA branching.

The most proximal portion of the MCA is termed the M1 segment which extends from the ICA bifurcation, laterally and horizontally for 1–2 cm through the lateral cerebral fissure (Fig. 9a). Multiple lateral lenticulostriate arteries which penetrate the inferior surface of the frontal lobe to supply portions of the basal ganglia, caudate nucleus, and internal capsule originate from the M1 segment. The M1 segment may also give rise to anterior temporal branches (which may alternatively originate from the proximal M2 portion) which supply the temporal tip cortex (Fig. 9b, c). In its most distal portion, the M1 segment curves posterosuperiorly to the insular cortex (island of Reil) where it bifurcates into major anterior and posterior cortical branches. Approximately 20 %

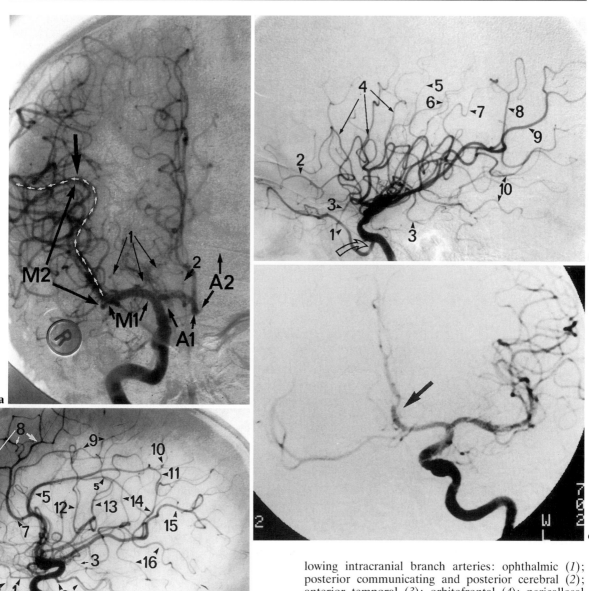

Fig. 9. a Normal right internal carotid frontal subtraction arteriogram demonstrating the M1 and M2 segments of the right middle cerebral artery as well as the A1 and A2 segments of the right anterior cerebral artery. Also note the course of angular branch of the middle cerebral artery within the sylvian fissure (*small white arrows*), sylvian point (*large arrow*), medial and lateral lenticulostriate arteries (*1*), and the recurrent artery of Heubner (*2*). **b** Normal right internal carotid lateral subtraction arteriogram demonstrating the following intracranial branch arteries: ophthalmic (*1*); posterior communicating and posterior cerebral (*2*); anterior temporal (*3*); orbitofrontal (*4*); pericallosal (*5*); frontopolar (*6*); callosal marginal (*7*); anterior, middle, and posterior internal frontal (*8*); paracentral (*9*); superior internal parietal (precuneal) (*10*); inferior internal parietal (*11*); precentral (prerolandic) (*12*); central (rolandic) (*13*); anterior and posterior parietal (*14*); angular (*15*); posterior temporal (*16*). **c** Normal left internal carotid lateral subtraction arteriogram in a patient with marked hypoplasia of the left A1 segment (as a result, no opacification of left anterior arterial branches during this injection) demonstrating the following intracranial branch arteries: ophthalmic (*1*); lateral orbitofrontal (*2*); anterior temporal (*3*); ascending frontal (candelabra) (*4*); precentral (prerolandic) (*5*); central (rolandic) (*6*); anterior parietal (*7*); posterior parietal (*8*); angular (*9*); posterior temporal (*10*). Also note the variant origin of the ophthalmic artery from the cavernous internal carotid artery (*open arrow*). **d** Left internal carotid frontal digital arteriogram revealing a single azygous anterior cerebral artery (arrow)

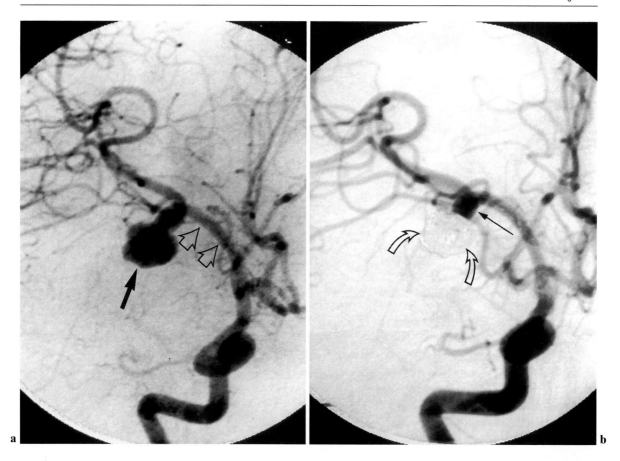

a   b

Fig. 10. a Slightly LAO right internal carotid digital arteriogram in an elderly man with an inoperable right M1 bifurcation aneurysm (*arrow*). The aneurysm is much larger than its angiographic appearance would suggest due to extensive mural thrombus. Note how mass effect from the lesion has elevated the right M1 segment (*open arrows*). **b** Repeat right internal carotid digital arteriogram following transcatheter embolization of the aneurysm sac with multiple electrolytically detached platinum coils (*open arrows*). Note the small residual aneurysm neck (*thin arrow*)

of intracranial aneurysms occur at the M1 bifurcation (Fig. 10a, b).

The insular cortex is covered by the frontoparietal and temporal opercula which coapt to form the sylvian fissure. The MCA branches that course over the insular cortex and contours of the frontoparietal operculum (forming the M2 portion of the MCA) follow a complex, sinusoidal course as they travel posterosuperiorly to the superior margins of the insular cortex and then pass inferolaterally on the internal and inferior surfaces of the frontoparietal operculum (Fig. 9a). These multiple cortical branches then emerge from the Sylvian fissure to again course superiorly over the frontoparietal cortex (Fig. 9c).

On frontal angiographic images the most superior M2 arterial loop (usually formed by a branch of the angular artery) at the superior margin of the insula is called the Sylvian point (Fig. 9a). On lateral angiographic images this complex array of MCA cortical branches extending over the insular and opercular cortices roughly forms a triangular shape (the Sylvian triangle) with its base in the frontosellar region and apex in the parietal region (Fig. 7b). Intracranial mass lesions may cause distortions and displacements of the Sylvian triangle.

A common branching order of the anterior cortical branches of the M2 portion is: lateral orbitofrontal, operculofrontal (also called ascending frontal or "candelabra" branch), and central sulcus arteries (Fig. 9b, c). The central sulcus arteries, usually called precentral (prerolandic) and central (rolandic) branches supply the motor and sensory cortical strips. The posterior M2 cortical branches include the anterior and posterior parietal, angular, and posterior temporal arteries (Fig. 9b, c).

The M2 cortical branches provide vascular supply to the cerebral centers of speech, comprehension, and calculating ability (dominant hemisphere) as well as the motor and sensory functions of the contralateral face, neck, upper extremities, thorax, and abdomen. Acute M1 occlusion results in contralateral hemiplegia, hemianesthesia, and hemianopsia, global aphasia (with dominant hemisphere involvement), and may cause coma or death. Nondominant hemisphere ischemic injuries are frequently associated with apraxia, problems with spatial orientation and dressing, and neglect of contralateral limbs (anosognosia). Temporal lobe ischemic injuries may be associated with cortical deafness, disturbances of short-term memory and learning, olfactory hallucinations, behavior changes, or damage to the optic radiation.

Occlusion of a specific M2 branch is usually associated with characteristic neurologic deficits. Lateral orbitofrontal artery occlusion may result in expressive aphasia. Isolated precentral arterial blockage causes weakness in the contralateral lower face and tongue (and motor aphasia if occlusion is in the dominant hemisphere). Rolandic arterial occlusion leads to contralateral hemiplegia or hemiparesis (more prominent in the upper extremity). Anterior parietal artery occlusion frequently causes astereognosis of the contralateral side. Contralateral hemianopsia can occur with posterior parietal, angular, or posterior temporal artery occlusions. Aphasia can result from dominant hemisphere posterior temporal artery blockage.

Atherosclerosis is the most common cause of MCA and other intracranial arterial stenoses. Other causes of intracranial stenoses and occlusions include arteritis (Fig. 11a, b), radiation changes, drug abuse (methamphetamine and cocaine), vasospasm following subarachnoid hemorrhage (Fig. 11c, d), dissections (Fig. 11e, f), sickle cell disease, neurofibromatosis, Menkes' kinky hair syndrome, idiopathic progressive arteriopathy of childhood, metabolic disorders (e.g., homocystinuria), and basal meningitis (especially due to tuberculosis).

High-grade stenosis or occlusion of the supraclinoid ICA and M1 and A1 segments due to one of the above disorders may result in a pseudoangiomatous or "puff of smoke" angiographic appearance of multiple lenticulostriate, thalamoperforating, choroidal, and leptomeningeal collateral vessels providing collateral flow to M2 and A2 branches (Fig. 11g). The term moyamoya (Japanese for "puff of smoke") syndrome is applied to this angiographic pattern.

Vertebrobasilar Circulation

The VAs originate from the subclavian arteries adjacent to the origins of the internal maxillary arteries and just proximal to the thyrocervical and costocervical trunks (Fig. 12a). In approximately 5% of cases the VA (usually on the left) arises directly from the aortic arch. The thyrocervical and costocervical trunks may have anastomoses with the extracranial portion of the VA and provide branches to the anterior and posterolateral spinal arteries (along with the VA).

One of the two VAs may be dominant in size (usually left greater than right); sometimes one of the VAs may be so diminutive in diameter as to appear threadlike. A high-grade stenosis or segmental occlusion near the subclavian artery origin may result in retrograde flow within the ipsilateral VA. If vertebrobasilar insufficiency results, this is called subclavian steal syndrome (Fig. 12b, c).

As the vertebral artery ascends, it enters the transverse foramen of C6 and passes superiorly through the transverse foramina of C5-1. After emerging from the transverse foramen of C1, the VA courses posteriorly around the atlantooccipital joint and then ascends through the foramen magnum, penetrating the atlanto-occipital membrane and dura. The origin of the posterior meningeal artery usually marks the dural penetration point of the VA (Fig. 13b). The intradural VA then travels superiorly around the lateral aspect of the medulla. In about 1% of angiograms, the VA terminates in the posterior inferior cerebellar artery (PICA).

AVFs of the extracranial VA (with or without VA transection) uncommonly occur. They may be the result of penetrating injuries, congenital or spontaneous, or associated with disorders such as FMD or neurofibromatosis. Presenting symptoms may include bruit, pain, mass effect, and spinal cord or vertebrobasilar ischemia (due to vascular steal). Endovascular therapy with detachable balloons or coil embolization is the treatment of choice (Fig. 12d, e). However, closure of such fistulas, especially ones of a long-standing nature, should be accompanied by measures to lower

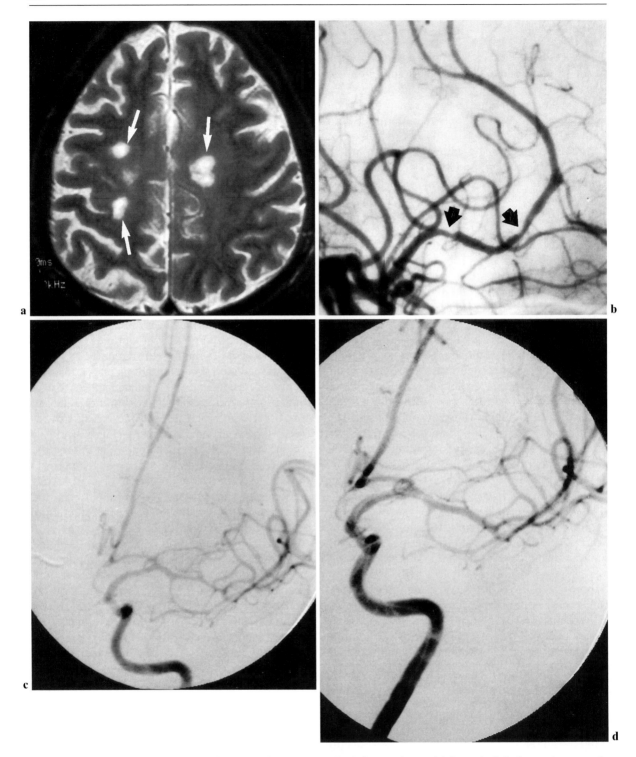

Fig. 11. a Axial T2-weighted spin-echo magnetic resonance brain image in a child demonstrating high signal zones (*arrows*) consistent with multiple deep white matter infarctions. **b** Same pateint as in **a**. A right internal carotid lateral subtraction arteriogram revealing multiple focal arterial stenoses along the course of the right anterior cerebral artery (*arrows*) caused by arteritis.

c Left internal carotid frontal digital arteriogram obtained in this comatose middle-aged woman 1 week following a subarachnoid hemorrhage showing diffuse luminal narrowing affecting the distal internal carotid artery as well as the middle and anterior cerebral arteries due to posthemorrhagic vasospasm. **d** Same patient as in **c**. Repeat left internal carotid arteriography fol-

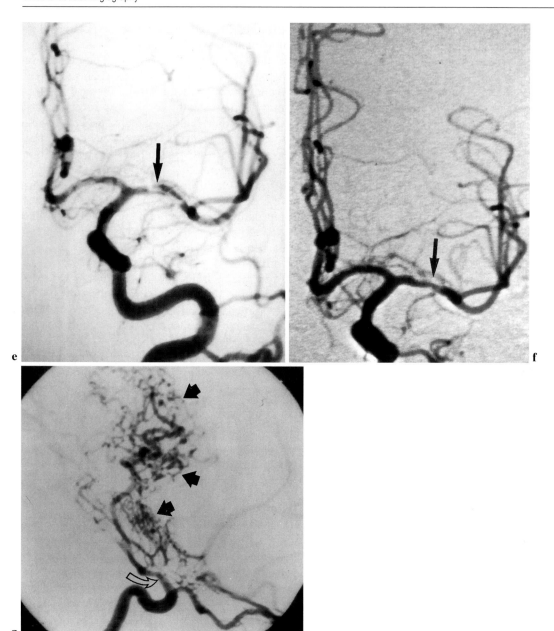

lowing transluminal balloon angioplasty of the distal internal carotid artery as well as the A1 and M1 segments. Note the significantly improved luminal caliber and opacification of the more distal A2 and M2 segments following angioplasty. The patient's mental status rapidly improved. **e** Left internal carotid frontal digital arteriogram obtained in a hypertensive elderly woman with a recent history of transient ischemic attacks. Note the focal linear M1 intraluminal filling defect due to a vascular dissection (*arrow*). **f** Same patient as in **e**. Following a 2-month course of oral anticoagulation therapy, a repeat internal carotid arteriogram reveals marked improvement in the appearance of the M1 segment (*arrow*) consistent with healing of the dissection. **g** Right internal carotid lateral digital arteriogram in this child with left hemiparesis showing occlusion of the supraclinoid internal carotid artery (*open arrow*) due to moya-moya disease. Collateral flow to the more distal middle cerebral arterial branches is via multiple lenticulostriate vessels (*solid arrows*) which have a pseudoangiomatous or "puff of smoke" appearance

blood pressure and thus reduce the risk of post-embolization normal perfusion pressure break-through (with attendant posterior fossa hemorrhage). Irregular fusiform aneurysms of the intra-dural portion of the VA are typically dissecting aneurysms and are usually the result of atherosclerosis and or hypertension. These lesions may present with subarachnoid hemorraghe (SAH) and may cause posterior circulation embolization. The proximal PICA (Fig. 13a,b) follows an inferiorly then superiorly looping course (caudal and cranial loops, respectively). These loops are formed by the anterior, lateral, and posterior medullary segments of the proximal PICA. These proximal PICA segments, and at times the distal VA, provide crucial branches to the medulla, the occlusion of which can cause the lateral medullary syndrome (ipsilateral Horner's syndrome, facial pain/temperature sensory loss, and pharyngeal/laryngeal paralysis as well as contralateral pain and temperature sensory loss in the limbs and trunk) or occasional pyramidal tract ischemia (with resultant hemiparesis or hemiplegia).

The apex of the PICA cranial loop (the choroidal point) roughly defines the floor of the fourth ventrical on lateral vertebral arteriograms (Fig. 13b) and gives rise to fourth ventricular choroidal branches. Just distal to the choroidal point is the supratonsillar segment of the PICA from which originate tonsillohemispheric and inferior vermian branches. The inferior vermian artery anastomoses distally with the superior vermian branch of the superior cerebellar artery (SCA) providing a major posterior fossa collateral pathway. Occlusion of the PICA supratonsillar segment may present as dysarthria, ipsilateral limb ataxia, vertigo, and nystagmus.

The anterior spinal arteries originate from the VA, just distal to the PICA origin, and in approximately 50 % of cases course inferomedially to join with their contralateral mate along the anterior cord. There may normally be a variable degree of hypoplasia of the VA distal to the PICA origin.

Near the pontomedullary junction, the two VAs coalesce to become the BA (Fig. 13a) which courses anterosuperiorly over the ventral pons. Both the VAs and BA may be fenestrated, i.e., they may divide into two parallel channels over short distances (Fig. 13c). Multiple small pontine perforating branches arise from the BA supplying the pyramidal tracts, medial lemnisci, red nuclei, respiratory centers, and nuclei for cranial nerves III, VI, VII, and XII.

Prodromal symptoms of impending BA thrombosis may include visual defects, diplopia, paresthesias, paresis, ataxia, and vertigo. The clinical severity of BA occlusion varies based on the extent of available collateral pathways. Acute thrombosis may lead to death, coma, respiratory arrest, cerebellar and cranial nerve signs, as well as bilateral motor and sensory dysfunction. Local intra-arterial thrombolysis should be initiated as soon as possible (generally, within 6 h of the onset of symptoms). Occlusion of pontine perforators during BA angioplasty may cause "lockend-in" syndrome manifested by loss of speech and quadraplegia, although spinothalamic sensation and at times some facial and eye movements are preserved.

The first major branches of the BA distal to the joining of the VAs are the paired anterior inferior cerebellar arteries (AICAs; Fig. 13a,b) which course around the pons toward the cerebellopontine angle and the internal auditory canal, to distally supply the anterior cerebellar hemispheres. The AICA also supplies lateral pontine structures, and gives rise to the labyrinthine artery (which originates directly from the basilar artery 15 % of the time). Occasionally, the PICA and AICA originate from the BA as a common trunk. The labyrinthine artery travels with cranial nerve VIII through the internal auditory canal and supplies the inner ear. Besides ipsilateral hearing loss, AICA occlusion may result in ipsilateral limb

Fig. 12. a Frontal digital arteriographic image with con- ▶ trast injection into the right subclavian artery demonstrating: right vertebral artery (*1*), right internal mammary artery (*2*), right thyrocervical trunk (*3*), right costocervical trunk (*4*), inferior thyroidal branch of thyrocervical trunk (*5*), right deep cercial artery (*6*), and ascending cervical branch of thyrocervical trunk (*7*). **b** LAO arch arteriogram in patient with proximal left subclavian arterial occlusion (*arrow*). **c** Delayed images from study in **b** demonstrating retrograde left vertebral artery flow (*open arrow*) providing blood supply to left subclavian artery (*arrows*) distal to occlusion (subclavian steal syndrome). **d** Left lateral digital vertebral arteriogram in an adolescent female demonstrating a high-flow, single-hole arteriovenous fistula (*arrow*) between an enlarged left vertebral artery (*open arrows*) and deep cervical vein (*curved arrows*). Note the diminutive caliber of the intracranial vertebral artery (*thin arrows*) and filling of the posterior inferior cerebellar artery (*curved open arrow*). **e** Same patient as **d** following placement of a detachable silicone balloon within the fistula (*arrow*). Repeat left vertebral arteriography shows obliteration of arteriovenous shunting

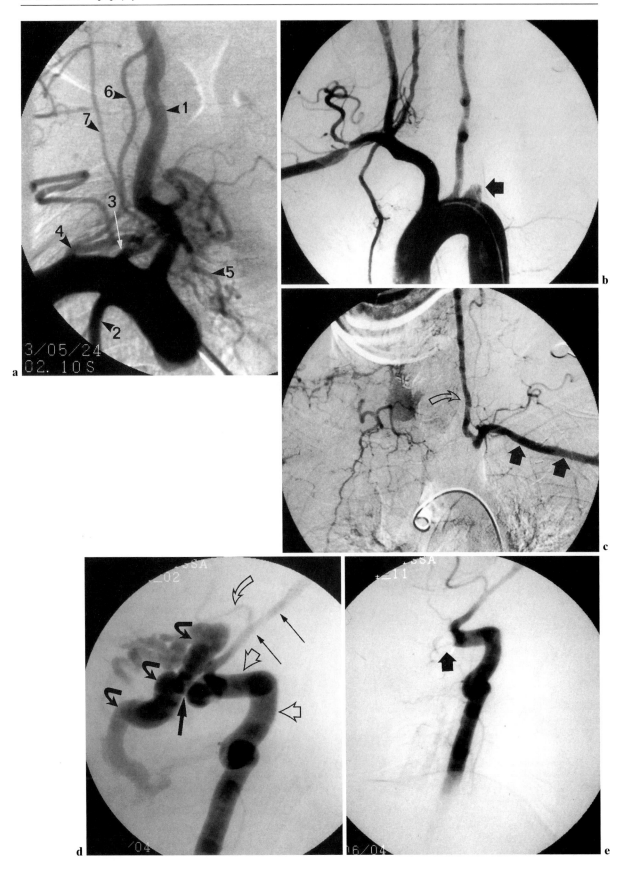

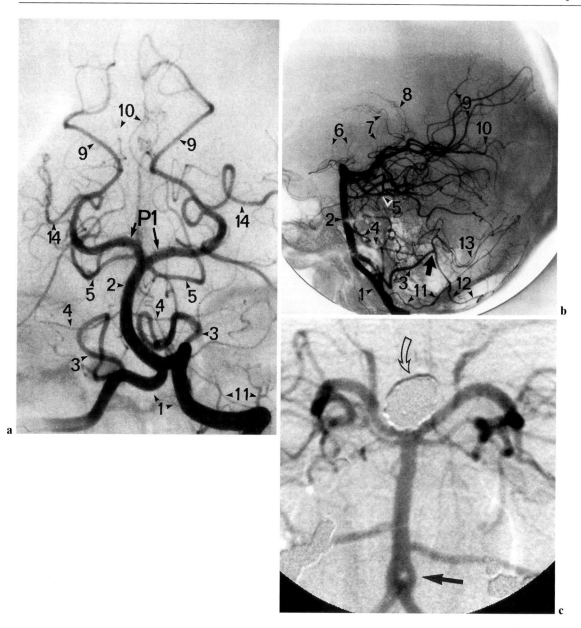

Fig. 13. a, b Normal left vertebral Towne's (**a**) and lateral (**b**) subtraction angiographic views of the skull. The following arteries are demonstrated: vertebral (*1*); basilar (*2*); posterior inferior cerebellar (*3*); anterior inferior cerebellar (*4*); superior cerebellar (*5*); anterior and posterior thalamoperforating (*6*); medial and lateral posterior choroidal (*7*); splenial (*8*); parieto-occipital (*9*); calcarine (*10*); posterior meningeal (*11*); tonsillo-hemispheric (*12*); inferior vermian (*13*); posterior temporal (*14*). Note the P1 segments of the proximal posterior cerebral arteries on the Towne's view. The cranial loop (choroidal point) of the posterior inferior cerebellar artery (*arrow*) is shown on the lateral view. **c** Frontal digital arteriogram with left vertebral injection demonstrating fenestration of the proximal basilar artery (*solid arrow*) in this middle-aged man who has undergone successful coil embolization of a basilar tip aneurysm (*open arrow*)

ataxia, Horner's syndrome, facial pain/temperature senory loss, cranial nerve X and XII dysfunction, and contralateral pain/temperature sensory loss of the limbs and trunk.

The last infratentorial branches of the BA are the paired SCAs (Fig. 13a,b). The SCA arises from the BA subjacent to the oculomotor motor nerve and travels above the trigeminal nerve in the perimesencephalic cistern around the brainstem. Proximally it provides vascular supply to lateral pontine structures including sympathetic and spinothalamic tracts. Distally, the SCA branches into cerebellar hemispheric branches (supplying portions of the cerebellar penducles, the dentate nucleus, and superolateral aspects of the cerebellar hemispheres) and the superior vermian artery. Occlusion of the SCA may be accompanied by disturbed gait, limb ataxia, ipsilateral Horner's syndrome, and contralateral pain/temperature sensory loss.

The paired PCAs arise from the basilar tip at the level pontomesencephalic junction, superior to the oculomotor nerve and tentorium (Fig. 13a). The tentorium separates the proximal PCA and SCA on both frontal and lateral vertebral arteriograms. The proximal PCA is divided into P1 and P2 segments at the junction point of the PCA with the PCOM (Fig. 8a). A filling defect is frequently seen at the transition between P1 and P2 during frontal VA angiograms due to the inflow of unopacified blood from the ipsilateral PCOM. In approximately 20 % of patients the PCA arises directly from the ipsilateral ICA (fetal origin of the PCA) with absence or marked hypoplasia of the proximal P1 segment (Fig. 8b, c). Uni- or bilateral absence of the PCA during vertebral arteriography should prompt one to first consider fetal origin of the PCA rather than its occlusion.

The proximal P2 segment gives rise to posterior thalamoperforating and thalamogeniculate arteries (supplying portions of the thalamus, geniculate bodies, posterior limb of the internal capsule, and optic tract), minute branches serving the cerebral peduncles, and provides vascular supply to the choroid plexus of the third and lateral ventricles via the medial and lateral posterior choroidal arteries (which collateralize with the anterior choroidal artery; Fig. 13b).

The major branches of the P2 segment and more distal PCA include: the splenial artery (coursing up and over the splenium of the corpus callosum and collateralizing with the distal ipsilateral peri-callosal artery), anterior and posterior temporal branches (supplying the undersurface of the temporal lobe), parieto-occipital artery (supplying the inner posterior cerebrocortical surface), and calcarine artery (traveling within the calcarine sulcus and supplying the visual cortex; Fig. 13a, b). The PCA courses posteriorly around the brainstem in the ambient cistern, traveling more medially in the quadrageminal plate cistern. The distal calcarine cortical branches of the two PCAs converge toward midline on a Towne's projection (with caudad angulation of the image intensifier) vertebral arteriogram, separated by the falx cerebri.

PCA cortical branch occlusions may result in varying degrees of contralateral homonymous visual field defects, depending on the extent of pial collateral pathways. P1 occlusion resulting in blockage of perforating branches, or an aneurysm involving the P1 segment with mass effect upon the adjacent cerebral peduncle and oculomotor nerve, may cause Weber's syndrome (ipsilateral third cranial nerve palsy together with contralateral hemiplegia). Occlusion of P1 perforators may also affect the reticular activating system and thus cause consciousness disturbances and coma. PCA embolization or occlussion may result in thalamic disorders including chorea, hemiballismus, contralateral hemisensory deficits, and thalamic pain syndromes.

Intracranial Venous Drainage Pathways

The following brief overview concentrates only on the most important venous pathways.

Cerebral Cortical Veins

These vessels run in highly variable superficial paths within the cortical sulci and drain the cerebral cortex and some white matter. Multiple cortical veins drain superiorly toward the superior sagittal sinus (SSS; Fig. 14a,b). The superficial middle cerebral vein is located within the sylvian fissure and receives drainage from the surrounding opercular cortical regions. It frequently courses anteromedially around the temporal tip to empty into the sphenoparietal or cavernous sinus (Fig. 6a). It may have anastomotic communications with the deep cerebral venous system and extracranial pterygoid venous plexus and facial veins.

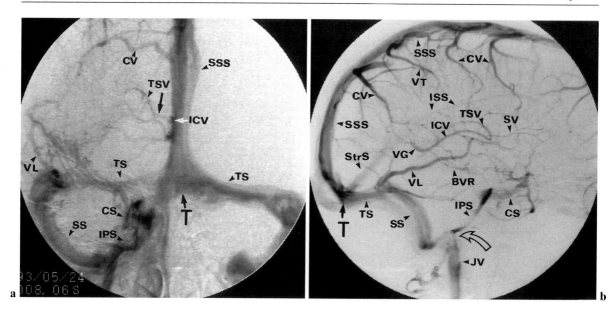

Fig. 14. Frontal (**a**) and lateral (**b**) late-phase digital skull images from right internal carotid arteriographic study demonstrating normal intracranial venous anatomy. Opacified sinuses and veins include: superior sagittal sinus (*SSS*); cortical veins (*CV*); vein of Trolard (*VT*); vein of Labbe (*VL*); inferior sagittal sinus (*ISS*); septal vein (*SV*); thalamostriate vein (*TSV*); internal cerebral vein (*ICV*); basal vein of Rosenthal (*BVR*); vein of galen (*VG*); straight sinus (*StrS*); torcula (*T*); cavernous sinus (*CS*); inferior petrosal sinus (*IPS*); transverse sinus (*TS*); sigmoid sinus (*SS*); internal jugular vein (*JV*). Note the jugular bulb (*open arrow*)

Posteriorly, the superficial middle cerebral vein communicates with the veins of Trolard (draining superiorly toward the SSS) and Labbe (draining inferoposteriorly toward the ipsilateral transverse sinus; Fig. 14a,b). Both the veins of Trolard and Labbe cross the subdural space to enter the dural sinuses. Accidental occlusion of the vein of Labbe or other cortical veins during endovascular or surgical procedures may result in cerebral venous infarction.

Deep Cerebral Veins

The paired septal veins run posteriorly near midline along the septum pellucidum (Fig. 14b). These veins drain the deep white matter of the anterior portions of the frontal lobes. The paired thalamostriate veins run in a subependymal course anteriorly and medially along the floor of the lateral ventricles, passing between the body of the caudate nucleus and thalamus. They drain the caudate nucleus, deep white matter of the parietal and posterior frontal lobes, and internal capsule, and pass anteriorly through the foramina of Monro where they join with the septal veins to form the paired paramedian internal cerebral veins. The internal cerebral veins run posteriorly within the velum interpositum, defining the roof of the third ventricle (Fig. 14a,b).

The paired basal veins of Rosenthal are formed by the confluence of the deep middle and anterior cerebral veins on the ventral surface of the brain and continue posteriorly around the cerebral peduncles (Fig. 14a,b). The basal veins also receive venous drainage from the insula and cerebral peduncles. The basal veins travel posteromedially and superiorly, coalescing with the internal cerebral veins (subjacent to the splenium of the corpus callosum) to form the vein of Galen (Figs. 14b, 15b). The midline vein of Galen travels posteriorly approximately 2 cm under the splenium of the corpus callosum within the quadrigeminal plate cistern. It receives the posterior, pericallosal, posterior mesencephalic, internal occipital, and several posterior fossa veins before it joins with the inferior sagittal sinus to form the straight sinus at the junction of the falx and tentorial incisura (Figs. 14b, 15b).

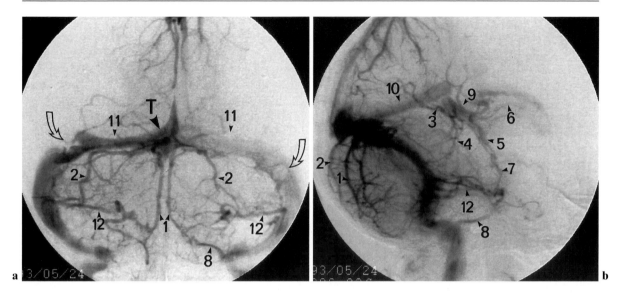

Fig. 15. Towne's (**a**) and lateral (**b**) late-phase digital skull images following contrast injection into the left vertebral artery demonstrating normal posterior fossa venous anatomy. The following sinuses and veins are displayed: inferior vermian vein (*1*); hemispheric vein (*2*); superior vermian vein (*3*); precentral vein (*4*); posterior mesencephalic vein (*5*); internal cerebral vein (*6*); anterior pontomesencephalic vein (*7*); inferior petrosal sinus (*8*); vein of Galen (*9*); straight sinus (*10*); transverse sinus (*11*); superior petrosal sinus (*12*); torcula (*T*). Note filling defects within the transverse sinuses (*open arrows*) caused by arachnoid granulations

Posterior Fossa Veins

The anterior pontomesencephalic vein, actually a network of multiple small veins along the ventral surface of the pons, provides drainage for this structure (Fig. 15b). Superiorly, it drains toward either the basal vein of Rosenthal or posterior mesencephalic vein (Fig. 15b). The precentral vein, providing drainage for a portion of the cerebellar hemispheres, runs just posterior to the roof of the fourth ventricle (Fig. 15b). The precentral vein courses superiorly behind the inferior coliculi to drain into the vein of Galen.

The superior and inferior vermian veins run along the superior and inferior surfaces of the vermis, respectively, and provide drainage for the cerebellar vermis and hemispheres (Fig. 15a,b). The superior vermian vein drains anterosuperiorly toward the vein of Galen. The paramedian inferior vermian veins usually drain posteriorly into the straight sinus.

Dural Sinus Network

The dura mater enveloping the central nervous system has two layers which form reflections known as the falx cerebri, tentorium, and the falx cerebelli separating the cerebral hemispheres, cerebrum from cerebellum, and cerebellar hemispheres, respectively. The layers of the dura separate to form venous drainage channels or dural sinuses for the brain. Some of these dural sinuses communicate with veins in the scalp and diploic space of the calvarium via emissary veins.

The SSS travels along the superior margin of the falx cerebri (Fig. 14a,b). It receives venous drainage from multiple cerebral cortical veins, vein of Trolard, and emissary veins. At times, the anterior one-third of the superior sagittal sinus may not opacifiy during late-phase cerebral angiography or may be congenitally absent. This midline sinus carries blood flow posteriorly and inferiorly in a cresentic course to the posterior junction point between falx and tentorium containing the confluence of sinuses (also known as the torcular Herophili or torcula) near the occiptial protuberance (Fig. 14, 15).

Multiple arachnoid invaginations are present along the superior sagittal as well as transverse sinuses known as arachnoid granulations which serve as the sites of cerebrospinal fluid resorption from the subarachnoid space. These structures may appear as filling defects during the venous phase of cerebral angiograms and should not be mistaken for intraluminal thrombi (Fig. 15b).

The inferior sagittal sinus is contained within the lower curvilinear edge of the falx where it receives venous drainage from the falx and the cerebral hemispheres (Fig. 14b). This dural channel drains posteriorly in the midline to join with the vein of Galen to form the straight sinus within the intersection between the falx cerebri and the tentorium (Figs. 14b, 15b). The straight sinus drains posteriorly toward the torcula. Occipital sinuses, of variable caliber, are frequently visualized during cerebral angiography, coursing supramedially within the dura of the posterior fossa, just lateral to the foramen magnum, draining toward the torcula.

The paired transverse sinuses follow a cresentic course, within the periphery of the tentorium, laterally and anteriorly from the torcula (Figs. 14, 15). Usually the right transverse sinus is dominant or larger than the left. Occasionally, one may be normally extremely hyposplastic. The transverse sinus receives drainage from the inferior cerebral veins and vein of Labbe and communicates with the cavernous sinus via the superior petrosal sinus which runs along the petrous ridge (Figs. 6a, 15). The transverse sinus, as it travels subjacent to the tentorium, becomes the sigmoid sinus. This sinus, contained within the dura of the posterior fossa, follows a curved course toward the jugular foramen where it empties into the internal jugular vein (Figs. 6a, 14). A bend in contour at this junction point is termed the jugular bulb (Fig. 14b). Other structures traversing the jugular foramen include cranial nerves IX through XI and small branches of the ascending pharyngeal and occipital arteries. The jugular bulbs communicate with the cavernous sinuses by means of the paired inferior petrosal sinuses, which ascend supramedially from the jugular foramen within the dural flanking the clivus (Figs. 6a, 14). The inferior petrosal sinuses interconnect through a clival venous plexus.

The structure and contents of the paired cavernous sinuses have been discussed above. The cavernous sinus receives venous drainage from the orbit and its contents via the superior and inferior ophthalmic veins (which in turn communicate with the angular, frontal scalp, and anterior facial veins; Figs. 6a, 14a). The cavernous sinus may also communicate with the pterygoid venous plexus, situated between the temporalis and lateral pterygoid muscles and supplying drainage for the IMAX distribution. This venous drainage pattern may allow intracranial spread of central and deep facial infectious processes.

Stenoses may occur within major dural sinuses causing varying degrees of cerebral venous obstruction. These stenoses may be associated with chronic headache syndromes. Dural sinus thrombosis may occur in hypercoagulable conditions (including pregnancy), mastoiditis, or dehydration. Increased intracranial pressure and venous infarctions (with or without intracranial hemorrhage) can result. Local thrombolysis using urokinase has shown some success in the management of these thromboses. The dural sinuses may also be invaded and occluded by tumors, especially meningiomas.

Selected Intracranial Vascular Lesions

Direct Carotid-Cavernous Fistulas

A direct carotid-cavernous fistula is an AVF between the cavernous ICA and the cavernous sinus through which it passes (Fig. 6a,b). This lesion is caused by a rent or tear in the cavernous ICA resulting from severe head trauma (e.g., a severe blow to the cranial region, deceleration injury, or basilar skull fracture), rupture of a cavernous ICA aneurysm, or site of arterial wall weakness due to an underlying disorder such as Ehlers-Danlos disease.

The fistula causes arterialization of the ipsilateral cavernous sinus and superior and inferior ophthalmic veins (draining the globe and orbital contents). Clinically, there are variable degrees of ipsilateral exophthalmus, scleral injection, chemosis, ptosis, and deficits of cranial nerves III, IV, and VI. The patient usually hears a loud bruit (which can be auscultated over the affected periorbital area).

ICA arteriography on the affected side reveals rapid cavernous sinus opacification, poor filling of the distal intracranial ICA branches, and engorgement of and retrograde flow within venous drainage pathways from the fistula site, including the superior ophthalmic vein (Fig. 6a). The presence of cortical draining veins denotes arterialization of these veins and a significant risk of intracranial hemorrhage. The mainstay of treatment of direct carotid-cavernous fistulas has been transarterial balloon embolization of the affected cavernous sinus.

Dural Arteriovenous Fistulas

Dural AVFs usually occur in elderly and postpartum women, although men may also develop such lesions. Their pathogenesis is not clearly understood, but it is theorized that they arise during the recanalization of a thromboses dural sinus with the formation of numerous small arterial channels between external carotid and dural branches and the effected dural sinus segment (usually cavernous, transverse, or sigmoid sinus; Fig. 4a–c). Dural AVFs chiefly affecting a cavernous sinus may be referred to as indirect carotid-cavernous fistulas.

These lesions may result in a disturbing intracranial bruit and arterialization of the intracranial and ocular venous systems with concomitant headache, ocular pain, scleral injection, chemosis, ptosis, proptosis, and/or ophthalmoplegia. The development of cerebral cortical or deep cerebral venous drainage pathways creates the risk of intracranial hemorrhage.

Treatment for these lesions consists of particle and/or liquid adhesive embolization of the involved external carotid branches and/or transvenous catheterization and embolization of the cavernous or other affected dural sinus with coils or, rarely, liquid adhesive. Dural AVFs with very slow flow may also be successfully treated in some cases by intermittent manual compression, by the patient of the involved CCA using their contralateral hand (contraindicated in cases of significant carotid bifurcation atherosclerotic disease or during Amicar therapy). Surgical therapy of dural AVFs involves "skeletonization" (obliteration of all small entering vessels) of the involved dural sinus segment.

Cerebral Arteriovenous Fistulas

Pial AVFs and vein of Galen vascular malformations (VGVM, also known as vein of Galen aneurysms) are less common than arteriovenous malformations (AVMs) and generally involve direct communications between arteries and veins without the interposed tangle of vessels (angioma or nidus) seen in AVMs.

AVFs typically consist of one or more major cerebral arteries directly connected with a prominent varix (Fig. 16a). Drainage is then to one of the dural sinuses involving a variable number of cortical veins. If the varix is located in the interhe-

mispheric and convexity regions, then drainage is usually to the superior sagittal sinus. In the neonatal period, such lesions usually cause congestive heart failure. This is usually an indication for emergent embolization of these lesions (if cardiac decompensation cannot be controlled medically). Infants, older children and adults usually present with mass effect, seizures, or intracranial hemorrhage.

VGVMs are actually not aneurysms and do not involve the vein of Galen. Instead, there has been absence of development of the normal vein of Galen. There is persistence and dilatation of an embryologic midline venous structure called the median prosencephalic vein of Markowsky which drains to the SSS via a falcine sinus (not the straight sinus; Fig. 16b). Multiple AVFs are associated with this postencephalic vein arising primarily from posterior choroidal and thalamoperforator arteries (Fig. 16b). The result is usually massive arteriovenous shunting that may be accompanied by cardiac anomalies, intracardiac shunts, and/or heart failure with or without pulmonary hypertension. Embolotherapy is generally regarded as the initial treatment of choice for VGVMs due to the poor results achieved with surgery in the management of these malformations.

In addition to presenting with cardiac decompensation, VGVMs may cause hydrocephalus, neuronal damage, encephalomalacia, and/or delayed brain development. Heart failure present at birth or discovered in utero is an indication for urgent embolotherapy. The aim of therapy should be primarily to stabilize the infant and to allow delay of further therapy until the child is physically larger. However, if most arteriovenous shunting can be eliminated during the initial procedure(s), this would be desirable. In general, embolotherapy should be preceeded by an echocardiogram to rule out significant right-to-left shunt.

Initial angiographic evaluation would consist of vertebral and carotid arteriography (performed via the transfemoral route or, if necessary, through the umbilical artery) to assess for feeding vessels as well as the size and configuration of the varix or venous aneurysm. Frequently a stenosis is observed in the draining falcine sinus (usually composed of mural thrombus). Initially, transarterial embolization of prominent feeding vessels may be undertaken (some authors recommend liquid adhesive as the embolic agent). More frequently, in our experience, we have utilized transvenous (Fig. 16c,d) and at times transtorcular routes (via an occipital surgical burr hole) for delivery of embolization coils to the prosencephalic varix.

Intracranial Aneurysms

Intracranial aneurysms (Figs. 7c–e, 10) may be caused by congenital processes, septic emboli, tumors, atherosclerosis, and trauma. They occur with increased frequency in polycystic kidney disease, FMD, collagen-vascular disease, Ehlers-Danlos syndrome, Marfan's syndrome, neurofibromatosis, and coarctation of the aorta. Generally, more peripheral aneurysms tend to be post-traumatic or mycotic. Dysplastic aneurysms (due to high-flow states) may occur in feeding vessels and the central nidus of approximately 7%–18% of patients with AVMs (see below). Congenital anomalies involving the circle of Willis (e.g., azygous and hypoplastic ACA; Fig. 9d) as well as the presence of a persistent trigeminal artery (Fig. 5) or basilar fenestration (Fig. 13c) are associated with a higher incidence of intracranial aneurysms. Rarely, intracranial aneurysms are familial.

Overall, the yearly risk of hemorrhage in intracranial aneurysms is about 1%. This risk significantly increases in aneurysms larger than 10 mm in diameter and in elderly patients. Giant aneurysms are at least 25 mm in diameter and have the greatest risk of hemorrhage. The risk of recurrent hemorrhage from an untreated aneurysm is over 20% within the first 2 weeks and approximately 50% within 6 months. The risk of death following intracranial subarachnoid rupture may be as high as 30%–40%. Of patients surviving the initial hemorrhagic incident as many as 50% suffer significant, long-term neurologic deficits. Aneurysms with a defined neck which are not amenable to surgical clipping may be treated by electrolytically detachable platinum microcoil embolization (Fig. 10).

Besides direct brain parenchymal disruption and mass effect from hemorrhage, the most deleterious effect of aneurysm rupture or leakage is the delayed onset of cerebral vasospasm due to the presence of subarachnoid blood. It typically presents within 3–14 days following the initial hemorrhage and is usually greatest in severity at 7 days posthemorrhage (Fig. 11c,d). It can result in extensive cerebral/brainstem infarction, and death. Prophylactically an oral calcium channel

Fig. 16. a Left lateral common carotid arteriogram in an infant with seizures and right-sided weakness. Multiple pial arteriovenous fistulas are present with large varicosities/venous aneurysms (*open arrows*) located at the connection sites between middle cerebral arterial branches and cortical veins. Venous drainage is to the dural sinuses (*solid arrows*). **b–d** Same patient. **b** Left vertebral frontal digital arteriogram in a neonate with severe cardiac failure at birth. Vein of Galen malformation (*arrows*) with massive arteriovenous shunting from multiple enlarged choroidal branches (off the posterior cerebral arteries; *curved arrows*). Drainage of the malformation is via an enlarged falcine sinus (*thin arrows*). **c** Lateral digital radiograph of skull following successful transvenous platinum coil embolization of the common venous drainage pouch of the malformation (*arrows*). **d** At 4 years of age, a repeat vertebral arteriogram in this patient reveals complete obliteration of the vein of Galen malformation. His neurologic development since embolotherapy has been normal

blocker, nimodipine, is given for 21 days following SAH to prevent vasospasm. If it occurs, the primary management of vasospasm includes blood volume expansion and pressor therapy. However, in the event of failure of this regimen, emergent balloon angioplasty of the affected cerebral vessels is indicated (Fig. 11c,d).

Arteriovenous Malformations

Congentital parenchymal (pial) AVMs are the most common symptomatic intracranial vascular malformations. They consist of a tightly packed mass of tortuous arteries and veins with no normal interposed capillary bed or brain tissue (Fig. 17a, b). The majority are supratentorial and become symptomatic before the age of 50 years. These lesions may present with intracranial hemorrhage, seizure, headache, or neurologic deficit. Overall, the risk of hemorrhage from AVMs is between 2% and 4% per year. However, AVMs that have previously bled are at increased risk for future hemorrhage. The risk of death during hemorrhage from an AVM is approximately 10%. Long-term morbidity resulting from their hemorrhage is as high as 25%.

The feeding vessels may be markedly enlarged, harbor dysplastic aneurysms (Fig 17e,f), and be derived from multiple pial and, at times, dural arteries. The central tangle of vessels is referred to as the nidus. One or more direct AVFs as well as aneurysms may be present within the nidus (Fig. 17f). The veins draining the nidus (carrying

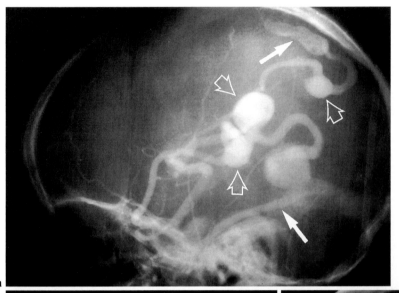

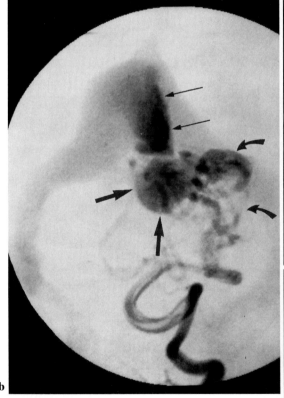

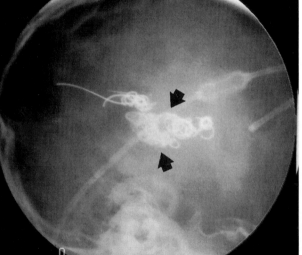

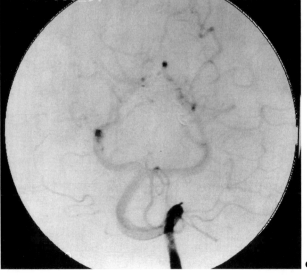

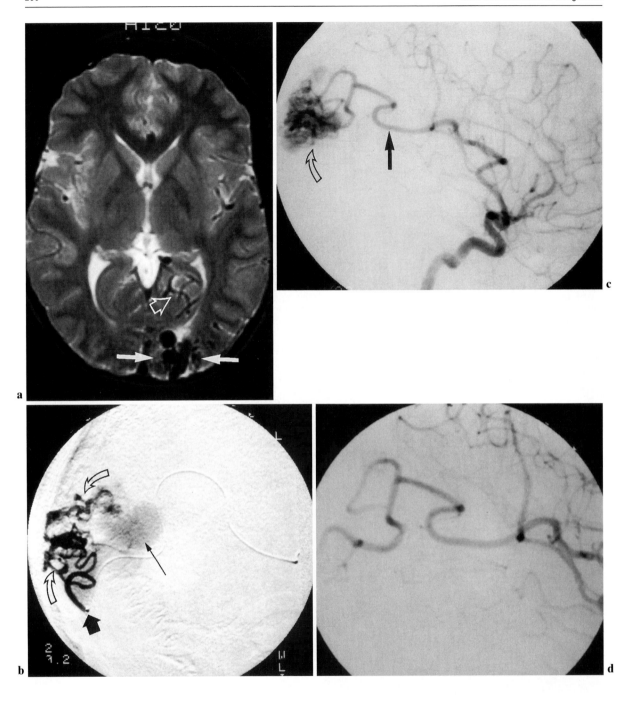

Fig. 17. a–d Same patient. **a** Axial T2-weighted spin-echo magnetic resonance brain image in a young woman with chronic headaches. There are multiple flow voids in the left occipital lobe (*solid arrows*) together with enlarged vessels medial to the trigone of the left lateral ventricle (*open arrow*), highly suggestive of a parenchymal arteriovenous malformation (AVM). **b** Left internal carotid arteriography confirms the presence of a left occipital AVM nidus (*open arrow*) fed by the angular branch (*solid arrow*) of the left middle cerebral artery. **c** A microcatheter was maneuvered into a distal feeding artery branch (*solid arrow*) where contrast injection again demonstrates the AVM nidus (*open arrows*) as well as an enlarged draining varix (*thin arrow*). **d** Following polyvinyl alcohol particle embolization within the distal left angular branch, repeat left internal carotid arteriography shows no filling of the nidus. The next day, the patient underwent successful surgical resection of the lesion.

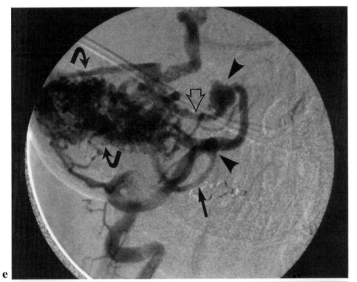

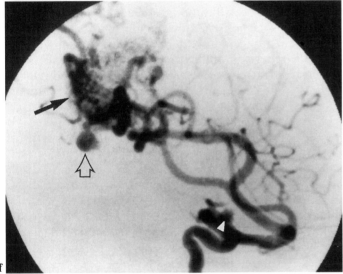

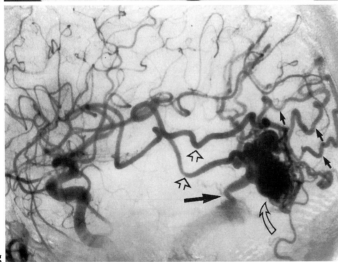

Fig. 17. e Left vertebral digital arteriogram in a 50-year-old woman who had suffered a recent subarachnoid hemorrhage. The angiogram reveals a large right cerebellar AVM nidus (*curved arrows*) supplied mainly by branches of the right posterior (*straight arrow*) and anterior (*open arrow*) inferior cerebellar arteries both of which display dyspastic aneurysms at their origins (*arrowheads*). **f** Young man with a right temporoparietal AVM (*solid arrow*), shown on this lateral right internal carotid digital arteriogram. A small nidus aneurysm (*open arrow*) and dysplastic aneurysm of the supraclinoid right internal carotid artery (*arrowhead*) are also seen. **g** Patient with a 4-cm left temporo-occipital AVM (*curved open arrow*) displaying marked venous outflow restrictive disease. Note the high-grade stenosis of the major draining vein as it joins the sigmoid sinus (*large straight arrow*). The enlarged, tortuous posterior temporal feeding arteries (*small open arrows*) must not be confused with the multiple draining cortical veins (*small solid arrows*) having a similar appearance

outflow to the dural sinuses and/or deep cerebral veins) may be quite enlarged and may have stenoses causing venous outflow restriction (Fig. 17g). AVMs with coexisting aneurysms and/or venous outflow restrictive disease are associated with a higher risk of intracranial hemorrhage.

Therapy of AVMs is usually aimed toward preexcisional particle or liquid adhesive nidus embolization (Fig. 17c,d) to reduce the risk of intraoperative blood loss. Definitive surgical therapy of these lesions would appear even more desirable in the face of previous AVM hemorrhage. However, with AVMs located in regions difficult or dangerous to surgically access, the size of the nidus may be reduced to 2.5–3 cm in diameter using liquid adhesive embolization, at which point the patient may then be a candidate for focused-beam radiation therapy. Dysplastic aneurysms of feeding vessels should be treated first (either by surgical clipping or endovascular means) as occlusion of the AVM nidus could induce hemodynamic changes that could lead to rupture of the aneurysm.

Embolotherapy of intracranial AVMs itself may result in hemorrhage, either from the nidus or surrounding brain parenchyma. Because of reduced flow through the AVM resulting from embolization, sluggish flow through a draining vein may be induced. This may in turn cause thrombosis of draining veins and acutely increased intranidus pressure and nidus rupture. Hemorrhage occurring within the parenchyma surrounding the nidus may be due to normal pressure perfusion breakthrough. In this condition, the existence of which is still considered to be contraversial, once the arteriovenous shunting within the AVM nidus has been reduced or obliterated by embolization, there would be increased perfusion directed toward surrounding parenchyma. This surrounding vascular bed may have lost its normal autoregulation due to the longterm effects of diverted flow through the AVM. When acutely exposed to this relatively higher perfusion pessure, vascular rupture within the surrounding parenchyma could ensue.

Appendix

Indications for carotid and cerebral angiography (adapted from Spies et al.)

Carotid arteriography
- Cerebrovascular insufficiency
    - Stroke, transient ischemic attack, or amaurosis fugax when other causes (hemorrhage, tumor, etc.) have been excluded; noninvasive testing is not required in symptomatic patients
    - Symptomatic and asymptomatic patients with severe carotid artery stenosis or ulcerated plaque at noninvasive testing when confirmation is required for surgical or medical management
    - Symptomatic patients with inconclusive or contradictory noninvasive testing results
- Suspected carotid dissection
- Diagnosis and evaluation of vascular trauma, head and neck tumors, and aneurysms

External carotid arteriography
- Diagnosis and evaluation of suspected tumors, recurrent epistaxis, trauma, vascular malformations, vasculitis, and other primary vascular abnormalities
- Evaluation for potential arterial bypass or of previous bypass

Cerebral arteriography
- Diagnosis and evaluation of primary vascular abnormalities (including aneurysms, vascular malformations, occlusive disease, and vasculitis), intracranial tumors, intracranial hemorrhage (including cases due to trauma), and suspected cerebral vasospasm
- Assessment of cerebral collateral flow
- Pre- and postoperative evaluation of neurosurgical and neurointerventional procedures

Vertebrobasilar arteriography
- Symptoms of vertebrobasilar insufficiency including episodic dizziness, vertigo, unsteadiness of gait, and/or ataxia
- Brainstem or cerebellar infarction
- With carotid arteriography, to evaluate intracranial occlusive disease and collateral flow
- Diagnosis and evaluation of subclavian steal, head and neck tumors, vascular malformations, and trauma

Suggested Reading

1. Artiola I, Fortuny L, Prieto-Valiento L (1981) Long term prognosis in surgically treated intracranial aneurysms. I. Mortality. II. Morbidity. J. Neurosurg 54: 26–43

2. Barnwell SL, Halbach VV, Higashida RT, Hieshima G, Wilson CB (1989) Complex dural arteriovenous fistulas. Results of combined endovascular and neurosurgical treatment in 16 patients. J Neurosurg 71: 352–358

3. Barr ML, Kiernan JA (1988) The human nervous system, 5th edn. Lippincott, Philadelphia

4. Brown RD, Wiebers DO, Forbes GS (1990) Unruptured intracranial aneurysms and arteriovenous malformations: frequency of intracranial hemorrhage and relationship of lesions. J Neurosurg 73: 859–863

5. Drumm DA, Green KA, Marciano FF, Prigatano GP, Spetzler RF (1993) Neurobehavioral deficits following rupture of anterior communicating artery (ACoA) aneurysms: the ACoA aneurysm syndrome. BNI 9: 2–12

6. Gilman S, Newman SW (1987) Manter and Gatz's essentials of clinical neuroanatomy and neurophysiology, 7th edn. Davis, Philadelphia

7. Guglielmi G, Vinuela F, Dion J, Duckwiler G (1991) Electrothrombosis of saccular aneurysms via endovascular approach, part 2: preliminary clinical experience. J Neurosurg 75: 8–14

8. Halbach VV, Hieshima GB, Higashida RT, Reicher M (1987) Carotid cavernous fistulae: indications for urgent treatment. AJNR 8: 627–633

9. Halbach VV, Higashida RT, Hieshima GB (1987a) Treatment of vertebral arteriovenous fistulas. AJNR 8: 1121–1128

10. Halbach VV, Higashida RT, Hieshima GB (1987b) Dural fistulas involving the cavernous sinus: results of treatment in 30 patients. Radiology 163: 437–442

11. Halbach VV, Higashida RT, Hieshima GB et al (1987c) Dural fistulas involving the transverse and sigmoid sinuses: results of treatment in 28 patients. Radiology 163: 443–447

12. Halbach VV, Higashida RT, Hieshima GB, Norman D (1987d) Normal perfusion pressure breakthrough occuring during treatment of carotid and vertebral fistulas. AJNR 8: 751–756

13. Higashida RT, Halbach VV, Tsai FY, Norman K, Pribram HF, Mehringer CM, Hieshima GB (1989) Interventional neurovascular treatment of traumatic carotid and vertebral artery lesions: results in 234 cases. AJR 153: 577–582

14. Higashida RT, Halbach VV, Hieshima GB (1991) Treatment of intracranial aneurysms by interventional neurovascular techniques. In: Kadir S (ed) Current practice of interventional radiology. Decker, Philadelphia, pp 150–154

15. Higashida RT, Tsai FY, Halbach VV, Dowd CF, Hieshima GB (1993) Cerebral percutaneous transluminal angioplasty. Heart Dis Stroke 2: 497–502

16. Lasjaunias P, Berenstein A (1987). Surgical neuroangiography, vol I–IV, 1st edn, Springer, Berlin Heidelberg New York

17. North American Symptomatic Carotid Endarterectomy Trial Collaborators (1991) Beneficial effect of carotid endarterectomy in symptomatic patients with high-grade carotid stenosis. NEJM 325: 445–453

18. Osborn AG (1980) Introduction to cerebral angiography. Harper and Row, Philadelphia

19. Serbinenko FA (1974) Balloon catheterization and occlusion of major cerebral vessels. J Neurosurg 41: 125–145

20. Spetzler RF, Wilson CB, Weinstein P et al. (1978) Normal perfusion pressure breakthrough theory. Clin Neurosurg 25: 651–672

21. Spetzler RF, Martin NA, Carter LP, Flom RA, Raudzens PA, Wilkinson E (1987) Surgical management of large AVM's by staged embolization and operative excision. J Neurosurg 67: 17–28

22. Spies JB, Bakal CW, Burke DR, et al. Standards for diagnostic arteriography in adults. JVIR 1993; 4: 385–395

23. Suzuki J, Takaku A (1969) Cerebrovascular "moyamoya" disease. Disease showing abnormal netlinke vessels in base of brain. Arch Neurol 20: 288–299

24. Theron J, Raymond J, Casasco A, Courtheoux P (1987) Percutaneous angioplasty of artherosclerotic and post-surgical stenosis of carotid arteries. AJNR 8: 495–500

25. Touho H, Karasawa J, Shishido H, Tazawa T, Yamada K, Kabayashi K, Asai M, Yasue H, Kagawa M (1988) Transbrachial artery approach for selective cerebral angiography in outpatients. AJNR 9: 334–336

26. Vinuela F, Dion JE, Duckwiler G et al. (1991) Combined endovascular embolization and surgery in the management of cerebral arteriovenous malformations: experience with 101 cases. J Neurosurg 75: 856–864

27. Vinuela F, Halbach VV, Dion JE (eds) (1992) Interventional neuroradiology: endovascular therapy of the central nervous system. Raven, New York

28. Weir B (1985) Intracranial aneurysms and subarachnoid hemorrhage: and overview. In: Wilkins RH, Rengachary SS (eds) Neurosurgery, vol 2. McGraw-Hill, New York, pp 1308–1329

29. Wilkins RH (1985) Natural history of intracranial vascular malformations: a review. Neurosurgery 16: 421–430

Coronary Angiography

J. Haase and N. Reifart

Since the introduction of percutaneous transluminal coronary angioplasty (PTCA) by Andreas Grüntzig in 1977, assessment of coronary artery morphology by contrast angiograms has represented the standard technique to visualize coronary artery stenoses before, during, and following any interventional procedure [1]. It has been well established that the angiographic appearance of coronary artery lesions does not directly reflect their hemodynamic significance as investigated by Doppler flow measurements [2]; in addition, it does not allow assessment of the atherosclerotic process within the arterial wall as demonstrated by intravascular ultrasound [3]. In spite of this, however, the angiographic approach is the most rapid technique for assessing the result of coronary angioplasty and provides the operator with the immediate information on lesion morphology following PTCA [4]. Optimal visualization of the coronary artery segment of interest in two orthogonal projections is the most important prerequisite for estimating the severity of the coronary artery lesion and for documenting the angiographic outcome of any intervention.

This chapter discusses a series of angiographic standard projections as used in the interventional laboratories of the Red Cross Hospital and Heart Center in Frankfurt for examining the left and right coronary arteries. The role of quantitative coronary angiography during coronary angioplasty as well as the indications for coronary angioplasty will be discussed. The role of angiographic lesion morphology in selecting among the currently available interventional techniques is highlighted, and the angiographic control of interventional procedures is explained. Finally, the angiographic outcome of coronary angioplasty is discussed, including potential complications and their management.

Angiographic Projections

Terminology

The terms used in the literature to describe radiographic projections in coronary arteriography (half axial, caudocranial, craniocaudal, right posterior oblique, etc.) are confusing [5–8]. This is due in part to the fact that radiologists and cardiologists use different nomenclatures. The radiologist defines X-ray beam orientation from the X-ray tube to the image intensifier. This terminology results in the posteroanterior chest X-ray. In most interventional coronary laboratories the same X-ray beam orientation is termed "anterior or frontal" view. Similarly, when the under-the-table X-ray tube is moved toward the feet and the overhead image intensifier toward the head (Fig. 1), the radiologist's term to describe this view is caudocranial, since the X-ray beam passes in a caudal to cranial direction. However, it appears simpler to indicate angulation of the X-ray beam in the sagittal plane by referring only to the location of the image intensifier. If the image intensifier is moved toward the head 30° from vertical as in Fig. 1, this

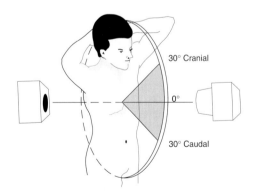

Fig. 1. Diagrammatic illustration of X-ray angulations in the sagittal plane. While the direction of the X-ray beam is posterior to anterior, the image intensifier is moved toward a cranial or caudal position, resulting in a cranial or caudal projection, respectively

may be described as a 30° cranial view (rather than caudocranial), and if moved toward the feet 30°, as a 30° caudal view.

This nomenclature has been adopted by the authors and others [8–11] and greatly simplifies terminology. The picture obtained is that which the viewer would have if his or her face were in the same position as the image intensifier. In the standard right anterior oblique (RAO) view the viewer looks at the right anterior chest, and in the left anterior oblique (LAO) cranial view the coronaries are viewed as if one were looking over the left sholder of the patient (Fig. 2). The cranial RAO view allows one to peer at the coronary arteries from a position over the right shoulder (Fig. 3), while the caudal RAO and caudal LAO are views from the liver and spleen, respectively. The degree of rotation in the transverse plane is measured from the midline (i.e., a left lateral projection is a 90° LAO) and angulation in the sagittal plane from the vertical as in Fig. 1. This simple

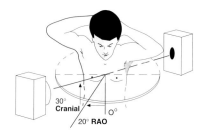

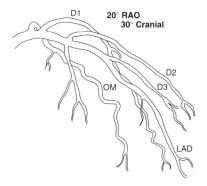

Fig. 3. RAO cranial view of the left coronary artery. In the 20° RAO projection with 30° cranial angulation the image intensifier is positioned over the patient's right shoulder. This projection is useful for imaging the middle segment of the LAD and is perfectly suited to visualizing the origin of the diagonal and septal perforating arteries. Overlap with diagonal branches is usually avoided. The origin of the circumflex artery is seen well, as in this illustration

terminology allows all coronary arteriography views to be described clearly by the location of the image intensifier alone.

Choice of Views

To achieve optimal visualization of a coronary arterial stenosis during angioplasty, it should be visualized perpendicular to the course of the arterial segment without overlap and circumferentially to detect maximal luminal reduction by an asymmetric lesion. In practice this can best be achieved by performing several routine views of the coronary arteries and then special views to highlight segments of interest or segments not adequately visualized. The routine views in our laboratories are as follows:

– Left coronary artery: 90° LAO, 50° LAO with 30° cranial angulation, frontal, and 20° RAO with 20° caudal angulation

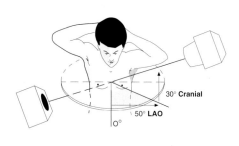

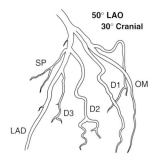

Fig. 2. LAO cranial view of the left coronary artery. In the 50° LAO view with 30° cranial angulation the image intensifier is positioned over the patient's left shoulder. This view is one of the most important projections of the left coronary artery during interventional procedures. Foreshortening of the left main and proximal LAD which impairs a regular LAO view (45° LAO), is overcome by the cranial angulation. The view is perfectly suited to controlling guidewire insertion into the distal segments of the LAD, since erroneous insertion of the wire into diagonal or septal branches can be clearly visualized

– Right coronary artery: 45° LAO, 45° LAO with 30° cranial angulation, and 30° RAO.

These projections are modified according to the anatomy of individual patients.

LAO projections are selected to avoid superimposing the coronary arteries over the spine and cranial LAO views, to display the coronary arteries between the spine and the right hemidiaphragm.

Depending on the clinical condition, some patients cannot tolerate a full coronary arteriogram, and procedures are tailored for the individual patient. In unstable patients the angiographer may choose the special views necessary to evaluate arterial segments of interest by making mini-injections (1–2 ml) in various views, finally settling on the optimal one, which is recorded with a full 4- to 8-ml injection of contrast medium. The choice of special views is influenced by the orientation of the heart (horizontal versus vertical), the complexity of the arterial tree, and the location of the disease. Our choice of views to evaluate problem areas in various arterial segments is indicated below.

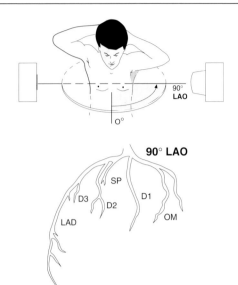

Fig. 4. Lateral view of the left coronary artery. In the 90° LAO projection the X-ray system is in a horizontal position, and the image intensifier is positioned at the left side of the patient. This view shows the entire course of the LAD without foreshortening and without overlap from diagonal and septal branches. Since diagonal and septal branches commonly take an inferior course from the LAD in this projection, the view is perfectly suited to controlling the angioplasty guidewire position in the distal segment of the LAD

Left Main Coronary Artery

Visualization of the left main coronary artery is most important and problematic. Pathological studies commonly confirm a significant underestimation of disease by angiography. The best views are frontal or shallow RAO projections during which forceful contrast injection produces reflux into the aorta thus visualizing the ostium. A second view is necessary, and depending on the position of the heart either the 45° LAO view with 30° cranial angulation or the 50° LAO projection with 30° caudal angulation ("spider view"), the latter displaying especially the bifurcation of the left main. When an eccentric distal left main stenosis is present, a frontal projection with 30° cranial angulation (view from the patient's chin) may be the only one to show the stenosis. In the presence of very early bifurcation of the left main coronary artery, a 20° RAO projection with 20° caudal angulation may elucidate the anatomy. Multiple injections may be needed at slightly different angles to evaluate difficult eccentric lesions.

Left Anterior Descending Coronary Artery

To visualize the entire course of the left anterior descending coronary artery (LAD) we generally use the 90° LAO view (Fig. 4). Imaging of the proximal and middle segments of the LAD as well as the origin of diagonal and septal branches may best be obtained using the 50° LAO with 30° cranial angulation (Fig. 2) or the 10°–20° RAO with 20°–30° cranial angulation (Fig. 3). Individual projections should be adapted to the patient's anatomy. When the heart is horizontal (e.g., in obese patients), and the proximal LAD has a cephaled direction, the LAO caudal view is better than the LAO cranial view [12]. When the middle LAD is tortuous with eccentric stenoses, the cranial 30° view may visualize the anatomy best. To evaluate diagonal branches one may need to perform multiple 30° RAO views with different amounts of caudal and cranial angulation to identify the various overlapping segments. By combining these RAO views with an LAO cranial view one can usually evaluate diagonal arteries, including branch points.

Circumflex Coronary Artery

There are several problem areas in evaluating the circumflex coronary artery. The origin of the circumflex is not well seen in the standard RAO view (RAO 30°) since this segment is visually foreshortened. RAO caudal views (Fig. 5) may permit better visualization of the proximal circumflex coronary artery when it has an initial caudal direction, but the RAO cranial view may be preferable when the circumflex is cranially directed (Fig. 3). The RAO caudal view is usually an excellent projection to visualize the proximal circumflex, origin of an intermediate branch, or origin of obtuse marginal branches arising from the proximal portion of the circumflex artery. The middle and distal portions of obtuse marginal branches are also usually well seen in RAO views. If the middle circumflex is tortuous, or lesions are visualized foreshortened using an RAO view, a 40°–90° LAO projection should be selected. To obtain a second view visualizing the middle and distal portions of obtuse marginal branches an LAO cranial projection may be helpful.

Right Coronary Artery

The most difficult segments to visualize in the right coronary artery are the orifice, especially when the origin is quite anterior, and the origin of the posterior descending artery or the left ventricular branches, especially when the heart is in a horizontal position. Baseline angiography is performed using the 45° to 60° LAO view displaying the proximal segments of the vessel (Fig. 6) and the standard RAO projection (30° RAO). When the origin of the right coronary artery is anterior, the ostium may be best visualized using a 90° LAO or a RAO cranial projection. To image the origin of the posterior descending artery or the left ventricular branches the LAO cranial projection (Fig. 7) or an RAO cranial view offer a means to avoid viewing segments foreshortened.

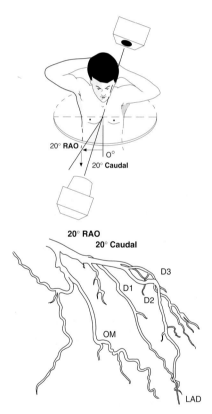

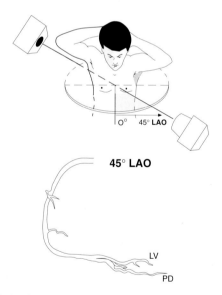

Fig. 5. RAO caudal view of the left coronary artery. In the 20° RAO projection with 20° caudal angulation the image intensifier is positioned over the patient's liver. This view is helpful in visualizing the proximal and middle segments of the circumflex coronary artery. The origin of marginal and posterolateral branches of the circumflex artery is normally imaged without overlap in this projection

Fig. 6. LAO view of the right coronary artery. The 45° LAO projection shows the course of the proximal and middle segments of the right coronary artery without foreshortening. If the proximal segment takes an anterior direction from the aorta, ostial lesions are not well visualized. This can usually be overcome by turning to a steeper LAO projection. The posterior descending and left ventricular branches may be severely foreshortened in this view

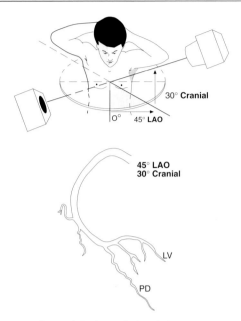

Fig. 7. LAO cranial view of the right coronary artery. The 45° LAO projection with 30° cranial angulation overcomes the problem of foreshortening of the posterior descending and left ventricular branches observed in Fig. 6. When the right coronary artery originates anteriorly from the aorta, the proximal portion of this vessel is frequently well seen in this projection

Quantitative Coronary Angiography

Although visual assessment of the severity of coronary artery stenoses remains the standard procedure in our daily practice, high interobserver and intraobserver variability has been well documented [13]. These observations have stimulated the development of computer-based systems for objective quantitative analysis of geometric parameters at the site of coronary artery lesions [14]. During the past decade quantitative coronary angiography (QCA) has become the reference technique for assessing coronary artery lesion geometry and is widely used in scientific research on progression and regression of coronary heart disease [15] as well as in evaluating the efficacy of new interventional devices [16].

During coronary angioplasty on-line digital assessment of vessel diameters and length of coronary artery stenoses enables the operator immediately to assess both the dimension of the device to be selected and the result of any intervention. In the interventional laboratories of the Red Cross Hospital and Heart Center in Frankfurt, the Automated Coronary Analysis (ACA) package of

the Philips Digital Cardiac Imaging system is used to assess directly the geometric dimensions of the coronary artery segment at which angioplasty is performed. The automated contour detection algorithm of the ACA package employs the first and second derivative functions applied to the brightness profile of scanlines perpendicular to a previously defined centerline within the coronary artery contrast image. The reliability of this software package for geometric coronary measurements has been evaluated by in vitro test series [17] and by an in vivo model involving percutaneous insertion of stenosis phantoms in porcine coronary arteries [18].

Calibration of the QCA System During Angioplasty

Whenever QCA measurements are used as an adjunct to peri-interventional coronary angiography, calibration procedures should be readily applicable and fast. While off-line analysis of digital or cinefilm-based angiographic recordings can rely on catheter calibration based on direct measurement of the angiographic guiding catheter with a precision micrometer, this procedure cannot be used during angioplasty unless the measurement can be carried out under sterile conditions. We therefore recommend using the catheter size indicated by the manufacturer, although the well-known variations in catheter dimensions remain uncorrected [19]. For the purpose of peri-interventional coronary angiography, however, these variations are negligible. Figure 8a illustrates the process of catheter calibration with the ACA package of the Philips Digital Cardiac Imaging system. The contour detection algorithm is applied to a nontapering part of the catheter tip, and the distance of both contours is assigned to the indicated size (French) resulting in a calibration factor (mm/pixel). As long as the operator uses the identical projection for QCA measurements, the same calibration factor can be applied. Different angiographic projections, however, require additional calibration, since out-of-plane magnification of the catheter tip may vary with various angulations of the X-ray system [20].

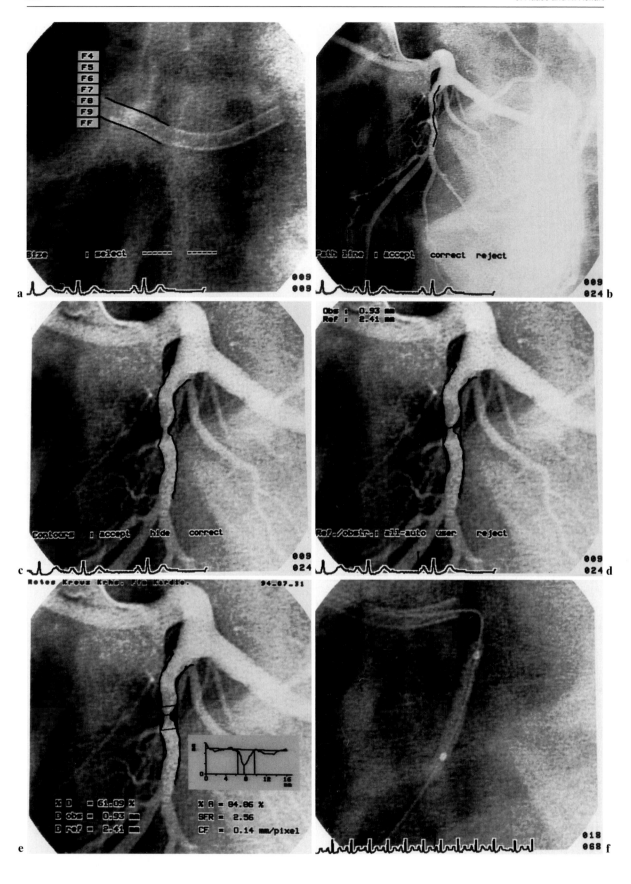

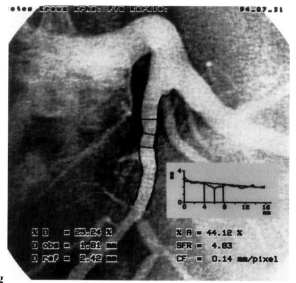

g

Fig. 8 a–g. On-line QCA measurements at the site of the proximal LAD during PTCA. **a** To calibrate the QCA system the contour detection algorithm of the ACA package is applied to a nontapering portion of the tip of the angioplasty guiding catheter, and the distance between the contours is assigned to the indicated size (French) resulting in a calibration factor (mm/pixel). **b** The user indicated the segment length by defining a beginning and an end-point within the contrast image of the coronary artery. A centerline is then traced automatically. **c** Based on the first and second derivative functions on the brightness profile of scanlines perpendicular to the previously defined pathline, the contour of the coronary artery lumen is detected automatically. **d** The reference contour is traced automatically by means of a linear regression technique, representing a computer-defined model of the prediseasel luminal contour. The location of the maximal percent diameter stenosis is indicated by a single scanline connecting the two reference contours. **e** The calculated values for percent diameter stenosis *(%D)*, obstruction diameter *(D obs)*, and reference diameter *(D ref)* are displayed together with a plot of the diameter function curve (see text for details). **f** Based on the calculation of a 2.41 mm reference diameter, a 2.5-mm angioplasty balloon catheter is selected and inflated within the coronary obstruction. **g** Following balloon angioplasty the QCA measurement is repeated, demonstrating an improvement of the obstruction diameter from 0.93 to 1.81 mm with a residual stenosis of 25 %

Geometric Measurements at the Coronary Artery Lesion

Following calibration the angiographic image is selected for QCA measurements. This selection should take into account that the coronary artery segment of interest is visualized without overlap of surrounding vessels or structures, preferably during the end-diastolic phase of the cardiac cycle. Whenever the length of the lesion is measured, the coronary artery segment must be imaged without foreshortening. The process of automated contour detection by the ACA package begins with the definition of a centerline within the coronary artery segment. The user defines a start and an endpoint within the vessel segment, and a centerline is then defined through the coronary artery segment automatically (Fig. 8b). The edge detection algorithm is carried out in two iterations and two spatial resolutions. In the first iteration the scan model is the initially detected centerline, and edge detection takes place at the 512×512 matrix resolution. Here the contours detected in the first iteration function as scan models. In the second iteration a region of interest centered around the defined arterial segment is magnified digitally by a factor of 2 with bilinear interpolation. The final contour detection takes place on the magnified image, and both the contour of the coronary artery lesion and an interpolated reference contour are displayed (Fig. 8c, d). This reference contour is defined by the so-called iterative linear regression technique [21]. This approach tapers the vessel to account for the decrease in arterial caliber associated with branches. The reference diameter (D_{ref}) is now taken as the value of the reference diameter function at the location of the minimal luminal diameter (MLD). Percent diameter stenosis (DS) is calculated from D_{ref} and MLD as follows: $DS = (1 - MLD/D_{ref}) \times 100\%$. The actual MLD is not displayed by the ACA package (Fig. 8e). The so-called obstruction diameter (D_{obs}) represents the vessel diameter at the site of maximal percent diameter stenosis and thus does not necessarily represent the absolute minimum of the diameter function curve [22]. Tapering of the vessel is again taken into account with this approach. The automated quantitative analysis of coronary artery lesions is carried out in less than 2 min and is therefore extremely suitable for on-line assessment of coronary artery dimensions during the angioplasty procedure.

The digital geometric coronary measurements described above are especially helpful in assessing borderline stenoses ($\pm 50\%$), where the uncertainties of visual assessment of lesion severity are most obvious. Furthermore, on-line QCA measurements may become extremely important when accurate matching of interventional devices is required, such as in the assessment of balloon sizes prior to stent implantation or the dimension of atherectomy or laser catheters. Finally, as illustrated by Fig. 8g, the result of the angioplasty procedure on lesion geometry can be objectively documented and used for comparison with angiographic follow-up.

Indications for Coronary Angioplasty

Continuous improvement in balloon catheters and new devices as well as increasing operator experience has extended the indications for interventional revascularization. These indications however, are only partially determined by the morphologic appearance of coronary artery lesions. The functional relevance of coronary lesions must be assessed before the revascularization procedure, potential contraindications and the relative risk of the procedure must be evaluated. To provide cardiologists with a guideline for the indications of coronary interventions the American Heart Association/American College of Cardiology task force has recently established the following classification [23]:
- Class I: conditions for which there is general agreement that coronary angioplasty is justified
- Class II: conditions for which there is divergence of opinion with respect to the justification for coronary angioplasty in terms of value and appropriateness
- Class III: conditions for which there is general agreement that coronary angioplasty is not ordinarily indicated

We have slightly modified these guidelines to match our experience and the more conservative approach of interventional cardiology in Germany than in the United States.

Single-Vessel Coronary Artery Disease

Mildly Symptomatic (Functional Class I) Patients With or Without Medical Therapy

Class I (Mild Symptoms, Single-Vessel Coronary Disease). This category applies to patients who have a significant lesion ($>50\%$ diameter stenosis) in a major epicardial artery that subtends a large area of viable myocardium, and who show evidence of myocardial ischemia induced by exercise. These patients should have a lesion or lesions associated with a high likelihood of success-

ful dilatation and be at low risk for morbidity and mortality.

Class II (Mild or No Symptoms, Single-Vessel Coronary Disease). This category applies to patients who have a significant lesion in a major epicardial artery that subtends at least a moderately sized area of viable myocardium, and who show objective evidence of myocardial ischemia and (a) have at least a moderate likelihood of successful intervention associated with (b) a high likelihood of achieving the result without the use of additional expensive interventions, and (c) a low risk for morbidity and mortality.

Class III (Mild or No Symptoms, Single-Vessel Coronary Disease). This category applies to all other patients with single-vessel disease and mild or no symptoms who do not fulfill the criteria for class I or II. It includes, for example, patients who (a) have only a small area of myocardium at risk, (b) do not manifest evidence of myocardial ischemia, (c) have borderline lesions ($50\%-60\%$ DS) and no inducible ischemia, or (d) are at moderate or high risk for morbidity or mortality.

Symtomatic Patients with Angina Pectoris Class II–IV With Medical Therapy and Single-Vessel Disease

Class I (Symptomatic, Single-Vessel Coronary Disease). This category applies to patients who have a significant lesion in a major epicardial artery that subtends at least a moderately sized area of viable myocardium and who (a) show evidence of myocardial ischemia while on medical therapy, (b) have angina pectoris that is inadequately responsive to medical treatment, or (c) are intolerant of medical therapy because of uncontrollable side effects. These patients should have at least a moderate likelihood of successful dilatation and be at low or moderate risk for morbidity or mortality.

Class II (Symptomatic, Single-Vessel Coronary Disease). This category applies to patients who have a significant lesion in a major epicardial artery that subtends at least a moderately sized area of viable myocardium, and who (a) show evidence of myocardial ischemia and (i) have one or more complex lesions in the same vessel or its branches and (ii) are at moderate risk for morbidity; (b) have disabling symptoms and a small area of viable myocardium at risk, and (i) at least a moderate likelihood of successful dilatation and (ii) are at low risk for morbidity and mortality; or (c) have at least moderately severe angina on medical therapy with equivocal or nondiagnostic evidence of myocardial ischemia on laboratory testing, and who prefer treatment with coronary angioplasty to medical therapy, and (i) have at least a moderate likelihood of successful dilatation and are (ii) at low risk for morbidity and mortality.

Class III (Symptomatic, Single-Vessel Coronary Disease). This category applies to all other symptomatic patients with single-vessel disease who do not fulfill the criteria for class I or II. It includes, for example, patients who (a) have no or only a small area of viable myocardium at risk in the absence of disabling symptoms, (b) have clinical symptoms not likely to be indicative of ischemia, (c) have a very low likelihood of successful dilatation, (d) are at high risk for morbidity and mortality, or (e) have no symptoms or objective evdence of myocardial ischemia during high-level stress testing.

Multivessel Coronary Artery Disease

Asymptomatic or Mildly Symptomatic Patients (Functional Class I) With or Without Medical Therapy

Class I (Mild to No Symptoms, Multivessel Coronary Disease). This category applies to patients who have one significant lesion in a major epicardial artery that could result in nearly complete revascularization because the additional lesion(s) subtends a small viable or nonviable area of myocardium. Additionally, patients in this category must (a) have a large area of viable myocardium at risk, and (b) show evidence of myocardial ischemia while on medical therapy during laboratory testing, or (c) be undergoing high-risk noncardiac surgery and demonstrate objective evidence of myocardial ischemia. These patients should have one or more lesions that would have a high success rate, the successful dilatation of which would provide relief of all major regions of ischemia, and be at low risk for morbidity and mortality.

Class II (Mild to No Symptoms, Multivessel Coronary Disease). This category applies to patients (a) who are similar to patients in class I, but who (i) have a moderately sized area of viable myocar-

dium at risk or (ii) have objective evidence of myocardial ischemia during laboratory testing; (b) who have significant lesions in two or more major epicardial arteries, each of which subtends at least a moderate-sized area of viable myocardium; (c) who have a subtotally occluded vessel requiring angioplasty in which the development of total occlusion of the vessel would result in severe hemodynamic collapse due to left ventricular dysfunction; (d) have chronic total occlusions in major epicardial vessels subtending moderate or large areas of viable myocardium with a moderate likelihood of successful dilatation. These patients should show evidence of myocardial ischemia during laboratory testing, have lesions with at least a moderate likelihood of successful dilatation, the successful dilatation of which would provide relief to all major regions of ischemia, and be at low or moderate risk for morbidity and mortality.

Class III (Mild to No Symptoms, Multivessel Disease). This category applies to all other patients with multivessel disease and mild or no symptoms who do not fulfill the criteria for class I or II. It includes, for example, patients who (a) have only a small area of viable myocardium at risk, (b) have chronic total occlusions with a low likelihood of successful dilatation, or (c) are at high risk for morbidity and mortality.

Symptomatic Patients with Angina Pectoris (Functional Classes II–IV) With Medical Therapy and Multivessel Disease

Class I (Symptomatic, Multivessel Disease). This category applies to patients who have significant lesions in two or more major epicardial arteries both subtending at least moderately sized areas of viable myocardium, and who (a) show evidence of myocardial ischemia while on medical therapy, (b) have unstable angina or angina pectoris that has proven inadequately responsive to medical therapy, or (c) are intolerant of medical therapy because of intolerable side effects. These patients should have lesion morphology associated with a high rate of successful dilatation, which would provide relief of all major regions of ischemia, and be at low risk for morbidity and mortality.

Class II (Symptomatic, Multivessel Disease). This category applies to patients who have significant lesions in two or more major epicardial arteries that subtend at least moderately sized areas of viable myocardium, and who (a) are similar to patients in class I, but who are at moderate risk for morbidity and mortality, or (b) have angina pectoris but do not necessarily show objective evidence of myocardial ischemia during laboratory testing. These patients should have lesion morphology associated with a high rate of successful dilatation, which would provide relief of all major regions of ischemia, and be at moderate risk for morbidity and mortality. Patients in this category also are those who (c) have disabling angina that has proven inadequately responsive to medical therapy and (i) are considered poor candidates for surgery because of advanced physiologic age or coexisting medical disorders, (ii) have lesions with at least a moderate likelihood of successful dilatation, and (iii) are at moderate risk for morbidity and mortality; or (d) have a subtotally occluded vessel requiring angioplasty, and the total occlusion of the vessel would result in severe hemodynamic collapse due to left ventricular dysfunction.

Class III (Symptomatic, Multivessel Coronary Disease). This category applies to all other symptomatic patients with multivessel disease who do not fulfill the criteria in class I or II. It includes, for example, patients who (a) have only a small area of myocardium at risk in the absence of disabling symptoms, (b) have lesion morphology with a low likelihood of successful dilatation and subtending moderate or large areas viable myocardium, or (c) are at high risk for morbidity or mortality, or both. It is to be stressed that risk assessment is different in patients with multivessel disease than in those with single-vessel disease. In the former group there should ideally be the opportunity for anatomically complete revascularization, although adequate functional revascularization can be achieved without necessarily being anatomically complete. In every instance the goal is to achieve relief of ischemia at a risk acceptable for the procedure. In estimating this risk in multivessel disease it is imperative that each lesion be considered in the context of all other lesions present. Some assessment must then be made of the likely consequences should any of the attempted dilatations fail and result in abrupt vessel closure. For example, there is an increased risk in dilating a left coronary artery lesion if it jeopardizes the entire collateral blood supply to a large area of viable myocardium in the distribution of a totally occluded, nondilatable, dominant right coronary artery [24].

Direct Immediate Coronary Angioplasty for Evolving Acute Myocardial Infarction

Class I. This category applies to the dilatation of a significant lesion in the infarct-related artery only in patients who can be managed in the appropriate laboratory setting, and who (a) are within 0–6 h of the onset of a myocardial infarction (the procedure is used as an alternative to thrombolytic therapy), (b) are within 6–12 h of the onset of a myocardial infarction but have continued symptoms of ongoing myocardial ischemia, or (c) are in cardiogenic shock due to myocardial infarction with or without previous thrombolytic therapy and are within 12 h of the onset of symptoms.

Class II. This category applies to patients who (a) are within 6–12 h of the onset of an acute myocardial infarction and have no symptoms of myocardial ischemia but have a large area of myocardium at jeopardy and/or are in a higher risk clinical category, (b) are within 12–24 h of the onset of an acute myocardial infarction but have continued symptoms of ongoing myocardial ischemia, or (c) have received thrombolytic therapy and have continuing or recurrent symptoms of active myocardial ischemia.

Class III. This category applies to (a) angioplasty of a non-infarct-related artery at the time of acute myocardial infarction and (b) patients who are more than 12 h after the onset of acute myocardial infarction at the time of admission and have no symptoms of myocardial ischemia. The role of direct angioplasty in the management of patients during the course of acute myocardial infarction is currently the subject of intense investigation [25]. A number of recent studies indicate that the procedure is most effective as a primary means of establishing reperfusion in the early hours of an evolving myocardial infarction [26–34]. The procedure is associated with the relief of acute symptoms and associated with acceptable mortality rates when the dilatation has been successful. Patients with cardiogenic shock complicating acute myocardial infarction appear to derive significant benefit from direct PTCA, particularly when it is done in conjunction with the use of the intra-aortic balloon pump for hemodynamic support [35–38]. Compared with the conventionally high mortality rate associated with cardiogenic shock (approximately 80 %), a relatively low in-hospital mortality (approximately 40%) has been observed in selected patients with cardiogenic shock treated with angioplasty [38–42].

Coronary Angioplasty After Acute Myocardial Infarction

Class I. This category applies to the dilation of any significant lesion(s) in patients who (a) have recurrent episodes of ischemic chest pain, particularly if accompanied by electrocardiographic changes (postinfarction angina), (b) show objective evidence of myocardial ischemia before discharge from the hospital, or (c) have recurrent sustained ventricular tachycardia or ventricular fibrillation, or both, while receiving intensive medical therapy. These patients should have one or more lesions that predict a high (>90%) success rate and be at low risk for morbidity and mortality.

Class II. This category applies to the dilation of significant lesions in patients (a) who are similar to patients in class I but (i) have more complex lesions with at least a moderate likelihood of successful dilation, (ii) undergo multivessel angioplasty, or (iii) are at moderate risk for morbidity or mortality or both; (b) who have survived cardiogenic shock in the period before discharge; (c) who are asymptomatic but have a significant residual lesion in the infarct-related artery supplying a large or moderate area of angiographically functioning myocardium; or (d) who have a non-Q-wave myocardial infarction or (i) a large area at risk or objective evidence of myocardial ischemia, (ii) single-vessel disease with noncomplex lesion morphology, and (iii) are at low risk for morbidity and mortality.

Class III. This category applies to all other patients in the immediate postinfarction period (during initial hospitalization) who do not fulfill the criteria for class I and II, for example, (a) dilatation of borderline residual lesions (50%–60%) in the absence of spontaneous or stress-induced ischemia, (b) dilatation of chronic total occlusions subtending nonviable myocardium, and (c) angioplasty in patients at high risk for morbidity and mortality.

Angiographic Lesion Characteristics

Although the emergence of new interventional techniques has altered our approach to coronary angioplasty and improved initial success rates even in complex lesions, the traditional angiographic classification of lesion morphology remains an important element of preprocedural stratification for the expected interventional success and the selection of new devices.

Angiographic Lesion Morphology

Angiographic evaluation of lesion morphology is based on a "lumenogram" of coronary artery stenosis yielding little information on surface morphology and plaque composition. Despite this limitation, several angiographic lesion characteristics have been identified which provide important clinical and prognostic information in patients undergoing coronary angioplasty [43, 44].

On the basis of these lesion-specific characteristics the following three types can be defined:

Type A lesions (minimally complex)
Discrete (length <10 mm)
Concentric
Readily accessible
Nonangulated segment (<45°)
Smooth contour
Little or no calcification
Less than totally occlusive
Not ostial in location
No major side branch involvement
Absence of thrombus

Type B lesions (moderately complex)
Tubular (length 10–20 mm)
Eccentric
Moderate tortuosity of proximal segment
Moderately angulated segment (>45°, <90°)
Irregular contour
Moderate or heavy calcification
Total occlusions <3 months old
Ostial in location
Bifurcational lesion requiring double guidewires
Some thrombus present

Type C lesions (severely complex)
  Diffuse (length >2 cm)
  Excessive tortuosity of proximal segment
  Extremely angulated segments >90°
  Total occlusions >3 months old and/or bridging collaterals
  Inability to protect major side branches
  Degenerated vein grafts with friable lesions

When conventional balloon angioplasty is applied, the highest primary success rate and lowest complication rate is found in type A lesions, characterized by a short stenosis length (<10 mm), concentric morphology with smooth contours in a readily accessible, nonangulated segment (<45°). Type A lesions show little or no calcium during fluoroscopy, are free of thrombi and do not involve the coronary ostium or major sidebranches. Lesions with two or more type B characteristics entail an intermediate risk between lesions with one type B characteristic and type C lesions. Specific lesion characteristics associated with an adverse outcome include chronic total occlusion, high-grade stenoses, stenoses on a bend greater than 60°, and lesions located in vessels with proximal tortuosity [43].

Angiographic Flow Patterns Across Stenotic Lesions

Apart from the geometric estimation of the severity of a coronary artery stenosis, its functional significance during physical rest can be roughly assessed using the following angiographic flow pattern established by the Thrombolyis In Myocardial Infarction (TIMI) Study Group [45]:

Grade 0 (no perfusion): No contrast flow through the stenosis.

Grade 1 (penetration with minimal perfusion): A small amount of contrast flows through the stenosis, but fails to opacify the artery beyond.

Grade 2 (partial perfusion): Contrast flows through the stenosis to opacify the terminal artery segment. However, contrast enters the terminal segment perceptibly more slowly than the terminal segments of a comparable artery without stenosis. Alternatively, contrast material clears from a segment distal to a stenosis noticeably more slowly than from a comparable segment not preceded by a significant stenosis.

Grade 3 (complete perfusion): Anterograde flow into the terminal coronary artery segment through a stenosis is as prompt as anterograde flow into the terminal segment of a comparable coronary artery without preceding stenosis. Contrast material clears as rapidly from the distal segment as from a comparable uninvolved segment.

Impact of Lesion Morphology on the Choice of Interventional Techniques

Although a variety of new interventional devices have become available during the past few years, none of these new technologies has proven definitely superior to balloon angioplasty with respect to restenosis. Even in a high-volume center such as the Red Cross Hospital and Heart Center at Frankfurt, where approximately 5000 angioplasty procedures are performed annually, a second-generation device is selected as the primary approach in only 20 % of procedures. At the present time new interventional technologies remain an alternative approach for the treatment of complex coronary lesions.

In our laboratories type A lesions are usually treated with conventional balloon angioplasty, which yields primary success rates of approximately 96 %. However, eccentric and irregular lesions as well as bifurcational lesions may also be adequately dilated using balloon angioplasty, with similar rates of procedural success. In ostial lesions or highly eccentric stenoses with slight to moderate calcification, directional coronary artherectomy can be performed with excellent primary results (Fig. 9) as long as the lesion is located in the proximal or middle segment of the large coronary arteries [46]. Despite recent technical improvements aiming at enhanced flexibility of the device, its relative stiffness and high profile remain important limitations when coronary arteries with proximal tortuosity must be passed, or the device is to be advanced to more distally located coronary segments. Calcification, however, may also impair the primary success of directional coronary artherectomy.

Both ostial lesions and the protected main stem, where balloon angioplasty seldom yields acceptable results, can also be treated with excellent primary success using rotational coronary atherectomy [47] (Fig. 10). We prefer this approach to alternative techniques such as directional coronary artherectomy, excimer laser angioplasty [48,

49], and stenting especially if the lesions are calcified, ostial in location, tortuous, long and, located in vessels less than 3 mm in diameter.

In a large randomized trial comparing procedural and angiographic results of excimer laser angioplasty, rotational atherectomy, and balloon angioplasty for complex lesions (ERBAC) we found rotational artherectomy associated with superior procedural outcomes to balloon angioplasty and eximer laser angioplasty [49]. In our experience rotational coronary artherectomy improves the initial result of angioplasty especially in lesions that are of type B or C, eccentric, long and irregular, subtotal (>80 %) or located on a bend greater than 45°. Among the currently available second-generation technologies, the importance of eximer laser angioplasty as an alternative approach to balloon angioplasty seems questionable. At least, ERBAC did not demonstrate any relevant advantage of excimer laser angioplasty over conventional balloon angioplasty. However, in selected cases of subtotal or total thrombotic coronary occlusions [50] excimer laser angioplasty followed by balloon dilation may be performed with excellent angiographic results (Fig. 11).

Angiographic Strategies During Angioplasty

Once the severity and morphology of the coronary obstruction is evaluated, the indication for angioplasty is established, and the interventional technique is selected coronary angiography in conjunction with on-line digital imaging techniques have substantially improved the ability of the operator to control individual steps in the interventional procedure and to modify the manuevers according to intermediate angiographic results.

Baseline Angiography

Based on the above explanation of angiographic views for diagnostic coronary angiography, a minimum of two representative radiographic projections of the segment of interest should be selected. One of these projections should visualize the tightest view of the coronary lesion to allow quantitative assessment of lesion severity before PTCA if desired. Another projection should show the coronary artery segment without foreshortening to allow the assessment of the true length of the lesion. At this stage of peri-interventional coronary angiography QCA measurements may be performed on-line. Exact angulations of the angiographic views must be documented to allow corresponding quantitative assessments at the end of the procedure and at follow-up (Fig. 9).

Angiographic Control of Guidewire Insertion

The correct positioning of the angioplasty guidewire may require additional angiographic projections visualizing the course of the target coronary artery by repeated injection of small amounts of contrast medium.

If the target vessel is the LAD, an LAO 50° projection with 30° cranial angulation is normally sufficient to control guidewire positioning and to correct erroneous insertion of the wire in diagonal or septal branches (Fig. 2). If the guidewire cannot be advanced into the LAD in this projection, an LAO 50° projection with 30° caudal angulation may be helpful to visualize the bifurcation of left anterior descending and circumflex coronary artery ("spider view"). Occasionally the position of the guiding catheter must be corrected in this angiographic projection (counterclockwise rotation, deep insertion) to allow engagement of the angioplasty guidewire in the LAD. Potential mismatch of the guiding catheter as a reason for unsuccessful guidewire insertion into the LAD ostium is easily recognized in this angiographic view. The best view to prevent erroneous entering of side branches in the mid LAD is a frontal view or an RAO projection with cranial angulation (Fig. 3).

If the target vessel is the circumflex coronary artery, an RAO 20° projection with 20° caudal angulation facilitates guidewire positioning (Fig. 5). For insertion of the angioplasty guidewire into the right coronary artery an LAO 45° view is normally sufficient (Fig. 6). For insertion of the wire into the right posterior descending artery, a 20°–30° cranial angulated LAO view is superior if the patient is able to take a deep breath to lower the diaphragm (Fig. 7).

To ascertain a distal position of the angioplasty guidewire tip in the target vessel, one angiographic projection visualizing the coronary artery of interest without foreshortening should be recorded as soon as the procedure of guidewire insertion has been completed.

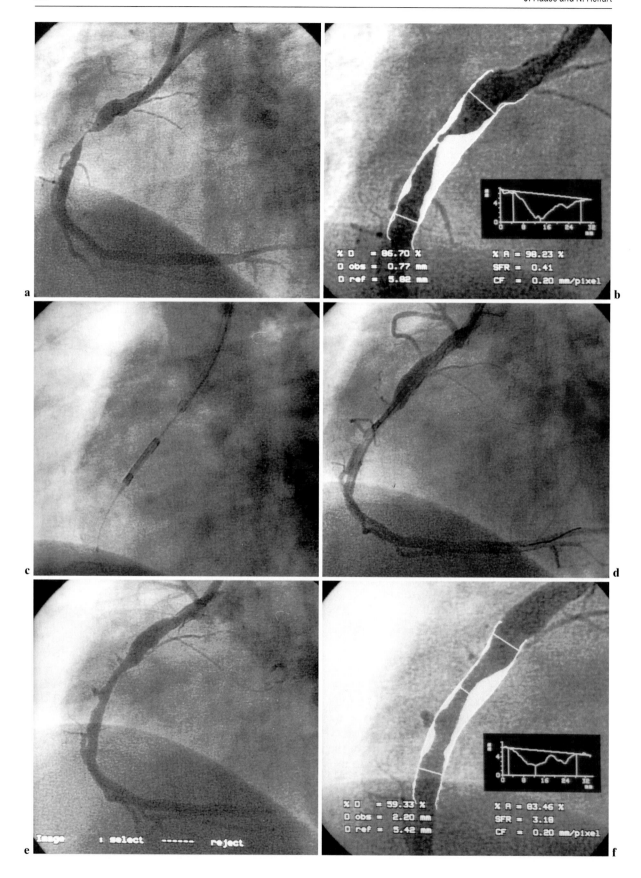

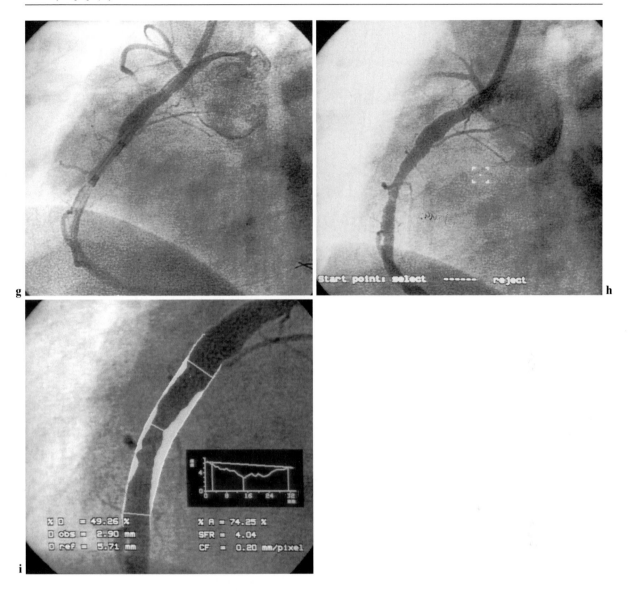

Fig. 9a–i. Angiographic control of directional coronary artherectomy (DCA) at the proximal right coronary artery. **a** A highly eccentric lesion in the proximal right coronary artery is visualized angiographically following insertion of the atherectomy guiding catheter. **b** On-line QCA measurement is performed using the ACA package of the Philips Digital Cardiac Imaging system. **c** The atherectomy device is advanced to the lesion, and the housing is first oriented to the inferior plaque. **d** Following atherectomy from the inferior portion of the plaque, the device is turned upward and contrast medium is injected to control the position of the housing with respect to the remaining atheroma. **e** An intermediate result of directional coronary atherectomy is recorded demonstrating a "borderline" residual stenosis. **f** The intermediate result of DCA is analyzed by on-line QCA measurements, showing a 59% residual stenosis. **g** Based on the suboptimal result additional cuts with the DCA device are carried out to remove material from the inferior portion of the plaque. **h** The final result following directional coronary atherectomy is recorded angiographically. **i** At the end of the procedure the on-line QCA measurement is repeated demonstrating a residual stenosis <50% ("suboptimal result")

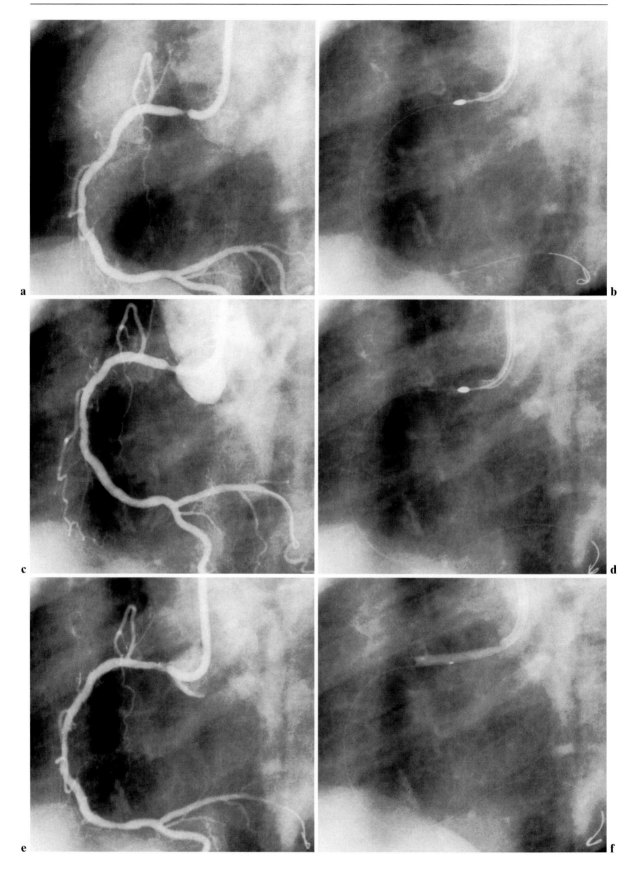

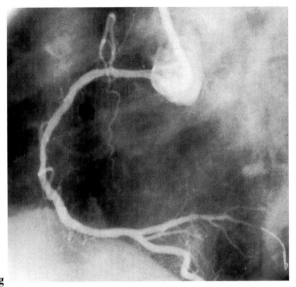

g

Fig. 10 a–g. Rotational coronary atherectomy of a right coronary ostial stenosis. A high-grade ostial stenosis of the right coronary artery is visualized angiographically using a 9-F Hokey Stick angioplasty guiding catheter. **a** The guiding catheter is positioned in front of the ostium without engagement. **b** Following insetion of a 0.009-in. rotablator wire type C, a 1.5-mm-diameter burr rotating at 190 000 rpm is advanced through the ostium. **c** The primary result is recorded angiographically to exclude the occurrence of intimal dissections. **d** A second run is made, with a 2.0-mm-diameter rotablator burr. **e** The result is again documented. **f** Final balloon dilatation is performed. **g** The final result is again recorded with an injection of contrast medium, keeping the tip of the guiding catheter in front of the coronary ostium

Angiographic Control of the Dimension and Position of Interventional Devices

Angiographic control of the dimension and intracoronary position of interventional devices facilitates accurate matching to vessel diameter and length of the lesion or dissection. For routine visual estimation of balloon diameters the known diameter of the guiding catheter may serve as a guideline. Optimal matching of the diameter of the interventional device to vessel diameter can be achieved by QCA analysis of the coronary artery segment in which angioplasty should be performed. The "reference diameter" as obtained at the location of the coronary artery lesion by the automated contour detection algorithm provides the most accurate measure for the balloon or stent diameter (Fig. 8). Definite matching of balloon length and accurate matching of intracoronary stents are obtained during insertion of the device by injecting small amounts of contrast medium with simultaneous fluoroscopic digital imaging to compare the geometric dimension of the coronary lesion directly with the device to be applied (Fig. 9).

Geometric matching of lesion dimension with the size of the interventional device is also crucial when rotational coronary atherectomy is used (Fig. 12). In our experience a stepwise increment of burr sizes starting with small diameters oriented at the obstruction diameter up to burr sizes at a maximum of two-thirds of the reference diameter provides optimal results in conjunction with final balloon angioplasty directly matched to the full reference diameter at the site of the coronary lesion. In rotational coronary atherectomy, however, accurate geometric matching of burr size and the obstruction diameter is only one important prerequisite for optimal angiographic results. More important is that any force is avoided when the rotating burr is advanced through the lesion. Spontaneous decrease in the rotational speed of more than 10 % in conjunction with resistance that can be felt manually indicates either that the device has been advanced too rapidly, or that the burr diameter is oversized. This may result in intimal dissections or even vessel wall perforation.

When excimer-laser angioplasty is used, simultaneous angiographic control during the process of catheter insertion is necessary to allow positioning of the laser catheter tip exactly in front of the lesion before the laser energy is applied (Fig. 11). Exact angiographic measurement of the lesion length is required to avoid any laser energy being applied to areas beyond the lesion, which may also result in intimal dissections or vessel wall perforation.

Following each balloon inflation or passage of an interventional device through the coronary artery lesion, angiographic control of the dilation or debulking effect is required. This allows immediate recognition of potential complications such as spasm, intimal dissections, and vessel wall perforations, and the interventional strategy can then be modified immediately if necessary. The stepwise increment of burr sizes is stopped, for example, as soon as an intimal dissection is visualized angiographically, and the procedure is completed with a final balloon inflation, by which small dissections may be sealed.

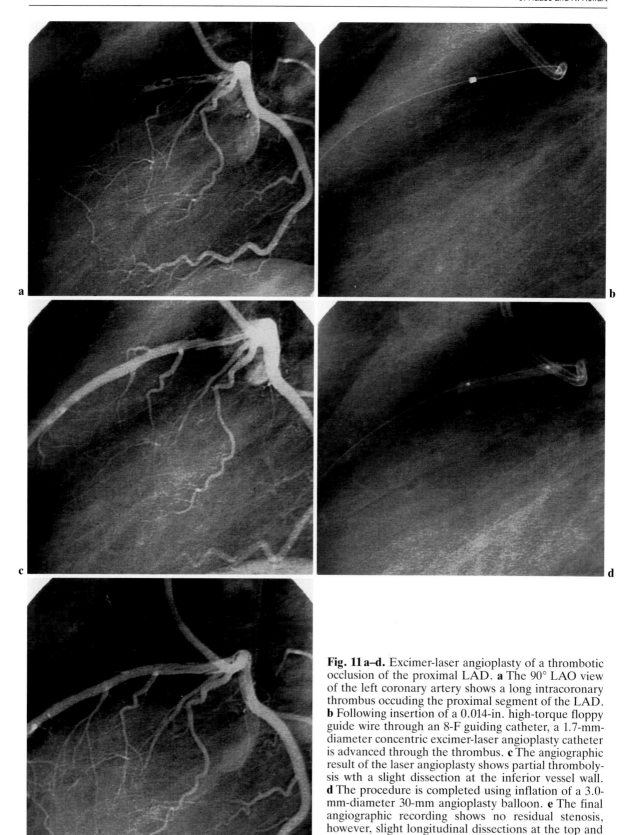

Fig. 11 a–d. Excimer-laser angioplasty of a thrombotic occlusion of the proximal LAD. **a** The 90° LAO view of the left coronary artery shows a long intracoronary thrombus occuding the proximal segment of the LAD. **b** Following insertion of a 0.014-in. high-torque floppy guide wire through an 8-F guiding catheter, a 1.7-mm-diameter concentric excimer-laser angioplasty catheter is advanced through the thrombus. **c** The angiographic result of the laser angioplasty shows partial thrombolysis wth a slight dissection at the inferior vessel wall. **d** The procedure is completed using inflation of a 3.0-mm-diameter 30-mm angioplasty balloon. **e** The final angiographic recording shows no residual stenosis, however, slight longitudinal dissections at the top and at the bottom of the proximal segment

Angiographic Outcome of Coronary Angioplasty

As soon as the interventional procedure is completed, the device is removed from the coronary artery under fluoroscopic control while the angioplasty guidewire remains in place and a postprocedural angiographic evaluation is carried out. For this purpose, the baseline coronary angiography is repeated using the identical projections that have been selected before the angioplasty procedure. Angiographic evaluation of the results of interventional procedures examines (a) the luminal dimensions at the site of the lesion (either visual estimation or quantitative geometric measurements), (b) the vessel wall morphology following angioplasty, and (c) the run-off of contrast medium (grading of flow pattern).

While the primary success of coronary angioplasty is defined as a stenosis reduction to less than 50% diameter stenosis with complete restoration of blood flow in the absence of major complications, the aim of any interventional procedure is to dilate an obstructive lesion to less than 30% diameter stenosis and to achieve angiographically smooth vessel contours. Due to a varying degree of plaque calcification and to elastic recoil following angioplasty diameter stenosis values of up to 50% or 60% are rather frequent (10%–20%) and are considered an acceptable result with regard to lesion geometry and the potential risk of a more aggressive dilation. Since intimal disruption is an inherent mechanism of balloon dilatation, a varying degree of vessel wall dissection is to be expected following angioplasty. The angiographic morphology of coronary dissections can be classified as follows:

Type A: small radiolucent area within the lumen of the vessel
Type B: linear, nonpersisting extravasation of contrast
Type C: extraluminal, persisting extravasation of contrast
Type D: spiral-shaped filling defect
Type E: persisting lumen defect with delayed anterograde flow
Type F: filling defect accompanied by total coronary occlusion

The angiographic appearance of small dissections includes "haziness" defined as a small radiolucent area within the lumen of the vessel and nonsharp wall contours. This type of dissection as well as a linear extravasation of contrast medium without significant (<50%) reduction in the free intracoronary lumen may also be tolerated as an acceptable angioplasty result. Spiral-shaped filling defects or persistent lumen defects with more than 50% diameter stenosis, however, must be regarded as "threatening closure" and requiring additional interventional treatment such as the use of perfusion balloons or stent implantation. In the presence of an acceptable morphologic appearance and complete restoration of coronary blood flow, the final angiographic evaluation is performed when the angioplasty guidewire has been removed from the coronary artery. Occasionally a vessel wall dissection previously deemed of low grade turns out to be occlusive when the scaffolding effect of the angioplasty guidewire is lost.

Control of Interventional Complications

Peri-interventional coronary angiography represents the fastest approach to assess complications due to angioplasty procedures and allows immediate control of adjunctive interventions. The most frequent complication following coronary angioplasty is threatened closure or complete vessel occlusion due to intimal dissection. Immediate repeat PTCA with either long balloons or perfusion balloons are used to seal occlusive dissections, with 80%–90% success rates [51]. However, when long inflations fail to restore coronary blood flow, intracoronary stents should be implanted at the site of occlusive vessel wall dissections [52–56]. Alternatively, a primary stent implantation may be justified. A 24-h "interventional stand-by" of an experienced team with special training in the field of coronary stent implantation guarantees the optimal outcome of these high-risk patients. The goal of the stent implantation is complete sealing of the entire dissection [57], with a close to 0% residual narrowing (Fig. 13). Occasionally, multiple stents are necessary to seal an intimal dissection completely.

A relatively rare but dangerous complication of percutaneous coronary angioplasty is the perforation of a coronary artery, which can be detected angiographically by extravasation of contrast medium into the pericardial space. Immediate sealing of the respective coronary artery with a perfusion balloon in conjunction with pericardiocentesis may be used as an emergency procedure to prevent cardiac tamponade until definite surgical repair is carried out.

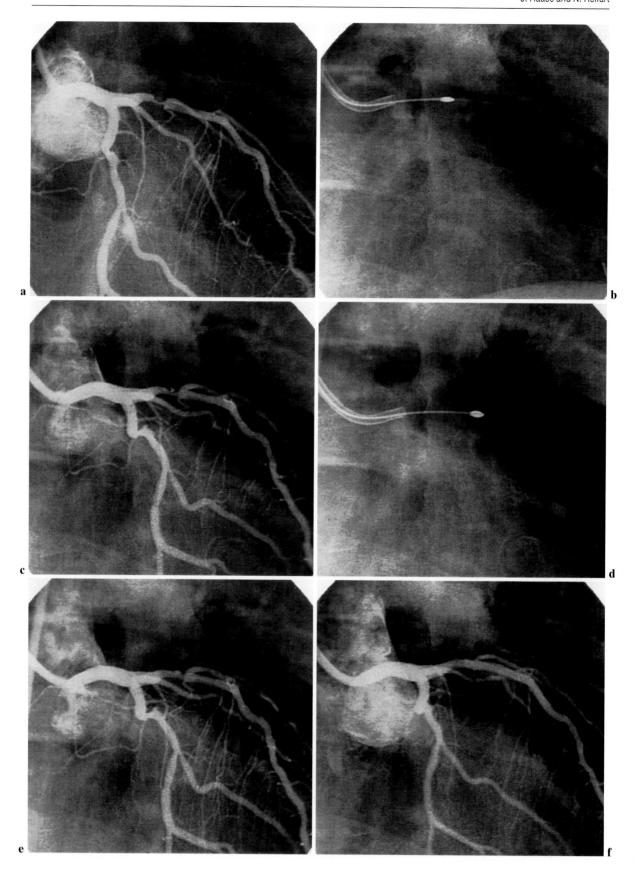

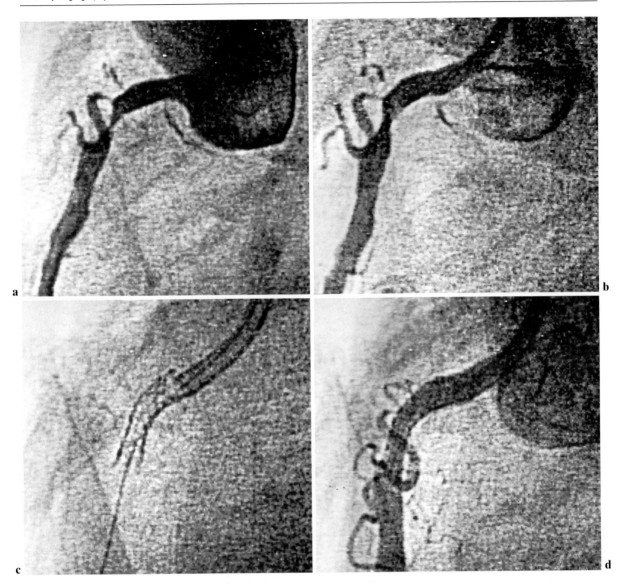

Fig. 12 a–f. Rotational coronary atherectomy of the proximal LAD. **a** An RAO view of the left coronary artery shows the high-grade eccentric lesion in the proximal segment of the LAD. **b** A 1.5-mm-diameter rotablator burr is advanced slowly through the lesion. **c** Angiographic control following the first rotational atherectomy reveals a plaque ulceration which is now filled with contrast medium. **d** A 2.0-mm-diameter rotablator burr is then advanced through the lesion. **e** The result is documented by contrast injection. **f** Following adjunctive inflation of a 3.0-mm-diameter angioplasty balloon the vessel contour is smoothened without residual stenosis

Fig. 13 a–d. Implantation of a Strecker stent in the right coronary artery. **a** A high-grade stenosis in the proximal segment of the right coronary artery is first treated with a 3.0-mm angioplasty balloon. **b** This results in an intimal dissection with threatened closure that cannot be sealed adequately using long inflation (10 min) with a 3.5-mm perfusion balloon. **c** Subsequently a 25-mm Strecker stent mounted at a 3.5-mm angioplasty balloon is inserted. **d** The final coronary angiography demonstrates complete sealing of the intimal dissection

Follow-Up Coronary Angiography

Angiographic follow-up after successful coronary angioplasty is required in patients at high risk for restenosis or reocclusion. This is relevant especially if major dissections remain following angioplasty since more than 60 % of these patients experience early restenosis [58], or if angioplasty was performed at chronic total coronary occlusions, where early restenosis occurs in 55 % and early reocclusion in about 20 % of patients [59]. For these subgroups angiographic follow-up is recommended within 6–8 weeks. When recurrent angina occurs following angioplasty, follow-up coronary angiography must be carried out immediately, since repeat PTCA may be performed with high success rates at low risk.

References

1. Grüntzig AR, Senning A, Siegenthaler WE (1979) Nonoperative dilatation of coronary artery stenosis: percutaneous transluminal coronary angioplasty. New Engl J Med 301: 61
2. Vogel RA (1993) Transcatheter assessment of coronary blood flow and velocity. In: Vogel JHK, King SB III (eds) The practice of interventional cardiology, 2nd edn. Mosby, St. Louis, p 19
3. Nissen SE, Gurley JC, Grines CL, Booth DC, McClure R, Berk M, Fischer C, DeMaria AN (1991) Intravascular ultrasound assessment of lumen size and wall morphology in normal subjects and patients with coronary artery disease. Circulation 84: 1087
4. Baim DS (1991) Coronary angioplasty. In: Grossman W, Baim DS (eds) Cardiac catheterization angiography and intervention, 4th edn. Lea & Feibiger, Philadelphia, p 441
5. Bunell IL, Greene DG, Tandon RN, Arani DT (1973) The half-axial projection. A new look at the proximal left coronary artery. Circulation 48: 1151
6. Lesperance J, Saltiel J, Peticlerc R, Bourassa MG (1974) Angulated views in the sagittal plane for improved accuracy of cine coronary angiography. Am J Roentgenol 121: 575
7. Aldridge HE, McLoughlin MJ, Taylor KW (1975) Improved diagnosis in coronary cinearteriography with routine use of 110 oblique views and cranial and caudal angulations. Am J Cardiol 36: 468
8. Grover M, Slutsky R, Higgins C, Atwood JE (1984) Terminology and anatomy of angulated coronary arteriography. Clin Cardiol 7: 37
9. Elliott LP, Bream PF, Soto B, Russell RO jr, Rogers WJ, Mantle JA, Hood WP jr (1981) Significance of the caudal left-anterior-oblique view in analyzing the left main coronary artery. Radiology 139: 39
10. Gomez A, Esposito V, Grollman J, O'Reilly R (1983) Angled views in the evaluation of the right coronary artery. Cathet Cardiovasc Diagn 8: 71
11. King SB III, Douglas JS jr, Morris DC (1981) New angiographic views for coronary arteriography. In: Hurst JW (ed) Update IV: the heart. McGraw Hill, New York, p 193
12. Arani DT, Bunnell IL, Greene DG (1975) Lordotic right posterior oblique projection of the left coronary artery: a special view for special anatomy. Circulation 52: 504
13. DeRouen TA, Murray JA, Owen W (1977) Variability in the analysis of coronary arteriograms. Circulation 55: 324
14. Serruys PW, Booman F, Troost J, Reiber JHC, Gerbrands JJ, Brand M van den, Cherrier F, Hugenholtz PG (1982) Computerized quantitative coronary angiography applied to percutaneous transluminal coronary angioplasty: advantages and limitations. In: Kaltenbach M, Grüntzig A, Rentrop K, Bussman WD (eds) Transluminal coronary angioplasty and intracoronary thrombolysis – heart disease IV. Springer, Berlin Heidelberg New York, p 110
15. De Feyter PJ, Serruys PW, Davies MJ, Richardson P, Lubson J, Oliver MF (1991) Quantitative coronary angiography to measure progression and regression of coronary atherosclerosis: value, limitations and implications for clinical trials. Circulation 84: 412
16. Strauss BH, Escaned J, Foley DP, DiMario C, Haase J, Keane D, Hermans WRM, De Feyter PJ, Serruys PW (1994) Technological considerations and practical limitations in the use of quantitative angiography during percutaneous coronary recanalization. Progr Cardiovasc Dis 5: 343
17. Reiber JHC, van der Zwet PMJ, Koning G, von Land CD, Padmos I, Buis B, van Bethem AC, van Meurs B (1991) Quantitative coronary measurements from cine and digital arteriograms; methodology and validation results. 4th International Symposim on Coronary Arteriography, Rotterdam, June 23–25, 1991. Erasmus University Press, Rotterdam, p 36
18. Haase J, Di Mario C, Slager CJ, van der Giessen WJ, den Boer A, De Feyter PJ, Reiber JHC, Verdouw PD, Serruys PW (1992) In vivo validation of on-line and off-line geometric coronary measurements using insertion of stenosis phantoms in porcine coronary arteries. Cathet Cardiovasc Diagn 27: 16
19. Reiber JHC, Kooijman CJ, den Boer A, Serruys PW (1985) Assessment of dimensions and image quality of coronary contrast catheters from cineangiograms. Cathet Cardiovasc Diagn 11: 521
20. Wollschläger H, Zeiher AM, Lee P, Solzbach U, Bonzel T, Just H (1988) Optimal biplane imaging of coronary segments with computed triple orthogonal projections. In: Reiber JHC, Surruys PW (eds) New developments in quantitative coronary arteriography, 1st edn. Kluwer, Dordrecht, p 13
21. Reiber JHC, Zwet PMJ van der, Land CD von, Koning G, Loois G, Zorn I, Brand M van den, Gerbrands JJ (1989) On-line quantification of coronary angiograms with the DCI system. Medica Mundi 34: 89

22. Haase J, Nugteren SK, van Swijndregt EM, Slager CJ, Di Mario C, De Feyter PJ, Serruys PW (1993) Digital geometric measurements in comparison to cinefilm analysis of coronary artery dimensions. Cathet Cardiovasc Diagn 28: 283

23. Ryan TJ, Bauman WB, Kennedy JW, Kereiakes DJ, King SB III, McCallister BD, Smith SC, Ullyot DJ (1994) Guidelines for percutaneous transluminal coronary angioplasty – a report of the AHA/ ACC Task Force on Assessment of Diagnostic and Therapeutic Cardiovascular Procedures (Committee on Percutaneous Transluminal Coronary Angioplasty). Circulation 88: 2987

24. Teirstein P, Giorgi L, Johnson W, McConahay D, Rutherford B, Hartzler G (1990) PTCA of the left coronary artery when the right coronary artery is chronically occluded. Am Heart J 119: 479

25. Eckman MH, Wong JB, Salem DN, Pauker SG (1992) Direct angioplasty for acute myocardial infarction: a review of outcomes in clinical subsets. Ann Intern Med 117: 667

26. O'Keefe JH jr, Bailey WL, Rutherford BD, Hartzler GO (1993) Primary angioplasty for acute myocardial infarction in 1000 consecutive patients – results in an unselected population and high-risk subgroups. Am J Cardiol 72: 107G

27. Elizaga J, Garcia EJ, Delcán JL, Garcia-Robles JA, Bueno H, Soriano J, Abeytua M, Lopez-Bescós L (1993) Primary coronary angioplasty versus systemis thrombolysis in acute anterior myocardial infarction – in-hospital results from a prospective randomized trial. Circulation 88: 1–411

28. Stone GW, Grines CL, Browne KF, Rothbaum D, O'Keefe J, Hartzler GO, Overlie P, Donohue B, Chelliah N, Puchrowicz-Ochocki S, Timmis G (1993) Primary angioplasty reduces recurrent ischemic events compared to tPA in myocardial infarction – implications for early discharge. Circulation 88: 1–105

29. O'Neill WW, Zijlstra F, Suryapranata H, Timmis GC, Grines CL (1993) Meta-analysis of the PAMI and Netherlands randomized trials of primary angioplasty versus thrombolytic therapy of acute myocardial infarction. Circulation 88: 1–106

30. O'Keefe JH jr, Rutherford BD, McConahay DR, Ligon RW, Johnson WL jr, Giorgi LV, Crockett JE, McCallister BD, Conn RD, Gura GM jr, et al. (1989) Early and late results of coronary angioplasty without antecedent thrombolytic therapy for acute myocardial infarction. Am J Cardiol 64: 1221

31. Kander NH, O'Neill W, Topol EJ, Gallison L, Mileski R, Ellis SG (1989) Long-term follow-up of patients treated with coronary angioplasty for acute myocardial infarction. Am Heart J 118: 228

32. Rotbaum DA, Linnemeier TJ, Landin RJ, Steinmetz EF, Hillis JS, Hallam CC, Noble RJ, See MR (1987) Emergency percutaneous transluminal coronary angioplasty in acute myocardial infarction: a 3 year experience. J Am Coll Cardiol 10: 264

33. Brodie BR, Weintraub RA, Stuckey TD, LeBauer EJ, Katz JD, Kelly TA, Hansen CJ (1991) Outcomes of direct coronary angioplasty for acute myocardial infarction in candidates and non-candidates for thrombolytic therapy. Am J Cardiol 67: 7

34. O'Keefe JH jr, Rutherford BD, McConahay DR, Johnson WL jr, Giorgi LV, Shimshak TM, Ligon RW, McCallister BD, Hartzler GO (1992) Myocardial salvage with direct coronary angioplasty for acute infarction. Am Heart J 123: 1

35. Moosvi AR, Khaja F, Villanueva L, Gheorghiade M, Douthat L, Goldstein S (1992) Early revascularization improves survival in acute myocardial infarction. J Am Coll Cardiol 19: 907

36. Lee L, Bates ER, Pitt B, Walton JA, Laufer N, O'Neill W (1988) Percutaneous transluminal coronary angioplasty improves survival in acute myocardial infarction complicated by cardiogenic shock. Circulation 78: 1345

37. Klein LW (1992) Optimal therapy for cardiogenic shock: the emerging role of coronary angioplasty. J Am Coll Cardiol 19: 654

38. Lee L, Erbel R, Brown TM, Laufer N, Meyer J, O'Neill W (1991) Multicenter registry of angioplasty therapy of cardiogenic shock: initial and long-term survival. J Am Coll Cardiol 17: 599

39. Hibbard MD, Holmes DR jr, Bailey KR, Reeder GS, Bresnahan JF, Gersh BJ (1992) Percutaneous transluminal coronary angioplasty in patients with cardiogenic shock. J Am Coll Cardiol 19: 639

40. Gacioch GM, Ellis SG, Lee L, Bates ER, Kirsh M, Walton JA, Topol EJ (1992) Cardiogenic shock complicating acute myocardial infarction: the use of coronary angioplasty and the integration of the new support devices into patient management. J Am Coll Cardiol 19: 647

41. Seydoux C, Goy JJ, Beuret P, Stauffer JC, Vogt P, Schaller MD, Kappenberger L, Perret C (1992) Effectiveness of percutaneous transluminal coronary angioplasty in cardiogenic shock during acute myocardial infarction. Am J Cardiol 69: 968

42. O'Neill WW (1992) Angioplasty therapy of cardiogenic shock: are randomized trials necessary? J Am Coll Cardiol 19: 915

43. Ellis S, Vandormael M, Cowley M, et al. (1990) Coronary morphologic and clinical determinants of procedural outcome with angioplasty for multivessel coronary artery disease. Implications for patient selection. Circulation 82: 1193

44. Savage M, Goldberg S, Hirschfeld J, et al. (1991) Clinical and angiographic determinants of primary coronary angioplasty success. J Am Coll Cardiol 17: 22

45. The TIMI Study Group (1989) Comparison of invasive and conservative strategies after treatment with intravenous tissue plasminogen activator in acute myocardial infarction: results of the Thrombolysis in Myocardial Infarction (TIMI) phase II trial. N Engl J Med 320: 618

46. Safian RD, Gelbfish JS, Erny RE, Schnitt SJ, Schmidt DA, Baim DS (1991) Coronary atherectomy. Clinical, angiographic, and histologic findings and observations regarding potential mechanisms. Circulation 82: 69

47. Sterzer SH, Rosenblum J, Shaw RE, Sugeng I, Hidalgo B, Ryan C, Hansell HN, Murphy MC, Mylert RK (1993) Coronary rotational ablation: initial experience in 302 procedures. J Am Coll Cardiol 21: 287

48. Popma J, et al. (1991) Atherectomy of right coronary ostial stenoses: initial and long-term results, technical features and histologic findings. Am J Cardiol 67: 431

49. Vandormael M, Reifart N, Preusler W, Schwarz F, Störger H, Hofman M, Klöpper JW, Müller S (1994) Comparison of excimer-laser angioplasty and rotational atherectomy with balloon angioplasty for complex lesions: ERBAC study final results. J Am Coll Cardiol 23: 57 A

50. Gregory KW (1993) Laser thrombolysis. In: Vogel JHK, King SB III (eds) The practice of interventional cardiology, 2nd edn. Mosby, St. Louis, p 273

51. Reifart N, Langer A, Störger H, Schwarz F, Preusler W, Hofmann M (1992) Strecker stent as a bail-out device following transluminal coronary angioplasty. J Interven Cardiol 5: 79

52. Sigwart U, Puel J, Mirkovitch V, Joffre F, Kappenberger L (1987) Intravascular stents to prevent occlusion and restenosis after transluminal angioplasty. N Engl J Med 316: 701

53. Roubin GS, Cannon AD, Subodh KA, Macander PJ, Dean LS, Baxley WA, Breland J (1992) Intracoronary stending for acute and threatened closure complicating percutaneous transluminal coronary angioplasty. Circulation 3: 916

54. De Feyter PJ, DeScheerder I, van den Brand M, Laarman GJ, Suryapranata H, Serruys PW (1990) Emergency stenting for refractory acute coronary artery occlusion during coronary angioplasty. Am J Cardiol 66: 1147

55. Haude M, Erbel R, Straub U, Dietz U, Schatz R, Meyer J (1991) Results on intracoronary stents for management of coronary dissections after balloon angioplasty. Am J Cardiol 67: 691

56. Reifart N, Haase J, Massa T, Preusler W, Schwarz F, Störger H, Vandormael M, Hofmann M (1994) Randomaized trial comparing two devices: the Palmaz-Schatz and the Strecker stent in bail-out situations. J Interven Cardiol (in press)

57. Colombo A, Goldberg SL, Almagor Y, Maiello L, Finci L (1993) A novel strategy for stent deployment in the treatment of acute or threatened closure complicating balloon coronary angioplasty. J Am Coll Cardiol 22: 1887

58. Waller B, Orr C, Pinkerton C, Van Tassel J, Peters T, Slack J (1992) Coronary balloon angioplasty dissections: "The good, the bad and the ugly." J Am Coll Cardiol 20: 701

59. Ishizaka N, Issiki T, Saeki F, Ishizaka Y, Ikari Y, Abe J, Soumitsu Y, Hashimoto H, Masaki K, Yamaguchi T (1994) Angiographic follow-up after successful percutaneous coronary angioplasty for chronic total coronary occlusion – experiences in 110 consecutive patients. Am Heart J 127: 8

Quantitative and Qualitative Coronary Angiography

J. B. Hermiller, E. T. Fry, T. Peters, C. M. Orr, J. Van Tassel, and C. A. Pinkerton

Although the technical quality of coronary angiographic images has dramatically improved, the method by which the great majority of clinical cardiac catheterization laboratories estimate coronary lesion severity has remained essentially unchanged. Most laboratories continue to rely on visual assessments of percent diameter stenosis, so called "eyeball" estimates, to define lesion severity. Unfortunately, these visual estimates are neither accurate nor precise [1–3]. Created to circumvent the weaknesses of "eyeball" measurements, quantitative coronary angiography (QCA) was developed to more reproducibly and accurately guage the magnitude of coronary obstructions [4–6]. Hand-held calipers were the first form of QCA. Subsequently, computer-assisted, quantitative angiographic systems were introduced. Although QCA significantly enhances the accuracy of measuring percent stenosis, the biologic behavior of an atherosclerotic lesion often depends not on the degree of lumen area reduction, but rather on qualitative angiographic factors, such as lesion ulceration and overlying thrombus [7–9]. To fully describe a lesion, these qualitative, morphologic attributes must be determined. Finally, these qualitative descriptors of vessel morphology are particularly important in predicting the outcome of percutaneous coronary interventions [10].

Visual Methods

The poor reproducibility of "eyeball" measures of percent diameter stenosis were first reported over two decades ago [11]. Recent publications continue to demonstrate the inherent biases of visual measures. For example, Beauman and Vogel compared visual analysis, derived from 11 angiographers, with computer-assisted QCA [12]. Seven phantom stenoses and 11 randomly chosen coronary lesions were analyzed. QCA was substantially more accurate. A phantom image with a 50% stenosis was visually read over a range from 30% to 95% stenosis with a standard deviation of 17%. More severe lesions, those over 50%, were systematically overestimated and those less than 50% were systematically underestimated. Fleming et al. analyzed visual readings of phantom stenoses by both novices and experienced angiographers [13]. No difference in precision and accuracy was noted between the novice and experienced readers; however, moderately severe lesions were overestimated by 30%. The visual readings corresponded more closely to true percent area stenosis than to diameter stenosis. Because of increased geometric complexity, the visual estimation of lumen size and percent stenosis following coronary interventional therapy is even less reliable [14]. Fleming and colleagues demonstrated that the preinterventional percent stenosis was systematically overestimated, while the postinterventional percent stenosis was underestimated [13].

Quantitative Methods

Calipers

Gensini and colleagues were the first to introduce quantitative angiography. In 1971 they reported their experience with an electronic caliper system which defined the reference and lesion diameters by manually driven cursors [15]. The advantages of the caliper system is its simple and low-cost implementation; however, compared to computerized systems, the caliper is suboptimal. Kalbfleisch and colleagues compared electronic calipers with a validated QCA system in 155 coronary lessions [16]. Although there was moderately good correlation between the two methods, the results from electronic calipers were less reproducible. For example, interobserver variability was much greater for the calipers than for quantitative angiography ($r = 0.63$ for calipers and $r =$

0.95 for QCA). In addition, calipers overestimated stenoses which were greater than 50 % and underestimated stenoses that were less severe, much like "eyeball" estimates. Although calipers are an improvement over simple visual estimates by a single observer and likely provide adequate precision when large changes in vessel geometry occur, such as in angioplasty, the caliper is not reproducible enough to allow measurement of small changes over time, such as might be expected in trials of atherosclerotic disease progression and regression [17].

Beyond the Caliper: Computerized Quantitative Angiography

Brown and colleagues at the University of Washington pioneered the first computerized QCA system [18, 19]. For Brown's method, orthogonal images from 35-mm cinefilm are projected at high (×5) magnification, and vessel edges are hand traced. The orthogonal hand-traced borders are corrected for pincushion distortion and combined to form a three-dimensional representation that assumes an elliptical lesion geometry. Quite accurate and precise, this method has been utilized in a large number of angiographic trials [20–22]. It suffers from being labor intensive and consequently slow, and also edge detection relies on the human eye.

Subsequent QCA systems incorporate automatic, computerized contour detection algorithms to locate vessel edges and do not rely on manually defining the vascular silhouette. Examples of such systems include the Cardiovascular Angiographic Analysis System (CAAS), developed by Reiber and associates at Erasmus University, and ART-REK (ADAC), developed by Lefree et al. at the University of Michigan, USA [23, 24]. Coronary analysis with these systems is divided into three major steps: (1) film digitalization (2) calibration, and (3) contour detection. Although these systems can be applied to direct digital images, more frequently a cinefilm image is employed that must first be converted to a digital image. For this, the cinefilm is projected into a high resolution camera attached to a cinevideo converter. Calibration of the image allows for absolute dimension analysis. Typically, the catheter is used as the scaling device. Following digitization and calibration, edge detection is performed. The operator selects a region of interest, consisting of an area that encloses the stenosis and proximal and distal reference zones. Videodensity data are then sampled along the vessel length and a centerline generated. From this initial centerline, perpendicular scanlines are produced. The videodensity profile along each scanline is computed and the first and second derivatives of this profile are calculated. The vessel edge is then defined as a point lying between the maximum first and second derivatives of the scanline videodensity profile. After the edges are smoothed, the diameters of the lesion and selected reference segments are generated, and subsequently percent diameter stenosis and percent area stenosis are calculated. An example of an output from the CAAS system is shown (Fig. 1). These systems are precise and accurate. The overall accuracy (average difference of computed results from true values) and precision (pooled standard deviation of the differences) of the CAAS system for percent diameter stenosis was found to be 2 % and 2.7 %, respectively, and for the absolute diameters 0.003 and 0.09 mm, respectively [25].

The above methods calculate lesion severity based on edge detection methodologies. Most QCA systems are also capable of performing videodensitometric analysis. Videodensitometry is based on the Beer-Lambert law, which states the

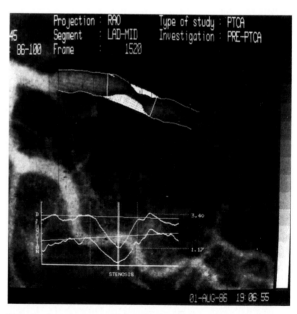

Fig. 1. A representative ouput from the CAAS systems applied to a left anterior descending coronary artery obstruction. The computer generated vessel and plaque outlines are shown. (From [25])

logarithmic attenuation of an X-ray beam through a vessel is proportional to the thickness of the contrast medium inside that vessel. Conveniently, the photographic grain density of exposed film is a logarithmic function of incident light intensity. Consequently, there should ideally be a linear relationship between vessel thickness and film density. Videodensitometry utilizes standard QCA algorithms to first determine vessel edges. Subsequently, brightness profiles are generated along scanlines perpendicular to the centerline, and the background brightness is subtracted, resulting in an intensity profile due solely to the vessel of interest. After this procedure is repeated for each scanline, a cross-sectional area function is generated by summing all scanlines. Percent area reduction is calculated by comparing the area function from the reference segment with the minimal stenosis area function. By assuming circular geometry, the area function can be converted to absolute area, and minimal lesion diameter can be generated.

Theoretically, videodensitometry is an attractive method, because it is independent of vessel geometry. Unfortunately, there are many practical problems with videodensitometry. Results are often unreliable because developed film is in the nonlinear range of exposure. Although the Beer-Lambert law applies only to monochromatic X-rays, X-ray generators for cardiac catheterization produce polychromatic radiation. X-ray scatter interferes with the analysis as well. Doriot et al. have shown in phantom models that videodensitometry measurements were dependent on lesion shape, vessel size, and orientation [26]. When Sanz and coworkers compared the densitometric area of lesion pre- and post-angioplasty in orthogonal views, they found a poor correlation both for the pre- and post-angioplasty images [27]. As a consequence of these limitations, there is no validated, practical system currently available.

Optimizing QCA Results

Obtaining reliable quantitative angiographic results requires meticulous radiographic technique. Compared to visual analysis, QCA requires *greater* attention to angiographic methods. A large number of variables can affect QCA quality. For example, vessel overlap and lesion foreshortening may produce significant errors. It is essential that the coronary artery be maximally opacified. Although some authors have suggested that ECG-triggered power injectors be utilized, hand injections, accompanied by reflux of contrast into the aortic root, are generally adequate. The end-diastolic frames should be selected to minimize artifact due to vessel motion. Digitally averaging multiple frames of a stenosis, as suggested by some authors, is unnecessary [28]. Reproducibility of QCA over time is enhanced by controlling vasomotor tone. Typically, intracoronary nitroglycerin is administered prior to angiographic investigation. There are a number of other radiographic parameters that may impair reproducibility and accuracy. For example, through the imaging chain, veiling glare, pincushion distortion, and spherical aberration can distort the radiographic image. Because the focal spot of the X-ray tube is finite rather than a point, edges are redundant leading to penumbra. Random statistical variation of low levels of transmitted γ radiation provoke focal anomalies, so-called quantum mottling. If the exposure is not in the linear range of the cinefilm, then the image be "burned away" or "whited out."

Along with radiographic parameters, the underlying plaque geometry determines the accuracy of quantitative methods. The majority of atherosclerotic lesions are non-cylindrical. Many QCA systems attempt to correct for this geometry by assuming an elliptical shape, derived from orthogonal views. Unfortunately, this simplification is often inadequate. For example, acceptable orthogonal views are obtainable in only 50 % – 60 % of angiograms [4]. Spears utilized mathematical modeling to demonstrate the potential errors associated with estimating cross-sectional area based on arbitrary orthogonal views [29]. In his study, the maximal error for two arbitrary orthogonal views was small only for mild degrees of ellipticity (major/minor axis <2); however, this error increased significantly as the views were less than orthogonal and as ellipticity increased. Thus, on a theoretic basis, arbitrary orthogonal views do not prevent inaccurate measurements of truly elliptical lesions, and furthermore, area measurements of lesions that deviate from an eliptical geometry are even more inaccurate. Lespereance examined the utility of orthogonal views immediately after and 6 months after angioplasty [30]. He found a high correlation between lumen diameters derived from the average of two orthogonal views and the worst view. This study and

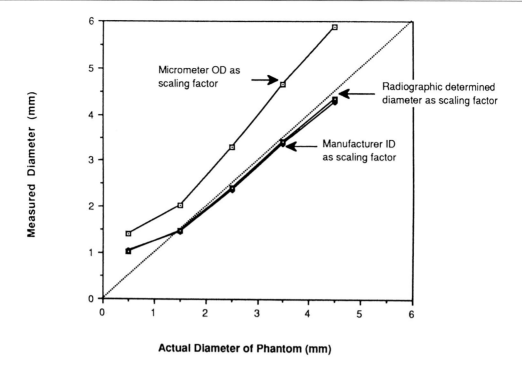

Fig. 2. Catheter calibration can significantly affect absolute lesion and reference diameters. The effect of assumed catheter size on measured phantom diameter is shown. Using the micrometer outer diameter *(OD)* as the scaling for this 8F catheter, significantly increases the QCA-measured phantom dimater. The manufacture internal diameter *(ID)* of the radiographic determined diameter, however, led to close approximations of the true phantom size *(small dotted line)*. (From [31])

others suggest that for routine clinical assessment, QCA measurements in the one worst view are adequate.

Even if excellent angiographic and radiographic techniques are employed, QCA can still fail if accurate calibration is not available. Typically, the coronary catheter is employed as the scaling device for calibration. It is essential that during coronary angiography, the angiographic catheter be included in the angiographic shot. Fortin and coworkers examined the effects of scaling parameters on QCA accuracy [31]. X-ray images of a variety of contrast and air-filled catheters were acquired atop a calibration grid, and vessel phantoms were imaged simultaneously. QCA was used to determine the edges of both the catheters and phantom. Calibrations were calculated using various measures, which included the manufacturer's specified value for the inside diameter (ID), the catheter French size, a micrometer measurement

of the outer diameter (OD), and the radiographic determined diameter (based on the grid calibration). Figure 2 demonstrates the effects of the various calibration factors on estimates of phantom size. For this 8F catheter (Baxter), it is evident that the best fit is obtained from a calibration using either the manufacturer's internal diameter or the calibration grid. Employing the outer diameter as the calibration factor significantly overestimates phantom size. It appears that the X-ray intensity profile used to determine the catheter edges differs in shape from one catheter to another, depending on the amount of radioopaque material in the walls of the catheter. Consequently, calibrations obtained from two different 8F guiding catheters can vary by as much as 25%. As a result, representative catheter dimensions for each catheter should be employed in calibrating quantitative coronary measures.

Qualitative Descriptors of Lesion Severity

The methods outlined above focus on determining the magnitude of lumen narrowing. Even if vessel and obstructive dimensions were determined quantitatively with complete accuracy and reproducibility, the description would be incomplete. Recent observations have shown that quantitative descriptors may predict the presence of stable, flow-limiting angina but are less useful in predicting the presence of unstable syndromes. It has become clear that qualitative morphologic descriptors, which describe the underlying complexity of the coronary stenosis, better predict unstable outcomes.

Utilizing postmortem arteriography, Levin and Fallon outlined the angiographic features of complex coronary lesions [32]. Composed of fatty or fibrous plaques with intact internal surfaces, uncomplicated lesions histologically had no superimposed thrombus. Angiography of these lesions, classified as type I stenoses, revealed smooth borders with an hourglass configuration, and no intraluminal lucencies. In contrast, type II complicated lesions demonstrated histologic evidence of plaque rupture, plaque hemorrhage, and superimposed thrombus. The corresponding angiograms demonstrated irregular borders and intraluminal lucencies. This study suggested that angiography did correlate with underlying lesion complexity.

Ambrose and coworkers subsequently demonstrated that these qualitative angiographic features of lesion complexity predicted clinical outcome [33]. They studied 47 patients with stable angina and 63 patients with unstable syndromes. Angiographic morphology was classified as concentric, smooth eccentric (type I), ulcerative eccentric (type II), or as multiple irregularities. Those with stable syndromes had predominantly concentric or type I morphologies, while those with unstable syndromes had type II ulcerative lesions or multiple irregularities. Angiographic evidence of thrombus is the most predictive feature of instability [34]. Angioscopy has demonstrated the nearly universal presence of thrombus in patients with unstable coronary syndromes [35].

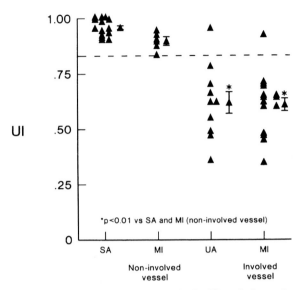

Fig. 4. The ulceration index *(UI)* is significantly lower in stable angina *(SA)* and the noninfarct coronary artery than in unstable angina *(UA)* or the infarct related artery. (From [8])

In patients with acute myocardial infarction, Little and colleagues demonstrated no relationship between quantitative measures of lesion severity, such as percent stenosis, and time to myocardial infarction; however, lesion irregularity was noted in all [36]. Freeman et al. found similar results in their study of 42 patients in whom coronary angiography was performed before and after myocardial infarction [37]. They found that in the great majority of their patients, the artery that subsequently occluded had less than a 50% stenosis. What did predict infarction was coronary thrombus (77%), complex morphology (55%), and multivessel disease (58%). Ellis et al. examined 259 patients from the CASS (Coronary Artery Surgery Study) registry to determine predictors of subsequent acute anterior wall infarction during the 3 years following catheterization [38]. Multivariate analysis found that lesion roughness and left anterior descending >50% stenosis predicted future infarction. Univariate analysis revealed that the probability of a myocardial infarction was 4.5 times greater if lesion roughness was present.

Quantifying these qualitative morphologic attributes has been somewhat ellusive. Wilson and coworkers described an ulceration index [8]. The ulceration index equals the diameter of the least severe stenosis within the lesion divided by the maximum intralesional diameter (Fig. 3). The less ulcerated the lesion, the closer the index to one.

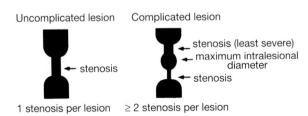

Ulceration Index

diameter of least severe stenosis within lesion
──
maximum intralesional diameter

Fig. 3. This diagram defines ulceration index. See text for discussion. (From [8])

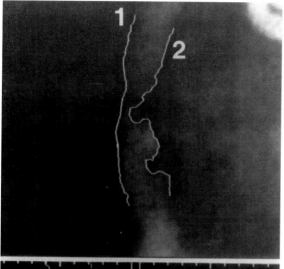

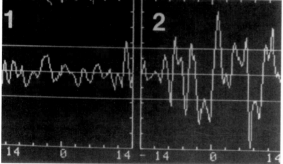

Fig. 5. The *top* of figure is the outline of a complex coronary lesion; the edges determined by an automatic edge detection QCA algorithm. *Below* is the curvature signature of edge *1* and edge *2*. Edge *2*, more irregular visually, has a corresponding curvature signature that is significantly more complex. This complex signature pattern correlates with an unstable clinical course. (From [39])

Utilizing this semiquantitative approach, these investigators demonstrated that low ulceration indices were associated with unstable syndromes (Fig. 4). In a more sophisticated approach, Kalbfleisch et al. used vector analysis to derive a curvature signature for both the angiographic catheter (which is smooth) and the coronary artery [39]. The curvature signature of vessel edges is normalized by dividing by the standard deviation of the catheter curvature signature. Complex features are represented by large curvature peaks, which quantify the degree of irregularity present (Fig. 5). This method was studied in 59 patients with unstable angina and 17 with stable angina pectoris. Neither luminal narrowing nor prior indices of lesion complexity, such as the ulceration index, correlated with unstable symptoms. In contrast, four of five indices derived from the curvature signature were observed in the unstable group but not in the stable group. Further efforts to quantify lesion morphology based on this method seem warranted.

Qualitative Characteristics Relevant to Coronary Interventional Therapy

As noted above, morphology is an essential factor in predicting lesion behavior. In addition, qualitative morphologic attributes are critical predictors of acute and long-term outcome following coronary interventional therapy. Qualitative characteristics determine the suitability for angioplasty and ultimate success.

Table 1. The American College of Cardiology/American Heart Association Joint Task Force classification of type A, B, and C lesions

Type A (high success, >85 %; low risk)

Discrete (<10 mm)	Little or no calcification
Concentric	Less than totally occlusive
Readily accessible	Not ostial in location
Smooth contour	No major branch involvement
Absence of thrombus	Nonangulated segment (<45°)

Type B (moderate success, 60 % – 85 %; moderate risk)

Tubular (10–20 mm in length)	Moderate to heavy calcification
Eccentric	Total occlusions <3 month old
Moderate tortuosity proximally	Ostial location
Irregular contour	Bifurcation lesions, requiring double guidewires
Some thrombus present	Moderately angulated segments (>45° but <90°)

Type C (low success, <60 %; high risk)

Diffuse (>2 cm in length)	Inability to protect major side branches
Excessive tortuosity proximally	Degenerated vein grafts with friable lesions
Total occlusions >3 months old	Extremely angulated segments, >90°

The American College of Cardiology/American Heart Association (ACC/AHA) Joint Task Force, in 1988, defined three categories of coronary lesions based on their qualitative/morphologic characteristics [40] (Table 1). Type A lesions have a high success rate (>85%) and low risk of acute complication. Type B lesions have a lower success rate (60% – 85%) and moderate rate of acute vessel closure. Type C lesions have the highest risk and lowest success rate. The various descriptors are defined in Table 2. Although when these guidelines were published they were based simply on the author's impressions and clinical experience, subsequent studies have demonstrated the predictive value of this stratification scheme.

Ellis et al. studies 350 patients undergoing coronary angioplasty [41]. Qualitative morphologic analysis was performed on all lesions based on modified ACC/AHA guidelines. Group A and C lesions were defined as they are in Table 1, but type B lesions were subclassified into B1 and B2 lesions. B1 lesions had only one B characteristic, while B2 lesions had two or more B characteristics. Procedural success and complication rates were 92% and 2%, respectively for type A lesions, and 84% and 4% for lesions with B1 morphology, 76% and 10%, respectively, for B2 lesions and 61% and 21% for C lesions. Substantially more predictive information was gained by dividing the B lesions into B1 and B2 subsets. Individual descriptors that were particularly predictive of poor outcomes included chronic total occlusion, high-grade stenosis (80% – 99% diameter stenosis), stenosis bend of more that 60°, and excessive tortuosity. Ellis and coworkers found similar results when this modified ACC/AHA classification was applied to directional coronary atherectomy [42]. Multivariate analysis suggested that for directional atherectomy, stenosis angulation, proximal tortuosity, and calcification were particularly predictive of an unsuccessful result or an acute complication.

Despite the predictive value of these descriptors, the reproducibility is at best fair. Ellis and colleagues found that when independent observers examined 57 angiograms, they agreed on the ACC/AHA class in only 30 (58%) and disagreed by two classification units in four (7%) [42]. Kleiman et al. found interobserver agreement on ACC/AHA grade in only 61% of the lesions analyzed. Variability was particularly high when lesion length, eccentricity, angulation, and tortuosity were examined [43].

Table 2. American College of Cardiology/American Heart Association Joint Task Force qualitative descriptors and their definitions

Stenosis angle	Formed by a centerline through the lumen proximal to the stenosis and a second centerline in the straight portion of the artery distal to the stenosis
Thrombus	Present if an intraluminal filling defect largely separated from the adjacent wall is clearly definable
Vessel tortuosity	Moderate tortuosity of the proximal segment is present when the stenosis is distal to two bends and is defined as excessively tortuous when it is distal to three or more bends
Bifurcation stenosis	Present if a medium or large branch vessel originates within the stenosis and if the side branch is completely surrounded by stenotic portions of the lesions to be dilated
Chronic occlusion	Defined by TIMI-0 flow and is chronic if judged to be present for more than 3 months, duration
Calcification	Moderate to heavy calcification is present if readily apparent densities are seen within the vessel wall at the lesion site
Eccentric stenosis	Present when the lumen is within the outer one-quarter diameter of the apparent normal lumen
Irregular contour	Defined by the presence of a rough or "sawtooth" appearance of the vascular margin
Lesion length	Measured by calipers or quantitative angiography: lesion length is defined as the distance from the proximal to distal shoulder of the lesion in the least foreshortened view; discrete = <10 mm; diffuse = >20 mm
TIMI flow	
TIMI-0	*No perfusion:* no antegrade flow beyond occlusion
TIMI-1	*Partial opacification:* contrast passes beyond occlusion but fails to opacify distal bed
TIMI-2	*Partial perfusion:* antegrade, complete filling of artery after three or more cardiac cycles
TIMI-3	*Complete perfusion:* antegrade, complete filling within three cardiac cycles

TIMI, thrombolytics in myocardial infarction

Summary

Selective coronary angiography continues to play an essential role in the mangagement of ischemic heart disease. Although many improvements have been made in the images produced, the method for analyzing lesion severity remains unchanged in the majority of clinical catheterization laboratories. Most angiographers continue to rely on "eyeball" estimates of percent diameter stenosis. These visual estimates are inaccurate and imprecise. Computerized systems that quantify reference and lesion diameters have substantially improved the reproducibility and accuracy of coronary angiographic interpretation. Although these computerized systems enhance angiographic analysis, they are not without a price. Quantitative coronary angiography requires rigorous attention to angiographic technique, more so than with visual "eyeball" analysis. Despite improvements in measuring percent stenosis and minimal lesion diameter, these quantitative measures are inadequate descriptors of lesion prognosis. Qualitative, morphologic attributes are as, or more, important in defining lesion instability. These qualitative descriptors have been extended to not only define the risk of a subsequent unstable syndromes but have also been successfully employed in predicting the success of percutaneous coronary interventional therapy.

References

1. Zir LM, Miller SW, Dismore RE, Gilbert JP, Harthorne JW (1976) Interobserver variability in coronary angiography. Circulation 53: 627–632
2. Galbraith JE, Murphy ML, de Soyza N (1978) Coronary angiography interpretation: interobserver variability. JAMA 240: 2053–2056
3. Fisher LD, Judins MP, Lesperance J, Cameron A, Swaye P, Ryan T, Maynard C, Bourassa M, Kennedy JW, Gosselin A, Kemp H, Faxon D, Wexler L, Davis KB (1982) Reproducibility of coronary arteriographic reading in the coronary artery surgery study (CASS). Cather Cardiovasc Diagn 8: 565–575
4. Hermiller JB, Cusma JT, Spero LA, Fortin DF, Harding MB, Bashore TM (1992) Quantitative coronary angiographic analysis: review of methods, utility, and limitations. Cathet Cardiovasc Diagn 25: 11–131
5. Brown BG, Bolston EL, Dodge HT (1986) Quantitative computer techniques for analyzing coronary arteriograms. Prog Cardiovasc Dis 18: 403–418
6. Mancini JGB (1988) Quantitative coronary arteriography: development of methods, limitations and clinical applications. Am J Cardiac Imag 2: 98–109
7. Ambrose JA, Tannenbaum MA, Alexopoulos D, Hjemdahl-Monsen CE, Leavy J, Weiss M, Borrico S, Gorlin R, Fuster V (1988) Angiographic progression of coronary artery disease and the development of myocardial infarction. J Am Coll Cardiol 12: 56–62
8. Wilson RF, Holida MD, White CW (1986) Quantitative angiographic morphology of coronary stenoses leading to myocardial infarction or unstable angina. Circulation 73: 286–293
9. Ambrose JA, Hjemdahl-Monsen CE, Borico S, Gorlin R, Fuster V (1988) Angiographic demonstration of a common link between unstable angina pectoris and non-Q wave acute myocardial infarction. Am J Cardiol 61: 244–247
10. Black AJR, Namay DL, Niederman AL, Lembo NJ, Roubin GS, Douglas JS, King SP (1989) Tear or dissection after coronary angioplasty: morphologic correlates of an ischemic complication. Circulation 79: 1035–1042
11. Detre KM, Wright E, Murphy ML, Takaro T (1975) Observer agreement in evaluating coronary angiograms. Circulation 52: 979–986
12. Beauman GJ, Vogel RA (1990) Accuracy of individual and panel visual interpretations of coronary arteriograms: implications for clinical decisions. J Am Coll Cardiol 16: 108–113
13. Fleming RM, Kirkeeide RL, Smalling RW et al. (1991) Patterns in visual interpretation of coronary arteriograms as detected by quantitative coronary arteriography. J Am Coll Cardiol 18: 945
14. Rensing BJ, Hermanns WRM, Deckers JW et al. (1992) Lumen narrowing after percutaneous transluminal coronary balloon angioplasty follows a near gaussian distribution: a quantitative angiographic study in 1445 successfully dilated lesions. J Am Coll Cardiol 19: 939
15. Gensini GG, Kelly AE, DaCosta BCB, Huntington PP (1971) Quantitative angiography: the measurement of coronary vasomobility in the intact animal and man. Chest 60: 522–530
16. Kalbfleisch SJ, McGillem MJ, Pinto IMF, Kavanaugh KM, DeBoe SF, Mancini GBJ (1990) Comparison of automated quantitative coronary angiography with caliper measurements of percent diameter stenosis. Am J Cardiol 65: 1181–1184
17. Brown G, Albers JJ, Fisher LD, Schaefer SM, Lin J-T, Kaplan C, Zhao X-Q, Bisson BD, Fitzpatrick VF, Dodge HT (1990) Regression of coronary artery disease as a result of intensive lipid-lowering therapy in men with high levels of Apolipoprotein B. N Engl J Med 323: 1289–1298
18. Brown BG, Bolson E, Frimer M, Dodge HT (1977) Quantitative coronary arteriography: estimation of dimensions, hemodynamic resistance, and atheroma mass of coronary artery lesions using the arteriogram and digital computation. Circulation 53: 329–337
19. Brown BG, Bolson EL, Dodge HT (1982) Arteriographic assessment of coronary arteriosclerosis: review of current methods, their limitations, and clinical applications. Arteriosclerosis 2: 1–15
20. Badger RS, Brown BG, Kennedy JW, Mathey C, Gallery CA, Bolson EL, Dodge HT (1987) Useful-

ness of recanalization of 0.6 millimeter or more with intracoronary streptokinase during acute myocardial infarction in predicting normal perfusion status, continued arterial patency and survival at one year. Am J Cardiol 59: 519–522

21. Brown BG, Bolson EL, Peterson RB (1981) The mechanisms of nitroglycerin action: stenosis vasodilation as a major component of the drug response. Circulation 64: 1089–1097

22. Brown BG, Lee AB, Bolson EL (1984) Reflex constriction of significant coronary stenosis as a mechanism contributing to ischemic left ventricular dysfunction during isometric exercises. Circulation 70: 18–24

23. Reiber JHC, Serruys PW, Kooijman CJ, Slager CJ, Schuurbiers JHC, den Boer A (1986) Approaches towards standardization in acquisition and quantitation of arterial dimensions from cineangiograms. In: Reiber JHL, Serruys PW (eds) State of the art in quantitative coronary arteriography. Nijhoff, Boston, pp 145–172

24. Lefree MT, Simon SB, Mancini GBJ, Vogel RA (1986) Digital radiographic assessment of coronary arterial diameter and videodensitometric cross-sectional area. Proc SPIE 626: 334–341

25. Reiber JHC (1988) Morphologic and densitometric analysis of coronary arteries. In: Heintzen PH, Bursch JH (eds) Progress in digital angiocardiography. Kluwer, London, pp 137–158

26. Doriot PA, Pochon Y, Welz R, Rutishouser W (1988) Non-linearity by densitometric measurements of coronary arteries. In: Heintzen PH, Bursch JH (eds) Progress in digital angiocardiography. Kluwer, London, pp 173–180

27. Sanz ML, Mancini GBJ, LeFree MT, Mickelson JK, Starling MR, Vogel RA, Topol EJ (1987) Variability of quantitative digital subtraction coronary angiography before and after percutaneous transluminal coronary angioplasty. Am J Cardiol 60: 55–60

28. Reiber JHC, Van Eldik-Helleman P, Visser-Akkerman N, Kooijman CJ, Serruys PW (1988) Variabilities in measurement of coronary arterial dimensions resulting from variations in cineframe selections. Cathet Cardiovasc Diagn 14: 221–228

29. Spears JR, Sandor T, Baim DS, Paulin S (1983) The minimum error in estimating coronary luminal cross-sectional area from cineangiographic diameter measurements. Cathet Cardiovasc Diagn 9: 119–128

30. Lesperance J, Hudson G, White CW, Laurier J, Walters D (1989) Comparison by quantitative angiographic assessment of coronary stenosis of one view showing the severest narrowing to two orthogonal views. Am J Cardiol 64: 462–465

31. Fortin DF, Spero LA, Cusma JT, Santoro L, Burgess R, Bashore TM (1991) Pitfalls in the determination of absolute dimensions using angiographic catheters as calibration devices in quantitative angiography. Am J Cardiol 68: 1176–1182

32. Levin DC, Fallon JT (1982) Significance of angiographic morphology of localized coronary stenoses: histopathologic correlations. Circulation 66: 316–320

33. Ambrose JA, Winters SL, Stern A, Eng A, Teichholz LE, Gorlin R, Fuster V (1985) Angiographic morphology and the pathogenesis of unstable angina pectoris. J Am Coll Cardiol 5: 609–616

34. Cowley MJ, DiSciascio G, Rehr RB, Vetrovec GW (1989) Angiographic observations and clinical relevance of coronary thrombus in unstable angina pectoris. Am J Cardiol 63: 108E–113E

35. Sherman CT, Litvack F, Grundfest W, Lee M, Hickey A, Chauz A, Kass R, Blanche C, Matloff J, Morgenstern L, Ganz W, Swan HJC, Forrester J (1986) Coronary angioscopy in patients with unstable angina. N Engl J Med 315: 913–919

36. Little WC, Constantinescu M, Applegate RJ, Kutcher MA, Burrow MT, Kahl FR, Santamore WP (1988) Can coronary angiography predict the site of subsequent myocardial infarction in patients with mild-to-moderate coronary artery disease? Circulation 78: 1157–1166

37. Freeman MR, Williams AE, Chisholm RJ, Armstrong PW (1989) Intracoronary thrombus and complex morphology in unstable angina. Relation to timing of angiography and in-hospital cardiac events. Circulation 80: 17–23

38. Ellis S, Alderman E, Cain K, Fisher L, Sanders W, Bourassa M and the CASS Investigators (1988) Prediction of risk of anterior myocardial infarction by lesion severity and measurement method of stenoses in the left anterior descending coronary distribution: a CASS Registry study. J Am Coll Cardiol 11: 908–916

39. Kalbfleisch SJ, McGillem MJ, Simon SB, DeBoe SF, Pinto IMF, Mancini GBJ (1990) Automated quantitation of indexes of coronary lesion complexity: comparison between patients with stable and unstable angina. Circulation 82: 439–447

40. ACC/AHA Task Force (1988) Guidelines for percutaneous transluminal coronary angioplasty. A report of the American College of Cardiology/American Heart Association Task Force on Assessment of Diagnostic and Therapeutic Cardiovascular Procedures (Subcommittee on Percutaneous Transluminal Coronary Angioplasty). J Am Coll Cardiol 529

41. Ellis SG, Cowley MJ, DiSciascia G, et al. (1991) Determinants of 2-year outcome after coronary angioplasty in patients with multivessel disease on the basis of comprehensive preprocedural evaluation. Circulation 84: 1905

42. Ellis SG, DeCessare NB, Pinkerton CA, et al. (1991) Relation of stenosis morphology and clinical presentation to the procedural results of directional coronary atherectomy. Circulation 85: 644

43. Kleiman NS, Rodriguez AR, Raizner AE (1992) Interobserver variability in grading coronary arterial narrowings using the American College of Cardiology/American Heart Association grading criteria. Am J Cardiol 69: 413

Quantitative Coronary Angiography in Interventional Cardiology

V.A.W.M. Umans, B. H. Strauss. D. Keane, J. Haase, P. de Jaegere, and P. W. Serruys

Introduction

Quantitative coronary angiography (QCA) has had a major impact in the field of interventional cardiology. Due to its superior accuracy objectivity and improved interobserver and intraobserver variability it has supplanted visual and hand-held caliper assessments of coronary arteriograms [1–3]. QCA is now the gold standard for assessing the coronary tree in the context of scientific research. It has not yet gained widespread appeal for routine clinical use because of expense and time constraints. To date there are two different techniques for measuring quantitative angiographic stenosis. One is based on the detection of luminal borders from orthogonal images to create a three-dimensional approximation of the diseased vessel, and the other uses videodensitometry of the stenosis to extract three-dimensional information from a single angiographic view. Although the latter approach has particular advantages, we favor the edge detection method because it provides absolute measurements that are relatively insensitive to the image quality.

From a clinical viewpoint the objectives of quantitative angiography are to obtain information that (a) contributes to the understanding of clinical syndromes, (b) facilitates decision making, (c) helps to forecast future events (e.g., subacute occlusion, restenosis), and (d) guides invasive therapy. It has been particularly useful in interventional cardiology as the only reliable means of assessing the short- and long-term effects of coronary interventions. In particular, the phenomenon of restenosis has been described primarily and researched most extensively on the basis of sequential QCA studies. At the Thoraxcenter in Rotterdam we have advocated QCA since the first publication of its use by our group in 1978 [4], particularly since our initial experience with QCA in the assessment of coronary interventions, as reported in 1982 [5]. The system developed at the Thoraxcenter by Reiber and colleagues, the cardiovascular angiographic analysis system (CAAS), has been extensively and rigorously validated [6–8]. In our database we have now collected information from 4662 patients who have undergone several different forms of nonoperative coronary revascularization [1]. We have had to adapt the principles of QCA, which were initially designed for diagnostic studies to assess the extent of coronary artery disease, to more complicated and complex situations related to either the presence of a device or the effect of an intervention on the angiographic appearance of a damaged vessel. The introduction of several newer devices in the past 6 years has presented a number of unique unforeseen problems in image analysis and subsequent interpretation of important quantitative data. The emergence of digital subtraction angiography has allowed the on-line performance of QCA measurements in the catheterization laboratory, so that a technique previously confined to research applications has been transformed into a powerful analytical tool, directly applicable to clinical decision making [9–12]. The immediate availability of QCA measurements during interventional procedures provides a unique opportunity for more accurate selection of appropriate interventional devices (e.g., balloon ar atherotome dimension) and for continuous monitoring and immediate evaluation of the result obtained.

This chapter highlights the basic features of and information provided by these two automatic computer-assisted angiographic analysis systems and discusses some of the benefits and limitations of QCA in the analysis of the angiographic short- and long-term sequelae of the various devices for interventional cardiology. Only close scrutiny of the analytical results combined with ongoing communication between the angiographer, the analyst, and the programmer ensures that meaningful and useful data to emerge from the use of QCA.

What Information Can Be Obtained from the Use of Automatic Computer-Assisted Angiographic Quantitative Analysis Systems?

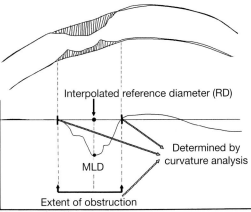

Fig. 1. Schematic representation of the diameter function of a coronary artery stenosis. Interpolated reference diameter, minimal luminal diameter (*MLD*), and lesion lenght or extent of the stenosis are determined by the curvature analysis

The primary aim of QCA is to provide precise and accurate measurements of coronary anatomy. The CASS system can provide this information by two different methods: (a) detection of luminal borders (so-called edge detection), preferably in two orthogonal projections (to provide a three-dimensional approximation of the diseased segment) which can then be converted into absolute values after calibration with an object of known diameter, such as the shaft of the guiding catheter; and (b) videodensitometry, an approach which assesses the relative area stenosis by comparing the density of contrast in the diseases and "normal" segments. The method by which the relative area stenosis is converted to absolute area stenosis measurements is explained below. The advantage of the information acquired by the densitometric method is that meaningful data can be obtained in a single projection even if the cross-sectional shape is highly asymmetrical or eccentric. In contrast, area measurements derived from edge detection data (and specifically from minimal luminal diameter values) by definition assume a circular cross-sectional lumen in the diseased arterial segment, which is at odds with the observations of several pathology studies [13, 14]. The limitations of both techniques are discussed below, as are differences in the results of the two methods following coronary interventions.

Edge Detection

In our laboratory the quantitative analysis of the stenotic coronary segments uses the computer-assisted (CAAS), described in detail elsewhere [2–7]. To analyze a coronary arterial segment a 35-mm cine frame is selected. Electronically a region of interest (512×512 pixels) encompassing the arterial segment to be analyzed, is digitized with a high-fidelity videocamera. Contours of the arterial segments are detected automatically on the basis of the weighted sum of the first and second derivative funcitons applied to the digitized brightness profile. From these contours the vessel diameter functions are determined by computing the shortest distance between the left and right contour positions (Fig. 1). A computer-derived es-timate of the original arterial dimension at the site of the obstruction is used to define the interpolated reference diameter. This technique is based on a computer-derived measurement of the original diamter values over the analyzed region (assuming absence of disease) according to the diameter function. Conversion of the diameter measurements of the vessel to absolute values is achieved by using the angiography catheter as a scaling devise, after correction for pin-cushion distortion. The minimal cross-sectional area of the narrowed segment and the interpolated percentage area stenosis are then derived by assuming a circular vessel cross-section and comparing the observed stenosis dimensions to the reference values.

The plaque area is a measure of the atherosclerotic plaque in this angiographic view, expressed in square milimeters. This area is calculated as the sum of pixels between the computer-estimated predisease reference contours and the actually detected luminal contours of the obstructive lesion. Since measurement of plaque area depends strongly on the length of the stenosis (which is subject to considerable variation) and the determination of the reference contours of the artery in the presumed prediseased state, the usefulness of this parameter is debatable.

The symmetry value is a measure of the eccentricity of a particular lesion. A symmetry measure of 1 denotes a concentric obstruction; the number decreases (down to 0) with increasing asymmetry or eccentricity of the obstruction. Unfortunately this parameter has not yet been validated against pathology, and thus the pathologist and angiographer may not be referring to the same feature.

The curvature value is measured to assess the bend of the coronary segment analyzed. The view in which the vessel appears to be the least foreshortened (i.e., the segment lenght is longest) is chosen for the curvature analysis. The inflow and outflow angles are derived from the slope of the diameter function at the descending and ascending limb of the diameter function curve at the defined site of the obstruction.

The CAAS and the Philips digital cardiac imaging system (DCI) have also attempted to convert information on angiographic parameters into functional data based on well-known fluid-dynamic equations [7].

The angiographic analysis is performed whenever possible using the average of multiple matched views with orthogonal projections.

Videodensitometry

Determining the changes in cross-sectional area of a coronary segment from the density profile within the artery requires calibration of the brightness levels in terms of the amount of X-ray absorption (Lambert Beer's law). The videodensitometric method used with our system corrects for spatially variant responses in the imaging chain and for daily variations in the cine film processing. Details of this technique have been described elsewhere [2–7]. Contours of the artery are detected by automated contour detection with the CASS system, as previously described. The diameter data described above are derived from the measured diameters along the analyzed segment. A profile of brightness is measured on each scan line perpendicular to the center line of the vessel. This profile is transformed into an absorption profile by means of a simple logarithmic transfer function. The background contribution is estimated by computing the linear regression line through the background points directly left and right of the detected contours. Subtraction of this background portion from the absorbed profile within the arterial contours yields the net cross-sectional absorption profile. Integration of this function gives a measure for the cross-sectional area at the particular scanline. The cross-sectional area function is obtained by repeating this pro-

cedure for all scan lines. A reference densitometric area is obtained following the same principles as described above for the diameter functions. Calibration of the densitometric area values is accomplished by comparing the reference area calculated from the diameter measurements (assuming a circular cross-section) with the corresponding densitometric area value.

This method makes no assumption about the cross-sectional shape of the lesion in the most severely diseased segment of the vessel. Although densitometry is extremely attrative on a theoretical basis, numerous technical problems have limited its use. The major limitations are the strict requirement of an angiographic projection perpendicular to the long axis of the vessel (to prevent oblique cuts which would lead to overestimation of the luminal area) and the absence of overlapping or closely parallel side branches of other vessels in the segment to be analyzed (which would interfere with the density of the lesion due to background subtraction). Densitometry is also more sensitive than edge detection to densitometric nonlinearities (X-ray scatter, veiling glare, and beam hardening) and to inhomogenous contrast filling of vessels.

Despite these limitations the results of a recent in vivo validation study suggest that videodensitometry can reliably measure vascular dimensions, provided (a) sufficient care is taken to obtain a perpendicular incidence of the X-ray beam onto the examined coronary segment, and (b) a homogeneous contrast filling of the vessel is obtained. The method was thoroughly validated in a porcine model in which precisions-drilled circular coronary stenosis phantoms (with diameters of 0.5–1.9 mm) and angiograms were analyzed using the edge detection and the densitometric technique of the CAAS system [5–8]. In this experimental application simulating diagnostic coronary angiography, both analysis techniques showed a high accuracy and precision in the automatic measurement of the stenosis phantoms. In particular, the mean difference between minimal cross-sectional area, measured with videodensitometry, and true stenosis cross-sectional area was $0.12 \pm 0.31\,\text{mm}^2$. A limitation of videodensitometry, however, was its inability to distinguish accurately the very low density of some of the stenosis phantoms with the smallest diameter stenosis from the background density.

Comparison of Various Digital and Cine Frame QCA Measurement Systems

Recent developments in digital cardiac imaging systems have been directed towards on-line stenosis measurements during the procedure from video digitized images. In this approach the system guides the operator in selecting the appropriate interventional technique (balloon, stent, atherectomy) in selecting the appropriate size of the device, and in assessing the effect of the intervention it helps to determine whether a better result may be achieved. Substantial clinical experience has been accumulated a the Thorxcenter over the past 5 years with the Philips DCI automated coronary analysis system [10, 11]. A recent in vivo study of stenosis phantoms placed in porcine coronary arteries has confirmed that the accuracy, and precision, of the DCI on-line measurements are closely comparable to those obtained off-line using the CAAS system, with a mean difference between true phantom stenosis diameter and DCI measurements of minimal luminal density of 0.08 ± 0.15 mm, for stenosis diameters of 0.5–1.9 mm [12]. We therefore believe that the data presented here, derived mainly from the analysis of cine film images, can now be used immediately to guide the operator during diagnostic and interventional procedures.

Over the past few years there has been substantial progress in the field of quantitative angiography. In particular, several new measurement system have been developed and will be introduced into clinical practice in the near future. At the Thoraxcenter we have validated three systems with the cine film approach and one digital angiography system [12].

Technical Considerations and Limitations of QCA in Clinical Practice

First, the use of the catheter as a scaling device has certain limitations, such as those due to the out-of-plane position of the catheter with respect to the measured coronary segment, which require complex corrections. We believe, however, that many possible sources of inaccuracy can be easily minimized with use of a strict protocol of calibration, including the measurement with a micrometer of the true size of the catheter, the avoidance of catheters with excessive tapering or poor radiopacity, and the acquisition before coronary angiography of the catheter image (saline or blood filled) in the same projection and field of view [15], positioning the catheter in the center of the radiographic image and a correction for pincushion distortion.

A second important technical point for all serial studies is the requirement of coronary vasodilation using agents of comparable efficacy for every study. In a recent study [16] the mean diameter of a normal segment of a nondilated vessel before and after percutaneous transluminal cororary angioplasty (PTCA) and at follow-up was analyzed in 202 patients. Of these, 34 who received intracoronary nitrate pre-PTCA but not prior to post-PTCA angiography exhibited a decrease in diameter of 0.11 mm versus the small increase of 0.02 mm in the group who did receive post-PTCA nitrate. Lack of control of vasodilator therapy at follow-up angiography may also partially explain an earlier observation by our group of a significant deterioration in the mean reference diameter 4 months after angioplasty, with several subsequent studies employing coronary vasodilators have produced contradictory information [17, 18]. However, we still believe that in certain patients the reference segment is involved in the restenotic process, invalidating the use of percentage diameter stenosis as an accurate measurement of lesion severity at follow-up.

Third, the computer-generated interpolated measurements may be unreliable for ostial lesions or lesions located at side branches. Manual contour correction may also be necessary when the angiogram is of poor technical quality, which fortunately is relatively infrequent, with only 0.9 % of films from multicenter trails being rejected due to poor technical quality [19].

A major *limitation* of edge detection (aside from the technical quality of the cine film) is its difficulty to analyze accurately the post-PTCA result. In particular, dissections are a frequent occurrence following PTCA, and the resulting haziness, irregular borders, or extravasation of contrast medium makes edge detection difficult. There is no ideal solution to this problem. If a dissection is present on the post-PTCA angiogram, the analyst must decide whether to include or exclude the extraluminal filling defect in the analysis. As advised by the Mercator Angiographic Committee, the computer should determine whether to include or exclude the extraluminal defect in the analysis, thereby avoiding subjective bias. If there is no clear separation between the

the lumen and the extravasation (large communicating channel), the computer includes the dissection in the analysis as the interpolated edge detection technique detects a small although not significant difference in brightness. However, in casses in which the extravasation is distinctly separate from the true vessel lumen (small communicating channel), the computer excludes the dissection from the analysis as there is a steep difference in brightness between the extravasation and the true lumen

QCA and Coronary Interventions

Prior to a discussion of the various devices used for coronary intervention the utility of the information generated by QCA in general (and the CAAS system specifically) must be addressed. Anatomic information, such as minimal luminal diameter, reference diameter, and percentage diameter stenosis, represent the most useful and relaible information obtained by this system. The physiologic and clinical significance of any individual value cannot be inferred, although the CAAS system can generate theoretical measures of resistance based on the lesion characteristics and assumed coronary flow rates. Angiographic features of a particular lesion which may be important to the clinical outcome such as ulceration or complex, ragged morphology have not been a focus of our research in terms of their natural history in large populations undergoing coronary interventions.

Although the absolute minimal luminal diameter is one of the parameters of choice for describing changes in the severity of an obstruction as a results of an intervention, percentage diameter stenosis is a convenient parameter with which to work in individual cases. The conventional method of determining the percentage diameter stenosis of a coronary obstruction requires the user to indicate a reference position. It is clear that this computed percentage diameter stenosis depends heavily on the position of the selected reference. In arteries with a focal obstructive lesion and a clearly normal proximal arterial segment the reference region is straightforward and simple. However, in cases in which the proximal part of the arterial segment shows combinations of stenotic and ectatic areas the choice may be very difficult. To minimize these variations we developed many years ago an *interpolated* technique, which is op-

erator independent, to determine the reference diameter at the actual stenosis site without operator interference. The basic idea of this technique is the computer estimation of the original diameter at the site of the obstructive region (assuming no coronary disease to be present) based on the diameter function. In this approach the reference diameter is taken as the value of the polynomial at the positon of the minimal luminal diameter. The interpolated percentage diameter stenosis is then computed by comparing the minimal diameter value at the site of the obstruction with the corresponding value of the reference diameter function. Avoidance of the arbirary choice of the reference, either proximal or distal to the stenosis, is a major practical advantage particularly in the analysis of repeated angiograms. On the other hand, this technique requires the coronary segments to be analyzed in a standard manner, i.e. from branch point to branch point, so that the length of segments are approximately equal in repeated analyses.

Although different approaches to the analysis of a coronary artery obstruction have been described, it is impractical to compare the various systems quantitatively. In particular, the lack of data about accuracy and precision and the use of different parameters to describe the validation make such comparisons difficult. It goes without saying that comparisons of angiographic data in studies performed in various core laboratories must use a properly standardized and validated procedure.

QCA and Specific Coronary Devices

Percutaneous Transluminal Coronary Angioplasty

The largest experience in the Thoraxcenter databank is in serial angiographic studies in patients treated before and after PTCA. In 1988 our group as well as Noboyushi et al. [20] demonstrated in a quantitative angiographic study that restenosis is a time-related phenomenon. Furthermore, it became apparent that the lack of agreement between different restenosis criteria applied affirmed the arbitrary nature of the categorical restenosis definitions used. At that time we stated the necessity to assess restenosis by repeat angiography, ascertained preferably according to the changes in minimal luminal diameter. Following this observation Beatt et al. [17] demonstrated that reference diameter may be involved in the dilating process and could be therefore subject to the same renarrowing process that takes place at the angioplasty site. Accordingly, percentage diameter stenosis measurements would underestimate the luminal change when there is a simultaneous reduction in the reference diameter. Also, these and subsequent studies revealed that the reproducibility of the CAAS system is high. Several large trials have obtained comparable values for the minimal luminal diameter pre-PTCA, post-PTCA, and at 6-month follow-up [21–23]. Based on data obtained from these studies it has become apparent that restenosis is not an all-or-nothing phenomenon, as is the conventional clinical belief. On the contrary, the distributions of minimal lumen diameter pre-PTCA (1.03 ± 0.37 mm), post-PTCA (1.78 ± 0.36 mm), at 6-month follow-up (1.50 ± 0.57 mm), as well as the percentage diameter stenosis at 6-month follow-up follow approximately a normal distribution [19]. Restenosis can therefore be viewed as the tail end of a phenomenon with an approximately gaussian distribution, with some lesions crossing a more or less arbitrary cut off point (depending on the particular arbitrary, categorical cutoff point applied) rather than a separate disease entity occurring in some lesions but not in others (i.e., a bimodal distribution), as suggested by the Emory group [9, 22]. This has quite profound significance for the design of trials (pharmacologic or specific devices) to inhibit the restenotic process since a normal distribution is a prerequisite for the use of parametric statistical tests (e.g., t test, analysis of variance) and perhaps more importantly, calls into question the current perception of the restenosis phenomenon and invalidates the use of the term "restenosis rate" to describe long-term outcome following intervention.

Insights into Mechanisms of Dilatation

The immediate result of PTCA is influenced by both "plastic" (dissections, intimal tears) and "elastic" changes in the vessel wall. Experimental studies have shown that part of the angioplasty mechanism consists of stretching the vessel wall with a resulting fusiform dilation or localized aneurysm formation [25]. To evaluate elastic changes from our angiographic studies we have defined elastic recoil as the difference between the minimal luminal diameter or cross-sectional area after PTCA and the mean balloon diameter

or cross-sectional area at the highest inflation pressure. We have observed that elastic recoil after PTCA results in a mean decrease of almost 50% in luminal cross-sectional area immediately after balloon deflation [26]. A follow-up study has shown that asymmetric lesions, lesions located in less angulated parts of the artery, and lesions with a low plaque burden show a more pronounced elastic recoil [27]. Furthermore, lesions located in distal parts of the coronary tree are also associated with a greater elastic recoil, likely due to relative balloon oversizing. Our initial analytical approach to serial angiographic studies in patients treated by balloon angioplasty was restricted to repeated measurements of the lesion site. The improved understanding of the mechanisms of balloon dilatation required extension of our measurements to include the inflated balloon. The now extended analyses include measurements of *stretch* (theoretical maximal gain in diameter or area during the angioplasty procedure), *elastic recoil* (which appears to affect the immediate post-PTCA result), and *relative balloon size* (which affects the incidence of dissection), Prior to these assessments the inflated balloon was used as a scaling device and (incorrectly) assumed to be uniform along the entire balloon lenght at a diameter according to the manufacturer's specifications. However, we recently measured the balloon diameter over its entire length in 453 patients [28]. During an average inflation pressure of 8.3 ± 2.6 atm we observed a difference of 0.59 ± 0.23 mm in diameter between the minimal and maximal balloon diameter. This difference results in large variations in the calculated stretch, elastic recoil, and balloon-artery ratio depending on the site of the balloon chosen for the assessment.

Angiographic Outcome after Conventional Balloon Dilatation

QCA has been useful to clarify conflicting data in the literature regarding angiographic risk factors associated with restenosis. In a recent report describing the restenosis rates in diverse segments of the coronary tree in 1234 patients no differences were observed between coronary segments using a definition of either 50% diameter stenosis at follow-up or a continuous approach comparing absolute changes in minimal luminal diameter adjusted for the vessel size [29].These results suggest that restenosis is a ubiquitous phenomenon without any predilection for a particular site in the coronary tree. A second study reported a larger "relative gain" in minimal luminal diameter at angioplasty (post-versus pre-PTCA, adjusted for vessel size); the lesion length (≥ 6.8 mm) and total occlusion pre-PTCA were independent predictors of restenosis [30]. Our interpretation of these data is that overstretching during PTCA, causing deeper arterial injury, may adversely stimulate the fibroproliferative vessel wall reaction. Although elastic recoil (described further below) may adversely affect the initial result, this study revealed no relationship between the extent of elastic recoil at the time of PTCA and late luminal renarrowing.

In an effort to determine which angiographic parameter best describes the functional status 6 months after balloon angioplasty, Rensing et al. [30] studied 350 patients with single-vessel coronary artery disease who underwent single site balloon dilatation. The diagnostic accuracy of the minimal luminal diameter at follow-up was similar to that of percentage diameter stenosis. However, because the minimal luminal diameter is the most unambiguous, directly obtained measurement of stenosis severity, this measure can be a more reliable surrogate for clinical outcome than the classical percentage stenosis measurement.

Finally, in an attempt to assess predictors of luminal renarrowing after successful PTCA, six parameters were retained in the multivariate model: diabetes mellitus, duration of angina less than 2.3 months, large luminal gain at PTCA, pre-PTCA minimal luminal diameter, lesion length of at least 6.8 mm, and thrombus post-PTCA. Although several QCA variables were independent predictors of luminal renarrowing, this process cannot be accurately predicted by clinical, morphologic, or lesion characteristics.

Densitometry may be more reliable for assessing PTCA outcome than edge detection since it is theoretically independent of the projection chosen. A study published in 1984 assessed agreement between edge detection and densitometry by the standard deviation of the difference of percentage area stenosis since absolute measurements of area by densitometry were not yet possible [18]. Prior to PTCA reasonable agreement existed between the densitometric percentage area stenosis and the circular percentage area stenosis (standard deviation of the mean difference was 5%). However, important discrepancies between these two types of measurements were observed after PTCA (standard deviation 18%). This discrepancy suggested the creation of asymmetric lesions after angioplasty and consequently cast doubt on the validity of the assumption of a circular cross-sectional stenosis area for the calculation of luminal dimensions by the edge detection technique.

Stenting

Three types of coronary stents have been employed in multicenter European clinical studies with angiographic follow-up and subsequent detailed QCA analysis at the Thoraxcenter Core Laboratory [31–35]. Two of these stents, the Wallstent and the Palmaz-Schatz stent, are composed primarily of radiolucent stainless steel, whereas radiopaque tantalum is the principle constituent of the Wiktor stent (Fig. 2). The main problem with radiolucent stents is their poor radiographic visibility while the radiopaque property of the Wiktor stent severely limits the assessment of follow-up studies by the CAAS system. Several cases have now been documented in which the contour detection program traces the radiopaque stent wires instead of the arterial borders of the narrowed intrastent segment. This invalidates the computer-derived data and requires manual correction of the contours by the analyst, which is also difficult in a segment containing radiopaque wires.

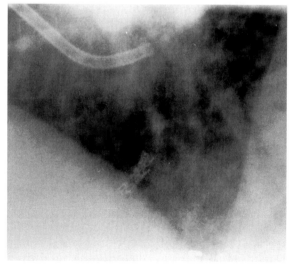

Fig. 2. Implanted Wiktor stent in the left anterior descending coronary artery

A second problem with angiographic analysis of stented vessels is due to the superior angiographic result immediately after stenting compared with following PTCA alone. Consequently, the "obstruction segment" may be completely corrected or in some cases overdilated in comparison to the reference diameter before stenting. This causes particular problems in measureing the length of obstruction and the reference diameter. We arbitrarily define the length of the obstruction after stenting to be the actual lenght of the stent (which requires manual selection of the stent boundaries). Thus the extent of the stented segment is defined for future follow-up analyses. We perform each stent analysis either by stent or by vessel. In the former the length of the lesion is the length of the stent, as previously described. In the latter there is no user interaction with the choice of computer-detected contours, and the minimal luminal diameter may then be located outside the stent. In reporting our angiographic studies we chose the pre-and post-PTCA frames to be analyzed by vessel, and the poststent and follow-up films according to the stent. This ensures that we obtain information related to the stent and its immediately adjacent segment rather than describing a more severe stenosis at a separate site in the coronary vessel.

Stenting has also highlighted a limitation of the CAAS system in the measurement of the reference diameter in an overdilated segment. Theoretically this should result in a negative value for diameter stenosis since the minimal luminal diameter (which, as noted above, was defined within the boundaries of the stent) was actually larger than the reference diameter, which is determined according to the diameter of the proximal and distal segments. However, for reasons still unclear, a negative diameter stenosis never occurred, and the reference diameter always remained larger than the minimal luminal diameter. A further confounding factor in determining the reference diameter after stenting is the marked vasospasm occasionally seen immediately proximal and distal to the stent, which persists despite nitrate administration.

Insights into the Mechanism of Stenting

Data from normal and atherosclerotic arteries of animals and humans in autopsied hearts have shown that balloon angioplasty may split the athe-

rosclerotic plaque and create tears in the intima and media. Frequently damage to the arterial media with overdistension and splitting also occurs. Therefore the main rationale for stenting these vessels is optimalization of the post-PTCA result by scaffolding the irregular surface of the atherosclerotic plaque created by the disruptive action of the balloon. Secondly, the recoil effect described above may be prevented by stent implantation. In addition, stent may have a smoothing effect which reduces the turbulent and laminar resistances and may be beneficial in preventing restenosis. All of these potential favorable actions have been addressed in quantitative angiographic studies. In 1988 Juilliere et al. [36] demonstrated the continuous radial force which has the effect of increasing luminal diameter until a balance is reached between the expanding force of the stent and the circumferential compliance of the vessel. The same study clearly demonstrated that stent implantation indeed improves the immediate post-PTCA result, producing a smooth appearance of the vessel wall. In addition, this visual impression has been confirmed by quantitative angiography using both edge detection and videodensitometry techniques. These results suggest that the self-expanding stent used had a dilating function in addition to its stenting role. This dilating sction of the stent was confirmed in a study by Beatt et al. [37] and appeared to continue up to 24 after implantation, resulting in continued improval in vessel wall geometry.

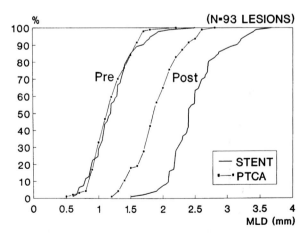

Fig. 3. Cumulative frequency of the immediate results of coronary stenting and balloon angioplasty in 93 matched lesions. *PTCA*, angioplasty; *Pre*, before intervention; *post*, after intervention

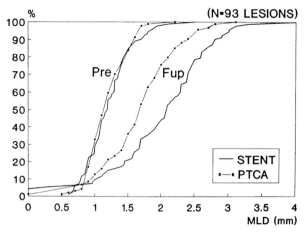

Fig. 4. The cumulative frequency of the long-term results of coronary stenting and angioplasty in this matched population. *MLD*, minimal luminal diameter; *PTCA*, angioplasty; *Pre*, before intervention; *Fup*, at follow-up

Our group has demonstrated superior immediate luminal improvement after stenting compared to balloon angioplasty [37]. Stenting induced a luminal gain of 1.4 ± 0.4 mm compared with a gain of 0.7 ± 0.4 mm after balloon angioplasty (Fig. 3, 4). This technique and directional coronary atherectomy were equally effective in luminal improvement. These favorable results have subsequently been confirmed [39].

Long-Term Outcome After Stenting

Restenosis following stenting has been extensively studied by quantiative coronary analysis. In particular, most of our corrent knowledge comes from Wallstent experience. Previous publications from our group report the late angiographic and clinical follow-up of 256 patients with 383 implanted stents. The stents were implanted in native and venous bypass grafts. In the overall group angiographic follow-up was obtained in 216 patients (82 %). Follow-up angiograms were analyzed quantitatively in 176 patients of the 225 patients (78 %) who were discharged from the hospital without known occlusion. These reports assessed restenosis by the categorical approach, and two different criteria were applied. We found a change in minimal luminal diameter of 0.72 mm or more to be a reliable indicator of angiographic progression of vessel narrowing and by no means to imply functional or clinical significance [4–8]. This value

takes into account the limitations of coronary angiographic measurements and represents twice the long-term variability for repeated measurements of a coronary obstruction using CAAS. The other criterion chosen for restenosis was an increase in diameter stenosis of less than 50 % after stent implantation to greater than or equal to 50 % at follow-up. This criterion was selected since common practice continues to assess lesion severity by percentage stenosis. The two criteria were assessed within the stent and in the segment immediately adjacent to the stent. In native vessels there was a mean increase in minimal luminal diameter from 1.17 ± 0.52 to 2.53 ± 0.53 mm immediately after stenting but a late luminal loss to 1.99 ± 0.81 mm when early occlusions we excluded. Similar changes have been observed in venous bypass grafts [40]. Detectable angiographic renarrowing (0.72 mm luminal loss) in the overall group was 42 % lesion and 43 % by patient. Using the 50 % diameter stenosis criterion, restenosis occurred in 27 % of lesions and patients. Restenosis according to either definition was assessed by calculating the relative risk ratios (RR) with 95 % confidence intervals (CI). The variables with statistically significant associations with restenosis using the 0.72-mm criterion were multiple stents and oversizing the stent (unconstraint diameter) with respect to reference diameter by more than 0.70 mm, which had a RR (and 95 % CI) of 1.56 (1.08–2.25) and 1.64 (1.10–2.45), respectively. The second criterion, at least 50 % diameter stenosis at follow-up, was associated with oversizing by 0.70 mm (RR 1.93, 95 % CI 1.13–3.31), bypass grafts (RR 1.62, 95 % CI 0.98–2.66), multiple stents (RR 1.61, 95 % CI 0.97–2.67), and residual diameter stenosis greater than 20 % after stenting (RR 1.51, 95 % CI 0.91–2.50).

The realization that the restenosis process has a gaussian distribution and thus does not represent an "all-or-nothing" phenomenon has exposed many of past efforts as being inaccurate and may explain why some of the early expectations have not been realized. A recent contribution by Kuntz et al. [41] has confirmed that restenosis after newer interventions can be described as a continuous (nondiscrete) process. Analytical methods based on such a continuous approach might be more sensitive to potential differences in restenosis tendencies among different therapies. Recent observations from their group and ours have demonstrated that stenting indeed results in better luminal gain than does balloon angioplasty [38, 39, 41]. Furthermore, a linear relationship between (relative) luminal gain and (relative) luminal loss was found, implying that part of the luminal improvement achieved at the intervention is lost during follow-up. A multivariate analysis to predict late luminal diameter supported the fundamental finding of Kuntz et al. that "bigger is better" in that more luminal gain at stenting translates into greater angiographic lumen at follow-up. Whether these particular favorable features of stenting indeed reduce the renarrowing process and beneficially influence long-term clinical outcome after stenting remains to be determined in a randomized trial.

Densitometry. In contrast to the situation after PTCA, there is excellent agreement between minimal luminal cross-sectional areas determined by edge detection and densitometry after stent implantation with the Wallstent [42]. The standard deviations of the mean differences between edge detection and densitometric determination of minimal luminal cross-sectional area were 0.51 mm^2 pre-PTCA, 1.22-mm^2 post-PTCA, and 0.79 mm^2 after coronary stenting [19]. This improvement is probably due to smoothing of the stent and remodeling of the stented segment into a more circular configuration. Therefore we believe that both methods are appropriate to assess the immediate results after stenting. In a separate in vitro study in which stents were placed in known stenoses within plexiglass phantoms, the Wallstent and Palmaz-Schatz stents caused minor and probably clinically insignificant interference with the densitometric determination of minimal luminal cross-sectional area within the known stenoses [43]. Conversely, the radiopacity of the tantalum Wiktor stent led to overestimation of minimal luminal cross-sectional area measurements in the same narrowings by 10%–56%, depending on the concentration of contrast and specific stenosis. Therefore, the follow-up assessment of a lesion containing a Wiktor stent is limited by both methods.

Directional Atherectomy

Few problems have been encountered in the angiographic analysis of lesions treated by directional atherectomy [44]. The radiopacity of the device, particularly when the support balloon is inflated, allows excellent visualization of the position of the eccentric cutting apparatus. The vessel luminal contours are typically smooth and much less ragged than after PTCA, facilitating the edge detection program. Despite the apparently smooth contours, however, a similar discrepancy exists between analyses performed by edge detection and those performed by densitometry as occurs post-PTCA [45], which suggests that the vessel wall assumes a less circular configuration as a result of atherectomy. As Baim's group has suggested, this may be due to preferential expansion of the bases of the atherectomy cuts [46].

Insights into the Mechanism of Atherectomy

Using directional atherectomy, the atherosclerotic plaque is selectively removed as the cutting device is directed towards the protruding plaque. With plaque removal instead of plaque disrupture observed with balloon angioplasty it was initially hypothesized that a greater gain in luminal area can be achieved and may account for the main mechanism of action. In recent years QCA of atherectomy-treated lesions has provided some insight into the mechanisms of lesion improvement. Penny et al, have shown that an average of approximately 28% of the effect of atherectomy can actually be attributed to tissue removal, although the individual values had a wide range (7%–92%) [46]. The correlation between the volume of tissue retrieved and the change in luminal volume was poor. The authors concluded that the major component of luminal improvement is due to "facilitated mechanical angioplasty" resulting from the high profile of the device and the low-pressure balloon inflations. Data from our angiographic core laboratory seems to support this hypothesis. The "dottering effect" of the device accounted for 65% of the luminal improvement [47] in ten patients who had QCA performed preatherectomy after crossing the stenosis with the device and after directional atherectomy (Fig. 5).

Long-Term Outcome After Directional Atherectomy

In experimental work Schwartz and colleagues have demonstrated that a relationship between vessel wall injury induced by an intervention is related to a reparative process. This approach has become known as the biological approach and can

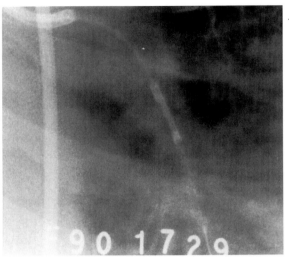

Fig. 5. Operational directional atherectomy device in a left circumflex coronary artery

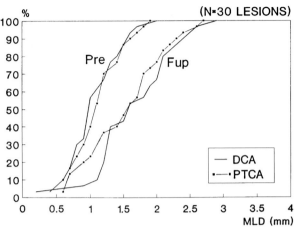

Fig. 7. The cumulative frequency of the long-term results of directional atherectomy and angiplasty in the matched population. At 6-month follow-up the initial favorable result of atherectomy is lost when compared to balloon angioplasty. *MLD*, minimal luminal diameter; *DCA*, atherectomy; *PTCA*, angioplasty; *Pre* before intervention; *Fup* at follow-up

be readily studied by QCA using the loss in minimal luminal diameter as the angiographic parameter. In a matched comparative study [48, 49] we found that atherectomy indeed results in a larger immediate gain than balloon angioplasty (1.17±0.29 to 2.44±0.41 mm versus 1.21±0.38 to 2.00±0.36 mm; *p*<0.001; Fig. 6). During follow-up, however, this immediate favorable acute result is partially lost by a larger luminal loss so that at 6 months follow-up the minimal luminal diameter was not significantly different in the atherectomy group compared with the PTCA group (1.76±0.62 versus 1.77±0.59 mm; Fig. 7). In this series of patients a linear relationship between relative gain (an index for wall injury) and relative loss (an index

for the healing response) was observed, but the slope of the regression line was steeper for atherectomy, suggesting that the relative loss after atherectomy is proportionally even larger for a given relative gain compared with that in the angioplasty population. Others have analyzed long-term results from a clinical perspective taking the final minimal luminal diameter as the ultimate clinical endpoint. In their analyses, Kuntz et al. [39, 41] concluded that a large postprocedural lumen is the principle determinant for the best angiographic result (i.e., large lumen at lollow-up) at 6 months. The observations made by Kuntz et al. [39, 41] that achieving greater luminal gain with newer devices may reduce angiographic restenosis is not

Fig. 6. The cumulative frequency of the immediate results of directional atherectomy and balloon angioplasty in 30 matched lesions. Directional atherectomy resulted in an increase in minimal luminal diameter (*MLD*) from 1.08 mm to 2.61 mm while angioplasty induced an increase from 1.15 to 1.92 mm. *DCA*, atherectomy; *PTCA*, angioplasty; *Pre*, before intervention; *Post*, after intervention

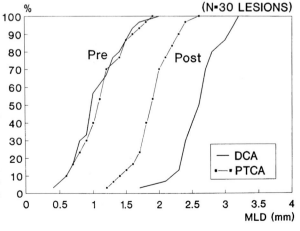

completely in agreement with the finding that a greater luminal gain results in greater luminal loss. While the clinical studies of our group focus mainly on the degree of renarrowing as a measure of the extent of the biological process, i.e., the development of intimal hyperplasia, others focus on the angiographic outcome, i.e., final minimal luminal diameter. This is the difference, as has been expressed by Schwartz et al. [50], between the "doughnut and the doughnut hole." There is little doubt that a larger lumen at follow-up may be clinically "better" for the patient, and that this parameter is of great importance in assessing the long-term outcome of therapy. However, in large clinical trials directed at the prevention of renarrowing, the effect of therapy must be measured by its restricting effect on the thickness of the "doughnut," which we believe is best expressed angiographically by the relative luminal loss during follow-up. As recently described, we believe that application of the two approaches (angiographic outcome and biological process) to the same population yields similar findings, and that the diverse interpretations arise from methodological differences [51].

Rotational Abrasion

The Thoraxcenter experience to date has been limited with this device (11 procedures) [52], a unique feature of which is its usefulness as a calibration unit as an alternative to the guiding catheter (Fig. 8). The Rotablator contains a burr of known size, and there is no question of completeness of expansion as with stents and PTCA catheters of specified size. Precise measurement of the device at the lesion site has been useful to assess the extent of elastic recoil, which appears to be an important phenomenon, since the luminal dimension immediately following rational abrasion is always smaller than the diameter of the burr used. A unique feature of the Rotablator is that the optimal angiographic result is not realized until 24 h later since due to the intense and prolonged vasoconstriction induced by the burr.

Excimer Laser

Excimer laser have presented an attractive alternative to other forms of coronary interventions on the basis of the experimental finding that a

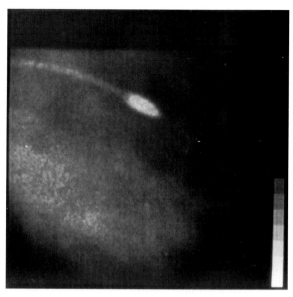

Fig. 8. On-Line quantitative measurement of the operational rotational abrasion device (Rotablator)

focused, pulsed, UV laser beam in air can ablate tissue with minimal adjacent tissue injury. The ability of pulsed UV laser light to ablate atherosclerotic tissue has been investigated in vitro an in vivo on human and porcine aorta [53, 54]. Considerable heat accumulation and expansion of evaporating debris trapped under the tip of the delivery system causes thermal and mechanical vessel wall injury, with subsequent pressure build up and expansion of a vapor cavity within adjacent tissue [54, 63]. The angiographic correlate of this phenomenon appears to be haziness of the contours of lesions treated with the excimer laser, which makes the immediate postprocedure analysis more difficult. The lased lesion typically has a "roughened" appearance which may lend itself to the detailed analysis of lesion morphology [55]. Whether videodensitometry should be preferred to edge detection for assessing the specific effects of the excimer laser in coronary interventionsis under investigation.

How Should We Use QCA Data to Compare Interventional Devices?

The safety and favorable clinical results of a number of interventional procedures have been demonstrated [30–41, 46–49]. The next step is to compare the relative efficacy of the devices in a particular clinical situation.

Immediate Results Postprocedure: The Expansion Ratio

The expansion ratio is a useful concept for assessing the immediate results of an intervention [48, 56]. It relates the final effect of the device on the luminal diameter to the size of the catheter required to deliver this effect. A favorable ratio is best examplified by a small catheter delivery system which can traverse severely narrowed segments and yet optimally dilate the stenosis. However, the maximum effect of the device may be partially lost due to the elastic recoil of the vessel. Current interventional devices may have differential effects in these two areas: the acute result, when the device is initially used, and the partial loss of the initial gain after the device has been removed. We have attemped to separate these two effects by subdividing the expansion ratio into the *theoretical* expansion ratio, which is a measure of the effect while the device is operational, and the *functional* expansion ratio, which takes into account vasoconstriction and the elastic recoil phenomenon. For example, a fully expanded 4 mm diameter angioplasty balloon catheter should achieve a luminal diameter of 4 mm at the time of balloon inflation, but the minimal luminal diameter may be considerably less after deflation, due primarily to the elastic recoil of the vessel. Balloon angioplasty and stenting yield extremely favorable theoretical *and* functional expansion ratios since they may be delivered on low-profile catheters. Although directional atherectomy is effective against elastic recoil, the bulky profile of the device restricts its use and limits the theoretical expansion ratio. The dimensions of the rotational atherectomy device and the excimer laser do not change while in operation, and therefore both exhibit lower theoretical expansion ratios. However, physically removing or vaporizing tissue diminishes the potential elastic recoil effect by atherectomy and excimer laser devices.

Late Results

Few randomized trials have been reported to date comparing the efficacy of the various interventional devices. In an early study we compared available data using three different methods. First, we compared pathological findings in an animal model; second, we distiguished the static clinical outcome after an intervention from the

dynamic biological process during follow-up; and third, we introduced matching as a surrogate for randomized trials.

Relative Gain as "Injury score", Relative Loss as an Index of Neointimal Hyperplasia. The important observation that a greater gain in lumen (i.e., injury) is associated with a greater loss (i.e., repair) during follow-up has been described by Schwartz et al. [57, 58]. In a domestic swine stented model, which accurately mimics the proliferative nature of human restenosis, the extent of proliferative response was strongly associated with rupture of the internal elastic lamina as induced by oversized and overpressurized balloon inflations, with or without coil implantation. To test this hypothesis in a clinical setting we substituted the concepts of injury score and neointimal hyperplasia as observed in the animal model with the angiographically derived parameters of relative gain and relative loss. Quantitative angiographic analysis of 522 coronary artery lesions treated by balloon angioplasty with a 95% angiographic follow-up revealed a linear relationship between relative gain and relativ loss, although the coefficient of relation was low (0.4). Another comparative study indeed confirmed these observations for balloon angioplasty but found a stronger correlation between relative gain and relative loss for atherectomy than in balloon angioplasty [49]. More importantly, the slope of the regression line was steeper in the atherectomy group than in the angioplasty group, implying that not only is the relative gain greater in the atherectomy group, but also that the reactive response (i.e. relative loss) was more pronounced after atherectomy than following angioplasty. The slope of the regression line between relative gain and relative loss, which reflects the inherent relationship between the degree of wall injury and the degree of repair, represents an index of luminal renarrowing specific for each treatment modality (atherectomy, balloon angioplasty).

Multivariate Analysis of the Renarrowing Process and Late Outcome. While examining the long-term results of intracoronary interventions, two aspects should be considered: (a) the clinical approach in which the determinant of the long-term angiographic *outcome* (minimal luminal diameter at follow-up) is characterized and (b) the biological approach which describes the determinants of the dynamic *process* (late luminal loss) which is initiated by the injury inflicted to the vessel wall during intervention. Initially these two viewpoints appear contradictory but on deeper examination it may be possible to reconcile the assessment of *outcome* and *process* and find that each view may in its own way be correct, although not considering the entire picture. We sought to reconcile the clinical and bilogical views (i.e., long-term angiographic *outcome* and the dynamic *process* of renarrowing which occurs during follow-up) in a consecutive series of patients treated by atherectomy [51]. We concluded that in analyzing the long-term results of interventional techniques the biological *process* (luminal loss during follow-up) — which characterizes the traumatizing nature of the intervention — should be *dissociated* from the clinical *outcome* (minimal luminal diameter at follow-up). It is clear that whereas improved clinical outcome is associated with larger vessel size and postprocedural luminal diameter, greater relative gain at intervention is strongly predictive of more extensive luminal renarrowing.

Matching. We have employed the technique of "matching" [38, 48, 49], which is based on three priciples: (a) the angiographic dimensions of matched lesions are assumed to be "identical," (b) the observed difference between the two "identical" lesions must be within the range of the CAAS analysis reproducibility of 0.1 mm ($\pm 1\,\mathrm{SD}$), and (c) the reference diameter of the potentially "matched" vessels are selected within a range of $\pm 0.3\,\mathrm{mm}$ ($\pm 3\,\mathrm{SD}$, i.e., 99 % confidence limits). The appropriate lesions are selected by an independent observer who is unaware of the 6-month angiographic outcome. Subsequent refinement of this technique also allowed the incorporation of clinical variables, thereby creating similar patient groups with identical lesion and clinical characteristics. Matching may eventually be used as a surrogate for randomized trials and may serve as a predictor of the outcome in such trials.

How Should Future Trials Be Designed To Compare Devices Using Angiographic Endpoints?

Of all the measurements directly acquired by QCA the absolute value of minimal luminal diameter has been shown to be the greatest single determinant of the hemodynamic consequences of a stenosis since this parameter affects blood flow by

a fourth-power term [59–62]. This parameter is therefore the only nonambiguous, objective, and reproducible parameter with which to describe the caliber of coronary vessels and changes it in resulting from interventions. All important multicenter trials examining the impact of various pharmacologic agents on restenosis post-PTCA are now assessed in a core laboratory [16] using quantitatively derived parameters, particularly minimal luminal diameter.

Restenosis Rates

A categorical approach using various "restenosis rates" is, in our view, inherently misleading and inaccurate since the figures quoted are by definition derived from and dependent on arbitrary criteria (which have little or no functional/physiologic basis) and have no relevance in the description of the continuous process of restenosis. They should no longer be the main focus of important scientific studies or discourse in this vital area. We believe that results of intervention trails may now be presented much more elegantly in graphic form, using cumulative distribution curves to display change minimal luminal diameter during follow-up for treated versus placebo populations or indeed for PTCA versus stent, atherectomy, or laser [32].

Minimal Luminal Diameter at Follow-Up, the Quantitative Angiographic Endpoint

In placebo-controlled restenosis prevention trials following PTCA the change in minimal luminal diameter during follow-up has traditionally been used to assess the value of a new pharmacologic strategy, and this approach is justified since the luminal enlargement observed in the two arms of the trial were by definition comparable. Due to the different nature of the interventions (e.g., atherectomy versus angioplasty), the immediate postprocedural results are different and no longer comparable. This is clearly shown in the cumulative distribution curve: atherectomy induces a larger gain in minimal luminal diameter than angioplasty, which makes the immediate postprocedural characteristics dissimilar so that the loss during follow-up is no longer a helpful comparison of the long-term benefit. The most valid parameter for the comparison of two interventional devices is the minimal luminal diameter *at* follow-up because this *static parameter*, it itself, represents the final luminal improvement at follow-up. Moreover, the minimal luminal diameter at follow-up may have a *functional component*. This information suggests that the absolute value of the minimal luminal diameter at follow-up may prove to be an even more useful parameter than those obtained by clinical examination or exercise testing.

The relative long-term benefits of the various treatment modalities are now under study in randomized clinical trails. The innate intertreatment modality differences with regard to relative gain and loss, as described above, suggest that it may be fallacious to continue assessing and using the „within–patient change in minimal luminal diameter" (i.e., the change from immediately postintervention to follow-up, measured by QCA), as the measurement of choice. To asses the relative value of the various interventions or indeed to judge the relative merits of new pharmacologic approaches to prevent restenosis, the most objective and meaningful parameter to use is minimal luminal diameter at follow-up as the primary angiographic endpoint.

Conclusion

The introduction of new devices for nonoperative coronary revascularization has exposed previously unknown limitations of computer-assisted CAAS, in addition to the well-known drawbacks of expense and analysis time (approximately 30 min per lesion for two projections selected at any stage of the procedure). However, thanks to rapid advances in computer technology in recent years second-generation systems based on powerful personal computers and workstations [63] are now available. These systems are characterized by improved contour detection with correction for the limited resolution of the X-ray imaging chain, automated path line tracing, lower costs, and significantly reduced processing time (complete analysis of coronary arterial segment can be performed in less than 10–12 s).

QCA, as the most objective and reproducible technique currently available, is still the gold standard for the study of coronary artery disease and accurate assessment of the immediate and long-term angiographic results of intervention, by a variety of different modalities. Through the analysis of data provided by QCA our group has developed a number of pertinent and contribu-

tory concepts to the *unfolding philosophy* of "restenosis." We believe that further progress in this relatively unexplored teritory will be accelerated by the universal adoption of the type of philosophy described here, as will the continued application and further development of QCA.

References

1. Mancini GBJ. Quantitative coronary arteriographic methods in the interventional catheterization laboratory: an update and perspective. J Am Coll Cardiol 91: 17 (6 Suppl B): 23B–33B.
2. Zir LM, Miller SW, Dinsmore RE, Gilbert JP, Harthorne JW. Interobserver variability in coronary angioggraphy. Circulation 76; 53: 627–32.
3. Goldberg RK, Kleiman NS, Minor ST, Abukhalil J, Raizner AE. Comparison of quantitative coronary angiography to visual estimates of lesion severity pre and post PTCA. Am Heart J 90; 1: 178–84.
4. Reiber JHC, Booman F, Tan HS, et al. A cardiac image analysis system. Objektive quantitative porcessing on angiocardiograms. Comput Cardiol 78; 239–242.
5. Serruys PW, Booman F, Troost GJ, Reiber JHC, Gerbrands JJ, van den Brand M, Charrier F, Hugenholtz PG. Computerized quantitative coronary angiography applied to percutaneous transluminal coronary angioplasty: advantages and limitations. In: Kaltenbach M, Gruntzig A, Rentrop K, Bussman WD Ceds) Transluminal coronary angioplasty. Advantages and limitations, p. 110–124, Springer Verlag, Berlin – Heidelberg – New York, 82.
6. Reiber JHC, Serruys PW, Kooijman CJ, et al. Assessment of short-, medium-, and long-term variations in arterial dimensions from computer-assisted quantitation of coronary cineangiograms. Circulation 85; 71: 280–8.
7. Reiber JHC, Serruys PW, Slager CJ. Quantitative coronary and left ventricular cineangiography: methodology and clinical applications. Boston: Martinus Nijhoff Publishers, 86.
8. Reiber JHC, Kooijman CJ, Slager CJ, et al. Coronary artery dimensions from cineangiograms: methodology and validation of a computer-assisted analysis procedure. IEEE Trans Med Imaging 84; 3: 131–41.
9. Mancini GB. Digital coronary angiography: advantages and limitations. In: Reiber JHC, Serruys PW (eds) Quantitative coronary angiography. p. 23–42, Kluwer Academic Publishers, Dordrecht – Boston – London, 81.
10. Reiber JHC, van Zwet CD, Koning G, Loois G, Zorn I, van den Brand M, Gerbrands JJ. On-line quantification of coronary angiograms with the DCI system. Medicamundi 89; 34: 89–98.
11. Nutgeren SK, Haase J, Rensing BJ, Di Mario C, Serruys PW. Can on-line quantitative analysis accurately measure vascular dimensions? A comparison with off-line cineangiographic measurements (abstract). J Am Coll Cardiol 92.

292

V.A.W.M. Umans et al.

12. Haase J, Di Mario C, Slager CJ, Reiber JHC, Serruys PW, et al. Accuracy and relevance of angiocardiographic coronary measurements. In: Heintzen PH, Brenneke R (eds) Digital maging in cardiovascular radiology. Georg Thieme Verlag, Stuttgart – New York, 92.

13. Vlodaver Z, Edwards JE. Pathology of coronary atherosclerosis. Prog Cardiovasc Dis 71; 14: 256–74.

14. Saner HE, Gobel FL, Salomonowitz E, Erlien DA, Edwards JE. The disease-free wall in coronary atherosclerosis: its relation to degree of obstruction. J Am Coll Cardiol 85; 6: 1096–9.

15. Di Mario C, Hermans W, Rensing BJ, Serruys PW. Calibration using angiographic catheters as scaling devices. Importance of filming the catheter not filled with contrast medium (letter). Am J Cardiol 1992.

16. Hermans WRM, Rensing BJ, Pameyer J, Reiber JHC, Serruys PW. Experiences of a quantitative coronary angiographic core laboratory in restenosis prevention trials. In: Reiber JHC, Serruys PW (eds) Quantitative coronary arteriography 92. Dordrecht: Kluwer Academic Publishers. In press.

17. Beatt KJ, Luijten HE, de Feyter PJ, van den Brand M, Reiber JHC, Serruys PW. Change in diameter of coronary artery segments adjacent to stenosis after percutaneous transluminal coronary angioplasty: failure of percent diameter stenosis measurement to reflect morphologic changes induced by balloon dilatation. J Am Coll Cardiol 88; 12: 315–23.

18. Seeruys PW, Reiber JHC, Wijns W, et al. Assessment of percutaneous transluminal coronary angioplasty by quantitative coronary angiography: diameter versus densitometric area measurements. Am J Cardiol 84; 54: 482–8.

19. Rensing BJ, Hermans WRM, Deckers JW, de Feyter PJ, Tijssen JGP, Serruys PW. Luminal narrowing after percutaneous transluminal coronary balloon angioplasty follows a near gaussian distribution. A quantitative angiographic study in 1445 successfully dilated lesions. J Am Coll Cardiol 1992.

20. Nobuyoshi M, Kimura T, Ohishi H, Horiushi H et al (1991) Restenosis after percutaneous transluminal coronary angioplasty: pathologie observations in 20 patients. I Am Coll Cardiol 17: 433–439.

21. Serruys PW, Luijten HE, Beatt KJ, et al. Incidence of restenosis after successful coronary angioplasty: a time-related phenomenon. A quantitative angiographic study in 342 consecutive patients at 1, 2, 3, and 4 months. Circulation 88; 77: 361–71.

22. Serruys PW, Rutsch W, Heyndrickx GR, et al. Prevention of restenosis after percutaneous transluminal coronary angioplasty with thromboxane A2 receptor blockade. A randomized, double-blind, placebo controlled trial. Circulation 1991; 84: 1568–80.

23. The Mercator Study Group. Does the new angiotensin converting enzyme inhibitor cilazapril prevent restenosis after percutaneous transluminal coronary angioplasty? In press.

24. King SB III, Weintraub WS, Xudong T, Hearn J, Douglas JS Jr. Bimodal distribution of diameter stenosis 4 to 12 months after angioplasty: implication for definitions and interpretation of restenosis (abstract). J Am Coll Cardiol 91; 17 (2 Suppl A): 345A.

25. Sanborn TA, Faxon DP, Haudenschild CG, Gottsman SB, Ryan TJ. The mechanism of transluminal angioplasty: evidence for information of aneurysms in experimental atherosclerosis. Circulation 83; 68: 1136–40.

26. Rensing BJ, Hermans WRM, Beatt KJ, et al. Quantitative angiographic assessment of elastic recoil after percutaneous transluminal coronary angioplasty. Am J Cardiol 90; 66: 1039–44.

27. Rensing BJ, Hermans WRM, Strauss BH, Serruys PW. Regional differences in elastic recoil after percutaneous transluminal coronary angioplasty: a quantitative angiographic study. J Am Coll Cardiol 91; 17 (6 Suppl B): 34B–38B.

28. Hermans WRM, Rensing BJ, Strauss BH, Serruys PW. Methodological problems related to the quantitative assessment of stretch, elastic recoil and balloon-artery ratio. Cathet Cardiovasc Diagn. In press.

29. Hermans WRM, Rensing BJ, Kelder JC, de Feyter PJ, Serruys PW. Postangioplastytransluminal angioplasty: evidence for formation of aneurysms in experimental restenosis rate between segments of the major coronary arteries. Am J Atherosclerosis. Circulation 83; 68: 1136–40. Cardiol. In press.

30. Rensing BJ, Hermans WRM, Vos J, et al. Quantitative angiographic risk factors of luminal narrowing after coronary balloon angioplasty using balloon measurements to reflect stretch and elastic recoil at the dilatation site. Am J Cardiol. In press.

31. Serruys PW, Strauss BH, Beatt KJ, et al. Angiographic follow-up after placement of a self-expanding coronary-artery stent. New Engl J Med 91; 324: 13–7.

32. Serruys PW, Juilliere Y, Bertrand ME, Puel J, Rickards AF, Sigwart U. Additional improvement of stenosis geometry in human coronary by stenting after balloon dilatation. Am J Cardiol 88; 61: 71G–76G.

33. Puel J, Juilliere Y, Bertrand ME, Rickards AF, Sigwart U, Serruys PW. Early and late assessment of stenosis geometry after coronary arterial stenting. Am J Cardiol 88; 61: 546–53.

34. Serruys PW, Strauss BH, van Beusekom HM, van der Giessen WJ. Stenting of coronary arteries. Has a modern Pandora's box been opened? J Am Coll Cardiol 91; 17 (6 Suppl B): 143B–154B.

35. Serruys PW, de Jaegere P, Bertrand M, et al. Morphologic change of coronary artery stenosis with the Medtronic Wiktor stent. Initial results from the core laboratory for quantitative angiography. Cathet Cardiovasc Diagn 91; 24: 237–245.

36. Jullier Y, Serruys PW, Beatt KJ, Sigward U. Contribution of self expansion of stent and additional endoluminal dilatation within the stent on patency of human coronary arteries. Eur Heart J 1988: 9 (Suppl I) 56.

37. Beatt KJ, Bertrand M, Puel J, Rickards T, Serruys PW, Sigward U. Additional improvement in vessel lumen in the first 24 hours after stent implantation due to radial dilating force. JACC 1989: 13; 224A.

38. Umans VAWM, Strauss BH, Rensing BJWM, de Jaegere P, de Feyter PJ, Serruys PW. Comparative angiographic quantitative analysis of the immediate efficacy of coronary atherectomy with balloon angioplasty, stenting, and rotational ablation. Am Heart J 91; 122: 836–43.

39. Kuntz RE, Safian RD, Carrozza JP, Fishman RF, Mansour M, Baim DS. The importance of acute luminal diameter in determining restenosis after coronary atherectomy or stenting. Circulation 1992; 86: 1827–35.

40. Strauss BH, Serruys PW, Bertrand ME, Puel J, Meier B, Goy J-J, Kappenberger L, Rickards AF, Sigwart U. Quantitative angiographic follow-up of the coronary Wallstent in native vessels and bypass grafts: the European experience March 86–March 90. Am J Cardiol 1991.

41. Kuntz RE, Safian RD, Levine MJ, Reis GJ, Diver DJ, Baim DS. Novel approach to the analysis of restenosis after the use of three new coronary devices. J Am Coll Cardiol 1992; 19: 1493–1500.

42. Strauss BH, Julliere Y, Rensing BJ, Reiber JHC, Serruys PW. Edge detection versus densitometry for assessing coronary stenting quantitatively. Am J Cardiol 91; 67: 484–90.

43. Strauss BH, Rensing BJ, den Boer A, van der Giessen WJ, Reiber JHC, Serruys PW. Do stents interfere with the densitometric assessment of a coronary artery lesion? Cathet Cardiovasc Diagn 91; 24: 259–264.

44. Serruys PW, Umans VAWM, Strauss BH, van Suylen RJ, de Feyter PJ. Quantitative angiography after directional coronary atherectomy. Br Heart J 91; 66: 112–9.

45. Umans VA, Strauss BH, de Feyter PJ, Serruys PW. Edge detection versus videodensitometry for quantitative angiographic assessment of directional coronary atherectomy. Am J Cardiol 91; 68: 534–9.

46. Penny WF, Schmidt DA, Safian RD, Erny RE, Baims DS. Insights into the mechanism of luminal improvement after directional coronary atherectomy. Am J Cardiol 91; 67: 435–7.

47. Umans VA, Haine E, Renkin J, de Feyter PJ, Wijns W, Serruys PW. On the mechanism of directional coronary atherectomy. Eur Heart J 1993.

48. Umans VAWM, Beatt KJ, Rensing BJWM, Hermans WRM, de Feyter PJ, Serruys PW. Comparative quantitative angiographic analysis of directional coronary atherectomy and balloon angioplasty: a new methodologic approach. Am J Cardiol 91; 68: 1556–63.

49. Umans VA, Hermans W, Foley DP, Strikwerda S, van den Brand M, de Jaegere P, de Feyter PJ, Serruys PW. Restenosis following directional coronary atherectomy and balloon angioplasty: a comparative analysis based on matched lesions. J Am Coll Cardiol 1993; 21; 1382–1390.

50. Schwartz RS, Huber KC, Murphy JG, Edwards WD et al. Restenosis and the proportional neointimal response to coronary artery injury. J Am Coll Cardiol 1992; 19: 267–275.

51. Umans V, Robert A, Foley D, Wijns W, Haine E, de Feyter P, Serruys PW. Clinical, histologic and quantitative angiographic predictors of restenosis following directional coronary atherectomy: a multivariate analysis of the renarrowing process and late outcome. JACC in press.

52. Laarman GJ, Serruys PW, de Feyter PJ. Percutaneous coronary rational atherectomy (Rotablator). Neth J Cardiol 90; 3: 177–83.

53. Gijsbers GHM, Spranger RLH, Keijzer M, et al. Some laser-tissue interactions in 308 nm excimer laser coronary angioplasty. J Intervent Cardiol 90; 3: 231–41.

54. van Leeuwen TG, Motamedi M, Meertens JH, van Erven L, Velma E, Post MJ, Borst C. In vivo tissue damage by excimer, holmium (?) and thulium laser ablation of porcine aorta. (abstract). Circulation 1991; 84 (supl. II): II–360.

55. Kalbfleisch SJ, McGillem MJ, Simon SB, Deboe SF, Pinto IMF, Mancini GBJ. Automated quantitation of indexes of coronary lesion complexity. Comparison between patients with stable and unstable angina. Circulation 90; 82: 439–47.

56. Beatt KJ, Serruys PW, Strauss BH, Suryapranata H, de Feyter PJ, van den Brand M. comparative index for assessing the results of interventional devices in coronary angioplasty (abstract). Eur Heart J 91; 12 Abstract Supplement: 395.

57. Schwartz RS, Murphy JG, Edwards WD, Carmrud AR, Vlietstra RE, Holmes DR. Restenosis after balloon angioplasty. A practical proliferative model in porcine coronary arteries. Circulation 1990; 82: 2190–220.

58. Schwartz RS, Koval TM, Edwards WD, Camrud AR, et al. Effect of external beam irradiation on neointimal hyperplasia after experimental coronary artery injury. J Am Coll Cardiol 1992; 19: 1106–1114.

59. Kirkeeide RL, Gould LK, Parsel L. Assessment of coronary stenoses by myocardial perfusion imaging during pharmacologic coronary vasoldilatation. Validation of caronary flow reserve as a single integrated functional measure of stenosis severity reflecting all its geometric dimensions. J Am Cardiol 86; 7: 103–13.

60. Zijlstra F, van Ommeren J, Reiber JHC, Serruys PW. Does quantitative assessment of coronary artery dimensions predict the physiological significance of a coronary stenosis? Circulation 1987; 75: 1154–61.

61. Klocke FJ: Measurements of coronary blood flow and degree of stenosis: current clinical implications and continuing uncertainties. J Am Coll Cardiol 1983; 1: 31–41.

62. Gould KL: Identifying and measuring severity of coronary stenosis. Quantitative coronary arteriography and positron emission tomography. Circulation 1988; 78: 237–245.

63. Reiber JHC, van der Zwet PJM, von Land CD, et al. Quantitative coronary arteriography: equipment and technical requirements. In: Reiber JHC, Serruys PW, (eds) Quantitative coronary arteriography 92. Dordrecht: Kluwer Academic Publishers. In press.

Thoracic and Upper Extremity Arteriography

R. Reyes, J.M. Pulido-Duque, E. Gorriz, P.J. Rubio, J. Carreira, C. Gervás, and M. Maynar

Introduction

The use of conventional angiography of the thorax and upper extremities has, as with other vascular regions diminished due to the development of noninvasive techniques such as ultrasound, computerized tomography, and magnetic resonance. However, in planning and performing percutaneous interventions, X-ray angiography still remains the diagnostic method of choice.

Arteriography of the Upper Extremities

Indications and Techniques

The main indications for angiography of the upper extremities are: (a) arterial occlusive diseases, (b) arteriovenous malformations, (c) thoracic outlet syndrome, (e) trauma, and (f) access for hemodialysis [1].

The femoral artery approach is the most frequently used and allows complete study of the extremities. The axillary approach is reserved for those cases in which femoral catheterization is not possible. Retrograde brachial artery puncture is the method of choice with angiography for hemodialysis access, as it allows the necessary hemodynamic evaluation of flow across the fistula. Both subclavian arteries can be catheterized with a 5F multipurpose catheter in younger patients. In elderly patients with tortuous vessels either a Sidewinder or Simmons catheter may be preferable. The Simmons and Sidewinder catheters are also used for contralateral axillary or brachial artery catherization. The guide wire facilitates safe advancement of the catheter to the desired vesel. New digital angiography equipment makes high-resolution images possible, saving 30% contrast medium compared with conventional cut film angiography [2–4].

Images are obtained with the arm in the neutral position (adducted) in the PA projection. Oblique views may be necessary in some cases. In patients with suspected thoracic outlet compression, additional arteriograms are obtained with the arm in 90° and 180° abduction.

Angiographic Findings

Arterial Occlusive Diseases

In atherosclerosis the most frequently affected parts are the proximal segments of the extremity vessels. Atherosclerosis of the forearm and hand vessels occurs less frequently [4]. The subclavian steal syndrome is due to severe stenosis or occlusion of the subclavian artery, proximal to the origin of the vertebral artery. Reversal of blood flow through the circle of Willis from the carotid artery to the vertebral artery provides collateral flow to the affected extremity. Arteriography is indicated to show the extent of the disease and the pattern of blood flow. Thromboembolism is the most frequent cause of acute vascular insufficiency of the upper extremities in elderly people. The diagnosis is established with noninvasive methods but arteriography is useful for determining the exact location of the embolic occlusion, for the evaluation of the underlying disease, and treatment. The arteriogram shows an abrupt cutoff with a convex meniscus in the involved vessel.

Arteriovenous Malformations

Angiography is indicated to determine the location of the fistula and to evaluate the feeding vessels, the shunting, and the venous drainage. The main angiographic findings are: (a) enlargement of the feeding artery or arteries with a network of abnormal vessels, (b) rapid arteriovenous shunting with tortuous and enlarged venous drainage, and (c) multiple arterial or venous aneurysms. The vessels feeding the malformation must be dis-

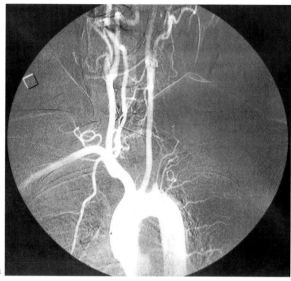

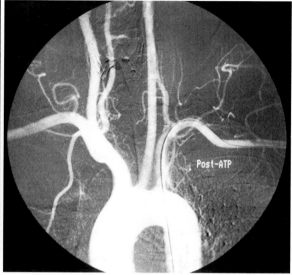

a   b

Fig. 1 a, b. Angiography shows total occlusion of the left subclavian artery. Total patency was achieved after PTA

tinguished from the normal vessels when a therapeutic embolization is planned, to avoid the risk of inappropriate embolization and to choose the optimum embolic material.

Thoracic Outlet Syndrome

Angiography may show: (a) mild dilatation of the distal subclavian or proximal axillary artery, this being the most common finding; (b) focal stenosis; (c) aneurysm; (d) occasionally no arterial abnormality is present with the arm in the neutral position.

Trauma

Arteriography prior to surgery for suspected vascular injury can decrease the number of negative explorations. The angiographic findings are: (a) arterial narrowing due to posttraumatic spasm or extrinsic compression by hematoma, (b) arterial occlusion, (c) false aneurysm, (d) arteriovenous fistula, (e) localized intimal defects, and (f) contrast medium extravasation.

Hemodialysis Access

Oblique and lateral projections are necessary to uncover any lesion that may be occult in the standard PA projection. The study must also include evaluation of the venous outlet up to the subclavian vein. The main angiographic findings are stenosis or thrombosis at the site of anastomosis or at the venous outflow. Arterial lesions are less frequent [5].

Interventional Procedures

The most commonly performed interventional procedure in the upper extremity is percutaneous angioplasty (PTA) for brachiocephalic and subclavian arterial stenoses, with a technical success rate of between 88% and 93% and a long-term clinical success rate of 80%–96% [6, 7]. In contrast, PTA of subclavian artery occlusions gives poor results, with a technical success rate of 53% and undefined long-term results [8] (Fig. 1). The most frequent complications of PTA are, as in other vascular areas dissection and distal embolization. Dissection with occlusive flap may be solved with a Simpson atherectomy catheter [9]. Special attention must be paid to distal embolization when performing PTA in the subclavian artery proximal to the origin of the vertebral artery. Stenotic of hemodialysis access lesions may be treated by percutaneous revascularization techniques such as PTA, fibrinolytic therapy, and

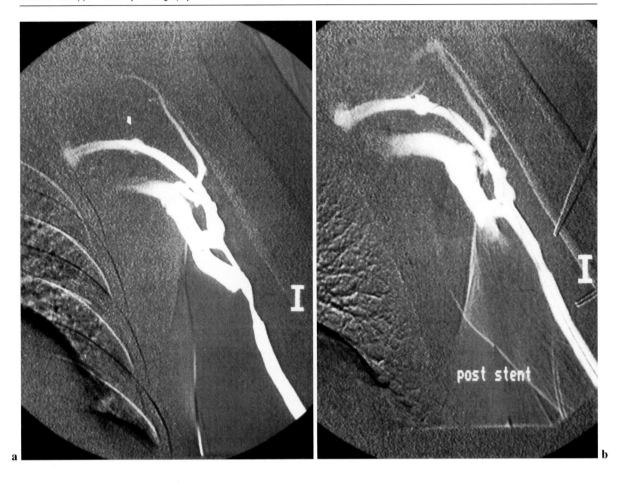

Fig. 2 a, b. Patient with loop PTEF graft between the brachial artery and vein. Digital subtraction angiography (DSA) shows: **a** high-grade cephalic vein stenosis; **b** result after PTA and stenting

vascular endoprostheses. Stenosis may recur within 6 months of dilatation; however, PTA can be repeated with a high success rate because the goal is to keep the fistula as long as possible. Local fibrinolysis is an alternative to surgical thrombectomy of occluded arteriovenous fistula. It also allows detection of the underlying cause, generally a stenosis, which can be treated percutaneously [10, 11] (Fig. 2a). Nowadays the mechanical thrombolytic catheter can offer a new alternative in the management of hemodialysis access fistulas [12].

Pulmonary Angiography

Indications

Thromboembolic disease is the most common indication for pulmonary arteriography. Other indications include the evaluation and treatment of pulmonary arteriovenous malformations [4].

Technique

Pulmonary arteriography is performed most frequently from the femoral approach, but the cephalic, basilic, and internal jugular veins may also be used when necessary. The study must be performed under continuous electrocardiographic monitoring. Right atrial and right ventricular, as well as pulmonary artery, pressures are recorded prior to contrast medium injection. In our experience the most commonly used catheter is the Grollman cather, essentially a pigtail-shaped ca-

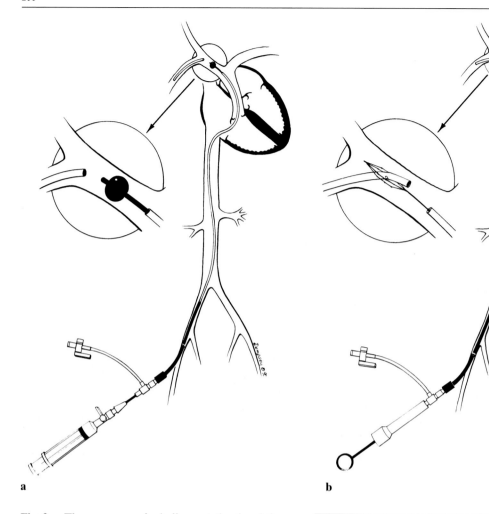

a   b

Fig. 3. a The presence of a balloon at the tip of the catheter facilitates the advancement of the long introducer sheath into the pulmonary artery. **b** The catheter fragment in the pulmonary artery is trapped with a Dormia basket

theter with as sharp distal curve in the terminal 5–7 cm. The catheter is inserted into the right atrium, then advanced into the right ventricle, where it is gently pushed with a counterclockwise rotation into the pulmonary artery. The first angiographic series is obtained in the anteroposterior projection, with the catherer tip in the main pulmonary artery. Contrast medium is injected at a rate of 25–35 ml/s, filming two images per second for at least 10 s. After selective catheterization of each pulmonary artery, oblique projections are performed at an injection rate of 20–25 ml/s, obtaining two images per second for at least 12 s.

Angiographic Findings

Pulmonary Thromboembolism (PTE)

An intraluminal defect is the most frequent and most specific arteriographic abnormality. Other abnormalities that may be encountered are: parenchymal hypovascularity, absence of a draining vein from the affected segments, and demonstration of large collaterals.

Arteriovenous Malformations (AVM)

There are two types of AVM according to their angiographic appearance: simple and complex types. The simple AVM presents a direct artery to vein communication, with a dilated fusiform or saccular vein. The complex type, which is rarer, presents several feeding arteries and multiple draining veins.

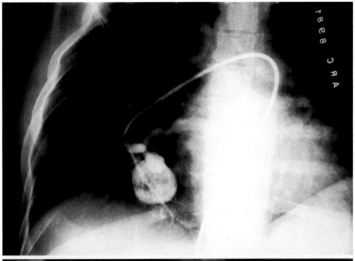

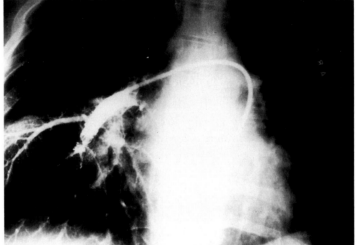

Fig. 4. a Pulmonary angiography shows a large arteriovenous fistula. The selective catheter has been advanced through the previously prepositioned sheath.
b Follow-up pulmonary angiography shows total occlusion of the arteriovenous fistula

Interventional Procedures

Thrombolytic therapy is indicated in those patients with PTE and angiographically demonstrated occlusion of more than 40%–50% of the lung arterial bed [13]. Thrombolysis must be performed as quickly as possible to avoid right heart failure and cardiogenic shock. Intrathrombus local perfusion of the fibrinolytic agent accelerates thrombolysis. AVM embolization is performed through selective catheterization of the feeding arteries. The most frequently used embolic material is the Gianturco spring coils. Knowledge of the diameter of the arteriovenous communication is important to avoid coil migration (Figs. 3, 4).

Bronchial Arteriography

Indications

The number and origin of the bronchial arteries varies widely. Between 21% and 38% of individuals have two bronchial arteries (one on each side). There are three bronchial arteries, two left and one right artery in 40%–50% of cases, and 25% have four bronchial arteries, two left and two right arteries. A single right bronchial artery is multiple in 70% of cases. Twenty percent of bronchial arteries have an anomalous origin from the subclavian artery, internal mammary artery, brachiocephalic artery, inferior thyroidal artery, inferior phrenic arteries, etc. [14, 15]. The main indication for bronchial arteriography is for the evaluation of a patient with hemoptysis. In chil-

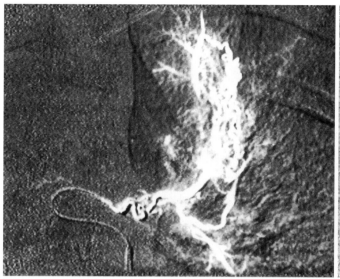
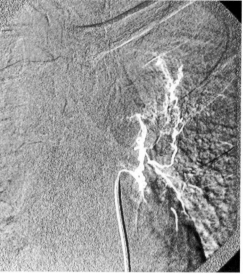

Fig. 5. a Left apical bronchial angiography shows tortuosity of the vessel and hypervascularity. **b** Control angiography reveals total occlusion of the apical vessels

dren with pulmonary atresia, it helps to define pulmonary artery anatomy prior to surgery.

Technique

Bronchial arteriography is performed via the femoral approach in most cases. Catheter selection depends on the anatomic characteristics of the patient. The multipurpose catheter is the one most frequently used, but the Cobra, Headhunter, and Sidewinder catheters are also useful. Selective catheterization of the right bronchial artery is performed, advancing the catheter tip along the right posterolateral wall of the thoracic aorta between T4 and T7. The left bronchial arteries are catheterized, advancing the catheter tip along the left anterolateral wall of the arota. Digital substraction arteriography with a manual injection of 6–8 ml non-ionic contrast medium, at a filming rate of two images per second, offers good diagnostic images.

Angiographic Findings

In the normal individual, the bronchial arteries are of small caliber and the peripheral branches are not visualized. In patients with disease (bron-

chiectasis, granulomatous infection, neoplasms), the arteries are enlarged and their peripheral branches are visualized. Other pathologic findings include peribronchial hypervascularity, bronchopulmonary artery communication, and contrast medium extravasation.

Interventional Procedures

Bronchial artery embolization is indicated for the treatment of massive or recurrent hemoptysis, with severe respiratory compromise. Immediate control of bleeding is achieved in 50% of cases, with long-term control in 82% of cases [16, 17]. Stability of the catheter in the artery must be assured prior to performing embolization to avoid reflux of embolization material. The most serious complication that can arise is spinal cord ischemia following inadvertent occlusion of the anterior spinal artery. Careful localization of this artery and advancement of the catheter distal to its origin is necessary to perform the embolization safely [18] (Fig. 5).

Upper Limb Venography

Indications

The main indications for upper limb venography are: deep venous thrombosis, venous obstruction secondary to trauma, neoplasm, or lymphadenopathy, and the thoracic outlet syndrome [19].

Technique

Venipuncture of a dorsal vein of the hand is performed when all the extremity has to be studied. For the evaluation of the axillary or more central venous structures, the proximal forearm veins (cephalic, basilic) are used. A torniquet is placed several centimeters above the puncture site to opacify the deep venous system. A total of 20 ml contrast medium is injected at a rate of 5 ml/s, with a filming rate of one film per second for a total of 12–15 films. In addition to the standard PA projection with the arm in the neutral position, images must be obtained with the arm abducted to 90° and 180° when thoracic outlet syndrome is suspected.

Angiographic Findings

An intraluminal filling defect outlined by a thin layer of contrast medium is visualized in acute thrombosis. As the thrombus ages, it becomes adherent to the vein wall and is no longer outlined completely by contrast medium. The next step is complete occlusion of the vein and diversion of blood flow through the collaterals. When the thrombus recanalizes, the vein presents an irregular and streaky appearance. Venography may be normal in venous compression due to the thoracic outlet syndrome when the arm is in the neutral position, with signs of extrinsic compression appearing when the arm is abducted to 90° and 180°.

Interventional Procedures

The most frequently performed interventional procedure in this area is fibrinolysis of the axillary and subclavian vein [20]. The introduction of an angiographic catheter through the cephalic or basilic vein allows accurate diagnosis of the extent of the occlusion and direct perfusion of the fibrinolytic agent. Once patency of the occluded segment is reestablished, any stenosis that may be uncovered can be treated percutaneously or surgically.

Superior Venacavography

Indications

The main indications are superior vena cava (SVC) syndrome and studies of anatomic variants. Compression or complete obstruction of the SVC is malignant in 80%–90% of cases. Lung cancer is the most frequent etiology (50%). The frequency of iatrogenic SVC thrombosis is currently increasing due to the use of central venous catheters, parenteral nutrition catheters, and pacemakers [20].

Technique

The SVC can be evaluated by simultaneous bilateral cubital vein injection or by venous catheterization. The introduction of a multihole catheter through the forearm veins, to the subclavian or brachiocephalic veins, allows an increased contrast flow rate and reduces the risk of contrast medium extravasation. A total of 25–30 ml contrast medium is injected at a rate of 8–10 ml/s, between both arms when simultaneous later injections are performed, at a filming rate of two images per second for the first 4 s, and one image per second for 10 c. Anteroposterior and lateral projections are obtained. Oblique views are usually not necessary.

Angiographic Findings

The most frequent pathologic findings are extrinsic compression and thrombosis. The compressed vena cava appears narrowed, with smooth undulating contours. Occlusion may present with or without the presence of a proximal thrombus. In chronic occlusions, dilated collaterals may be demonstrated, the extent of which depends upon the duration and severity of the obstruction.

Interventional Procedures

Superior vena cava stenosis due to extrinsic compression, which presents clinically with an SVC syndrome, can be treated by the placement of an endoprosthesis. The most frequently used endoprosthesis in this territory is the Gianturco-Rösch prosthesis, due to its strong radial force. When there is superimposed thrombosis, fibrinolysis may be performed prior to stent deployment [21, 22].

References

1. Kadir S (1986) Arteriography of the upper extremities. In: Kadir S (ed) Diagnostic angiography. Saunders, Philadelphia, pp 127–206
2. Wilking RA, Garwey CJ (1986) The role of digital subtraction angiography in interventional radiology. J Intervent Radiol 1: 3–8
3. Charing R, Kaufman SL, Kadir S, et al. (1984) Digital subtraction angiography in interventional radiology. AJR 142: 363–366
4. Turski PA, Stieghorst MF, Strother CM et al. (1982) Digital subtraction angiography „road map". AJR 139: 1233–1234
5. Glanz S, Bashit B, Gordon DH, Butt K, Adamsons R (1982) Angiography of upper extremity access fistulas for dialysis. Radiology 143: 45
6. Standards of Practice Committee of the Society of Cardiovascular and Interventional radiology (1990) Guidelines for percutaneous transluminal angioplasty. Radiology 177: 619–626
7. Selby JB, Matsumoto AH, Tegtmeger CJ et al. (1993) Balloon angioplasty above the aortic arch: immediate and long-terms results. AJR 160: 631–635
8. Duber C, Klose KJ, Kopp H et al. (1992) Percuataneous transluminal angioplasty for occlusion of the subclavian artery: short- and long-term results. Cardiovasc Intervent Radiol 15: 205–210
9. Maynar M, Reyes R, Cabrera V et al. (1989) Percutaneous atherectomy as an alternative treatment for postangioplasty obstructive intimal flaps. Radiology 170: 1029–1031
10. Gordon DH, Glanz S, Butt K, Adamsons R, Koenig MA (1982) Treatment of stenotic lesions in dialysis access fistulas and shunts by transluminal angioplasty. Radiology 143: 53–58
11. Glanz S, Gordon DH, Butt K, Hong J, Adamsons R, Sclafani SJA (1985) Stenotic lesions in dialysis-access fistulas: treatment by transluminal angioplasty using high-pressure balloons. Radiology 156: 236
12. Valji K, Bookstein J, Roberts AC, Davis GB (1991) Pharmacomechanical thrombolysis and angioplasty in the management of clotted hemodialysis grafts: early and late clinical results. Radiology 178: 243–247
13. Petitpretz P, Simmoneau G, Cerrina J et al. (1984) Effects of a single bolus of urokinase in patients with life-threatening pulonary emboli: a descriptive trial. Circulation 70: 861–866
14. Kadir S (1986) Arteriography of the thoracic aorta. In: Kadir S (ed) Diagnostic angiography. Saunders, Philadelphia, pp 124–171
15. Tadavarthy SM, Klugman J, Casteñeda-Zúñiga WR, Nath PH, Amplatz K (1982) Systemic-to-pulmonary collaterals in pathological states. Radiology 144: 55–59
16. Stoll F, Bettman A (1988) Bronchial artery embolization to control hemoptysis: review. Cardiovasc Intervent Radiol 11: 263–269
17. Uflaker R, Kaermmerer A, Picon PD et al. (1985) Bronchial artery embolization in the management of hemoptysis; technical aspects and long-term results. Radiology 157: 637–644
18. Ivanich MJ, Thorwarth W, Donohue J, Mandell V, Delany D, Jaques PF (1983) Infarction of the left main stem bronchus: a complication of bronchial artery embolization. AJR 141: 535–537
19. Kadir S (1986) Venous system. In: Kadir S (ed) Angiography. Saunders, Philadelphia, pp 536–583
20. Reed JD, Harman JF, Harris V (1992) Regional fibrinolytic therapy for subclavian vein thrombosis. Semin Intervent Radiol 9: 183–189
21. Putman JS, Uchida BT, Antonovic R, Rösch J (1988) Superior vena cava syndrome associated with massive thrombosis: treatment with expandable wire stents. Radiology 167: 727–728
22. Irving JD, Dondelinger RF, Reidi JF, Schild H, Dick R, Adam A, Maynar M, Zollikofer O (1992) Gianturco self-expanding stents: clinical experience in the vena cava and large veins. Cardiovasc Intervent Radiol 15: 328–333

Abdominal Arteriography

R. R. Saxon, R. E. Barton, J. Rösch, and F. S. Keller

Introduction

The success of most interventional procedures is largely determined through careful planning and preparation before they begin. High-quality diagnostic arteriography that clearly demonstrates the pathologic vascular anatomy is an integral part of this preparation (Fig. 1). Abdominal aortography prior to an interventional procedure requires an examination that is tailored to the clinical question at hand. Consequently, the request for angiography and intervention in patients with probable disease involving the abdominal aorta or its branches should be considered a request for consultation. The clinical situation, including any prior arteriograms, cross-sectional imaging studies, and noninvasive vascular assessment, must be carefully evaluated by the angiographer so that the diagnostic arteriogram can be planned in a manner that will obtain the maximum amount of information.

For vascular occlusive disease diagnostic angiography is usually followed by some form of intervention. Often the diagnostic arteriogram and intervention are performed in two separate sittings, allowing time for a discussion of the findings with the referring service and minimizing the amount of contrast administered at one session. However, potential interventions are always discussed with the patient and the referring service prior to the diagnostic study so that the treatment plan is efficient in terms of time and cost. In some circumstances it makes more sense to perform both the diagnostic study and the intervention at the same time. For example, renal artery angioplasty can be performed in conjunction with a diagnostic arteriogram if the clinical history and previous imaging studies are carefully reviewed prior to arteriography, and the patient is agreeable to this approach. Since Dotter's first angioplasty in 1964 there have been dramatic improvements in imaging guidance for percutaneous intervention. Generally, a cut-film angiogram is obtained before and after intervention. Analog radiography is useful due to its large field of view, low susceptibility to motion artifacts, and excellent image quality. Digital subtraction angiography (DSA) can be used liberally for supplemental views to clarify anatomic questions. DSA has several advantages, especially during an intervention. These include a high signal to noise ratio allowing a decrease in the amount of contrast material required, shortened procedure time, and real-time DSA or "road mapping." Finally, recent advances in other imaging modalities, such as angioscopy and intravascular ultrasound, promise to improve the accuracy of vascular evaluation [1, 2]. However, until further research is carried out into the clinical efficacy of these promising technologies, cost considerations prohibit their routine use. This chapter discusses specific approaches to the diagnostic arteriogram in the setting of occlusive vascular disease of the aorta and its branches.

Angiography Prior to Aortic Angioplasty and Stenting

Abdominal aortography can be performed from either a femoral, axillary, or translumbar approach. The femoral approach is chosen unless the patient has severe occlusive vascular disease that precludes safe, percutaneous access to the aorta from the common femoral artery. Using the axillary artery as an access to the aorta prior to an intervention should be undertaken with caution. The larger sized catheters that must be used with certain interventions (i.e., stent placement) coupled with administration of heparin can lead to axillary hematomas with potential motor and sensory deficits from compression of the nerves that run in the axillary sheath.

Diagnostic abdominal aortography at our institution is performed using a 65-cm, 5-F pigtail cathe-

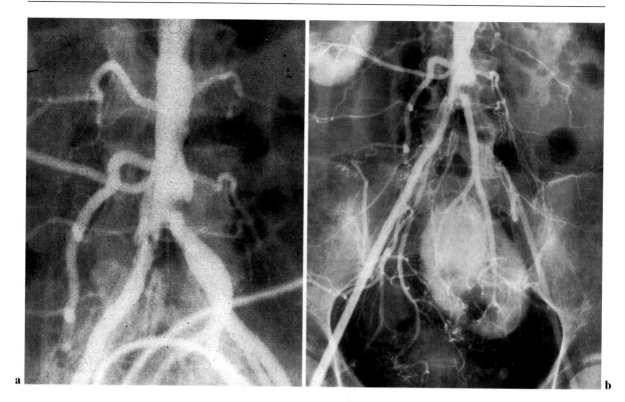

Fig. 1 a, b. Distal arotic disease with aberrant renal arteries and ectopic kidney. **a** A cine angiogram of the abdominal aorta obtained at the time of coronary arteriography demonstrates a distal aortic stenosis that extends into both common iliac arteries. The patient was referred for angioplasty. **b** A cut-film aortogram obtained prior to angioplasty shows a pelvic kidney with its artery originating from the abdominal aorta at the site of stenosis. A lower pole right renal artery also originates from the distal aorta. The left common iliac artery occluded after the cine angiogram. Due to the two renal artery origins arising from the site of aortic stenosis this patient was sent for surgical repair. This example graphically shows the need for an adequate field of view and a quality study when performing diagnostic arteriography

ter which is inserted into the abdominal aorta over a 0.035- in., 1.5-mm J guide wire. The pigtail is placed just above the level of the renal arteries. Our standard injection is 22 cc/s of 76 % diatrizoate meglumine for a total of 44 cc, with a filming rate of two films per second for 3 s and one film per second for 3 s. Prolonged filming is often required in the evaluation of stenosis and occlusions in order to adequately define collateral pathways and the distal vessels that they reconstitute. We continue to prefer cut film (analog) angiography for our initial study of the aorta. Our vascular surgeons prefer this format and cut film allows con-

sistent measurement of vessel size when selecting a balloon for angioplasty. We obtain an oblique or lateral digital aortogram in selected cases. This allows an accurate assessment of the degree of stenosis and the morphology of the lesion. Posterior atheromatous plaques or ulcerations that are associated with the "blue toe" syndrome can be detected with this view. In addition, a lateral aortogram detects stenoses at the origins of the celiac, superior mesenteric, and inferior mesenteric arteries. If the patient has significant celiac and superior mesenteric arterial disease, it is important to avoid compromising a large inferior mesenteric artery in the process of performing an aortic angioplasty. Although rarely a problem, if inferior mesenteric artery occlusion occurs in this setting, life-threatening visceral ischemia may result.

Just as a cardiologist should not perform an angioplasty of a right coronary artery stenosis without knowledge of the status of the left coronary artery and left ventricular function, one should not dilate an aortic stenosis without knowing the extent of disease in the patient's runoff vessels. Because many patients have multiple sites of disease that combine to produce symptoms of claudication or ischemia, aortoiliac revascularization often needs to be combined with an "outflow" procedure in order to adequately treat the patients symptoms. Therefore, unless contraindicated by poor renal function, an entire peripheral vascular study from the abdominal aorta to the feet should be performed and evaluated before intervention.

We complete our diagnostic study with a hemodynamic evaluation. A pressure gradient is measured across any apparent stenosis in the aorto-iliac system. If a patient does not have a significant pressure gradient (10 mmHg systolic) across a stenosis following administration of a vasodilator (tolazoline, 50 mg), we do not proceed with an intervention. The patient most likely has another site of disease accounting for the symptoms.

Angiography during aortoiliac intervention is usually performed in the anteroposterior projection

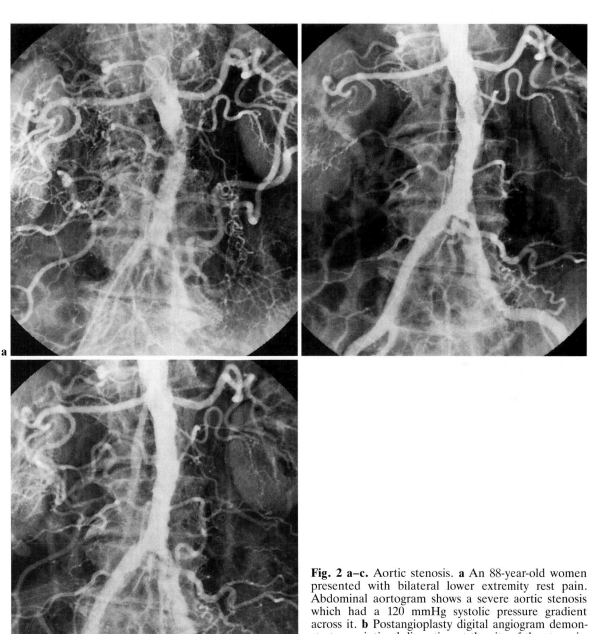

Fig. 2 a–c. Aortic stenosis. **a** An 88-year-old women presented with bilateral lower extremity rest pain. Abdominal aortogram shows a severe aortic stenosis which had a 120 mmHg systolic pressure gradient across it. **b** Postangioplasty digital angiogram demonstrates an intimal dissection at the site of the stenosis. A 50 mmHg gradient remained. **c** A single Palmaz stent was placed. The follow-up angiogram reveals no residual dissection or stenosis. There is also no gradient present

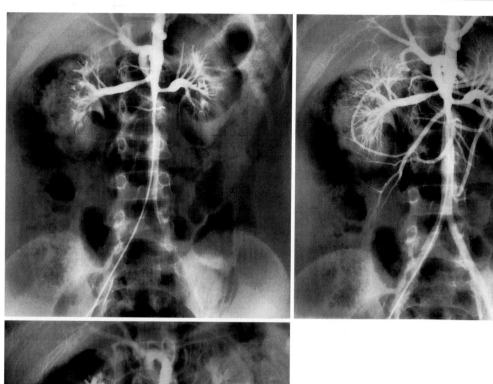

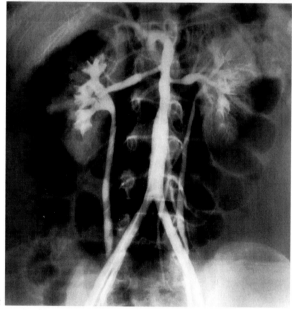

Fig. 3 a–c. Takayasu's aortitis. **a, b** Early and late films from an abdominal aortogram in a young, normotensive child with marked claudication demonstrate a severe abdominal aortic stenosis which extends into both renal arteries. Note the large arc of Riolan providing collateral flow from the superior mesenteric artery to the inferior mesenteric artery and down the aorta. These findings are classic for the "middle aortic syndrome". This child had Takayasu's aortitis. **c** Angioplasty was performed on the aorta. The follow-up arteriogram demonstrates a markedly improved appearance to the aorta. The child's claudication resolved

since this allows optimal evaluation of the aortic bifurcation. However, as a general rule, the view that best demonstrates the lesion on the preprocedure angiogram is chosen when performing the intervention and especially the follow-up arteriogram. Pressure gradients and repeat angiography determine whether the angioplasty result is adequate. If a significant gradient exists following the angioplasty, or significant dissection is identified, repeat balloon inflation or stent placement are indicated.

Abdominal aortic stenosis and occlusions present clinically with buttock, leg and thigh claudication, as well as impotence [3]. The vascular laboratory demonstrates decreased high thigh pressures. In older patients it is extremely unusual for aorto-iliac occlusive disease to have any other etiology but atherosclerosis. In some patients, however, aortic occlusion can be secondary to superimposed thrombus or embolus in addition to an underlying stenosis. It is important to look for signs of an acute process in these patients that might respond to thrombolysis. These include an intraluminal filling defect or meniscus, abrupt occlusion of the vessel with a "blind end", and a relative paucity of collateral vessels.

Angioplasty of the abdominal aorta has been evaluated by a number of recent investigators who have achieved uniformly excellent technical results as well as clinical success [4–6]. It has often been noted that focal isolated stenosis of the distal aorta tends to occur in relatively young female smokers [7]. The men in these studies were more likely to have disease extending into the iliac arteries [8]. The ideal lesion for angioplasty is a short, concentric, infrarenal stenosis. Eccentric, calcified lesions and diffuse aortoiliac disease have both been considered relative contraindications to percutaneous therapy. Extensive, long-segment disease of the abdominal aorta and iliac arteries may best be treated by surgery. However, Yakes et al. noticed no difference in technical success or midterm patency of aortic stenoses 4–7 cm in length compared to lesions less than 2 cm long that were treated with percutaneous angioplasty [9]. In addition, excellent results have been obtained using metallic stents in extensive disease of the iliac system [10]. Although the efficacy of intravascular stents in the abdominal aorta needs to be further evaluated, excellent results would be expected given the large size of the aorta. We have had significant success in selected cases (Fig. 2).

In younger patients abdominal aortic narrowing (the "middle aortic syndrome") can be caused by a number of unusual entities, including: vasculitis such as Takayasu's arteritis, neurofibromatosis, congenital rubella, and previous umbilical artery catheter placement. In most of these entities the angiogram demonstrates a smooth, concentric narrowing of the abdominal aorta that can involve origins of the visceral vessels (Fig. 3). The long-term efficacy of percutaneous intervention in most of these diseases is unknown. However, successful angioplasty has been described for Takayasu's arteritis after the disease had been brought under control with medical therapy [11].

Renal Artery Angiography/Renovascular Hypertension

Of all patients with hypertension, 4%–5% have a renovascular origin for their disease [12]. The noninvasive evaluation of renovascular hypertension includes a complex and confusing array of diagnostic tests, including peripheral renins, renal vein renins, radionuclide renograms, duplex ultrasonography, and magnetic resonance angiography. Unfortunately, none of these tests has proven sufficiently sensitive or specific enough to preclude renovascular hypertension in the setting of a patient who has appropriate risk factors [13, 14]. These risk factors include hypertension of sudden onset or which is difficult to control, hypertension without a family history, hypertension with a bruit over the renal artery, and the onset of renal insufficiency during medical therapy with an angiotensin-converting enzyme inhibitor. We generally proceed directly to diagnostic angiography in a patient suspected of having renovascular hypotension or an arterial cause of renal insufficiency.

Because the right renal artery usually arises slightly anterior on the aorta and the left renal artery arises slightly posterior, we begin our evaluation of the renal arteries with a 10°–15° (RPO) aortogram with the catheter positioned above the renal arteries. This position favors imaging of the renal artery origins in profile. Rapid filming (three or four films per second) is required to evaluate the renal artery origins for atherosclerotic disease. Such filming allows good visualization of the renal artery origins before they are obscured by contrast filling the overlapping superior mesenteric artery branches. A standard anteroposterior aortogram is also helpful because the location and number of renal arteries is highly variable and necessitates careful inspection of the entire abdominal aorta. We follow abdominal aortography with renal arteriography in selected cases only. If a renal angioplasty is not to be performed, it makes no sense to traverse a tight renal artery stenosis for a selective angiogram because the risk is not warranted. However, selective angiography is helpful at the time of angioplasty and to further evaluate the intrarenal branches. Our standard approach is to use a 5.5-F endhole catheter with an opened celiac curve. The catheter is placed in the proximal portion of the renal artery. However, in renal arteries that are caudally oriented and have a tight stenosis it is often helpful to use a "pull-down" or "sidewinder" catheter shape in order to engage the artery origin. Long tapered 0.035- or 0.018-in. guide wires can then be used to traverse the lesion. For a single, dominant renal artery we inject 5–6 cc/s for 2 s while filming at a rate of two films per second for 4 followed by one film every 2 s for 8 s. Contrast amounts must be decreased appropriately for the size of the individual artery being injected, especially when studying accessory renal arteries.

Although many recent studies have confirmed the efficacy of percutaneous transluminal angioplasty for the treatment of renovascular hypertension and azotemia [15, 16], a number of important questions must be answered when a renal artery stenosis is detected in order to optimize the results of intervention. What is the degree of the stenosis, and does it warrant intervention? Oblique DSA views are often helpful in unwinding complex renal artery anatomy. Renal artery stenosis which narrow the diameter of the vessel by 50% or more are hemodynamically significant. Although patients with lateralizing renal vein renins tend to respond more favorably to angioplasty, significant improvements can occur in hypertensive patients even in the absence of lateralizing renal vein renins [17]. Therfore we do not routinely obtain renin levels. In equivocal stenosis pressure gradients may be helpful. However, in the renal artery a catheter must cross the lesion in order to measure a pressure. Therefore, the presence of a gradient may be exaggerated due to the catheter falsely narrowing the lumen at the site of a stenosis. Are there multiple or intrarenal stenoses? Stenoses at branch points can significantly complicate an angioplasty and decrease the likelihood of success. What is the status of the renal parenchyma? A small, scarred kidney without signif-

icant functional tissue may cause hypertension but not respond to a successful angioplasty; embolization or nephrectomy may be indicated in such a case. On the other hand, a kidney that is relatively small with a functional nephrogram will likely benefit from angioplasty of a stenosis. Most importantly, one must be careful to evaluate the entire kidney angiographically and not overlook focal parenchymal lesions. A renal artery stenosis does not require dilation in the setting of an ipsilateral renal cell carcinoma! Finally, the etiology of the stenosis must be considered. Most often the disease is atherosclerosis; however, a number of other entities can cause renal artery stenosis, and each disease responds differently to angioplasty. Renal artery stenosis is caused by atherosclerotic disease in 70% of patients [18]. Atherosclerosis causes lesions at many locations in the kidney, including origin stenosis, focal or diffuse intrinsic stenoses of the main renal artery, branch stenoses, eccentric lesions, and densely calcified plaques (Fig. 4). The ideal lesion for angiplasty in the setting of renovascular hypertension is a focal, nonostial lesion with a normal contralateral renal artery [19]. The likelihood of improving azotemia is highest in patients with mild renal insufficiency and bilateral, nonostial renal artery stenoses [20]. A critical distinction that is sometimes difficult to make is whether the lesion is intrinsic to the renal artery itself or primarily involves the renal artery origin. If the lesion is predominately within or

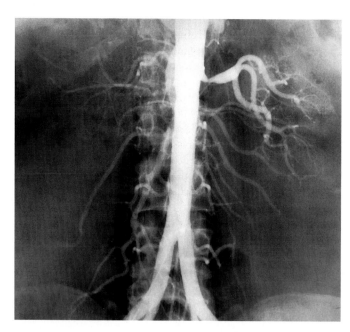

Fig. 4. Atherosclerotic disease. Abdominal arteriography in this patient with hypertension demonstrates a right renal artery occlusion and a left renal artery stenosis secondary to atherosclerotic disease

clearly intrinsic to the renal artery, angioplasty is definitely the treatment of choice. If the lesion is clearly ostial, it is often secondary to disease within the aortic wall and has a lesser chance of responding to angioplasty [21]. These lesions are often better treated with surgery. Presently the use of arterial stents is being evaluated for ostial lesions. Diffuse disease of the aortoiliac system requiring surgical repair can also be a contraindication to percutaneous intervention on the renal arteries. With such lesions the renal artery stenosis can be repaired at the time of aortic surgery, obviating the small but definite risk of significant complication that can occur at the time of angioplasty.

Fibromuscular dysplasia (FMD) causes renal artery stenosis in 25 % of patients with renovascular hypertension. Angiographic differentiation of FMD from atherosclerotic disease is important since FMD responds more favorably to angioplasty. FMD is most easily classified into three general types radiographically (although pathologically there are as many as six different types). Most common is the medial form of FMD, which responds extremely well to angioplasty. The intimal form and adventitial forms do not respond as well to angioplasty, but are fortunately less common. Medial FMD is classically described as a "string of beads" appearance with alternating areas of stenosis and aneurysmal dilatation (Fig. 5). The intimal form is usually secondary to a focal web, whereas the adventitial form is a long, smooth stenosis. Oblique views, usually the ipsilateral anterior oblique, demonstrates the length of the renal artery to best advantage.

When performing the diagnostic arteriogram, one should be aware of a number of diseases whose presence are a contraindication to renal angioplasty. For example, polyarteritis nodosa and other vasculitides can involve the renal arteries but should be treated medically, not with angioplasty. Polyarteritis involves the renal arteries in 80 % of patients and causes small vessel narrowing and microaneurysms (Fig. 6). The presence of a congenital renal artery aneurysm that is ipsilateral to a stenosis (Fig. 7) is also a contraindication to angioplasty, because there is significant risk of rupturing the aneurysm either during the procedure or after the stenosis is relieved due to the increased pressure within the artery. By carefully evaluating the diagnostic arteriogram, performing an angioplasty in inappropriate circumstances can be avoided.

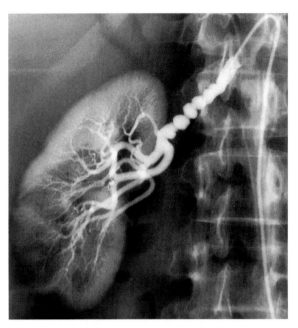

Fig. 5. Fibromuscular disease. Selective renal angiography in a patient with severe hypertension demonstrates the typical "string of beads" appearance of the artery with alternating areas of dilatation and stricture. These findings are diagnostic of the medial form of fibromuscular dysplasia

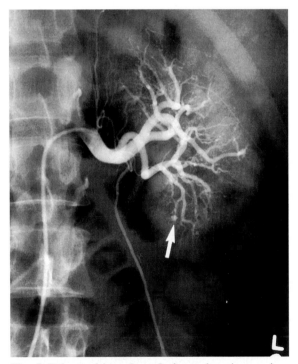

Fig. 6. Polyarteritis nodosa. Left renal angiogram in a patient with unexplained abdominal pain and hypertension demonstrates small vessel occlusion and microaneurysms diagnostic of polyarteritis nodosa

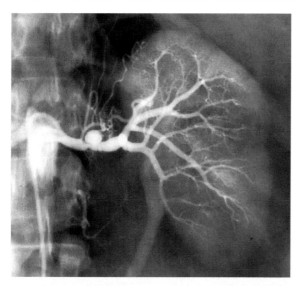

Fig. 7. Fibromuscular disease. This left renal arteriogram in a patient with medial fibromuscular dysplasia shows an eccentric aneurysm at the site of stenosis. Due to the large size of the aneurysm in comparison to that of the renal artery, angioplasty was not performed

Intestinal Ischemia

Visceral ischemia occurs in a number of different forms, many of which can be quite difficult to detect clinically. Consequently, the angiographer relies on an astute clinician to suspect acute or chronic visceral ischemia and to have the wisdom to order an angiogram. Only then does the angiographer have the opportunity to make the diagnosis and improve the patient's condition. Angiographic evaluation of the visceral vessels begins with a lateral aortogram. We often perform aortography in the frontal plane as well as selective visceral angiography, but this depends on the clinical situation. For example, a selective frontal superior mesenteric artery angiogram is most important in a patient with an embolus occluding the SMA distally. However, in a patient with acute or chronic disease involving the origin of the superior mesenteric artery we may perform only a lateral aortogram. For aortography a 5-F pigtail catheter is placed above the level of the celiac axis (usually at T12) and 22 cc/s is injected for 2 s. For the lateral aortogram rapid filming (at least three films per second) is required to evaluate the superior mesenteric and celiac artery origins. The lateral view is often performed using DSA. Prolonged filming (two films per second for 3 s and one film per second for 6 s) is most useful in frontal aortography to see delayed filling of obstructed vessels by collaterals. We use a series of selective catheters to complete a visceral study including 5.5- to 6.5 F celiac and inferior mesenteric artery catheters. The advent of hydrophilically coated guide wires has helped significantly with selective catheterization of visceral vessels, allowing peripheral catheter placement and evaluation of branch vessels.

Chronic visceral ischemia presents with abdominal angina, weight loss, and diarrhea. Due to extensive collateral circulation these vague clin-

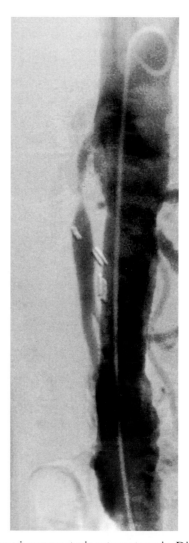

Fig. 8. Superior mesenteric artery stenosis. Digital lateral aortogram in a patient with chronic mesenteric ischemia demonstrates occlusion of the celiac axis at its origin and a severe intrinsic stenosis in the superior mesenteric artery secondary to atherosclerotic disease

ical symptoms are usually caused by severe stenosis of multiple visceral vessels that is almost always secondary to atherosclerotic disease [22, 23]. The lateral aortogram is the best study to document the lesions of chronic visceral ischemia since the stenoses are almost always close to the origins of the superior mesenteric, inferior mesenteric, and celiac arteries (Fig. 8). Selective angiography is useful to delineate the collateral circulation between these vessels, but catheterization of severely stenotic vessels should not be performed as a diagnostic exercise because of the risk of occlusion. Crossing these lesions should be limited to the time of intervention. The severity and location of stenosis should be fully evaluated prior to angioplasty. As with the renal arteries, stenoses intrinsic to the superior mesenteric artery tend to respond better to angioplasty than do lesions that involve predominately its origin. Finally, one should look for evidence of a median arcuate ligament extrinsically narrowing the origin of the celiac artery, as patients with this condition are not likely to respond to angioplasty [24].

Acute mesenteric ischemia is a life-threatening condition, with a number of nonspecific physical and laboratory findings that suggest impending bowel infarction [25]. These include abdominal pain (sometimes with peritoneal signs), fever, white count elevation, and abnormal lactate dehydrogenase levels. Due to an aggressive diagnostic and surgical approach, survival from this lethal entity has improved in recent years. Etiologies include acute embolic or thrombotic occlusion of the superior mesenteric artery (50 % of patients), nonocclusive mesenteric ischemia, and superior mesenteric vein thrombosis [26].

Diagnostic angiography generally begins with a lateral aortogram with the pigtail catheter above the celiac axis. This view excludes an acute thrombosis or embolus involving the origin of the celiac or superior mesenteric artery (SMA). This is followed by a selective SMA arteriogram and arterial portography (with intra-arterial vasodilator) to evaluate the superior mesenteric vein. For selective celiac and SMA arteriography we inject from 7–9 cc contrast per second depending on the size of the vessel and the rate of flow within it. Contrast amounts should be increased after administration of a vasodilator. Early and late filming is required to evaluate both the arterial and venous phase (one film per second for 7 films followed by one film per 2 seconds for 12 s). Embolic disease to the visceral vessels is usually seen in patients with underlying cardiac disease and the SMA is most commonly involved. Angiographically, emboli lodge anywhere along the SMA and often do not occlude the origin. The findings are a meniscus at the site of occlusion or an intraluminal filling defect in an incompletely obstructed artery (Fig. 9).

On the other hand, nonocclusive mesenteric ischemia generally occurs in patients with cardiovascular disease, hypotension and low cardiac output. Angiographically, these patients have diffusely narrowed mesenteric arteries without a mechanical obstruction (Fig. 10). The superior

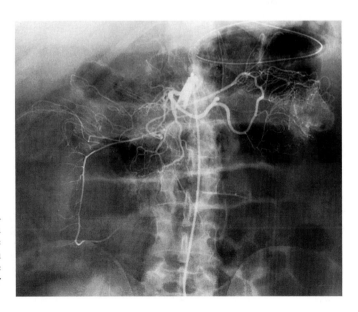

Fig. 9. Superior mesenteric artery embolus. Selective superior mesenteric arteriogram demonstrates an abrupt occlusion of the artery near its origin with a "meniscus sign" in a patient with acute mesenteric ischemia. The patient was found to have a cardiac source for emboli by echocardiography

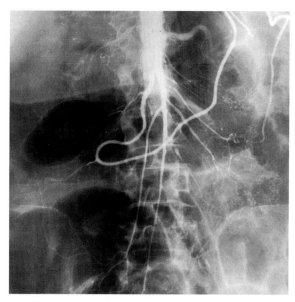

Fig. 10. Nonocclusive mesenteric ischemia. Selective mesenteric arteriogram in a patient with acute mesenteric ischemia demonstrates diffuse narrowing and spasm of multiple superior mesenteric branches, diagnostic of nonocclusive mesenteric ischemia

mesenteric vein is patent. This group of patients benefit from vasodilator therapy, whereas patients with embolic or thrombotic occlusion of the SMA require either lytic therapy (if they do not have signs of clear bowel infarction) or emergent surgical embolectomy and frequently concomitant bowel resection.

Thrombosis of the superior mesenteric vein can cause intestinal ischemia due to congestion. The diagnosis can be difficult to make on arterial portography. Patients have arterial vasoconstriction and, on the venous phase of the angiogram, an associated occluded vein or nonvisualization of the superior mesenteric and portal veins. Isolated cases of mesenteric vein occlusion have been recanalized transhepatically with and without the use of thrombolytics [27].

In this chapter we cover a disparate group of clinical entities that can all be treated with endovascular recanalization techniques. The reader should now have a greater appreciation for the importance of diagnostic angiography prior to the treatment of occlusive disease involving the abdominal aorta and its branches.

References

1. Katzen BT. Cuurrent status of intravascular ultrasound. Rad. Clinics of N. America 1992; 30 (5): 895–905.
2. Neville RF. Endovascular management of arterial intimal defects: an experimental comparison of arteriography, angioscopy, and intravascular ultrasound. J. of Vasc. Surg. 1991, 13 (4): 496–502.
3. Ravidmandalam K, Rao VRK, Kumar S, Gupta AK, Joseph S, Unni M, Rao AS. Obstruction of the infrarenal portion of the abdominal aorta: results of treatment with balloon angioplasty. AJR 1991; 156: 1257–1260.
4. Tegtmeyer CJ, Kellun CD, Kron IL, Mentzer RM. Percutaneous transluminal angioplasty in the region of the aortic bifurcation. Radiology 1985; 157: 661–664.
5. Odurny A, Colapinto RF, Sniderman KW, Johnston KW. Percutaneous transluminal angioplasty of abdominal aortic stenoses. CVIR 1989; 12: 1–6.
6. Yakes WF, Kumpe DA, Brown SB, et al. Percutaneous transluminal aortic angioplasty: techniques and results. Radiology 1989; 172 (3): 965–970.
7. Charlebois N, Saint-Georges G, Hudon G. Percutaneous transluminal angioplasty of the lower abdominal aorta. AJR 1986; 146: 369–371.
8. Morag B, Garniek A, Bass A, Schneiderman J, Walden R, Rubinstein ZJ. Percutaneous transluminal aortic angioplasty: early and results. CVIR 1993; 16: 37–42.
9. Yakes WF, Kumpe DA, Brown SB, et al. Percutaneous transluminal aortic angioplasty: techniques and results. Radiology 1989; 172 (3): 965–970.
10. Rees CR, Palmaz JC, Garcia O, et al. Angioplasty and stenting of completely occluded iliac arteries. Radiology 1989; 172 (3): 953–960.
11. Kumar S, Percutaneous transluminal angioplasty in nonspecific aortoarteritis (Takayasu's disease): experience in 16 cases. CVIR 1989; 12: 321–325.
12. Tegtmeyer CJ, Sos TA. Techniques of renal angioplasty. Radiology 1986; 161: 577–586.
13. Berland II, Koslin DB, Routh WD, Keller FS. Renal artery stenosis: prospective evaluation of diagnosis with color duplex US compared with angiography. Radiology 1990; 174: 421–423.
14. Debatin JF, Spritzer CE, Grist TM, et al. Imaging of the renal arteries: value of MR angiography. AJR 1991; 157: 981–990.
15. Martin LG, Casarella WJ, Gaylord GM. Azotemia caused by renal artery stenosis: treatment by percutaneous angioplasty. AJR 1988; 150: 839–844.
16. Sos TA, Pickering TG, Sniderman K, et al. Percutaneous transluminal renal angioplasty in renovascular hypertension due to atheroma or fibromuscular dysplasia. NEJM 1983; 309 (5): 274–279.
17. Martin LG, Price RB, Casarella WJ, et al. Percutaneous angioplasty in clinical management of renovascular hypertension: initial and long-term results. Radiology 1985; 155: 629–633.
18. Tegtmeyer CJ, Sos TA. Techniques of renal angioplasty. Radiology 1986; 161: 577–586.

19. Martin LG, Casarella WJ, Alspaugh JP, Chuand VP. Renal artery angioplasty: increased technical success and decreased complications in the second 100 patients. Radiology 1986; 159: 631–634.

20. Martin LG, Casarella WJ, Gaylord GM. Azotemia caused by renal artery stenosis: treatment by percutaneous angioplasty. AJR 1988; 150: 839–844.

21. Cicuto KP, McLean GK, Oleaga JA, Freiman DB, Grossman RA, Ring EJ. Renal artery stenosis: anatomic classification for percutaneous transluminal angioplasty. AJR 1981; 137: 599–601.

22. Calderon M, Reul GJ, Gregoric ID, et al. Long-term results of the surgical management of symptomatic chronic intestinal ischemia. J Cardiovasc Surg 1992; 33: 723–728.

23. Golden DA, Ring EJ, McLean GK, Freiman DB. Percutaneous transluminal angioplasty in the treatment of abdominal angina. AJR 1982; 139: 247–249.

24. Odurny A, Sniderman KW, Colapinto RF. Intestinal angina: percutaneous transluminal angioplasty of the celiac and superior mesenteric arteries. Radiology 1988; 167: 59–62.

25. Ottinger LW. Acute mesenteric ischemia. NEJM 1982; 307 (9): 535–537.

26. Clark RA, Gallant TE. Acute mesenteric ischemia: angiographic spectrum. AJR 1984; 142: 555–562.

27. Yankes JR, Uglietta JP, Grant J, Braum SD. Percutaneous transhepatic recanalization and thrombolysis of the superior mesenteric vein. AJR 1988; 151: 289–290.

Peripheral Angiography

E. Zeitler

Indications

Angiography of the lower extremities is indicated whenever a definite diagnosis is required and/or revascularization therapy is planned [1–4]. The indications for peripheral diagnostic angiography include:

1. Peripheral occlusive disease with rest pain and necrosis/gangrene (Fontaine classification III and IV)
2. Severe intermittent claudication (Fontaine classification IIb, in selected cases IIa)
3. Critical limb ischemia (acute and chronic), e.g. embolization
4. Suspected femoropopliteal aneurysm
5. Suspected thromboangiitis obliterans
6. Suspected microembolizations, e.g. blue-toe-syndrome
7. Suspected arteriovenous (AV) malformations, e.g., congenital angiodysplasia
8. Suspected vascular trauma
9. Tumors of soft tissues and bones
10. Follow-up evaluations after revascularizations

In addition, peripheral angiography is performed in conjuction with peripheral vascular interventions to document lesions and show their morphology. The status of the distal vascular beds prior to and following the interventions should always be assessed.

Techniques

Selection of the angiographic approach depends on the clinical problem, the question to be answered, the results of noninvasive evaluations, and the status of the prospective puncture site. Basic angiographic approaches include (see also Fig. 1):

1. Selective femoral arteriography (Figs. 2, 3a–c)
   a) Retrograde ipsilateral or contralateral
   b) Antegrade ipsilateral

2. Abdominal aortography with peripheral arteriography
   a) Retrograde transfemoral (Figs. 4a–f, 5a–b)
   b) Retrograde transbrachial or transaxillary (Fig. 6)
   c) Translumbar
3. Intravenous digital subtraction angiography (DSA)
   a) Retrograde transfemoral
   b) Retrograde transcubital with catheterization of the vena cava inferior or of the right atrium
4. Transpopliteal retrograde arteriography

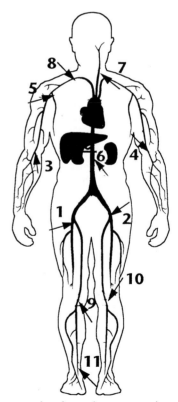

Fig. 1. Puncture sites for catheter access in arterial angiography. *1*, Transfemoral retrograde; *2*, transfemoral orthograde; *3*, transbrachial retrograde; *4*, transbrachial orthograde; *5*, transaxillary; *6* translumbar; *7* transcarotid; *8*, transsubclavian; *9*, transpopliteal retrograde; *10*, transpopliteal orthograde; *11*, transtibial retrograde

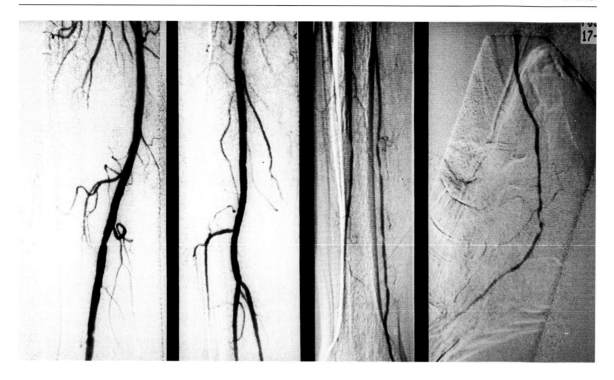

Fig. 2. Arteriography of the femoral arteries after retrograde needle puncture with the DSA technique. Stenoses of the tibial arteries and occlusion of the dorsal pedal artery are seen

In diagnostic angiography a retrograde transfemoral puncture is the preferred approach in the majority of patients [1, 6]. In patients with severe obstructive disease an alternative puncture site must be sought. In periinterventional angiography the puncture site is primarily determined by the location, extent, and distribution of the vascular pathology [5].

To ensure the angiographic examination is successfully performed and to minimize the risk of complications, it is recommended that the following basic rules be followed:

1. The physician is familiarized with the clinical situation.
2. The appropriateness of the indication is checked.
3. The optimum puncture site is determined.
4. The appropriate instrumentation (Table 1) is selected [3, 4].
5. The patient is adequately monitored.
6. Technically adequate and well-maintained angiography equipment is used.

7. The patient, the staff, and the physcician are protected from radiation.
8. Most importantly, the procedure is performed only if the physician has been adequately trained in percutaneous diagnostics and therapy, in interpretation of the results, and in treatment of complications.

Conventional and Digital Angiography

Whereas in peripheral diagnostic angiography both conventional and digital subtraction angiography (DSA) are frequently used, in periinterventional imaging DSA is much the preferred technique. The major advantages of DSA compared with conventional angiography include: higher image contrast resolution, rapid image availability, selective imaging, and direct control of the image acquisition by the operator, all particularly important in highly interactive and selective peri-interventional imaging. In addition, digitally based techniques such as "road mapping," "perivision," and "supervision" facilitate the operator's visual control over the intervention and the immediate evaluation of its morphologic and functional results. In addition, when using

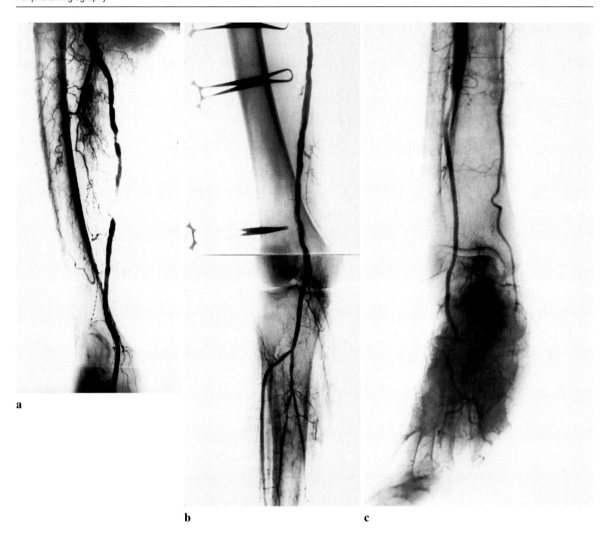

a

b   c

Fig. 3a–c. Orthograde femoral arteriography in a 77-year-old woman with rest pain and claudication. **a** Superficial femoral artery (SFA) occlusion shorter than 5 cm and a segmental stenosis. **b** SFA control angiography after successful angioplasty with the Dotter-Grüntzig technique. **c** Calf and foot arteries of the same patient

DSA, the contrast media load and the radiation exposure are usually reduced. Nevertheless, even the most sophisticated angiographic equipment is not a replacement for operator knowledge or compensation for lack of it. Optimum results are achieved only by a combination of medical expertise and a high level of imaging technology. With the imaging technology available today, misinterpretations of stenoses, artifacts, superpositons of vessels, and functional abnormalities can largely be avoided.

Angiographic Examination

With the exception of small children and critically ill patients, peripheral angiographies are performed with the patient under local anesthesia. Depending on the clinical setting, the majority of diagnostic procedures can be performed on an outpatient basis. In contrast, percutaneous interventions and associated angiographies are performed on an overnight or inpatient basis. In patients undergoing diagnostic and peri-interventional angiography the results of laboratory tests, including tests for creatinine, electrolytes, prothrombin partial thromboplastin time (PTT), and thrombocytes, should be available. Patients should fast for at least 4 h prior to examination, intravenous access should be in place, and i.v. fluids are started on the ward. In patients receiving i.v. heparin the infusion is stopped 4 h prior to

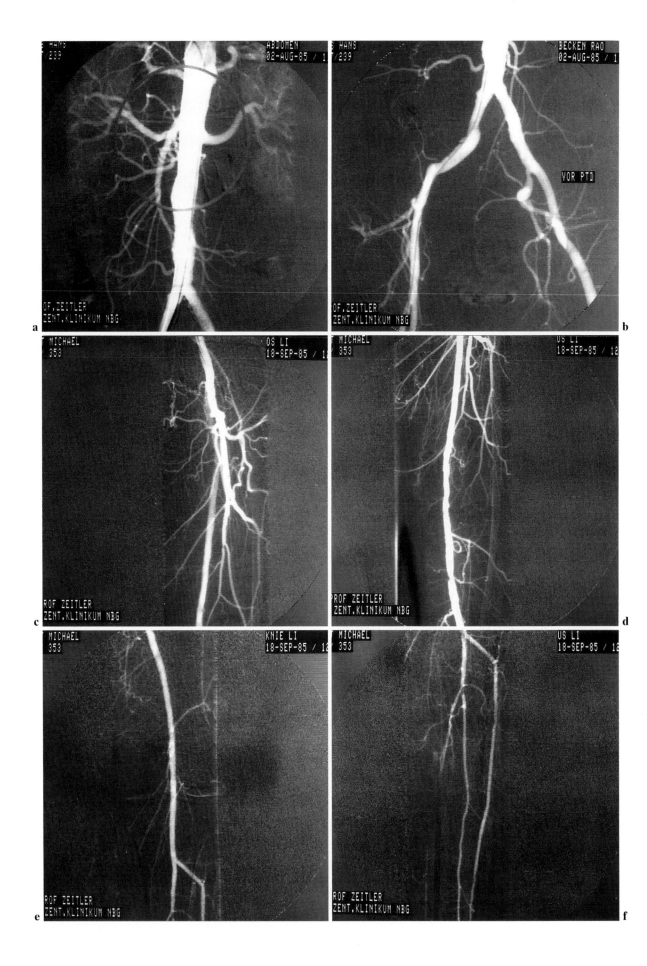

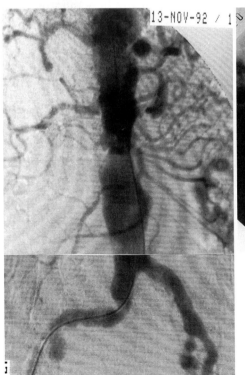

◀ **Fig. 4 a–f.** Arteriograms demonstrate the abdominal aorta, the pelvic arteries, and the arteries of the left leg

arterial puncture and restarted 6 h after the procedure. In patients receiving sodium warfarin (Coumadin), the drug is replaced by i.v. heparin at least 2 days prior to the procedure. In patients receiving insulin the regimen is adjusted to the fasting state. These patients are placed on the top of the schedule and studied first in the morning.

Patient Interview

Prior to the patients interview the angiographer studies the clinical history and reviews the results of the recent laboratory tests. During the interview the patient is informed about the procedure, procedural risks, outcomes, and possible therapeutic consequences. Informed consent is obtained and the date of the examination determined. If percutaneous revascularizations are planned in the same setting, informed consent for the revascularization procedure is also obtained.

Premedication

In patients with known allergies to contrast media or those with allergic diatheses premedication with corticosteroids and histamine H_1 and H_2 receptor antagonists at least 30 min prior to the contrast medium injection is obligatory. In patients with a history of a severe contrast media allergy 40 mg prednisolone daily for 2 days prior to the procedure is recommended. In some institutions allergic prophylaxis is given irrespective of history to all patients undergoing angiography. In the majority of patients preprocedural sedation is not required although depending on patient and physician preference it is often administered.

Procedure

After the patient has had the access site cleaned and shaved he or she is placed on the angiography table. Local anesthesia is given in our institution preferably using 1 % lidocaine without suprarenin. Using the Seldinger technique, retrograde catheterization of the femoral artery is performed. In patients with severe peripheral occlu-

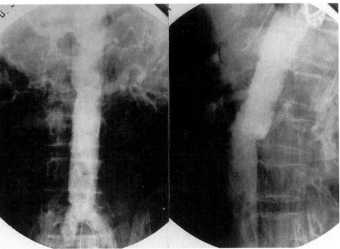

Fig. 5 a, b. Digital subtraction angiography of the abdominal aorta and the pelvic arteries. **a** Infrarenal abdominal aortic aneurysm, and stenosis of the left renal artery are seen. **b** Conventional aortography after surgical graft implantation and thromboendarterectomy of the left renal artery

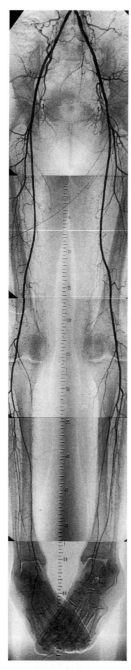

Fig. 6. Digital subtraction angiography of the abdominal and both leg arteries after transbrachial catheterization

In our laboratory a safety J-guide with a flexible tip and a 6-mm curve is used. As soon as the guide wire is securely placed in the vessel, the needle is withdrawn, the guide wire is cleaned with a saline solution, and the selected angiography catheter is inserted and positioned within the desired vessel. Generally, in diagnostic aortography with peripheral runoff a 5F pigtail catheter with multiple side holes is used. When the crossover approach has been chosen for selective angiography of the contralateral limb and renal, coeliac, and mesenteric arteries, the 5F–7F "sidewinder" or less frequently the "cobra" or the "head-hunting" catheters are used.

In peri-interventional angiography the target vascular segment is visualized via the sheath or a tapered 5F catheter. During the procedure the side arm of the Y-adapter or the guide wire port of the dilatation catheter often serve as injection site.

Whereas in diagnostic peripheral angiography the use of an introductory sheath is not obligatory, it is required in peri-interventional settings. For X-ray contrast the low-osmolality nonionic contrast agents are preferably used. In diagnostic procedures the contrast medium injections are performed depending on the vascular territory either manually or using a power injector. The total volume of the injection, the volumetric flow rates, and the imaging frame rates depend on the vascular bed studied, circulatory times, and other variables. Numerous recommendations have been given in the literature [1, 3, 7]. In peri-interventional angiography small-volume manual injections are usually sufficient to define the sites of vascular intervention. Larger volume injections might be needed to document the status of the peripheral runoff vessels.

Complications

The incidence of complications is dependent on the patient's age, severity of the peripheral disease, procedure time, operator experience, and other variables. Relevant data on complications related to the adverse reactions to contrast media, puncture site, catheter, and guide wire manipulations are cited in the literature [3, 7]. In peri-interventional angiography the complications are difficult to separate from those due to actual interventions and therefore are not usually indicated.

sive disease an alternative access, i.e. brachial, axillary, transpopliteal, or translumbar, may be necessary.

Following the correct arterial puncture a vigorous reflow of blood occurs. Using the Seldinger technique [6], a guide wire may be gently introduced.

Interpretation and Diagnosis

Irrespective of the specific vascular bed the pathomorphologic features of the angiographically documented peripheral lesions should be evaluated according to basic guidelines (see also Fig. 7), e.g.,

1. Stenosis — multiplicity, location, length, eccentricity, surface morphology (smooth/irregular/ulcerated)
2. Occlusion — length, collateralization, duration
3. Diffuse wall irregularities — extent, severity, ulceration
4. Dilatations — localized (aneurysm), diffuse (ectasia)
5. Arteriovenous shunts — singular (AV fistulas), multiple (AV malformation, angioma)
6. Mural defects — rupture, tear, dissection, involution

The severity of the stenosis and the length of the occlusion should be measured preferably against the skeletal background; and the shunt volume of the abnormal AV connections should be estimated. In addition, extended calcifications and collateral circulations (Fig. 8) including the runin and runoff vessels should be described. In cases of acute peripheral gangrene or necrosis the areas of hyper- or avascularization in peripheral runoff vessels should be evaluated. Patients with arterial bleeding and/or with tumors must be assessed regarding the degree of pathologic vascularization, the site of the feeding artery, infiltrations, and

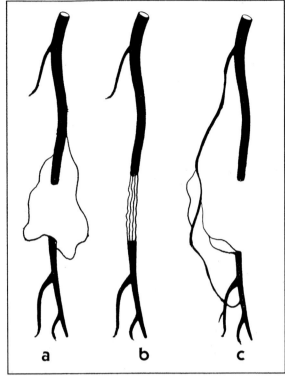

Fig. 8. Different types of collateralizations of arterial occlusions. *a*, Direct collateral vessel; *b*, adventitial collateral vessel; *c*, indirect collateral vessel

contrast pooling. In peri-interventional angiography the emphasis is on accurate definition of the lesions' surface morphology and close monitoring of the state of the peripheral runoff vessels.

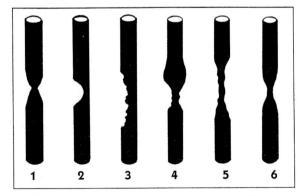

Fig. 7. Different types of arterial stenoses. *1*, Ring stenosis; *2*, smooth, eccentric stenosis; *3*, eccentric, verrucous stenosis; *4*, excentric, verrucous stenosis with poststenotic dilatation; *5*, band-shaped stenosis; *6*, hour-glass-shaped stenosis

Table 1. Peripheral percutaneous revascularization procedures and diagnostic devices

1. Low-speed rotating guide wire (Vallbracht)
2. High-speed rotating catheter (Kensey)
3. Laser application systems
4. High-frequency application catheter
5. Atherectomy devices
6. Different percutaneously applicable endoprostheses
   a) Balloon-expandable stents (Palmaz stent, Strecker stent, Gianturco-Roubin stent)
   b) Self-expanding stents (Wallstent, Cragg-Nitinol stent)
7. Diagnostic devices
   a) Intravascular angioscopy
   b) Intravascular ultrasound

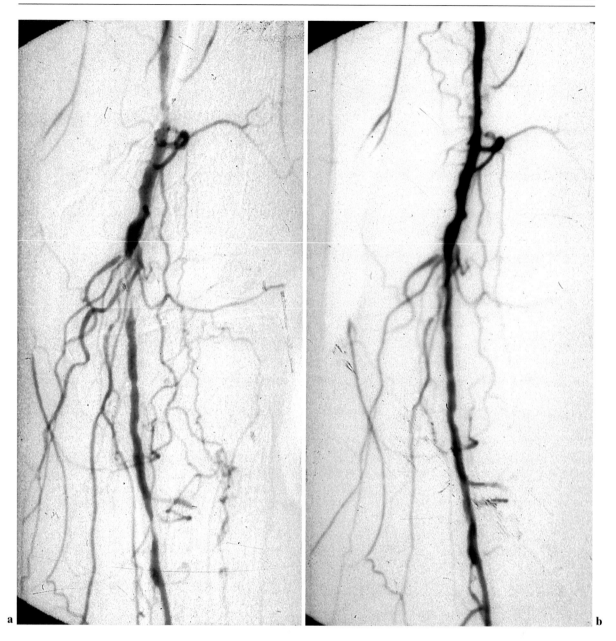

Fig. 9 a, b. Infrainguinal angioplasty; pre-PTA (**a**) and post-PTA (**b**) results are documented

Peri-interventional Angiography

The main percutaneous revascularization techniques include the Dotter technique using single or coaxial catheters, balloon dilatations according to Grüntzig known as percutaneous transluminal angioplasty (PTA), directional and rotational atherectomy, local and systemic thrombolysis, as-piration thrombectomy and embolectomy, stent implantation, and laser angioplasty (Table 1). Conventional angiographic images are evaluated to identify the lesions, to estimate the size of instrumentation required and to decide the specifics of the revascularization strategy. During the interventions fluoroscopy is employed to assist the operator in assessing the regions of the prospective interventions and to survey the state of the peripheral runoff vessels. External markers are helpful to locate the lesions against the background. "Road map" techniques are employed to

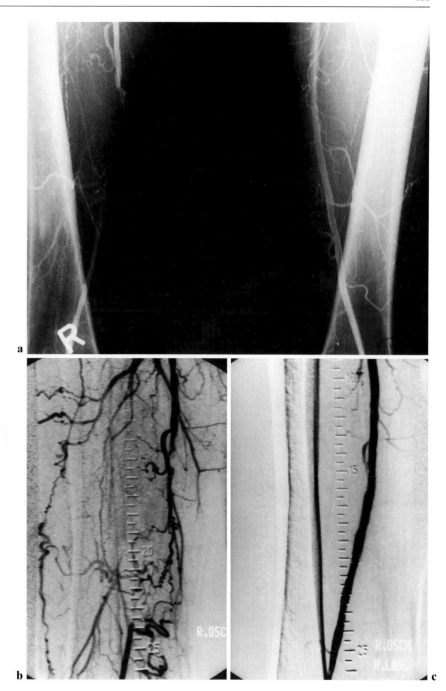

Fig. 10 a–c. Conventional angiography (**a**) showing a 12 cm segment occlusion of the right femoral superficial artery. Corresponding pre- and post- (**b, c**) interventional DSA images

facilitate the manipulation of the percutaneous hardware and to increase the precision of the hardware positioning. Brief contrast media injections allow close monitoring of the progress of the intervention as well as the DSA documentation of its results. Contrast media are used sparingly, and the imaging time is kept to a minimum.

The peri-interventional angiography begins with documentation and clear localization of the le-

sions for which intervention is required. Besides confirming the presence of a hemodynamically significant stenosis, the severity, length, and surface morphology of the lesion are defined. In lesions of questionable hemodynamic significance, particularly in the pelvis, the translesional pressure gradient can be measured. Spontaneous gradients or gradients induced by pharmacologic vasodilation greater than 20 mmHg are deemed to be signifi-

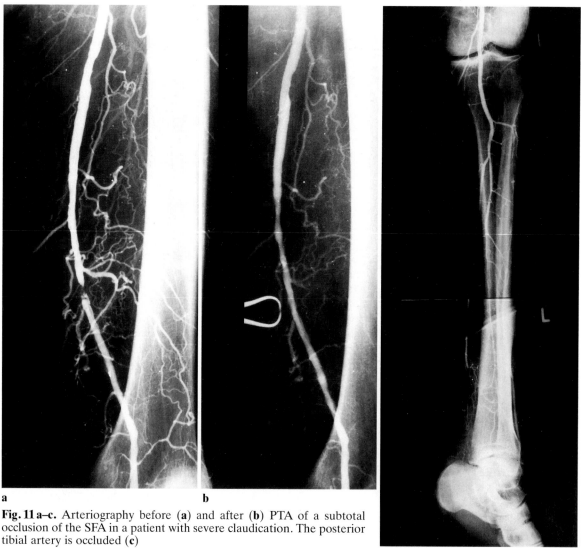

a   b

Fig. 11 a–c. Arteriography before (**a**) and after (**b**) PTA of a subtotal
occlusion of the SFA in a patient with severe claudication. The posterior
tibial artery is occluded (**c**)

c

cant. Markedly eccentric lesions, or those located
at branching points and bifurcations, are visualized
in at least two, preferably perpendicular, projections. The lesion's surface morphology is carefully
evaluated to assess the presence of thromboses,
ulcerations, dissections, calcifications, and vasa
vasorum collateralizations. It is essential to document the status of the peripheral runoff and of the
collateral vessels prior to each intervention.

During the interventions fluoroscopy and DSA
are used to guide the operator and to allow immediate assessment of the results of the performed percutaneous therapy. Based on the intrainterventional evaluations of the fluoroscopic
or DSA images, decisions are made as to the need
for repeat inflations, different instrumentation

sizing, or a change in revascularization strategy.
The morphologic appearance of the lesion is continuously monitored and the state of the dependent circulation is periodically monitored also to
allow immediate recognition of complications
such as dissections, extravasations, and closures.
Meticulous attention must be paid to the appearance of new dissection lines, intraluminal haziness, opacifications of extravascular structures,
and missing vascular opacifications. If dissection
lines are present, an attempt should be made to
assess their direction, extent, and severity. In contrast medium extravasations, circumscribed adventitial injuries and free perforations should be
differentiated. Closures of formerly present collaterals must be noted. Although frequent repeat

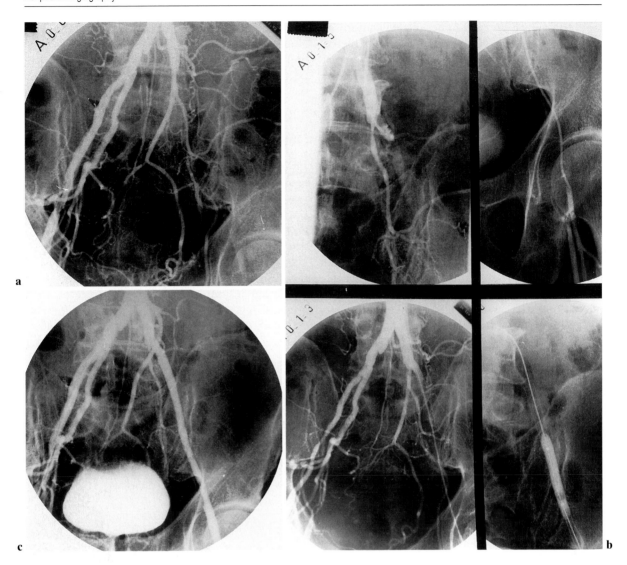

Fig. 12a–c. Combined percutaneous revascularization in a 54-year-old patient with severe claudication, 6 months after PTA of a high-grade external iliac stenosis on the left. **a** Angiography before treatment shows a total occlusion of the external iliac artery. **b** Sequential angiography showing the steps of the revascularization including thrombolysis with 250000IU urokinase, recanalization with a guide wire, balloon dilatation, and Wallstent implantation. **c** Pelvic angiogram showing the final result following combined revascularization of the left external iliac artery occlusion

injections may be necessary, contrast medium administration during interventions in particular balloon inflations should be avoided.

Following the percutaneous procedure the results are documented by angiography, angioscopy, intravascular ultrasound, or with color-coded duplex sonography, including the morphology of the revascularized arterial segments (Figs. 9a, b, 10a–c). The state of the entire runoff vessels must also be documented (Fig. 11a–c). Meticulous study of the images obtained is helpful to prevent acute complications. Although the ultimate goal of percutaneous revascularizations is complete removal of the flow obstructions, in reality this goal is not always achieved. In general, residual obstructions of up to 20 % represent an acceptable outcome. Residual stenoses of greater than 20 %, larger intimal flaps, and dissections usually require additional interventions such as directional atherectomy or stent implantation.

At present, the majority of peripheral percutaneous procedures are performed to revascularize single or multiple stenoses in one or more vascular territories. Less frequently, recanalizations of totally obstructed vessels with an obstructed segment longer than 10 cm are performed (Fig. 10a–c). The majority of procedures is currently performed using the standard PTA employing Teflon-coated safety J- or Terumo guide wires along with angioplasty balloon catheters selected for size and performance.

In complex stenoses and acute occlusions a combined approach consisting for example of intraarterial lysis, aspiration thromboembolectomy, angioplasty, and possibly stent implantation is selected (Fig. 12a–c). In highly eccentric, calcific, and diffuse stenoses in addition to chronic occlusions, additional angioplasty devices (Table 1) may improve the success rate [5]. However, the precise role and indications for the use of the devices, with the possible exception of stent implantation for the improvement of suboptimal angioplasty results in the abdominal aorta and in the iliac arteries, have not yet been established. Similarly, the diagnostic role of the peri-interventional use of intravascular ultrasonography and percutaneous angioscopy remains to be defined.

Perisurgical Angiography

Presurgical angiography is required to define accurately the vascular pathology and to provide the surgeon with a vascular "road map" to allow planning of the revascularization strategy. The status of the runin and runoff vessels must be defined. The presurgical angiogram answers a number of questions including the requirement for surgical or combined surgical and percutaneous revascularization, the optimum surgical strategy, and identification of the sites of the proximal and distal bypass anastomoses. In patients selected for femorocrural bypasses the foot arteries are also visualized. To estimate more accurately the spatial extent of the vascular pathology, in particular in patients with abdominal aortic aneurysms, tortuous arteries, and bifurcation lesions, additional oblique and lateral projections are often required. To allow the definition of slowly filling arteries distal to unilateral obstructions or multiple severe stenoses, additional correctly timed projections are obtained. In these instances DSA has proved particularly advantageous. Postsurgical angiography is required to document the morphologic and functional outcome of the operation. Particular attention must be paid to visualization of the anasto-

motic sites and of the body of the grafts to detect at an early stage anastomotic or clamping stenoses and suture dehiscences. If complications are suspected, additional projections are required for complete documentation.

Angiography in Specific Clinical Pictures

In patients with peripheral atherosclerotic vascular disease the distribution of lesions differs between smokers and diabetics. In the former, lesions in the femoral superficial arteries, in particular Hunter's canal, and in the iliac artery prevail, whereas in the latter the lesions are located primarily in the deep femoral, crural, and foot arteries, usually leaving the pelvic arteries free from significant lesions. In angiographies of the foot arteries, avascular and hypervascular diabetic macroangiopathies can be distinguished (Fig. 13).

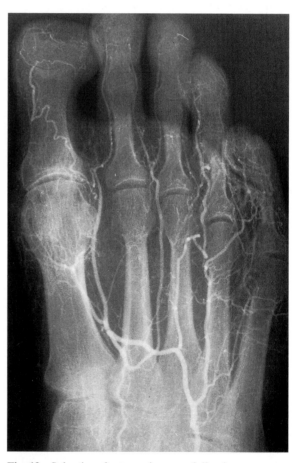

Fig. 13. Selective foot angiogram following an antegrade puncture of the ipsilateral SFA in a patient with diabetic micro- and macroangiopathy

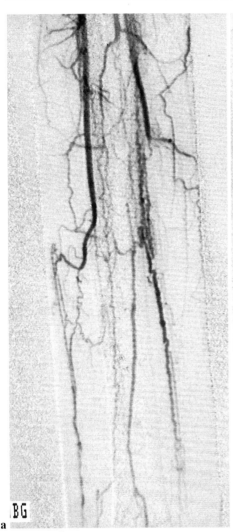

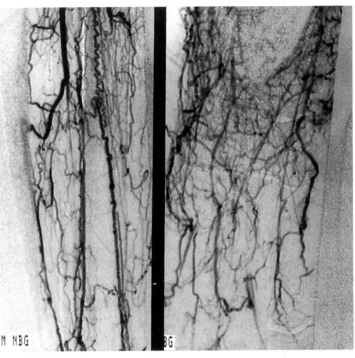

Fig. 14 a, b. Selective left leg arteriography via catheterization from the right groin demonstrating typical occlusions and collateralizations in a patient with Buerger's disease

Buerger's disease (thromboangiitis obliterans) more often affects the arteries of the lower legs and feet, but also of the forearms and hands. The lesions begin distally, involving larger and more central arteries in the later stages. Angiographic signs include segmental occlusions of the tibial and foot arteries and tightly coiled corkscrew-shaped collaterals of the vasa vasorum (Fig. 14 a, b). The majority of patients are men less than 45 years of age and heavy cigarette smokers. Accompanying superficial or migrating phlebitis is common. In patients with concomitant atherosclerotic disease superficial femoral and iliac artery lesions are also seen.

Peripheal embolizations of the lower extremities are typically found at bifurcations and branching points such as the popliteal trifurcation, femoral bifurcation, and muscular branching of the deep femoral artery. The corresponding filling defects display straight or concave edges, the interruption of blood supply to the distal circulation is usually complete, and the collateral circulation is typically absent (Fig. 15). Acute thrombosis often displays a convex delineation, occurring proximally to a chronic stenosis. Peripheral embolizations in small arteries of the digitis or toes such as those characteristic of blue-toe syndrome require high-quality angiograms and often the help of higher magnifications. Regardless of localization, proper management includes identification of the responsible thromboembolic source.

Aneurysms are detected as fusiform, saccular, false, or dissecting segmental arterial dilatations. Due to partial thrombosis with luminal obstruc-

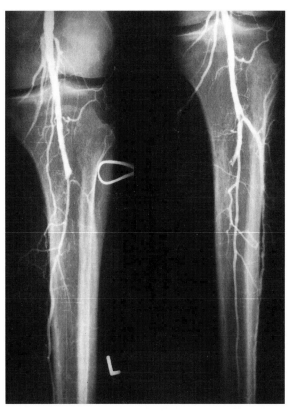

Fig. 15. Infrainguinal angiography in a patient with an embolic obstruction at the level of the trifurcation before (*left*) and after (*right*) percutaneous aspiration thrombembolectomy. Residual thrombus is visualized

tion, peripheral aneurysms can be missed on routine angiograms. In these cases, noninvasive vascular imaging techniques will establish the diagnosis. The pulsatile popliteal aneurysms are often accompanied by elongation of the superficial femoral artery and kinking or emoblizations in the tibioperoneal arteries. Popliteal artery entrapment is due to the abnormal insertion of the gastrocnemius muscle, causing medial displacement and external compression of the popliteal artery. Typical angiographic findings include poststenotic dilatation, stenoses, occlusions, and distal embolizations in a medially deviated artery. A more complete presentation of specific peripheral angiographic findings including pathologic arteriovenous communications and tumor vessels is available in the standard literature [3].

References

1. Zeitler E (1974) Aortoarteriographie. In: Heberer G, Rau G, Schoop W (eds) Angiologie. Thieme, Stuttgart, pp 243–298
2. Zeitler E, Grosse-Vorholt R (1980) Angiography in angiology. In: Vertraete M (ed) Methods in angiology. Martinus Nijhoff, The Hague, pp 303–333
3. Abrams HL (ed) (1983) Angiogaphy, 3rd. Little, Brown, Boston
4. Johnsrude IS, Jackson DC, Dunnick NR (1987) A practical approach to angiography. Little, Brown, Boston
5. Dondelinger RF, Rossi P, Kurdziel JC, Wallace S (eds) (1990) Interventional radiology. Thieme, Stuttgart
6. Seldinger SJ (1953) Catheter replacement of the needle in percutaneous arteriography. Acta Radiol 39: 368–376
7. Kandarpa K (1989) Handbook of cardiovascular and interventional radiologic procedures. Little, Brown, Boston

Section II
Radiographic Venography

Central and Peripheral Venography

P. C. Lakin and J. Rösch

Introduction

The role of contrast venography in the diagnosis of venous pathology has been reduced in recent years by the introduction of noninvasive vascular techniques including ultrasound, Doppler, nuclear imaging, computed tomography, and magnetic resonance imaging. In the diagnosis of acute deep vein thrombosis compression ultrasonography has all but replaced contrast venography [13, 16, 30, 37]. Computed tomography and duplex sonography have both been advocated in the diagnosis of Budd-Chiari syndrome and portal vein thrombosis [3, 34, 48, 50]. Magnetic resonance imaging has been recommended for the diagnosis of iliac and subclavian vein thrombosis [20] and renal vein compression [31]. Contrast venography is often still useful, particularly for the diagnosis of acute calf vein thrombosis, chronic deep vein thrombosis, and iliac vein thrombosis, where ultrasonography is less sensitive [12]. Contrast venography also remains the final diagnostic technique to confirm diagnoses suspected by other modalities. It is particularly important prior to percutaneous interventional therapy, which requires detailed definition of venous pathology in order to select the proper intervention and evaluate its outcome.

Technique

Contrast venography can be performed utilizing spot filming during fluoroscopy, standard or serial roentgenography, or digital substraction angiography (DSA). Depending on the examined area different imaging techniques are preferred.

Upper Extremity Veins

The upper extremity venogram is usually performed by injection of contrast medium into a hand or wrist vein entered by a 19-G needle or angiocath. For better visualization of the proximal arm veins or the subclavian and innominate veins, an injection into a median cubital vein which drains into the basilic vein is preferred. In the case of obstruction of central veins, catheterization of the median cubital vein with injection into the axillary or subclavian vein close to the obstruction gives the best results. Either ionic or nonionic contrast medium with lower iodine concentration (30%–40%) is used for the peripheral injections through a needle while the higher concentration (60%–70%) is utilized for central catheter injections. Either DSA or serial large film roentgenography are the preferred imaging techniques. Single film technique is unsatisfactory in the upper extremity because of flow dynamics.

Superior Vena Cava

The superior vena cava (SVC) and its innominate branches are best visualized by simultaneous contrast injections into the subclavian or axillary veins via catheters introduced through the cubital veins. To visualize the internal jugular veins and their drainage into the SVC, direct injections through percutaneously introduced catheters are necessary. The entire upper chest should be filmed in the frontal projection to identify collateral circulation. A lateral view is useful by providing further information about a SVC lesion. In the case of SVC occlusion the distal extent of the occlusion must also be defined in order to properly select the proper interventional treatment. A direct venogram is performed with a catheter introduced by the femoral approach and advanced through the right atrium to the occluding lesion. Imaging is performed with DSA or large rapid serial filming. The higher (60%–70%) concentraiton contrast medium is utilized. We prefer this concentration even for DSA.

Inferior Vena Cava and Pelvic Veins

The inferior vena cava (IVC) is best visualized with the direct injection of contrast through a catheter in its distal portion. The catheter can be introduced from either the femoral or jugular approach. The femoral approach is preferred, assuming there are no contraindications such as clinical or duplex evidence of iliac vein thrombosis or occlusion. Although either the left or right femoral vein can be utilized for diagnostic examinations, it is frequently easier to advance the more rigid sheaths required for filter or stent

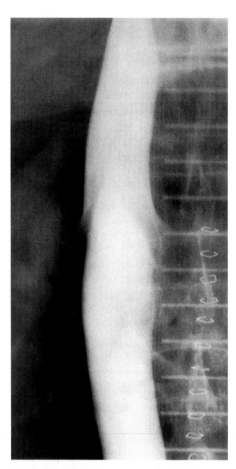

Fig. 1. Normal inferior vena cavogram performed prior to filter placement. Normal bilateral flow defects are evident from the inflow of nonopacified blood from the renal veins

placement through the right iliac veins. The transjugular approach is used when the femoral approach is not available because of iliac or distal IVC thrombus or precluding clinical circumstances.

The external and common iliac veins are visualized by the direct injection of contrast through a short catheter to evaluate the ipsilateral vein. If the iliac veins are to be evaluated bilaterally, both femoral veins need to be catheterized. Contrast is then injected simultaneously through both catheters utilizing a Y connector attached to the injector. Alternatively, four to six additional sideholes can be placed in the shaft of a multisidehole catheter approximately 20 cm from its end. When the catheter is advanced from the iliac vein over the IVC bifurcation into the contralateral iliac vein, sideholes are present in both iliac veins, thus allowing the bilateral examination to be performed from a unilateral approach. If evaluation of the internal iliac veins is needed, they must be selectively catheterized with the retrograde injection of contrast. However, adequate opacification beyond the catheter tip is difficult because of washout of the contrast by nonopacified blood. Either DSA or rapid serial roentgenography is utilized for visualization of IVC and pelvic veins. If intervention is planned, a ruler should be placed under the patient to be able to accurately measure the size of the IVC prior to filter or stent placement (Fig. 1). Contrast medium with high iodine concentration (76%) is used, and films are obtained in the frontal view. A lateral view of the IVC should also be obtained to evaluate the extent of extrinsic compression secondary to retroperitoneal or intrahepatic lesions or fibrosis.

Lower Extremity Veins

Lower extremity venography is performed with the patient in the semierect position (45°–60°) on a tilting radiographic table. The patient's uninvolved foot rests on a box 15–20 cm in height to allow the involved leg to be in a non-weight-bearing position. This is essential to prevent artifacts from muscular compression of the veins, especially the popliteal vein, and to obtain adequate opacification of the deep and muscular veins of the calf. Venipuncture is performed in a vein in the dorsum of the foot or the superficial vein of the great toe employing a 19- to 23-G butterfly needle, and the needle is secured in place. The di-

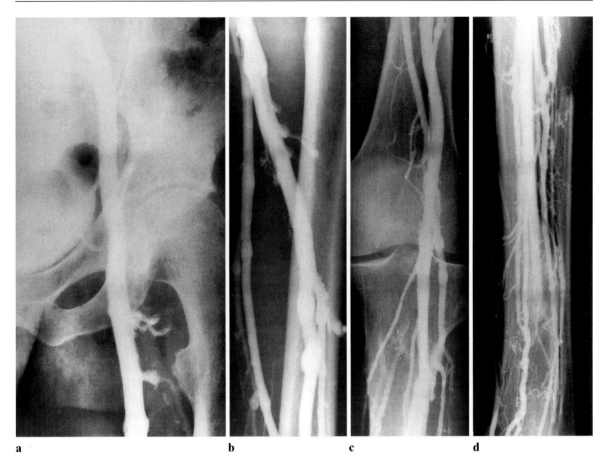

a   b   c   d

Fig. 2a–d. Normal left femoral venogram in a patient with a previous femoral-popliteal bypass graft

luted contrast medium (half contrast and half saline) is then injected, usually by hand, with a total of 100–150 cc injected. A tourniquet at the ankle frequently improves opacification of the deep veins. Either spot filming or standard large film roentgenography during the injection of contrast is performed although digital venography has also been advocated [40]. The first films of the calf (anteroposterior and roll-out lateral) and of the knee are obtained after the injection of 60–90 cc. Films of the thigh and pelvis follow after injection of additonal contrast medium. The patient is asked to forcibly dorsiflex the involved foot for these last two films by placing a box beneath the involved foot and having the patient step down onto the box at the time of the exposure. This causes the calf muscles to compress the deep veins in the calf and results in improved opacification of the femoral and iliac veins (Fig. 2).

Portal System

The portal system is most easily studied by visceral pharmacoangiography with the injection of contrast medium into the superior mesenteric or celiac artery. For better visualization of the portal venous phase of the angiogram we utilize an injection of the vasodilator tolazoline HCl (25–50 mg) 20 seconds prior to the contrast injection (Fig. 3). If portal intervention, for example, transjugular intrahepatic portosystemtic shunt (TIPS) placement or portal variceal embolization, is planned, the portogram can be performed by directly accessing the intrahepatic portal vein via a percutaneous transjugular transhepatic approach (Fig. 4).

Diagnosis

Even with excellent opacification of the venous system, flow defects secondary to the inflow of nonopacified blood appear under normal circumstances. In the evaluation of the venogram, nor-

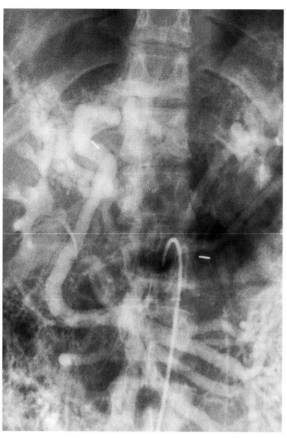

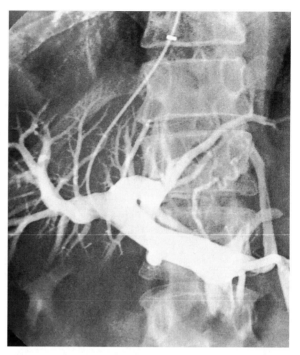

Fig. 4. Transhepatic portal venogram performed from the transjugular approach prior to a TIPS procedure. Excellent opacification of the portal system including gastric and esophageal varices is obtained

Fig. 3. Portal venogram obtained with superior mesenteric artery injection of contrast medium following intra-arterial tolazine HCl (50 mg) demonstrates portal vein thrombosis with extensive hepatopetal collateral circulation (cavernous transformation of the portal vein)

mal flow defects must be differentiated from defects caused by thrombus, extrinsic compression, or intraluminal neoplasm. Each of these lesions exhibit certain specific findings, and together with the evaluation of the clinical history and symptoms it is often possible to provide an accurate diagnosis.

Thrombosis

In *peripheral veins*, acute thrombus is frequently seen as a constant smooth intraluminal filling defect. With clot retraction, contrast may track between an occlusive clot and the wall of the vein resulting in a "railroad track" appearance (Fig. 5). Occasionally a meniscus appearance is evident between the column of contrast and the superior

or inferior margin of the clot, particularly in subacute thrombi. Extensive thrombosis usually causes complete occlusion of deep veins of an extremity. However, the nonvisualization of a vein(s) on a venogram, no matter how excellent the quality, is not a reliable indicator of deep vein thrombosis (DVT). Apparent venous obstruction on the venogram may be due to artifact from flow defects or extrinsic venous compression, either from technical factors (such as patient positioning or tourniquet placement) or from compressive syndromes [62]. Visualization of the trifurcation veins of the calf is particularly variable. The anterior tibial veins are frequently not seen, particularly if the injection is high in the dorsum of the foot.

In the chronic phase of DVT the veins appear irregular. When the acute thrombosis resolves by recanalization, the venous lumen is open but sometimes narrowed and does not exhibit any valves (Fig. 6). With healing by collateralization the venous lumen is replaced by irregular tortuous collaterals [55]. According to Hach [29], there is complete recanalization of the veins in 35.5% of patients, partial recanalization in 53.4%, and continued occlusion in the remaining 11.1%.

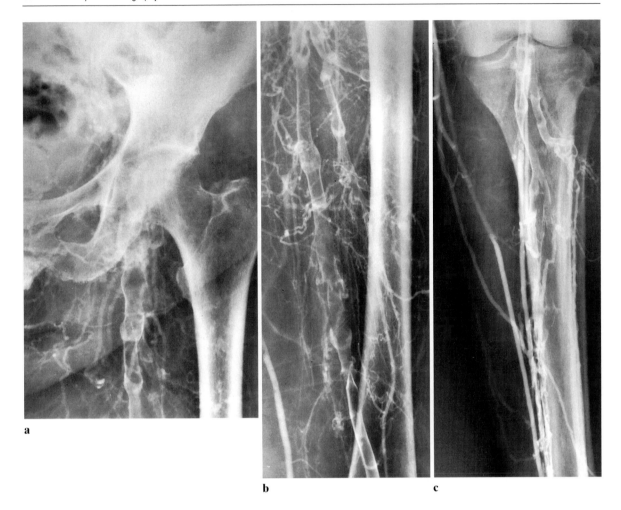

a b c

Fig. 5a–c. Extensive deep vein thrombosis of the left femoral system. Intraluminal thrombus extends from the calf veins through the iliac veins. Note the collateral flow to the contralateral obturator and pudendal veins

Venous thrombosis in the *upper extremity* is much less common than in the lower extremities and accounts for approximately 2% of patients presenting with DVT. It is usually secondary to peripheral line placement. Axillary and subclavian vein thrombosis are mostly associated with local trauma from central line or pacer placement [9, 23], compressive syndromes or neoplastic encasement. Pulmonary emboli from upper extremity thrombosis are rare but are reported from subclavian vein thrombosis [1].

Thrombosis in the *central venous system* is almost invariably associated with an underlying process such as compressive syndrome, venous web, stenosis, or malignant tumor invasion. Depending on the location of the thrombosis, these almost in-

evitably result in major obstructive symptoms such as profound upper or lower extremity edema, SVC or IVC syndrome, renal failure (either acute or chronic), or Budd-Chiari syndrome. Venographically, complete occlusion of the involved venous structure is often seen. With acute thrombosis only minimal collaterals are present. With chronic thrombosis or acute thrombosis superimposed on a chronic severe stenosis, extensive collaterals are seen.

With thrombosis of the *renal vein*, thrombus may be seen extending into the IVC or there may be only a lack of washout in the IVC from the renal vein (Fig. 7). Selective renal venography will confirm the thrombosis.

Portal vein thrombosis may be a sequelae of pancreatitis, portal phlebitis, sepsis, or trauma as well as neoplastic compression or invasion and results in extrahepatic portal hypertension. On the venous phase of a superior mesenteric or celiac angiogram there is lack of filling of the portal vein

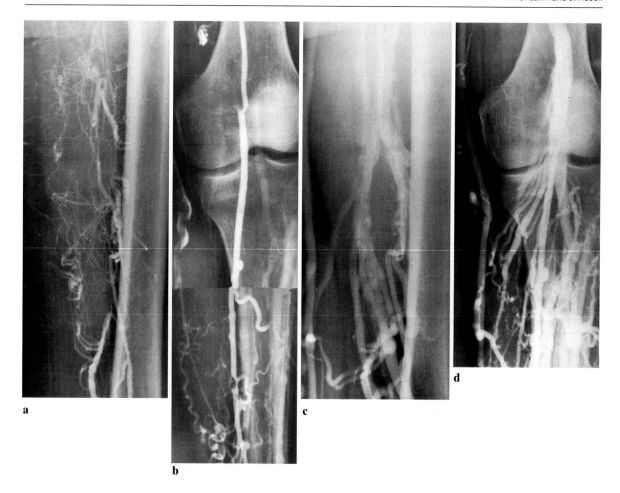

Fig. 6a–d. Extensive thrombosis of the deep and superficial left femoral systems with 4-year follow up. **a, b** Intraluminal thrombus is evident in the saphenous, posterior tibial, and peroneal veins with collateral flow about the occluded popliteal, femoral, and external iliac veins. **c, d** Repeat venogram 4 years later demonstrates venous recanalization. Note the absence of valves and the irregular lumen in the recanalized veins

with extensive portosystemic collaterals (Fig. 3). With chronic long-standing occlusion the hepatopetal collaterals often form a rich network which is called cavernous transformation of the portal vein. These collateral channels represent enlarged choledochal veins and other paraportal collaterals as well as the partially recanalized portal vein [36].

Thrombosis of the *splenic vein* results in segmental, left-sided portal hypertension. Patients often present with bleeding from gastric varices and normal hepatic function. The splenic vein thrombosis is usually secondary to pancreatic pathology [21]. The occlusion is best demonstrated angiographically by splenic artery injection with delayed filming of the venous phase. Occlusion of the splenic vein results in extensive hepatopetal collaterals, mainly gastric varices draining into the coronary and portal vein.

Benign Compressive and Obstructive Syndromes

Benign compression of the *subclavian vein*, which may be caused by several processes, results in swelling of the upper extremity. Pain, weakness, and paresthesia of the extremity may also be present. In females ipsilateral swelling of the breast may also be noted.

The *thoracic outlet syndrome* which may present with venous, arterial, or brachial plexus symptoms is caused by entrapment of these structures as they exit the thorax over the first rib and beneath the clavicle. The most common points of entrapment are (a) between the anterior and medial heads of the scalene muscles and the first rib

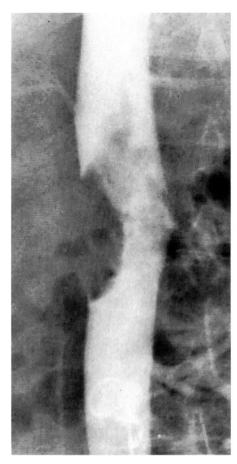

Fig. 7. Bilateral renal vein thrombosis in a 40-year-old man with recurrent nephrotic syndrome following membranous glomerulonephritis. Thrombus is evident extending into the IVC from the right and, to a lesser extent, the left renal veins

(scalenus anticus syndrome) [18, 47], (b) between the subclavian muscle, the clavicle, and the first rib, and (c) between an anomalous cervical rib and the scalene muscles. The compressive syndrome is often complicated by thrombosis. Although patients may not present until thrombosis occurs, a previous history of intermittent symptoms can frequently be elicited.

Effort (spontaneous) thrombosis, or Paget-Schroetter syndrome, also affects the subclavian vein and may extend into the axillary vein. It is frequently associated with transient compression of the subclavian vein between the subclavius muscle and the costocoracoid ligament during backward and downward bracing of the shoulders [22]. The syndrome occurs mainly in young males and is frequently seen after heavy exercise. The venogram may show occlusion of the subclavian

vein (Fig. 8). In patients with intermittent symptoms there may only be deformity of the subclavian vein as it passes over the first rib which becomes occlusion with arm elevation and hyperabduction. However, similar deformity can be identified in normal subjects with hyperabduction of the shoulder [22, 47].

Stenosis of the *subclavian or brachiocephalic* vein has become much more prevalent with the increased utilization of central lines, indwelling catheters such as Hickman and Groshong catheters and dialysis catheters [17, 18]. Permanent cardiac pacers have also been implicated as a cause for subclavian stenosis and thrombosis [9, 23].

In the lower extremities, extrinsic compression of the *popliteal vein* is seen in patients who do not completely relax the calf muscles during the injection of contrast. Deformity of the popliteal vein may also be seen due to compression of the vein by a Baker's cyst, popliteal artery aneurysm, or enlargement of the head of the gastrocnemius muscle due to trauma and/or hemorrhage [35]. Venous aneurysms of the popliteal vein are rare but can be the source of recurrent pulmonary emboli [28].

Budd-Chiari syndrome is an ambiguous term applied to the classic triad of ascites, hepatomegaly, and abdominal pain described by Budd in 1845 and further by Chiari in 1899 [49]. The syndrome may be due to an obstructive process either in the hepatic veins or in the intrahepatic IVC [45, 64, 65]. The process may be caused by thrombosis, compression, or weblike stenoses and has been associated with hypercoagulable states, neoplasms, trauma, medications, and congenital abnormalities. Venography demonstrates significant stenosis of the intrahepatic portion of the IVC, which is frequently better appreciated in the lateral view. Hepatic vein obstruction is seen only with selective catheterization of the hepatic veins (Fig. 9) [38]. Ludwig et al. [45] found in their series that large hepatic vein obstruction was more commonly thrombotic in origin while small hepatic vein or isolated IVC obstruction was usually nonthrombotic. With total venous occlusion a typical "spider web" appearance is often visualized.

Benign compression of the *infrahepatic IVC and iliac veins* may occur with retroperitoneal fibrosis or fibrosis associated with an abdominal aortic aneurysm or other retroperitoneal trauma [18]. Radiation therapy, particularly of pelvic tumors, may also result in diffuse narrowing of these veins. These compressions often progress and are

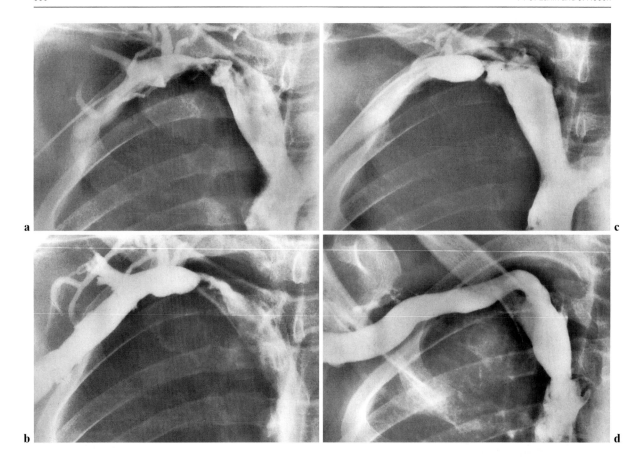

a   c

b   d

Fig. 8a–d. Paget-Schroetter syndrome with superimposed thrombosis in a 34-year-old man who presented with a painful and swollen arm. He was treated with local urokinase for 28 h with near complete thrombolysis. The underlying stenosis was surgically resected with transposition of the right jugular vein to the subclavian vein and resection of the first rib. **a** Initial venogram with thrombus extending from the left brachial through the subclavian vein. **b** Near complete clearing following 28-h urokinase infusion. **c** Five-week follow-up after fibrinolysis with persistent defect and no gradient at rest. Following exercise a 4 mmHg gradient in adduction and a 36 mmHg gradient in abduction was present. **d** One-year postsurgical follow-up venogram demonstrating the jugular vein transposition to the subclavian vein

complicated by secondary thrombosis of the iliac veins and/or IVC (Fig. 10).

Compression of the *left common iliac vein* secondary to pressure from the right iliac artery (iliac compression or Cockett syndrome) is thought to cause the increased incidence of deep venous thrombosis in the left lower extremity. A localized fibrous stricture which is present in some cases of this syndrome is thought to be a result of recanal-

ization of the iliac vein following iliac thrombosis [60]. In the May-Thurner syndrome the findings are similar, but extremity thrombosis is not present (Fig. 11). Focal spurs or webs present at the level of the junction of the left iliac vein and the IVC may be evident on phlebography and may demonstrate a pressure gradient, typically 2–4 cm water with exercise [60].

Fig. 9a–d. Budd-Chiari syndrome involving the hepatic ▶ veins and the IVC in a 26-year-old man presenting with severe ascites and lower extremity edema. Venography demonstrated right hepatic vein thrombosis, middle and left hepatic vein stenosis, and IVC compression. GRZ stents were placed in the left hepatic vein and the IVC with prompt and complete clearing and no recurrence until present (4 years). **a** Stenosis of the intrahepativ IVC is evident with a pressure gradient of 29 mmHg. Following PTA and GRZ stent placement the gradient was eliminated. **b** Severe stenosis of the left hepatic vein with a 26 mmHg gradient. This fell to 17 mmHg following PTA and was eliminated following GRZ stent placement. **c** Follow-up at 38 months reveals intimal hyperplasia without stenosis and with a 1 mmHg gradient in the IVC. **d** Left hepatic venogram at 38 months demonstrates continued patency of the vein, expansion of the stent, and a 1 mmHg gradient

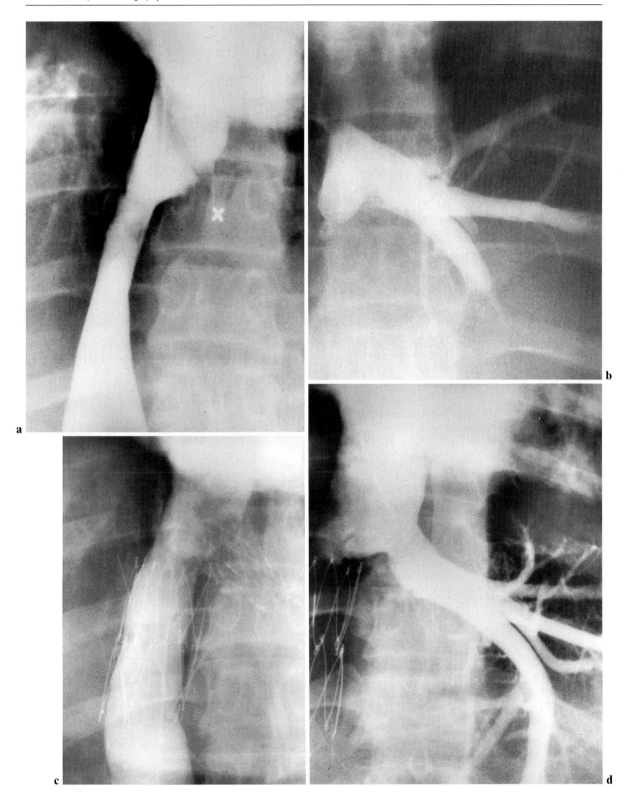

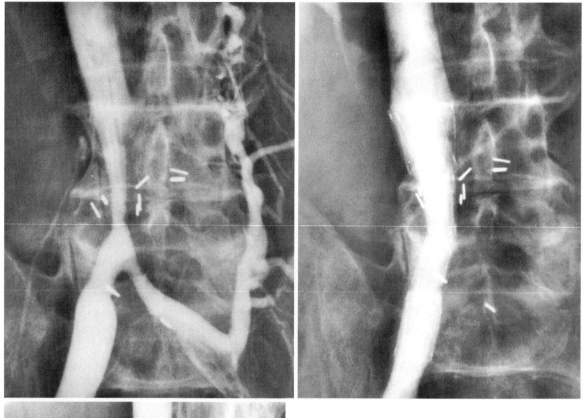

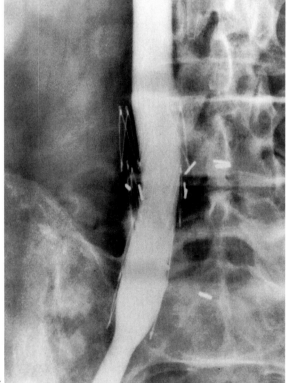

Fig. 10a–c. Severe stenosis of the IVC in a 71-year-old man due to fibrosis following IVC injury during aortic surgery with severe bilateral leg edema. Superimposed thrombosis of the left external iliac vein was present which was partially lysed with urokinase. Patency of the left external iliac vein could not be obtained, and GRZ stents were placed in the right common iliac vein and IVC. The edema on the right cleared promptly and after 34 months had not recurred. **a** Stenosis of the IVC and the common iliac veins at their confluence. **b** Venogram following stenting of the right common iliac vein and IVC. **c** Follow-up at 34 months demonstrates good vein patency, full expansion of the stent, and a 1 mmHg gradient

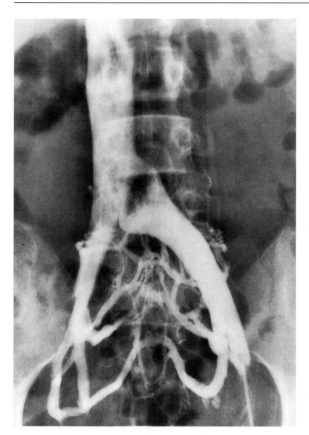

Fig. 11. May-Thurner syndrome with focal narrowing of the left common iliac vein

Renal vein compression secondary to entrapment of the renal vein between the aorta and the superior mesenteric vein (nutcracker syndrome) is often asymptomatic but may result in hematuria, particularly in younger patients. Phlebography of the left renal vein demonstrates the mesoaortic compression associated with the renal vein pressure gradient. Varicocele or pelviureteral varices may also be seen [4, 5, 31, 61].

Similar symptoms may occur with a retroaortic left renal vein (posterior nutcracker syndrome) which results from embryological obliteration of the left ventral renal vein and persistence of the dorsal left renal vein [6, 41]. The left renal vein has a distinctly caudal course prior to its entry into the IVC on venography and can be differentiated from mesoaortic compression [18].

Malignant Obstructive Syndromes

SVC syndrome presenting with head, neck, and upper extremity swelling, headache, dyspnea, and development of collateral veins in the thorax is most frequently caused by malignant mediastinal involvement. In the series reported by Yellin et al. [67] 47.6% had bronchogenic carcinoma and 20.6% lymphoma. Other primary and metastatic tumors of the mediastinum account for most of the remainder of the cases. In 10%–20% of patients the SVC syndrome is due to a benign etiology such as central venous lines, cardiac pacing wire, ascending aortic aneurysms, pericarditis, and mediastinitis. Venography demonstrates stenosis or occlusion of the SVC, frequently with superimposed thrombus which often will extend into the brachiocephalic veins (Figs. 12, 13). Extensive collateral circulation is usually present via intercostal and internal mammary veins to the azygous vein or, in a more central SVC occlusion, to the IVC.

IVC syndrome is most commonly due to malignant compression of the IVC. In our experience 72% of patients have the obstruction in the intrahepatic portion of the IVC secondary to hepatic metastasis or primary hepatic malignancy [39]. In the infrahepatic IVC, obstruction is most frequently due to paracaval adenopathy. Renal cell carcinoma is notorious for its direct intraluminal growth in the renal vein with IVC extension (Fig. 14). Benign etiologies include IVC filter placement and benign hepatic webs (Budd-Chiari syndrome). The patient presents with the onset of severe lower extremity and, in males, scrotal edema. Ascites is frequently present when the obstruction is in the intrahepatic portion of IVC. The onset is usually insidious but may be abrupt when secondary thrombosis occurs. Inferior vena cavography demonstrates either compression and narrowing or total occlusion of the IVC. Extensive collateral circulation may, again, be present with the ascending lumbar, azygous and hemiazygous, and anterior abdominal wall superficial veins being the most frequently filled collaterals.

Percutaneous Interventional Therapy

Percutaneous interventional therapy is extremely useful in the treatment of obstructions of large veins and may restore their patency with the re-

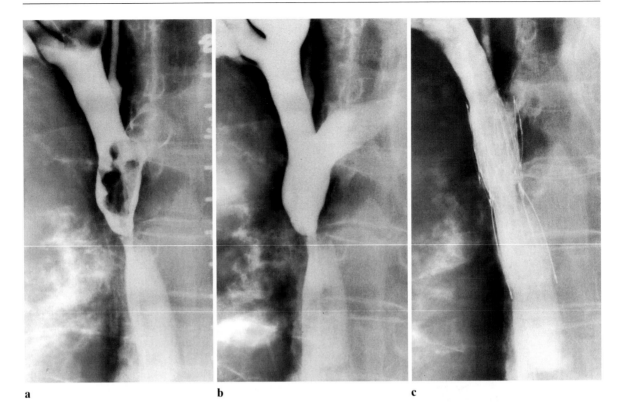

a   b   c

Fig. 12a–c. SVC stenosis with associated thrombosis in a 63-year-old man with severe SVC syndrome 6 years following hyperalimentation via a central venous catheter which became infected. Following fibrinolysis with urokinase and PTA, stents were placed in the SVC with complete relief of symptoms in 5 days. He remained asymptomatic until immediately prior to his death 1 year later. **a** Initial venogram reveals thrombus in the SVC above the stenosis as well as thrombi in the left brachiocephalic vein and the right internal jugular vein. **b** Complete lysis of all thrombi following 25-h local urokinase infusion. **c** Follow-up cavogram at 2 months with excellent flow in the SVC

versal of the congestive symptoms. As surgical repair or bypass of obstructed venous structures is frequently difficult or impossible, particularly in malignant obstructions, interventional therapy is crucial in these patients. It provides effective and long-term palliation in malignant obstructions and may provide the definitive therapy in benign obstructions. Three interventional modalities can be used for treatment of venous obstructions: percutaneous transluminal angioplasty, local thrombolytic therapy, and expandable stent placement. Although these modalities may be used alone, they are more often used in combinations.

Percutaneous Transluminal Angioplasty

Percutaneous transluminal angioplasty is considerably less effective in the venous than in the arterial system because of the difference in the character of the lesions involved. PTA is frequently initially successful in the treatment of benign subclavian vein stenoses. Glanz et al. [26] reported an initial 76 % success rate with the use of high pressure balloons, but they experienced a 65 % restenosis rate in the first year, although they maintained vein patency with repeated PTA. PTA may also be initially successful in focal uncomplicated SVC stenoses caused by an indwelling cath-

Fig. 13a, b. Right brachiocephalic and subclavian vein ▶ occlusion with superimposed thrombosis in a 58-year-old women with recurrent breast carcinoma in the mediastinum and severe right arm swelling. Following 26 h of local urokinase fibrinolytic therapy and PTA two GRZ stents were placed in the right subclavian and brachiocephalic veins and extended into the SVC. The edema cleared in 5 days and remained clear until her death 5 months later. **a** Right arm venogram demonstrates extensive thrombus extending from the brachial vein to the SVC. **b** Following local fibrinolysis and stent placement there is excellent flow through the stent to the SVC

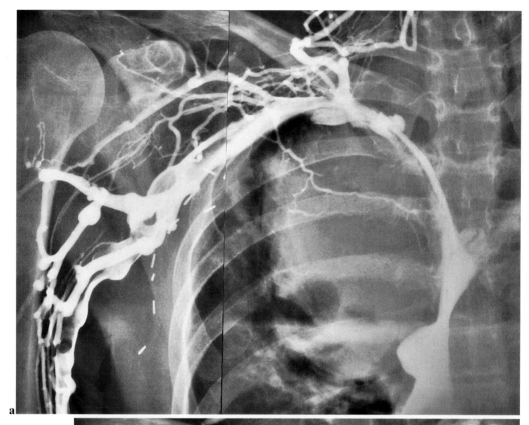

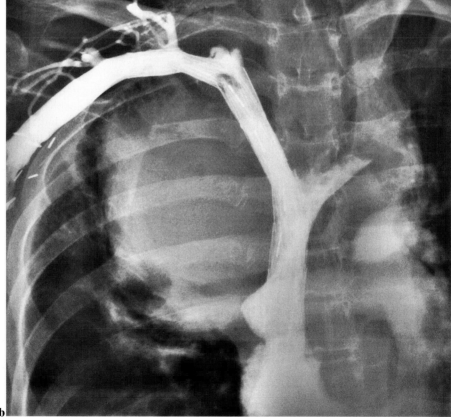

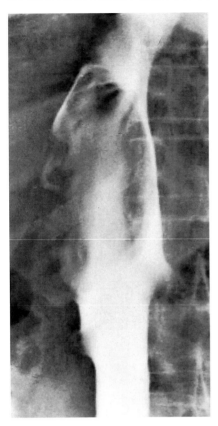

Fig. 14. Renal call carcinoma extending from the right renal vein into the IVC (compare Fig. 7)

eter, but its benefits are usually only short term, and early recurrences are frequent.

In patients with thoracic outlet syndrome PTA may also be useful following surgical decompression of the costoclavicular space. It can correct stenosis of the subclavian vein secondary to intrinsic venous changes such as fibrosis, intimal hyperplasia, and sclerosis [52].

In the treatment of Budd-Chiari syndrome PTA has been utilized successfully to disrupt the membrane or web found in the IVC and/or the hepatic veins [11, 43]. This results in the prompt regression of symptoms. Recurrence has, again, been a problem although repeat PTA can be utilized [46]. Furui et al. [25] reported improved patency in these patients with Nd-YAG assisted PTA.

The majority of patients with malignant obstruction and many with benign obstruction of major venous structures, however, fail to respond to PTA alone [58]. The stricture usually distends during balloon inflation but immediately recoils. In order to keep the lumen open, expandable stent placement is a much better therapeutic option for

these patients. Although Yellin et al. [67] reports a significant clearing of symptoms in patients with SVC syndrome following radiation therapy and/or chemotherapy, in our experience most patients with a limited life expectancy opt for a therapeutic option which provides prompt and persistent palliation with little morbidity [39].

Local Thrombolytic Therapy

Direct infusion of a thrombolytic agent through a catheter into a clot is an effective and relatively safe method for lysing clot associated with venous stenosis. However, for long-term success the underlying obstructive lesion needs to be corrected after thrombolysis by surgery, PTA or, stent placement, or the thrombosis will reoccur [17].

Urokinase is the fibrinolytic agent that we prefer although both urokinase and streptokinase produce clot lysis by converting fibrin bound plasminogen to plasmin. Urokinase has a biological half-life of 14 min and streptokinase a two-phase half-life totaling 100 min. Studies indicate that urokinase may be more effective than streptokinase in lysing clots, have a more rapid onset of action, and be associated with fewer bleeding episodes [8, 27, 59].

Local lytic therapy has been used successfully in the treatment of thrombosis of subclavian veins associated with thoracic outlet syndrome and Paget-Schroetter syndrome (Fig. 8) as well as secondary to indwelling catheters and pacer wires [7, 9, 17]. Local thrombolytic therapy has also been used in the treatment of acute renal vein thrombosis with the renal arterial infusion of urokinase as well as local lytic therapy in the renal vein [63].

Local thrombolytic therapy can also be effective in the thrombosis of major venous structures, i. e., the SVC and IVC. We have successfully treated 19 patients with thrombosis complicating major venous obstruction involving the SVC (15 patients) and the IVC (4 patients). The underlying obstruction was secondary to neoplastic encasement in 13 patients, radiation therapy in 2, and various benign etiologies in 2 [40]. Following venography the clot was partially disrupted with the passage of a guidewire and a catheter with multiple small sideholes was placed in the thrombus. An initial loading dose of 250 000–500 000 was then injected throughout the length of the clot with the larger dose utilized when the clot in the cava extends into the subclavian or iliac veins. One or two catheters, depending on the extent of the thrombosis, were then used to infuse urokinase at a rate of 50 000–100 000 U per catheter for 4 h. The patient was then reexamined and the dose adjusted with reexamination at 8- to 12-h intervals depending on the patient's clinical status. The dosage and position of the infusion catheters were adjusted depending on the status of the lysis. The patient was given a simultaneous systemic heparin infusion at a rate sufficient to maintain the partial thromboplastin time at $1.5 \times$ normal.

The length of the urokinase infusion varied from 20 min to 72 h, with a mean infusion time of 36.6 h. The dose similarly varied from 250 000 to 6 450 000 U, with a mean dose of 2 982 421 U. Upon completion of the lytic therapy and visualization of the underlying obstruction, all 19 of our patients were treated by expandable stent placement which corrected the obstruction and allowed good flow preventing recurrent thrombosis [40].

The possibility of pulmonary embolism following aggressive local thrombolytic therapy is a concern although none of our patients exhibited clinical signs of pulmonary embolism. The peripheral thrombus is intentionally lysed first, and the severe central venous obstruction probably functions as a barrier to the passage of large emboli. With the establishment of flow, smaller emboli probably occur, but these are partially lysed and are broken down in the lung and do not appear to cause clinical symptoms. The risk of pulmonary embolism is always considered and weighed against the benefits of fibrinolytic therapy. The severity of the patient's congestive symptoms is usually the decisive factor in our decisions.

Expandable Stent Placement

Placement of expandable metallic stents is the most effective interventional mode of treatment of large vein obstructions. Stent placement also offers long-term relief because expandable stents prevent recoil and recurrence of the stenosis is the majority of the cases.

The *Maass double-helix spiral prothesis* (Medivent, Zurich, Switzerland), was one of the first stents used clinically for venous obstructions. It used a large (7 mm diameter) introductory system and was usually introduced by cutdown in the jugular or femoral vein. It was employed successfully for treatment of obstruction of the IVC and iliac veins including left iliac thrombosis [69].

However, complications including perforation of the IVC due to the rigidity of the introductory system were reported, and this stent did not find a wider clinical use [33].

Other expandable stents have been developed which have an introductory system 3–4 mm in diameter, allowing easier and safer percutaneous introduction. The *balloon expandable Palmaz stent* (Johnson & Johnson Interventional Systems, Warren, NJ) has been used with very good success in stenoses of the subclavian and brachiocephalic veins related to hemodialysis shunts and catheters and also in stenoses in the SVC [19]. The *self-expandable Wallstent* (Schneider, Plymouth, MN) is available in the United States in smaller diameters (8–12 mm) but is available in Europe (Schneider, Bülach, Switzerland) in larger diameters (16 and 25 mm) as well. Its ease of introduction and flexibility are key advantages. It has been used with good success in obstructions of the vena cava and its branches [14, 15, 68, 69].

The *self-expandable Gianturco Z stent* (Cook Europe) has been the preferred stent for treatment of large venous obstructions because of its availability in large sizes (20–40 mm diameter), strong expansile force, and stability [10, 44, 51, 53, 56]. We have been using a second-generation modification of the Z stents, the *Gianturco-Rosch Z stents* (GRZ stent). The 8- to 12-mm diameter stents were obtained from Cook (Bloomington, IN; biliary GRZ stents). The larger sizes were handmade in our research laboratory with availability anticipated in the near future from Cook and Cook Europe. The individual stent bodies are 2 cm in length and connected with monofilament suture to limit the stent to the desired diameter and to connect the individual stent bodies together. We have used stents ranging from 4 to 10 cm in length and 8 to 25 mm in diameter. To obtain stable stent placement and to prevent its dislodgement and central migration, it is important to select a stent somewhat larger in diameter than the normal vein. We usually select a stent 20 % larger than the estimated normal diameter of the vein to be stented. The stents are all placed percutaneously, using a femoral on internal jugular approach with a 10- to 14-F Teflon introductory sheath.

All patients are heparinized during the stent placement. In our series the majority of the patients, except those receiving hemodialysis, are continued on anticoagulant therapy after stent placement. However, we no longer continue anticoagulant therapy after stent placement in patients with advanced abdominal malignancies because of possible complications related to anticoagulant therapy in these patients. In our patients who continue anticoagulant therapy following the stent placement, it is halted after 2 months when the stent is fully endothelialized [66] except in patients who require thrombolytic therapy to obtain or maintain patency.

Stent placement is very effective and provides rapid relief of congestive symptoms in the majority (70%–100%) of treated patients [2, 10, 15, 24, 32, 51, 57]. In our patients with major venous obstruction, stent placement was successful with the opening of even severe constrictions and resulted in the establishment of normal flow and symptomatic relief in all our 54 treated patients. In patients with SVC syndrome the facial cyanosis cleared immediately, and the facial edema and headache the following day with the upper extremity and truncal edema resolving in 2–3 days. In patients with IVC syndrome the lower extremity edema resolved much more slowly, usually in 3–7 days. Although the majority of patients with ascites improved markedly, 3 of the 15 patients (20%) with hepatic malignancy causing symptomatic intrahepatic caval occlusion had only limited improvement, with recurrence of the ascites prior to their death. Long-term results of stent placement depends on the nature of the obstructive lesion.

In obstruction secondary to *neoplastic lesions*, stent placement provides long-term palliation (Fig. 12, 13). In our 37 patients with neoplastic venous encasement, 83% were without symptom recurrence up to their death, with a mean survival of 4.2 months and patency as long as 27 months. Similar experiences have been reported by others [2, 10, 24, 32]. For the long-term palliation of obstructive lesions of the SVC and its branches in tumor patients and particularly in those receiving thrombolytic therapy prior to stent placement, it is essential to continue anticoagulation therapy. Our follow-up studies reveal that the tumor often grows slowly into the lumen through the stent, particularly with use of the Z stent. Continued anticoagulation prevents secondary thrombus formation and consequent stent occlusion. In our three patients with initial fibrinolytic therapy in whom anticoagulation was discontinued, thrombosis and symptom recurrence was noted in 1–3 days.

In patients with *benign lesions* causing large vein obstructions such as various types of fibrosis, congenital, or posttraumatic strictures and Budd-Chiari disease, stent placement provides long term treatment (Figs. 9, 10). This is particularly true in the SVC or IVC where the tendency to form abundant intimal hyperplasia is not exhibited. With the stenting of their branches, particularly of the subclavian veins where the stent is often placed at the site of a valve or in a vein curvature, intimal hyperplasia frequently develops and leads to obstruction and symptom recurrence in about 10 months. However, the recurrent lesion can effectively be treated with balloon dilation or the placement of another stent.

In our 15 patients with benign major vein obstruction, the 4 patients who died 2–26 months after stent placement and the 9 patients alive at follow-up after 8–42 months have not suffered symptom recurrence. Recurrent stenosis of the subclavian vein due to indwelling catheters in two patients was treated successfully by balloon dilation. Similar experience has been reported by others [2, 24, 68]. Very satisfactory long-term experience has been achieved particularly in patients with Budd-Chiari syndromes [24, 57].

In large vein stenosis related to *arteriovenous dialysis shunts*, particularly with those involving the subclavian and brachiocephalic veins, stent placement extends the life of the fistula [15, 54]. Increased flow from the fistula and probably stent placement across a venous valve leads to increased intimal proliferation with recurrence of stenosis and congestive symptoms. Stenosis recurrence has been observed from 6–10 months after stent placement and responds well to balloon angioplasty, endarterectomy, or new stent placement [2, 15, 68].

Complications may occur with venous stent placement and are usually related to improper stent selection (over or undersized), improper stent placement, insufficient or excessive thrombolytic and anticoagulation treatment, the puncture site, excessive contrast medium, or secondary infection. Chest pain has occasionally been reported with use of a large stent in the SVC but is usually only temporary. A small diameter stent was reported to migrate through the heart to the pulmonary artery without consequence. The placement of a short stent may fail to expand the obstructive lesion, and the placement of additional stents may be necessary. We always try to cover the obstructive lesion and, if possible, to extend the stent 2–4 cm above and below the lesion into the normal vein. With the use of fibrinolytic and anticoagulant therapy a fatal retroperitoneal hematoma occurred in one of our patients secondary to bleeding from tumor vessels. Major pulmonary hemorrhage occurred in another of our patients after we successfully treated a malignant SVC obstruction and continued local fibrinolytic therapy to lyse residual thrombus in an internal jugular vein. The risks of stent placement must always be considered and weighed against the benefits that may be achieved. In this group of patients where no other treatment can be offered the benefits usually predominate.

In summary, stents are effective devices for treatment of obstructions of larger veins, whether caused by malignant tumors, benign processes or related to dialysis shunts. They dilate venous obstructions by expanding to their given diameter, do not migrate, and exhibit long-term patency. Selective use of local fibrinolytic therapy is excellent adjunct treatment of superimposed thrombosis although it carried certain risks, particularly in patients with malignant disease.

References

1. Albertyn LE. Acute portal vein thrombosis. Clinical Radiology 1987; 38: 645–648.
2. Ameli FM, Minas T, Weiss M, Provan JL. Consequences of "conservative" conventional management of axillary vein thrombosis. Canadian Journal of Surgery 1987; 30: 167–169.
3. Antonucci F, Salomonowitz E, Stuckmann G, Stiefel M, Largiader J, Zollikofer CL. Placement of venous stents: clinical experience with a self-expanding prosthesis. Radiology 1992; 183: 493–497.
4. Ariyoshi A, Nagase K. Renal hematuria caused by "nutcracker" phenomenon: a more logical surgical management. Urology 1990; 35: 168–170.
5. Barnes RW, Fleisher HL 3d, Redman JF, Smith JW, Harshfield DL, Ferris EJ. Mesoaortic compression of the left renal vein (the so called nutcracker syndrome): repair by a new stenting procedure. Journal of Vascular Surgery 1988; 8: 415–421.
6. Batt M, Hassen-Khodja R, Bayada JM, Gagliardi JM, Daune B, Avril G, Serres JJ, LeBas P. Traumatic fistula between the aorta and the left renal vein: case report and review of the literature. Journal of Vascular Surgery 1989; 9: 812–816.
7. Becker GJ, Holden RW, Rabe FE, Castaneda-Zuniga WR, Sears N, Dilley RS, Glover JL. Local thrombolytic therapy for subclavian and axillary vein thrombosis: treatment of the thoracic inlet syndrome. Radiology 1983; 149: 419–423.
8. Bell WR. Update on urokinase and streptokinase: a comparison of their efficacy and safety. Hosp Form 1988; 230–241.
9. Bradof J, Sands MJ Jr, Lakin P. Sypmtomatic venous thrombosis of the upper extremity complicating permanent transvenous pacing: reversal with streptokinase infusion. American Heart Journal 1982; 104: 1112–1113.
10. Carrasco CH, Charnsangavej C, Wright KC, Wallace S, Gianturco C. Use of the Gianturco self-expanding stent in stenoses of the superior and inferior venae cavae. JVIR 1992; 3: 409–419.
11. Chan P, Lee CP, Lee YS. Budd-Chiari syndrome treated successfully by percutaneous transluminal balloon angioplasty: two cases follow-up for 6 years. Catheterization and Cardiovascular Diagnosis 1992; 27: 215–219.
12. Cronan JJ. Ultrasound evaluation of deep venous thrombosis. Seminars in Roentgenology 1992; 27: 39–52.
13. Cronan JJ, Dorfman GS, Scola FH, Schepps B, Alexander J. Deep venous thrombosis: US assessment using vein compression. Radiology 1987; 162: 191–194.
14. Dake MD, Semba CP. Stents for the treatment of venous obstruction. Abstract: 1993 Annual Meeting, Western Angiographic and Interventional Society. Portland, Oregon. p. 47.
15. Dondelinger RF, Goffette P, Kurdziel JC, Roche A. Expandable metal stents for stenoses of the venae cavae and large veins. Semin Intervent Radiol 1991; 8: 252.
16. Dorfman GS, Froehlich JA, Cronan JJ, Urbaneck PJ, Herndon JH. Lower extremity venous thrombosis in patients with acute hip fractures: determination of anatomic location and time of onset with compression sonography. AJR 1990; 154: 851–855.
17. Druy EM, Trout HH 3d, Giordano JM, Hix WR. Lytic therapy in the treatment of axillary and subclavian vein thrombosis. Journal Vascular Surgery 1985; 2: 821–827.
18. Kim D, Orron DE. Peripheral vascular imaging and intervention. 1992; Chap. 19. p. 269–350. Mosby Year Book, St. Louis, USA.
19. Elson JD, Becker GJ, Wholey MH, Ehrman KO. Vena caval central venous stenoses: management with Palmaz balloon-expandable intraluminal stents. J. Vasc Intervent Radiol 1991; 2: 215.
20. Erdman WA, Jayson HT, Redman HC, Miller GL, Parkey RW, Peshock RW. Deep venous thrombosis of extremities: role of MR imaging in the diagnosis. Radiology 1990; 174: 425–431.
21. Evans GR, Yellin AE, Weaver FA, Stain SC. Sinistral (left-sided) portal hypertension. American Surgeon 1990; 56: 758–763.
22. Falconer MA, Weddell G. Costoclavicular compression of the subclavian artery and vein. Lancet 1943; 2: 539–544.
23. Ferguson R, McCaughan B, May J, Waugh R. Venous occlusion: a rare complication of transvenous cardiac pacing. Australian and New Zealand Journal of Surgery 1992; 62: 977–980.
24. Furui S, Sawada S, Irie T, Makita K, Yamauchi T, Kusano S, Ibukuro K, Nakamura H, Takenaka E. Hepatic inferior vena cava obstruction: treatment of two types with Gianturco expandable metallic stents. Radiology 1990; 176: 665–670.

25. Furui S, Yamauchi R, Ohtomo K, Tsuchiya K, Makita K, Takenaka E. Hepatic inferior vena cava obstructions: clinical results of treatment with percutaneous transluminal laser-assisted angioplasty. Radiology 1988; 166: 673–677.

26. Glanz S, Gordon DH, Lipkowitz GS et al. Axillary and subclavian vein stenosis: percutaneous angioplasty. Radiology 1988; 168: 371.

27. Graor RA, Young JR, Risius B, Ruschhaupt WF. Comparison of cost-effectiveness of streptokinase and urokinase in the treatment of deep vein thrombosis. Annals of Vascular Surgery 1987; 1: 524–528.

28. Grice GD, Smith RB, Robinson PH, Rheudasil JM. Primary popliteal venous aneurysm with recurrent pulmonary emboli. Journal of Vascular Surgery 1990; 12: 316–318.

29. Hach W. Evaluation and management of postthrombotic syndrome. Herz 1989; 14: 287.

30. Hanrahan LM, Araki CT, Fisher JB, Rodriguez AA, Walker TG, Woodson J, LaMorte WW, Manzoian JO. Evaluation of the perforating veins of the lower extremity using high resolution duplex imaging. Journal of Cardiovascular Surgery 1991; 32: 87–97.

31. Hoehnfellner M, Steinback F, Schultz-Lampet D, Schantzen W, Walter K, Cramer BM, Thuroff JW, Hohenfellner R. The nutcracker syndrome: new aspects of pathophysiology, diagnosis and treatment. Journal of Urology 1991; 146: 685–688.

32. Irving JD, Dondelinger PF, Reidy JF, Schild H, Dick R, Adam A, Maynar M, Zollikofer L. Gianturco self-expanding stents: clinical experience in the vena cava and large veins. Cardiovasc Intervent Radiol 1992; 15: 328–333.

33. Jakob H, Maass D, Schmiedt W. et al. Treatment of major venous obstruction with an expandable endoluminal spiral prosthesis. J. Cardiovasc Surg 1989; 30: 112.

34. Jayanthi V, Victor S, Dhala B, Gajaraj A, Madanagopalan N. Pre-operative and post-operative ultrasound evaluation of Budd-Chiari syndrome due to coarctation of the inferior vena cava. Clinical Radiology 1988; 39: 154–158.

35. Kadir S. Diagnostic angiography. 1986. Chap. 19. p. 536–583. WB Saunders Co. Philadelphia, PA. USA.

36. Kadir S. Diagnostic angiography. 1986. Chap. 15. p. 377–444. WB Saunders Co. Philadelphia, PA. USA.

37. Killewich LA, Bedford GR, Beach KW, Strandness DE. Diagnosis of deep venous thrombosis. A prospective study comparing duplex scanning to contrast venography. Circulation 1989; 79: 810–814.

38. Klein AS, Cameron JL. Diagnosis and management of the Budd-Chiari syndrome. American Journal of Surgery 1990; 160: 128–133.

39. Lakin PC. Venous stents in the treatment of major venous obstruction. Abstract: 1993 Annual Meeting, Western Angiographic and Interventional Conference. Portland, OR. p. 52.

40. Lakin PC, Petersen BD, Barton RE, Keller FS, Rosch J. Combined local Urokinase thrombolysis with expandable Z-stents in the treatment of major venous obstruction. 18th Annual Scientific Meeting, Society of Cardiovascular and Interventional Radiology. New Orleans, LA. February 28 – March 4, 1993.

41. Lau JL, Lo R, Chan FL, Wong KK. The posterior "nutcracker:" hematuria secondary to retroaortic left renal vein. Urology 1986; 28: 437–439.

42. Lee KR, Templeton AW, Cox GG, Dwyer SJ, McClure CB. Digital venography of the lower extremity. American Journal of Roentgenology 1989; 153: 413–417.

43. Lois JF, Hartzman S, McGalde CT, Gomes AS, Grant EC, Berquist W, Perrella RR, Busuttil RW. Budd-Chiari syndrome: treatment with percutaneous transhepatic recanalization and dilation. Radiology 1989; 170 (3 pt 1): 791–793.

44. Lopez RR, Benner KG, Hall L, Rosch J, Pinson W. Expandable venous stents for treatment of the Budd-Chiari syndrome. Gastoenterology 1991; 100: 1435–1441.

45. Ludwig J, Hashimoto E, McGill DB, VanHeerden JA. Classification of hepatic venous outflow obstruction: ambiguous terminology of the Budd-Chiari syndrome. Mayo Clinic Proceedings 1990; 65: 51–55.

46. Martin LG, Henderson JM, Millikan WJ Jr, Casarella WJ, Kaufman SL. Angioplasty for long-term treatment of patients with Budd-Chiari syndrome. AJR 1990; 1007–1010.

47. McCleery RS, Kesterson JE, Kirtley JA, Love RB. Subclavius and anterior scalene muscle compression as a cause of intermittent obstruction of the subclavian vein. Ann Surg 1951; 133: 588–602.

48. Mori H, Hayashi K, Uetani M, Matsuoka Y, Iwao M, Maeda H. High-attentuation recent thrombus of the portal vein: CT demonstration and clinical significance. Radiology 1987; 163: 353–356.

49. Murphy FB, Steinbery HV, Shires GT 3rd, Martin LG, Bernardina ME. The Budd-Chiari syndrome: a review. AJR 1986; 147: 9–15.

50. Ohnishi K, Terabayashi H, Tsunoda T, Nomura F. Budd-Chiari syndrome: diagnosis with duplex sonography. American Journal of Gastroenterology 1990; 85: 165–169.

51. Oudkerk M, Heystraten FMJ, Stoter G. Stenting in malignant vena caval obstruction. Cancer 1993; 71: 142–146.

52. Perler BA, Michell S. Percutaneous transluminal angioplasty and transaxillary first rib resection: a multidisciplinary approach to the thoracic outlet syndrome. Am Surg 1986; 52: 485.

53. Putnam JS, Uchida BT, Antonovic R, Rosch J. Superior vena cava syndrome associated with massive thrombosis: treatment with expandable wire stents. Radiology 1988; 167: 727–728.

54. Quinn SF, Schuman ES, Hall L, Gross GF, Uchida BT, Standage BA, Rosch J, Ivancev K. Venous stenoses in patients who undergo hemodialysis: treatment with self-expandable endovascular stents. Radiology 1992; 183: 499–504.

55. Rosch J, Dotter CT, Seaman AJ, Porter JM, Common HH. Healing of deep venous thrombosis: venographic findings in a randomized study comparing streptokinase and heparin. Am J Roentgenol 1976; 127: 553–558.

56. Rosch J, Uchida BT, Hall LD, Antonovic R, Petersen BD, Invancev K, Barton RE, Keller FS. Gianturco-Rosch expandable Z-stents in the treatment of superior vena cava syndrome. Cardiovasc Intervent Radiol 1992; 15: 319–327.

57. Sawada S, Fujiwara Y, Koyama T, Kobayashi M, Tanigawa N, Iwamiya T, Katsube Y, Nakamura H, Furui S. Application of expandable metallic stents to the venous system. Acta Radiologica 1992; 33: 156–159.

58. Sherry CS, Diamond NG, Meyers TP, Martin RL. Successful treatment of superior vena cava syndrome by venous angioplasty. AJR 1986; 147: 834.

59. Sullivan KL, Gardiner GA Jr, Shapira MJ, Bonn J, Levin DC. Acceleration of thrombolysis with a high-dose transthrombus bolus technique. Radiology 1989; 173: 805–808.

60. Taheri SA, Williams J, Powell S, Cullen J, Peer R, Nowakowski P, Boman L, Pisano S. Iliocaval compression syndrome. American Journal of Surgery 1987; 154: 169–172.

61. Takahashi Y, Akaishi K, Sano A, Kuroda Y. Intra-arterial digital subtraction angiography for children with idiopathic renal bleeding: a diagnosis of nutcracker phenomenon. Clinical Nephrology 1988; 30: 134–140.

62. Vansant JP, Habibian RM, Melton RE. The effect of varying tourniquet applications of the flow pattern of lower extremity radionuclide venography. Clinical Nuclear Medicine 1990; 15: 783–786.

63. Vogelzang RL, Roel DI, Cohn RA, Donaldson JS, Langman CB, Nemcek AA Jr. Acute renal vein thrombosis: successful treatment with intra-arterial urokinase. Radiology 1988; 169: 681–682.

64. Wang ZG, Zhu Y, Wang SH, Pu LP, Du YH, Zhang H, Yuan C, Chen Z, Wei ML, Pu LQ, et al. Recognition and management of Budd-Chiari syndrome: report of one hundred cases. Journal of Vascular Surgery 1989; 10: 149–156.

65. Wang ZG. Recognition and management of Budd-Chiari syndrome. Experience with 143 patients. Chinese Medical Journal 1989; 102: 338–346.

66. Wright KC, Wallace S, Charnasangavej C. et al. Percutaneous endovascular stents: an experimental evaluation. Radiology 1985; 156: 69.

67. Yellin A, Rosen A, Reichert N, Lieberman Y. Superior vena cava syndrome. The myth – the facts. American Review of Respiratory Disease 1990; 141: 1114–1118.

68. Zollikofer CL, Antonucci F, Stuckmann G, Mattias P, Bruhlmann WF, Salomonowitz EK. Use of the Wallstent in the venous system including hemodialysis-related stenoses. Cardiovasc Intervent Radiol 1992; 15: 334–341.

69. Zollikofer CL, Largiader I, Bruhlmann WF, Uhlschmid GK, Marty AH. Endovascular stenting of veins and grafts: preliminary clinical experience. Radiology 1988; 167: 707–712.

Part III
Work-in-Progress

Section I
Vascular Magnetic Resonance

MR Principles and Technology

L. E. Crooks and N. M. Hylton

Introduction

This chapter provides a review of basic magnetic resonance imaging (MRI) principles with emphasis on the interactions with moving blood. An effort is made to help familiarize the reader with concepts and terminology unique to MRI. A glossary of conventional terms used in nuclear magnetic resonance has been prepared by the American College of Radiology and is recommended to the reader for standard definitions and conventions [1]. We approach this subject by first discussing the phenomenon of nuclear magnetic resonance. The topics that follow include relaxation parameters, Fourier transformation, spatial localization, the effects of imaging parameters on contrast, MR signal dependence on flow, MR angiographic techniques, instrumentation, quantitative image characteristics, and pulse sequences. The reader interested in a more thorough discussion of any of these subjects can refer to the texts referenced in the respective sections and listed at the end of the chapter.

How the Signal is Generated

The number value assigned to each pixel in the image is a measurement of the amount of signal generated by a small voxel (volume element) located at the corresponding position in the body. The magnitude of the signal is determined by properties of the tissue contained within the voxel, namely the number of nuclei in the element of interest (usually hydrogen), the T_1 and T_2 relaxation parameters that characterize how the nuclei respond to magnetic fields, chemical shift, diffusion, and motion. For flowing blood the phase of the signal is also important. Phase measures the direction of the voxel's nuclei. This depends mainly on field gradients and velocity.

Nuclear Magnetism

Nuclear magnetic resonance is the phenomenon that generates the signal for imaging [2, 3]. It is caused by the interactions between the nuclei of the atoms within the tissue and an external magnetic field. Two properties of the nucleus contribute to the effect; the fact that its subparticles, protons and neutrons, contain charges, and that they have a spinning motion (although neutrons have a net charge of zero, they consist of charged matter that is distributed unevenly along the radial direction). Any charged particle in motion produces a magnetic field. The circular motion of the nuclear particles causes them to generate a magnetic field with a north-south orientation along the axis of rotation, as that of a current loop. This field is referred to as a *magnetic dipole*, and the particles are said to possess a magnetic dipole moment, μ. The spinning motion of the nuclear particles gives them an angular momentum referred to as the *spin*, which depends on their mass and speed and how the mass is distributed. When a nucleus is placed in a magnetic field, B_0, the magnetic dipoles behave similarly to a bar magnet in the earth's magnetic field by tending to align with the field. Unlike the bar magnet which points in the direction of the field, because the charges are spinning, the magnetic dipole precesses as a top about the direction of B_0 (Fig. 1a). Every different species of nuclei precess with a unique frequency, called the *Larmor frequency*. The Larmor frequency depends on the strength of the field B_0 and a constant for the nuclei called the magnetogyric ratio, γ. The relationship between Larmor frequency, f_L and magnetic field strength B_0 is given by the following expression:

$$f_L = \gamma B_0 \qquad (1)$$

The angular momentum of a particle can be positive or negative depending on the two directions

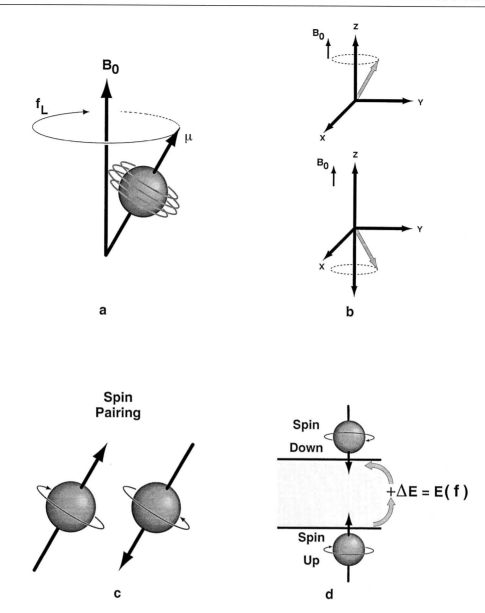

Fig. 1. a A magnetic dipole μ in magnetic field B_0 precesses about the direction of B_0 at the Larmor frequency f_L. **b** The two allowed orientations for a spin in a magnetic field. When the spin is aligned along the direction of B_0 it is in the lower energy, spin-up state. When aligned opposite the direction of B_0, it is in the higher energy or spin-down state. **c** Each pair of spins orient themselves in opposite directions, an energy-lowering process known as pairing. **d** A transition from the spin-up to the spin-down state requires the addition of an amount of energy exactly equal to the difference between the two energy states. This energy difference depends on the precession frequency of the spins, f_L. Electromagnetic energy must be at frequency f_L of the system to provide photons of this amount

of rotation, called spin up (aligned with B_0) and spin down (aligned opposite B_0; Fig. 1b). Each proton and neutron contributes its angular momentum to the total angular momentum of the nucleus. In nature, systems of particles orient themselves so as to lower the overall energy state of the system. In the nucleus this is done by pairing, in which every pair of like particles occupy opposing spin directions thus canceling each other's angular momentum and magnetic dipole contributions (Fig. 1c). It follows that if the nucleus has an even number of protons and an even number of neutrons, the net angular momentum and net magnetic dipole moment of the nucleus is zero. Only nuclei with a nonzero angular momentum and dipole moment can undergo nuclear magnetic resonance. The magnetic dipole of the nucleus is not free to assume any orientation with respect to the direction of the field B_0. It is restricted to occupy orientations that have certain exact energy levels. This implies that to change from one orientation to another energy must be absorbed or released in an amount exactly equal to the difference between the two energy states (Fig. 1d). The magnetic component of an oscillating electromagnetic field can be used to transfer energy to the magnetic dipole. To be exactly equal to the difference between the two energy states the electromagnetic field must be oscillating at the Larmor frequency of the nucleus. This is the phenomenon of *nuclear magnetic resonance*. If energy is added at a frequency other than the Larmor frequency, transitions are not made, and resonance does not occur.

A group of nuclei in a field B_0 at a given temperature form a natural distribution among their allowed orientations defined by the Boltzmann equation:

$$\frac{N_+}{N_-} = e^{(-\frac{E}{kT})} \qquad (2)$$

where N_+ and N_- are the relative numbers of spins in two allowed orientations, E is the energy difference between the two states, T is the absolute temperature, and k is Boltzmann's constant. If energy is added at the Larmor frequency using an oscillating field B_1, transitions to the higher energy states are made, and the distribution of energy states of the spins is shifted away from equilibrium. When B_1 is discontinued, nuclei return to the lower state by releasing energy, and equilibrium is reestablished. The released energy is transferred to the molecular lattice structure in which the nuclei are embedded and detected as a current oscillating at the Larmor frequency induced in a surrounding receiver coil.

The Hydrogen Nucleus

The simplest nucleus is that of the hydrogen atom. Hydrogen is the most commonly used nucleus for MRI because of its great abundance in water-containing soft tissue. It also generates the largest amount of nuclear magnetic resonance signal of all the stable elements. The hydrogen nucleus consists of a single proton, and therefore the

nucleus has a net angular momentum equal to that of the proton. The two spin states of the nucleus generate two allowable energy states in the magnetic field, one aligned with the field, the lower energy or parallel state, and one against the field, the higher energy or antiparallel state. Energy must be added at the Larmor frequency for hydrogen in order for resonance to occur. For a fixed field strength of 1 T, for example, and hydrogen's magnetogyric ratio of 4.258×10^7 Hz/T the Larmor frequency is 42.58 MHz. When a body in a magnetic field of 1 T is irradiated with a B_1 field of 42.58 MHz, only the hydrogen nuclei experience resonance. Because of their different magnetogyric ratios all other nuclei have Larmor frequencies different than 42.58 MHz and are therefore unaffectd by the B_1 field.

Radiofrequency Excitation

The B_1 field is generated using an oscillating electromagnetic field at the frequency f_L. The B_1 field must be directed perpendicular to the B_0 field and is turned on to create resonance and turned off to allow the system to return to equilibrium. Because we usually pulse the B_1 field, and since f_L is in the frequency range of radiowaves for typical whole-body imaging, the use of the B_1 field is generally referred to as the radiofrequency (RF) pulse [4, 5]. A common terminology with MRI is the phrase *90° pulse* (or any angle) to describe RF excitation sufficient in amplitude and duration to cause the net magnetic moment to rotate 90° away from the direction of B_0. A transmitter coil is usually placed in close proximity to the region being imaged and is designed to generate a B_1 field in the direction orthogonal to the main magnetic field.

The receiver coil is oriented along one axis in the plane transverse to the B_1 field. It samples one magnetic component of the spinning nuclei. A second coil can be placed orthogonal to this first coil to sample the complementary component of the nuclei. Phase shifting the second signal by 90° and adding it to the first improves the signal-to-noise value by $\sqrt{2}$. This is known as quadrature reception.

Magnetization Vector in a Rotating Frame of Reference

To facilitate our understanding of what happens in a magnetic resonance experiment, it is convenient to use the net magnetic moment vector **M** to represent the vector sum of all of the spins in a single voxel. Consider vector **M** in the frame of reference shown in Fig. 2a. The magnetic field B_0 is directed along the z-axis, also called the longitudinal direction. The plane formed by the x- and y-axes is called the transverse plane. As we mentioned above, the magnetic moments of individual nuclei precess about the direction of the magnetic field B_0. If we sum all of the magnetic moment vectors in the voxel, because of their distribution around the z-axis their components in the transverse direction cancel one another, leaving only a large longitudinal component **M** (Fig. 2a). If energy is added at the Larmor frequency using an oscillating magnetic field B_1 directed in the transverse plane, individual spins absorb energy and make transitions to the upper energy state. The effect on the vector sum **M** is for it to begin to move away from the z-axis towards the transverse plane while precessing about z. This spiraling motion (shown in Fig. 2b) continues as long as B_1 remains on. As **M** begins to move away from the z-axis, a component in the transverse plane appears. **M** can be represented by its two components M_z and M_{xy} is shown. We refer to the M_z component as the longitudinal magnetization and M_{xy} as the transverse magnetization. Because of the precessing motion of **M**, the transverse component M_{xy} rotates in the xy plane. The angle that M_{xy} makes with the y-axis (or any arbitary fixed direction in the plane) changes with time and is called the *phase angle* Φ. While the size of the vector M_{xy} ultimately determines the intensity of the pixel, the direction described by the phase angle is also important. The phase angle is shown in Fig. 2b.

It is convenient when describing the effect of the B_1 field to use a frame of reference [x'y'z], also rotating at the Larmor frequency (Fig. 2c). In this way B_1 appears to stay fixed on the x' axis in the same way that an object on a carousel appears to stand still if one is rotating with the platform. In the rotating frame, while B_1 is on, **M** rotates about the direction of B_1, shown along the positive x' axis in Fig. 2d. Depending on the strength and duration of the B_1 pulse, **M** rotates through an angle Θ known as the *flip angle* and shown in the figure. After the pulse, spin lattice relaxation allows the system to return to its equilibrium state (**M** aligned along positive z). While this happens, magnetic oscillations due to spin rotation at f_L induce current in the receiver coil generating the MR signal. The receiver coil is sensitive only to the transverse component of vector **M**. As the system relaxes and **M** realigns with the z direction, the transverse component decreases in size and eventually dies out. The signal decay over time is known as the *free induction decay* (FID).

Relaxation Parameters

The processes by which the signal decays and longitudinal magnetization is restored after RF excitation are characterized by two relaxation parameters. Both are exponential in nature. The high intrinsic contrast obtained with MRI arises mostly from its sensitivity to these relaxation parameters, T_1 and T_2 [6, 7]. Differences in T_1 and T_2 between neighboring tissues give rise to signal differences and may provide discrimination of disease states [8, 9].

T_1 Relaxation

Spin-lattice, or T_1, relaxation is the process by which equilibrium is reestablished after the absorption of RF energy. Following absorption energy can be released to the surrounding molecular structure or lattice. In the same way that RF energy is absorbed by a spin if the frequency matches its Larmor frequency, energy can be transferred from the spin to a neighboring process that is also oscillating at the Larmor frequency. As this happens, the excited spin system returns to its equilibrium distribution at a rate characterized by the relaxation constant T_1. The molecular makeup of different tissues give them characteristic values of T_1. T_1 also depends on the frequency of the applied external field and is known to increase with frequency [10].

T_2 Relaxation

A second process called *spin-spin*, or T_2 relaxation reduces the measurable transverse magnetization. To discuss T_2 and the idea of dephasing in general we need to remember that the magnetization **M** is

Voxel Magnetization in
Magnetic Field B_0

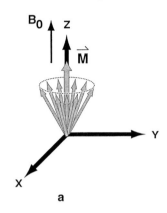

a

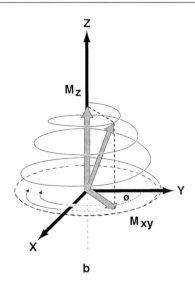

b

Rotating Frame Of Reference

Laboratory Frame X Y Z

Rotating Frame X' Y' Z
(moving at frequency f_L)

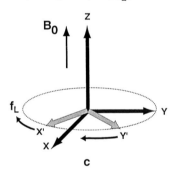

c

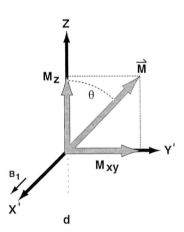

d

Fig. 2. a Vector **M** is used to represent the net magnetization of all the spins contained in one voxel in the field B_0. While all precessing at the same frequency, they are randomly distributed about B_0, causing cancellation of their transverse magnetization components and superposition of their longitudinal components. **b** When electromagnetic energy at the frequency f_L is added to the system in the form of an oscillating magnetic field B_1, vector **M** moves away from the direction of B_0 in a spiraling motion at frequency f_L. **c** Using a frame of reference x'y'z moving at the frequency f_L simplifies the motion of **M**. **d** In the rotating frame of reference, when B_1 is applied along the x'-axis, **M** rotates in the y'-z plane. Depending on the strength and duration T of B_1, **M** rotates through an angle of Φ degrees determined by $\Phi = 2\pi\gamma\int B_1(t)\,dt$, with the integral taken over the duration T

really the vector total of the magnetic moments of many individual nuclei. In a perfectly homogeneous magnetic field all of the nuclei precess at exactly the same frequency. They remain coherent, or in phase, meaning that as they rotate they always have the same phase angle. If, however, slight variations exist in the strength of the field from location to location, there also exist slight variations in the frequencies at which individual nuclei are precessing. If this happens, faster precessing nuclei begins to get ahead of slower nuclei, causing phase differences to appear (Fig. 3a). As the phase dispersion increases, cancellation of individual spin magnetic moment vectors causes a

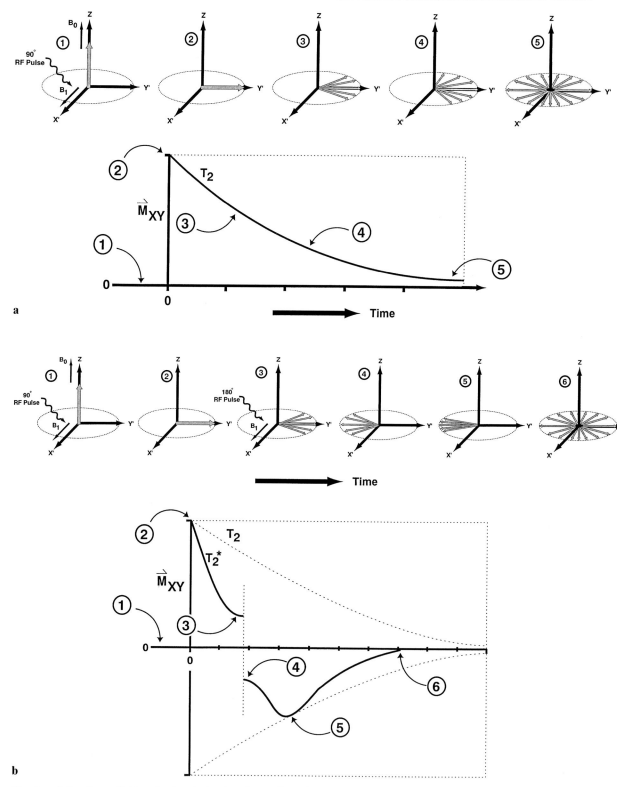

Fig. 3. a After B_1 excitation the free induction decay signal is measured in the receiver coil. The signal decays according to the relaxation constant T_2 as spin dephasing occurs. **b** Field inhomogeneity causes additional dephasing and results in signal decay at a faster rate given by T_2^*. The effect of inhomogeneity can be overcome using a 180° refocusing pulse to reverse the spin system and refocus the spins. This is known as a spin-echo technique

decrease in the net value M_{xy}, decreasing the signal detected by the receiver coil. When the nuclei are uniformly dispersed over 360°, no signal is measurable.

There are several sources of this loss of phase coherence. The first is the intrinsic, irreversible process of T_2 relaxation. Individual spins, being magnetic entities, themselves make small contributions to the total magnetic field. Each spin experiences the main static magnetic field plus small contributions from each of the spins around it. Since the configuration is slightly different from the vantage of each spin, the total magnetic field felt by a spin is slightly different from that of its neighbor. This creates a variation in field values over the voxel causing the value of $\mathbf{M}$ to decay over time at a rate described by the exponential constant T_2. For hydrogen in tissues the rate of T_2 decay is much faster than the rate at which longitudinal magnetization recovers as characterized by T_1. In other words, after RF excitation and the rotation of the net magnetization $\mathbf{M}$ into the transverse plane, signal in the receiver coil dies out as transverse magnetization dephases. However, although no longer measurable, transverse magnetization still exists. The T_1 relaxation process by which energy is transferred away from the spin system to the lattice and longitudinal magnetization is restored is still occurring.

Typical T_2 values for soft tissue in the human body range from 20 to 100 ms while typical T_1 values range from 200 to 1000 ms [11, 12]. Differences in the T_1 and T_2 values among body tissues is largely responsible for the contrast in MR images. Blood has relatively long T_1 and T_2 values. Many of the more successful angiographic techniques do not depend on the relaxation parameters to provide the contrast.

Phase Coherence and Dephasing

Other phenomena that can cause dephasing and signal loss are field inhomogeneity and magnetic field gradients. These are reversible to some extent and can be corrected. Added to spin-spin relaxation these effects cause the FID to decay at a rate faster than that given by T_2. The constant T_2^* is often used to describe the rate of decay due to the collective dephasing effects.

Inhomogeneities in the main magnetic field contribute frequency variations within a voxel in the same manner as described above. A spin located in a slightly higher field develops a phase lead over a slower moving spin, as described in Fig. 3b. By using a 180° RF pulse about the x-axis, the system of spins can be reflected about that axis as shown. The precession direction is still the same, but the faster moving spin is now situated behind the slower moving spin. In a time equal to that required to develop the phase lead, the faster spin catches up with the slower spin. A regrowth of the signal occurs as the spins rephase, creating a signal echo. This is known as a *spin-echo* technique [13]. Because of the dynamic nature of the T_2 dephasing process, it is not reversible as is the dephasing caused by field inhomogeneity. The peak of the echo created by the refocussing pulse still reflects T_2 decay.

Fourier Transform and Data Collection

The basic magnetic resonance experiment consists of a sample in a magnetic field. A transmitting coil excites the spin system with an RF pulse causing the net magnetization vector to rotate into the transverse plane. When the pulse ceases, the spin system begins to return to equilibrium. The receiver coil is turned on and measures the FID. One way to create an image would be to repeat this process at every location within the object. This is impractical for many reasons, particularly because of the excessive amount of time it would take to complete an image with, for example, 256 × 256 elements. The process is expedited by taking advantage of a mathematical tool known as the *Fourier transform* [14]. The principle behind the Fourier transform is that any signal can be represented as a sum of sine and cosine waves of many frequencies and can be decomposed into its individual frequency components. This is expressed in the following Fourier transform equation:

$$S(t) = C \int m(v)\, e^{i2\pi vt} dv \qquad (3)$$

where $S(t)$ is the signal at time t, $m(v)$ is the magnetization at frequency v, and C is a constant. In the case of MRI, if several voxels were placed in different field strengths and excited simultaneously, they would each generate an FID at a different Larmor frequency (Fig. 4). The signal measured by the receiver coil is the sum of these signals. This signal is processed by Fourier transform

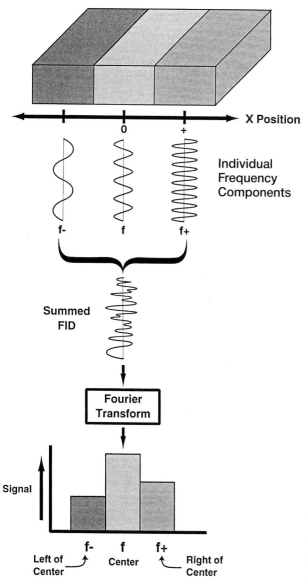

Fig. 4. In Fourier imaging the collective FID from spins with different Larmor frequencies is measured and processed by a Fourier transform to regain the individual frequency components of the input signal. By using magnetic field gradients to spatially vary the main field, frequency can be interpreted to give the location of the signal

and yields the distribution and content of the frequencies from each of the contributing voxels.

Furthermore, once we have the frequencies we can deduce the value of the field at each voxel due to the one-to-one relationship between frequency and field strength given in Eq. 1. If the spatial pattern of the field is known, the location of the voxel is known. In this way the signal values can be assigned to the appropriate location in the digital image. In practice this is accomplished by superimposing linear magnetic field gradients on the main magnetic field and exciting many frequencies simultaneously.

Many methods for data collection have been used successfully, including the sensitive point, line scan, and projection reconstruction techniques [15]. The method found on most commercial imagers today encodes position along rows and columns into the phase and frequency of the nuclear magnetic resonance signal. Spatial information is retrieved by performing a Fourier transform first along the columns of the image and then along the rows. This procedure is usually referred to as two-dimensional Fourier transform.

The MR signal is a complex valued signal. Ordinarily, it is the display of the magnitude of the signal that shows the soft tissue anatomy. Alternatively, the phase of the signal or the real or imaginary components of the signal can be displayed. Under ideal conditions for tissues with the same magnetic susceptibility values, the phase angle at every position in the image is the same and displaying phase values is uninformative. However, field inhomogeneity, an improperly tuned imaging sequence or disturbances such as flow can result in variations in the phase. Another cause of phase disturbance are differences in the magnetic susceptibilities of different tissue. This is seen particularly at boundaries between air and tissue or between tissue and blood. The phase image is frequently used to detect these occurrences. If desired, only the real or imaginary portion of the signal can be examined. These correspond to the signals measured by two orthogonal receiver demodulators. As we will see, phase can be made to depend on velocity. Alternatively, phase may be measured as a way to quantitate velocity.

In standard MRI data acquisition Fourier transform is an essential step in digital image processing before a recognizable image is obtained. Additional levels of digital signal processing are often used such as smoothing and edge enhancement to improve the appearance of the image. The image data can be manipulated to present a different form of the data, for example, an image composed of the T_1 or T_2 values at every pixel. There are an inexhaustible number of ways in which the data can be processed to provide different forms for display.

Spatial Localization

Throughout the development of MRI techniques there have been many methods used for data acquisition and image reconstruction, including the sensitive point and line methods and a number of variants of Fourier imaging. A number of texts provide details about the development and historical significance of each of these [16, 17]. We describe here the two-dimensional Fourier transform method that has become the standard for the majoritiy of commercial systems today. In this method the signal measured by the receiver has spatial information encoded into its frequency and phase. The "raw data" as collected (the FIDs or spin echoes) do not make a recognizable image until it is decoded by two-dimensional Fourier transform. In a typical data acquisition the position along the x direction is encoded into the frequency and position along the y direction into the phase.

Three steps are used to localize points spatially along the three axes in space. In two-dimensional data acquisition the first of these is the slice selection. Consider the following example of a transaxial slice acquisition. Slice selection is performed by turning on a magnetic field gradient in the slice direction, shown along the z axis in Fig. 5. A linear gradient G_z is used such that the field in the z direction has the form

$$B(z) = B_0 + G_z z \qquad (4)$$

With the z gradient on, every position along z has a different field value. The RF pulse used for excitation is tailored to contain frequencies corresponding only to the Larmor frequency of spins contained within the slice z. Only these spins are affected and experience rotation of their magnetization vectors. This is called *selective excitation*. These spins now have a transverse component to their magnetization and can generate signal.

Once a slice has been selected, phase encoding is used to provide differentiation along the y direction. It is convenient to first skip to the third axis of spatial localization and discuss frequency encoding. This is performed along the readout direc-

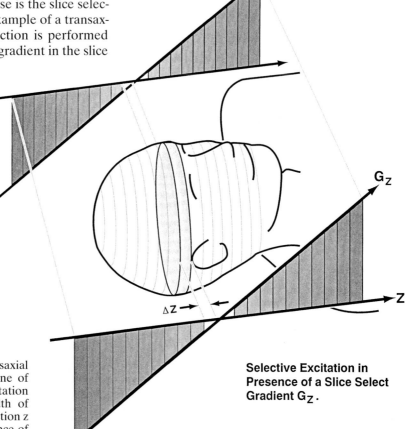

Fig. 5. In this example of a transaxial image acquisition, a selected plane of tissue is excited by using RF excitation that contains a narrow bandwidth of frequencies corresponding to a section z along the z direction in the presence of the gradient G_z

Selective Excitation in Presence of a Slice Select Gradient G_Z.

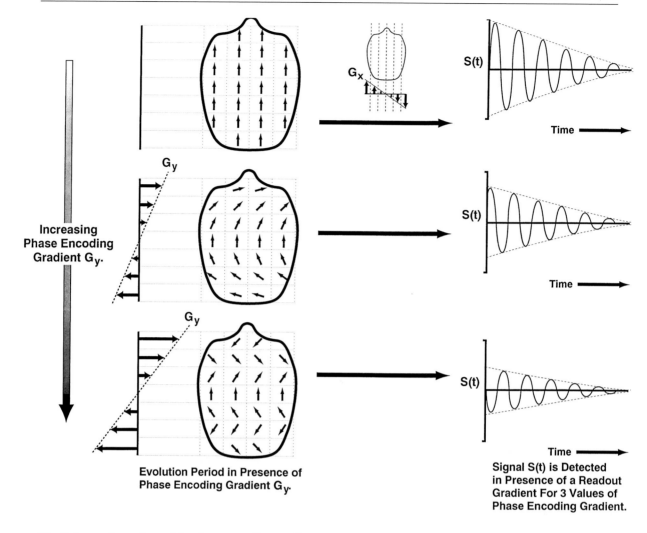

Evolution Period in Presence of
Phase Encoding Gradient G_y.

Signal S(t) is Detected
in Presence of a Readout
Gradient For 3 Values of
Phase Encoding Gradient.

Fig. 6. Increasing values of the phase-encoding gradient cause increasing distortions of the signal that is read out in the presence of an x gradient

tion, shown as x in Fig. 6. The readout gradient remains on while the FID is being sampled. The readout gradient is given by:

$$B(x) = B_0 + G_x x \qquad (5)$$

Spins at different positions along x generate signals at different frequencies. The combined FID is decomposed by Fourier transformation to give the individual frequency components. These correspond to x position.

Between the time of the RF excitation with slice selection and the time of the signal readout the phase-encoding gradient is turned on such that the field in the y direction has a linear dependence of the form

$$B(y) = B_0 + G_y y \qquad (6)$$

The phase encoding gradient is turned on for a short period of time and then removed. Slice excitation and signal readout is repeated for N_{pe} different values of the phase-encoding gradient. During the time that the phase-encoding gradient is on, spins in different rows along the y direction precess at different frequencies. When the phase encoding gradient is turned off, the spins are again in the same field B_0 and all return to the same precession frequency f_L. However, they have gained or lost a phase angle as a function of the y direction. In subsequent phase encoding cycles this is repeated but at increasing strengths of the phase-encoding gradient. Looking along each column, the combined FID is increasingly distorted with each phase-encoding step. The effect on the FID of a changing gradient over N_{pe} steps is the same as the effect of sampling the FID continuously in the presence of a constant gradient, as in the readout direction. Figure 6 demonstrates the effect of three increasing values of the phase-encoding gradient on the FID signal. Fourier transform along the y direction give the frequency components along y and thus position. The two dimensions of Fourier transform performed in x and y are identical.

The acquired data is in the form of rows of sampled FIDs with increasing phase-encoding gradient values. Because of the unique relationship between position and precession frequency, established by the use of the magnetic field gradients, the acquired data represent the spatial frequency contributions of the image and are therefore often referred to as k space data, where k is the wave number or value of the spatial frequency. In the majority of images encountered when imaging humans and animals with MRI, the largest contributions to the image are made by the low spatial frequencies with decreasing contributions at higher k values. The highest k values contribute details such as edges and features of small dimension.

The three gradients of the magnet can be used interchangeably to perform slice selection, phase encoding, or signal readout. This allows images of any orientation (transaxial, sagittal, coronal, or oblique) to be defined. There are often benefits to choosing one orientation over another. It is generally desirable to orient the readout direction along the long axis of the object (for example, the right-left axis through the chest in a transaxial image plane) and the phase-encoding direction along the short axis (anterior-posterior). The reason for this is that there is a time penalty incurred for increasing the number of phase-encoding cycles but not for increasing the number of samples taken along the readout direction. Another consideration when deciding the phase-encoding direction is to align it in the direction of least motion as this shows the greatest motion sensitivity.

An alternative to collecting slice images is three-dimensional data acquisition. A thick slab is excited rather than individual slices, and an additional dimension of phase encoding is used to spatially localize planes within the slab. There is an increase in imaging time proportional to the number of phase encoding steps used in the slice dimension with a concurrent improvement in signal-to-noise ratio (S/N). For this reason very short TR values are usually used in three-dimensional acquisitions to offset the increased imaging time.

Imaging Parameters

Relaxation Time Dependences

There are many adjustable parameters of an MRI procedure that can have an effect on image appearance. Three important parameters are the *pulse repetition interval* (TR), the *echo delay time* (TE), and the *flip angle* (Θ). TR is the time between successive RF excitations of a given slice. The intrinsic T_1 value of the tissue determines the rate at which longitudinal magnetization recovers. By choosing TR appropriately one can control whether a portion or all of that magnetization is allowed to recover. A long TR means a higher signal level but also lengthens the total imaging time. Since in most cases a heterogeneous group of tissues with a range of T_1 values are imaged simultaneously, TR must be chosen judiciously to best portray all the tissues of interest [18].

TE is the time delay between the RF excitation and the measurement of the signal. Transverse magnetization created by the RF pulse begins to dephase immediately after the pulse due to T_2 and other effects such as field inhomogeneity. A 180° refocusing pulse at time TE/2 creates a spin echo at time TE that is corrected for field inhomogeneity effects. If no spin echo is performed, the rate of signal decay is faster, as characterized by T_2^*. A short TE measures maximal signal early in the decay while a long TE measures less signal later in the decay.

The flip angle is the angle through which the magnetization vector **M** is rotated away from the longitudinal direction by the RF pulse. A 90° pulse maximizes the transverse component but also requires a long recovery time before the next excitation to fully restore longitudinal magnetization. Since the recovery rate varies for different tissues depending on T_1, a single choice of flip angle has a different effect on each tissue. Choice of TR, TE, and flip angle determines image contrast and S/N as well as the total imaging time and the ability to obtain multiple sections in a single experiment [19].

Image Contrast

Changing the above parameters gives MRI a powerful control of image contrast. Contrast is defined by the expression:

$$C = \frac{(I_A + I_B)}{I_B} \qquad (7)$$

where I_A is the feature signal, and I_B is the background signal. The MR image intensity depends not only on the hydrogen density distribution but on the relaxation characteristics of the nuclei. The intensity dependence in a spin-echo experiment is approximated by the following expression:

$$I = N(H) \frac{(1 - e^{-\frac{TR}{T_1}})\, e^{-\frac{TR}{T_2}} \sin \Theta}{1 - \cos \Theta \, e^{-\frac{TR}{T_1}}} \qquad (8)$$

Since water content in human soft tissue varies by only about 20 %, hydrogen density $N(H)$ accounts for only a small portion of the contrast seen with MRI. Certain pathological conditions, such as edema or fluid-contaning cysts, have a more marked increase in water content and may be detectable on this basis alone.

Most of the contrast is generated by T_1 and T_2 differences among tissues. The T_1 value of a tissue determines the rate at which its longitudinal magnetization M_z recovers after RF excitation. The TR value chosen determines how much recovered M_z is available to become transverse magnetization M_{xy} with the next RF excitation. Since signal intensity is determined by M_{xy}, we can control signal intensity by adjusting TR. A tissue with a long T_1 appears dark on a short TR image since little magnetization is allowed to recover. If the goal is simply to maximize signal, one should just allow a TR long enough for M_z to recover completely. However, considerations of contrast and imaging time often make it advantageous to shorten TR at the expense of signal. Adjusting TR is one strategy for improving the contrast between a feature and its surrounding tissue. The contrast between tissues is shown above to be proportional to the difference in signal intensity and therefore to the difference in M_{xy} values. Two tissues with different T_1 values recover at different rates, and a prudent choice of TR can maximize the difference in the amount of recovered M_z between the two.

TE is used to control contrast in a similar way. After M_{xy} is produced by RF excitation, it begins to dephase because of T_2 effects and field inhomogeneity. The size of the signal measured by the receiver decreases as the time delay TE increases. The rate of the signal decay is characterized by the T_2 value of the tissue. Signal can be maximized by using as short a TE value as possible. A long TE value makes tissues with a short T_2 appear dark. For two tissues with different T_2 values the difference in the amount of measurable M_{xy} can be improved by a longer TE value, improving contrast by sacrificing signal.

An addition to adjusting TR, the flip angle Θ can be used to affect T_1-related contrast. The optimal flip angle depends on the T_1 value of the tissue as well as the TR value used. At short TR values (TR $< T_1$) reduced flip angles can increase S/N as well. Figure 7 illustrates the behavior of the signal difference as a function of choice of TR and TE for tissues with different T_1 and T_2 values. Two tissues, A and B, have relative hydrogen density values reflected by M_{0A} and M_{0B}. After a 90° RF excitation T_1 relaxation occurs at different rates, T_{1A} and T_{1B} for the two tissues. The choice of the repetition time TR determines the relative amounts of magnetization M_{xyA} and M_{xyB} that become transverse magnetization. M_{xyA} and M_{xyB} decay with relaxation rates T_{2A} and T_{2B}, respectively. Choice of echo delay time TE determines the relative signal intensities I_A and I_B at the time of readout. It is clear from this example that the final intensity difference is affected by both TR and TE as well as the hydrogen density, T_1, and T_2 values of the tissues.

Vascular Contrast

Many of the procedures used for imaging blood rely on the inflow of spins, which have received no previous RF excitation, into a volume of stationary tissue that is darkened by frequent RF excitation (short TR value). Inflowing blood behaves as if it experiences an infinite TR. This gives a bright signal from blood while suppressing background signal [20, 21] an effect known as flow-related enhancement. In these techniques TR and flip angle must be selected to give sufficient background suppression while allowing enough time for fresh spins to enter the volume. By generating contrast in this way, T_1 effects become less important.

These are also referred to as time-of-flight (TOF) effects. Using this mechanism, vascular contrast is

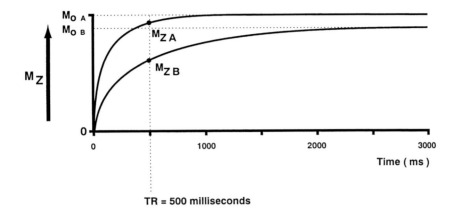

TR = 500 milliseconds

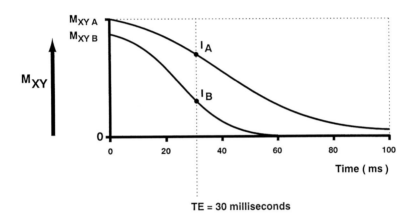

TE = 30 milliseconds

Fig. 7. The effect of choice of TR and TE on the relative signal intensities I_A and I_B of tissues A and B with hydrogen density, T_1 and T_2 values M_{0A}, T_{1A}, and T_{2A} for tissue A and M_{0B}, T_{1B}, and T_{2B} for tissue B

generated by creating large differences in longitudinal magnetization between stationary tissue and flowing blood.

It has recently been shown that the magnetization transfer effect [22] can help to improve vascular contrast in TOF MR angiography (MRA) [23]. Using this method, stationary tissue signal is affected by using an off-resonance RF excitation to reduce the longitudinal magnetization of immobile protons contained in macromolecular structures of the stationary tissue. Through chemical exchange of these immobile protons with the mobile water-based protons the reduced magnetization is transferred to the mobile protons. This reduces the detectable signal since signal comes mainly from mobile protons. The result is a further suppression of stationary tissue signal without a similar suppression of flowing blood's signal. This gives greater vascular contrast.

The other mechanism commonly used to generate vascular contrast uses differences in the phase of flowing and stationary spins. This is performed by using magnetic field gradients to introduce velocity-dependent phase changes. Stationary spins (zero velocity) acquire no phase angle. Moving spins acquire a phase angle that is proportional to their velocity.

Phase Dependences

When a nucleus moves through a field gradient, its frequency changes. For nuclei moving with constant velocity v along the gradient direction, their frequency in the rotating frame is:

$$f_v = \gamma\, G(t)\, v\, t \qquad (9)$$

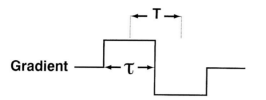

Fig. 8. Bipolar gradient pulse shifts spin phase in proportion to velocity

where G(t) is the gradient as a function of time, and t is time. If the gradient is on for some time Γ the phase accumulated is the area of this function. Thus the phase Φ is:

$$\Phi = \gamma \int_0^{\Gamma} G(t)\, v\, dt \qquad (10)$$

Figure 8 shows the common bipolar gradient waveform G(t) used for slice selection and signal readout. The phase accumulated by spins moving at a constant velocity v during this gradient waveform is:

$$\Phi = \gamma\, G\, v\, T\, \tau \qquad (11)$$

τ is the duration of each lobe of the bipolar waveform, and T is the time between centers of the positive and negative lobes. For stationary spins v = 0, and there is no phase accumulation.

When flow changes phase, if all of a sample moves at one velocity (as a plug pushed through a tube), all the nuclei have some phase change Φ. Thus, total signal would still be strong, only having a phase offset from zero. However, if there are many different velocities in the sample, as with laminar or turbulent flow, each velocity has a different phase. This distribution of phases reduces the signal. The distribution of phases is centered around the phase proportional to average velocity rather than zero.

Hahn first realized that one can find the average velocity of sea water by measuring the phase of a spin echo [24]. This experiment had no spatial resolution. In MRI, the phase distributions provide different effects. When there are many velocities in a voxel, the distribution of phase reduces signal. By repeating the measurement with many different values of gradient one can recover the velocity distribution [25–27]. On the other hand, if the voxel is made small enough, it includes only one velocity. There is then no destructive interference reducing the signal, and the phase gives the velocity. Velocity quantitation is thus possible with small voxels.

Magnetic Resonance Angiographic Techniques

MRA techniques utilize differences between flowing blood and stationary tissue to generate contrast that highlights the blood vessels. Relaxation differences and phase effects both contribute to such contrast. Most techniques attempt to maximize the contribution of one and suppress the other. TOF techniques depend mainly on relaxation times while phase-based techniques, including phase contrast (PC), use the velocity dependence of phase.

TOF angiograms use flow-related enhancement to obtain bright blood by one of two different methods: two-dimensional and three-dimensional. In the two-dimensional approach the imaging volume is limited to thin slices. Sequential slices are imaged to cover the structure of interest [28]. Because the slices are thin, the flowing blood does not stay in the slice long enought to loose longitudinal magnetization and remains bright throughout the slice. Two-dimensional imaging of thin slices limits S/N and coverage.

In three-dimensional TOF MRA a relatively thick slab is subdivided into thin slices by phase encoding [29]. Because the inflowing blood remains in the imaging volume for many times the TR time, it may loose longitudinal magnetization. This decreases the flow-related enhancement and results in decreased intensity of flowing blood relative to stationary tissues. The slower the blood flow, the more magnetization is lost, making three-dimensional TOF MRA somewhat insensitive to slowly flowing blood. The very thin partitions of three-dimensional TOF MRA improve spatial resolution with S/N kept up by the longer three-dimensional acquisition.

RF pulses applied outside the imaged region suppress the signal from blood flowing in from the pulsed region [30]. Such "presaturation" pulses can be employed to image selectively either the arteries or veins.

All TOF techniques generate images in which stationary tissues appear dark, and vessels containing flowing blood appear bright. To assist interpretation, computer postprocessing is used to create projection images in which the vessels are displayed in a format analogous to conventional angiography. The simplest and most popular method for producing such projections is the maximum-intensity projection (MIP) algorithm [31]. The three-dimensionally processed vessel data can be displayed at multiple projection angles with the signal intensity of the background tissues suppressed.

Angiography can exploit the signal loss in voxels that include a wide range of velocities. A spin-echo image can be made insensitive to velocity with the proper gradient pulses [32–36]. One angiographic approach is to acquire velocity insensitive (bright blood) and velocity sensitive (dark blood) images and then subtract the images. The stationary background is the same intensity in both images and cancels in the subtraction. Subtracting the dark flow regions from the bright flow regions leaves the flow bright. The resulting angiogram shows bright vessels. This approach has the usual registration problems of subtraction imaging but is the starting point for many newer techniques.

PC MRA relies directly upon phase shifts generated by the motion of flowing blood. In the simplest form pairs of bipolar gradient pulses of equal strength and duration but of opposite signs are applied. The phase shifts associated with these sequential acquisitions are then substracted. For stationary tissues the result is zero phase intensity because any phase shifts are equal and cancel one another when subtracted. Moving blood yields phase intensity proportional to its velocity.

This proportionality allows quantitation of blood velocity with PC MRA. Marked background tissue suppression is another advantage of this approach. As with TOF methods, computer post-processing with MIP and other algorithms produces MR angiograms that resemble conventional X-ray angiograms. Acquisition times are relatively long for PC MRA because multiple acquisitions along orthogonal flow directions are necessary to complete a volumetric data set.

One of the tradeoffs that must be made in vascular imaging techniques is between the precision of flow-sensitizing or flow-compensating gradient waveforms and minimizing TE. Both physiologic and abnormal flow exhibit speed and directional changes over the cardiac cycle. This flow is characterized by velocity and higher order motions, acceleration, pulsatility, etc. Gradient waveforms designed to compensate for, or be sensitive to, the higher order motions become increasingly complex, requiring longer times to execute and more gradient switching. The longer times result in longer TE values, which exacerbates the signal loss caused by uncompensated motion or other dephasing effects, such as inhomogeneity. In general, only first-order (velocity) compensation is used, keeping TE to a minimum. Other strategies that are used to minimize the amount of compensation necessary and thus reduce TE are the use of truncated RF excitation and asymmetric echo samples [37, 38].

Instrumentation

The whole-body MRI scanner has four major subsystems: the magnet, the gradient system, the RF transmitter/receiver system, and the computer system for data acquisition and display (Fig. 9) [16, 17, 39].

Magnet Subsystem

The magnet is the central component of the imaging system and can be permanent, resistive, or superconducting. The requirements for operating field strength and field homogeneity usually determine which magnet can be used. In general, for clinical imaging of hydrogen at a field strength greater than about 0.3 T a superconducting magnet is necessary. Resistive or permanent magnets perform adequately below this value. Some other considerations for magnet selection are the ease of access, cost, and siting.

Magnetic Field Gradients

The gradient subsystem provides the spatial dependence of the magnetic field needed for spatial localization. The simplest and most common design uses linear magnetic field gradients along each of three mutually orthogonal directions. While the actual physical design of each may differ to allow for patient access to the magnet, they perform identical functions and can be interchanged to acquire transaxial, sagittal, coronal, or oblique imaging planes. Some of the requirements on gradient design are the strength, linearity, and ability to switch rapidly. An increase in gradient strength is the easiest method of increasing spatial resolution. Gradient linearity assures that the pixel dimension is the same at every point in the image. Many imaging systems require the gradients to change values very rapidly. Fast switching allows a short TE and other factors needed for high-speed and angiographic imaging. The magnetic field exerts a force on the current-carrying wires of the gradient coil.

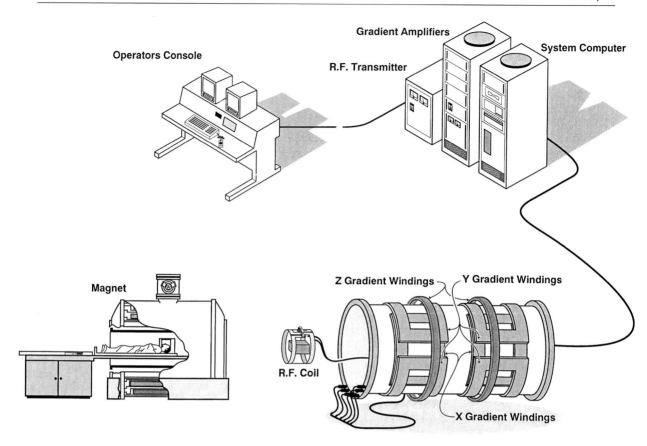

Fig. 9. Major components of MRI apparatus are the magnet, gradient subsystem, RF coils and associated electronics, and the computer system for data acquisition, processing, and display

When the gradients are switched, an audible knocking is heard as the coil reacts to the forces upon it. This is the source of the rhythmic pattern heard during an imaging procedure.

When a rapidly changing magnetic field intersects with a conductive surface, it induces currents in the conductor that oppose the change in magnetic field. These are called eddy currents. In an MR system the gradients produce changing fields that intersect with the magnet structure. The resulting eddy currents reduce the strength, rise time, and linearity of the gradient field. An effective way to eliminate this performance degradation is to use shielded gradient coils [40, 41]. These use pairs of concentric coils. The inner coil provides the gradient, and the outer coil cancels the fields outside that would reach the magnet structure. The shielding opposition of the outer coil reduces the gradient but by less than the eddy current's field

reduction. The shielded gradient coil thus improves imager performance.

The gradient subsystem is the most critical to the performance of vascular techniques. In flow imaging specialized gradient waveforms are used that compensate for phase differences accumulated by moving spins or, conversely, to introduce precise amounts of phase to moving spins. These waveforms are more demanding in terms of accuracy and speed than those used for conventional imaging. Another means of minimizing the phase accumulation is to reduce TE. Both of these procedures are limited by gradient performance. In general, stronger gradients and faster rise times improve the capability for vascular imaging. Strengths greater than 10 mT/m and rise times (5 %–95 % levels) of less than 1 ms are desirable.

Transmitter/Receiver

The transmitter coil provides the magnetic field B_1 in the form of an RF magnetic field oscillating in the transverse plane. The receiver coil detects the induced voltage during relaxation. Because of the intermittent nature of transmission and reception these two functions can often be served by the same coil. The performance of the receiver coil is strongly affected by how well the object fills the coil. For this reason special coils are built for almost every body part. Most coils surround the body to produce a uniform B_1 field. Surface coils that span only a limited area produce better S/N images for anatomy close to the body surface. The sensitivity of these surface coils falls off quickly with depth, and the images suffer from nonuniform intensity shading.

The requirements of coils to be used for vascular imaging are the same as for conventional imaging. The highest S/N obtainable must be weighed against the useful field of view (FOV) and homogeneity of the coil. Some usefulness has been shown for a specialized vascular coil for imaging the carotid arteries from their origin at the aorta through the bifurcation region and ending at the circle of Willis. Other areas of interest for vascular imaging, including the cerebral circulation, cardiac output, and peripheral flow, generally use standard imaging coils for their angiographic applications.

Computer System

The computer system is responsible for coordinating the entire system performance. Its function can be divided into two major areas. It is the controller for all hardware operation and maintains the timing of all events in the MRI pulse sequence. Once the data have been acquired, it also carries out all image manipulations including processing by two- or three-dimensional Fourier transform, disk storage, display, and archiving. These tasks are supported by at least two computers. Additional units, commonly in the form of workstations, provide for additoinal image processing and review.

The control computer times each event in the imaging sequence, such as the duration of the gradient and RF pulses. Digital-to-analog converters allow this computer to set the values of the gradients and to create modulated RF pulses. The computer operates switches in the receiver and transmitter that route the signals to and from the RF coil(s). The computer provides the frequency setting for the frequency synthesizer and also controls the digitization of the demodulated signal by setting the sampling rate and then turning on the analog-to-digital converters, which perform the digitization and send the results to the data acquisition system. Many different imaging sequences are stored in the computer's memory. To image a patient the MRI system operator, using the data acquisition computer, chooses a sequence, and the data acquisition system sends the choice to the control computer.

The MRI data acquisition and display processor system records the digitized MRI signal, performs any signal averaging needed to improve S/N, carries out Fourier transforms to create the images based on spectral information, displays the images for the physician, and provides for permanent archiving of the images. A minicomputer and array processor handle these tasks. The computer has a multitasking operating system that allocates time-critical resources to the averaging and storing of data during the imaging procedure. It has a large amount of disk storage available since 20-slice images typically have over 10 Mbyte of data. Once all the data are available from a patient, this minicomputer uses the array processor to perform the Fourier transforms. The resulting images are viewed while additional data is acquired, other patient protocols are selected, and images are archived to magnetic tape or optical disk. The processor speed and storage are large enough to hide most operations from the user. One sets up patient scans and reviews images. The reconstruction and archiving operations can be automated.

Resolution, Signal-to-Noise Ratio, and Imaging Time

Resolution and Field of View

Image quality is affected by its resolution, S/N ratio, and imaging time [42, 43]. The resolution in MRI is measured by the voxel dimensions used in the image. It is determined by the frequency bandwidth of the RF excitation and reception and by the strength of the magnetic field gradients. Achievable resolution in a whole-body image is $0.5 \times 0.5 \times 2$ mm. Despite increasing capabilities of the hardware there are other limitations to the minimum voxel dimension. As the voxel size decrease, signal strength decreases in proportion to the reduction in the number of nuclei it contains.

The S/N ratio becomes a practical limitation. Even with improvements in noise-reduction techniques, thermal motion and diffusion within a voxel may become a more fundamental constraint. Another consideration is the relationship between resolution, the size of the FOV, and the imaging time. For a fixed matrix size and imaging time the FOV is reduced in proportion to the reduction in voxel size. To maintain FOV at the higher resolution additional measurements would be necessary. If these are taken in the phase-encoding direction, the imaging time increases proportionally.

When the object size exceeds the imaging FOV, a condition known as *aliasing* results, whereby signal from tissue outside of the FOV is interpreted to be overlapping with tissue within the FOV. This occurs when the object contains frequencies above the maximum frequency f_{max} that can be unambiguously assigned.

$$f_{max} = \frac{1}{2T_s} \qquad (12)$$

where T_s is the sampling interval. The result is image wraparound. For example, in a head image for which the FOV in the anterior/posterior direction is smaller than the size of the head, signal from the anterior of the head that is above the FOV appears at the bottom of the image, overlapping the posterior segment of the image. This can be overcome by increasing the FOV either by increasing the number of samples at the same resolution or by decreasing the resolution for the same number of samples in that direction. An alternative is to eliminate outside tissue by selective excitation or presaturation.

Signal-to-Noise Ratio

The S/N ratio is another important contributor to image quality. Parameters of the imaging sequence such as TR, TE, and flip angle all affect the total signal. Increasing TR, decreasing TE, and using a flip angle of 90° with a long TR all increase the total signal but may be undesirable from the standpoints of contrast and imaging time. Reduction of the voxel size provides an improvement in resolution but proportionally reduces the number of signal-generating spins while noise remains the same. If more measurements are taken to provide the resolution, the additional measurements bring back some S/N. Another im-

portant determinant of signal is the frequency bandwidth of the voxel spectrum. Distributing the voxel signal over a larger bandwith reduces S/N by increasing the noise included in the image. Increasing FOV, total bandwidth, and number of elements by the same factor has no impact on S/N because individual voxel bandwidth does not change.

For a fixed imaging sequence the signal intensity is also affected by the operating frequency of the magnet. Signal increases as the square of frequency, ignoring variations in relaxation times. The noise dependence is not as easily quantified. Theory shows that a high frequency noise increases in proportion to frequency while at low frequency it is proportional to the square root of frequency. The dependence of S/N on operating frequency has been reported experimentally to vary to the first power or less. For a well-tuned system the body itself is the greatest noise source because random currents in the body are picked up as noise by the receiver coil.

Imaging Time

To acquire a full data set, excitation and readout are repeated after time TR for each value of the phase-encoding gradient. Repeated measurements at the same value of the phase encoding gradient may also be obtained to improve the S/N using signal averaging:

$$\text{Total time} = TR \, N_{pe} N_{acq} \qquad (13)$$

where N_{acq} is the number of repetitions at each phase-encoding step,

$$S/N \propto \sqrt{N_{acq}} \qquad (14)$$

Thus improving S/N by increasing N_{acq} requires a large increase in imaging time.

In general, the acquisition of multiple slices does not affect the imaging time. *Multislicing* is achieved by using the time between the completion of data acquisition and the start of the next excitation at TR to acquire data at additional slice locations. For example, for a double spin echo sequence with TE values of 30 and 60 ms and a TR value of 2000 ms, generously allowing 100 ms to complete data readout, an interval of 1900 ms is available before the next excitation occurs. During this time 19 additional slices can be acquired

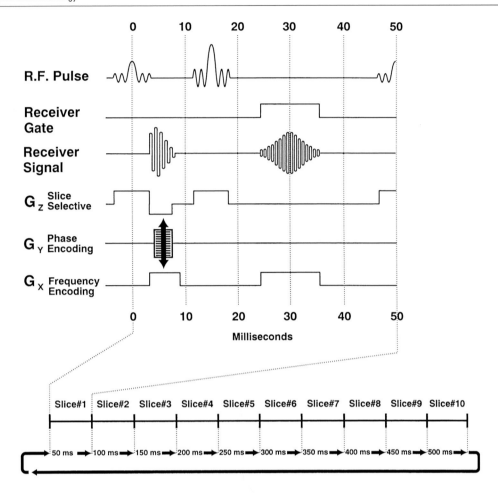

Fig. 10. A pulse timing diagram showing the strengths and timing of transmitted RF excitations, gradients G_x, G_y and G_z, and signal reception for a typical spin-echo data acquisition. In this example, data collection is complete in less than 50 ms. This allows excitation and data acquisition to be performed at nine other slice locations before the interval between excitations, TR = 500 ms elapses for slice number 1

by moving the slice selection to a new location that is parallel and usually contiguous to the previous slices. In this way multislicing improves the duty cycle of the acquisition without increasing the total imaging time.

Imaging Pulse Sequence

All of the necessary components are now in place to talk about the *pulse sequence*. All of the parameters of the imaging technique are specified with the pulse sequence and are often shown schematically in the pulse timing diagram. The number, strength, timing, and waveform of the RF excitations, the duration and strength of the three magnetic field gradients, and the length and sampling rate of the readout period are all selected to determine the TR, TE, resolution, FOV, S/N, and contrast for the tissues being imaged. A priori knowledge of the T_1 and T_2 values helps with the selection of these parameters. Figure 10

presents an example of a pulse timing diagram for a spin-echo pulse sequence with TR = 500 ms and TE = 30 ms. At the start of the experiment at $t = 0$, a 90° RF pulse is transmitted in the presence of a slice selection gradient along the z-axis. After the pulse is completed, the slice-select gradient is reversed to correct the phase dispersion caused by the slice selection. At the same time the phase-encoding gradient is turned on at its first value. The readout gradient (frequency encoding) also appears. This is a dephasing lobe used to dephase the spins so that a full gradient echo can be measured during readout. At time $t = 15$ ms, a 180°

RF pulse is transmitted in the presence of the slice-select gradient to create a spin echo. Because the 180° pulse creates a mirror image of the spin system, the slice-select gradient acts in a positive sense prior to the 180° pulse and in a negative sense afterwards. This is also why the dephasing lobe of the readout gradient is in the same direction as during readout. When the 180° pulse is completed, the readout gradient is turned on, and the signal is sampled symmetrically about the echo time $t = 30$ ms. After time TR the experiment is repeated for each new value of the phase-encoding gradient. In practice, because data acquisition is completed in less than 50 ms, the waiting time can be spent acquiring other slices until it is time to return to the first slice at TR = 500 ms. Many special-function pulse sequences have been developed to address specific imaging needs. The spin-echo pulse sequence has been a standard over the years, but it has some drawbacks. The time spent issuing 180° pulses to correct for field inhomogeneities also serves to prolong the TE value. If the 180° pulse is removed and a shorter TE is used, the loss of signal due to field inhomogeneity can be offset to some extent by the reduced T_2 decay. Sequences that create the signal echo by dephasing and rephasing the spins using the readout gradient rather than using 180° pulses are referred to as *gradient-reversal* or *gradient-echo* sequences.

Throughout the development of MRI technology, as methods for signal acquisition and noise reduction have improved, it has become possible to maintain more than adequate S/N ratios while increasing resolution, reducing scan times, and improving contrast. In addition to manipulating TR and TE for contrast, the angle of rotation of the magnetization vector **M** by RF excitation can also be adjusted. *Partial-flip* sequences, as they are called, create less transverse magnetization and therefore less signal but generate another degree of T_1 contrast. More importantly, by rotating the longitudinal magnetization vector only partway into the transverse plane, less time is required for it to recover. This allows TR to be reduced substantially and lowers the total imaging time. Many sequences combine these features, most notably the FLASH [44] or GRASS [45] sequences. These partial-flip, gradient-echo sequences have a unique image appearance due to their reduced flip angle, TR and TE. Two-dimensional multislice and three-dimensional sequences of this type are commonly used to perform MRA.

Summary

It is hoped that the reader is left considering the many parameters that are involved in defining an MRI procedure and how these interact with the physical properties of the tissues. Therein lies the flexibility of MRI as well as the frustration when faced with an overwhelming number of techniques from which to select. The considerations become greater with the imaging of blood flow.

The intent of this chapter has been to familiarize the reader with the essential components of MRI, emphasizing the technical needs for imaging flowing blood. It has not been possible to be exhaustive in the coverage; many important and interesting topics have been only briefly mentioned or omitted altogether. Topics such as fast imaging, use of contrast agents, and cardiac gating are relevant to the study of flow and can be studied in the texts listed in the references.

References

1. Axel L, ed. (1991) ACR glossary of MR terms, 3rd edn. Reston, Virginia: American College of Radiology.
2. Abragham A (1961) The principles of nuclear magnetism. Oxford: Clarendon.
3. Curry TS, Dowdey JE, Murry RC (1978) Nuclear magnetic resonance. In: Christensen EE, Curry TS, Dowdey JE (eds) Introduction to the physics of diagnostic radiology. Philadelphia: Lea and Febiger.
4. Farrar TC, Becker ED (1971) Pulse and Fourier transform NMR. New York: Academic Press.
5. Fukushima E, Roeder ED (1981) Experimental pulse NMR: a nuts and bolts approach. Reading, MA: Addison-Wesley.
6. Mansfield P, Morris PG (1982) NMR imaging in biomedicine. New York: Academic Press.
7. Crooks LE, Mills CM, Davis PL, et al (1982) Visualization of cerebral abnormalities by NMR imaging: the effects of imaging parameters on contrast. Radiology 144: 843–852.
8. Damadian R (1971) Tumor detection by NMR. Science 171: 1151–1153.
9. Davis PL, Kaufman L, Crooks LE, Margulis AR (1981) NMR characteristics of normal and abnormal rat tissues. In: Kaufman L, Crooks LE, Margulis AR (eds) Nuclear magnetic resonance imaging in medicine. New York: Igaku-Shoin, Inc., 71–100.
10. Koenig SH, Brown RD (1986) Relaxometry of tissue. In: CRC handbook on NMR in cells. Boca Raton: CRC Press.
11. Bottomly PA, Foster TH, Argersinger RE, Pfeifer LM (1984) A review of normal tissue hydrogen NMR relaxation times and mechanisms from 1–100

MHz: dependence on tissue type, NMR frequency, temperature, species, excision and age. Med Phys 11: 425–448.

12. Chen J-H, Avram HE, Crooks LE, Arakawa M, Kaufman L, Brito AC (1992) In vivo relaxation times and hydrogen density at 0.063–4.85 T in rats with implanted mammary adenocarcinomas. Radiology 184: 427–434.

13. Hahn EL (1950) Spin echoes. Phys Rev 80: 580–594.

14. Bracewell RN (1978) The Fourier transform and its applications. New York: McGraw-Hill.

15. Morris PG (1986) Nuclear magnetic resonance imaging in medicine and biology. Oxford: Clarendon.

16. Kaufman I, Crooks LE, Margulis AR (eds) (1981) Nuclear magnetic resonance imaging in medicine. New York: Igaku Shoin.

17. Partain CL, Patton JA, Kulkarni MV, James AE (eds) (1988) Magnetic resonance imaging, vol II. Philadelphia: Saunders.

18. Ortendahl DA, Hylton NM, Kaufman L, et al (1984) Analytical tools for magnetic resonance imaging. Radiology 153: 479–488.

19. Edelstein WA, Bottomley PA, Hart HR, Smith LS (1983) Signal-to-noise and contrast in nuclear magnetic resonance. J Comput Assist Tomogr 7(3): 391–401.

20. Kaufman L, Crooks LE, Sheldon PE, Rowan W, Miller T (1982) Evaluation of NMR imaging for detection and quantification of obstructions in vessels. Investigative Radiology 17: 554–560.

21. von Schulthess GK, Fisher M, Crooks LE, Higgins CB (1985) Gated MR imaging of the heart: intracardiac signals in patients and healthy subjects. Radiology 156: 125–132.

22. Wolff SD, Balaban RS (1989) Magnetization transfer contrast (MTC) and tissue water proton relaxation *in vivo*. Magn Reson Med 10(1): 135–144.

23. Pike GB, Hu BS, Glover GH, Enzmann DR (1992) Magnetization transfer time-of-flight magnetic resonance angiography. Magn Reson Med 25(2): 372–379.

24. Hahn EL (1960) Detection of sea-water motion by nuclear precession. J Geophys Res 65: 776–777.

25. Grover T, Singer JR (1971) NMR spin-echo flow measurements. J Appl Phys 42: 938–940.

26. Garroway AN (1974) Velocity measurements in flowing fluids by NMR. J Phys D: Appl Phys 7: L159–163.

27. Moran PR (1982) A flow zeugmatographic interlace for NMR imaging in humans. Magn Reson Imaging 1: 197–203.

28. Keller PJ, Drayer BP, Fram EK, Williams KD, Dumoulin CL, Souza SP (1989) MR angiography with two-dimensional acquisition and three-dimensional display: work in progress. Radiology 173: 527–532.

29. Ruggieri PM, Laub GA, Masaryk TJ, Modic MT (1989) Intracranial circulation: pulse sequence considerations in three-dimensional (volume) MR angiography. Radiology 171(3): 785–791.

30. Felmlee JP, Ehman RL (1987) Spatial presaturation: a method for suppressing flow artifacts and improving depiction of vascular anatomy in MR imaging. Radiology 164: 559–564.

31. Rossnick S, Laub G, Braeckle R, et al (1986) Three dimensional display of blood vessels in MRI. Proceedings of the IEEE Computers in Cardiology Conference, New York 193–196.

32. Constantinesco A, Mallet JJ, Bonmartin A, Lallot C, Briguet A (1984) Spatial or flow velocity phase encoding gradients in NMR imaging. Magn Reson Imaging 2: 335–340.

33. Nayler GL, Firmin DN, Longmore DB (1986) Blood flow imaging by cine magnetic resonance. J Comput Assist Tomogr 10: 715–722.

34. Nishimura DG, Macovski A, Pauly JM (1986) Magnetic resonance angiography. IEEE Trans Med Imag MI-5: 140–151.

35. Haacke EM, Lenz GW (1987) Improving MR image quality in the presence of motion by using rephasing gradients. AJR 148: 1251–1258.

36. Axel L, Morton D (1987) MR flow imaging of velocity compensated/uncompensated difference images. J Comput Assist Tomogr 11: 31–34.

37. Nishimura DG, Macovski A, Jackson JI, Hu RS, Stevick CA, Axel L (1988) Magnetic resonance angiography by selective inversion recovery using a compact gradient echo sequence. Magn Reson Med 8: 96–103.

38. Schmalbrock P, Yuan C, Chakeres DW, Kohli J, Pelc NJ (1990) Volume MR angiography: methods to achieve very short echo times. Radiology 175: 861–865.

39. Maudsley AA, Hilal SK, Simon HE (1984). Electronics and instrumentation for NMR imaging. IEEE Trans Nucl Sci NS-31: 990–993.

40. Turner R, Bowley RM (1986) Passive screening of switched magnetic field gradients. J Phys E 19: 876–879.

41. Mansfield P, Chapman B (1986) Active magnetic screening of gradient coils in NMR imaging. J Magn Reson 66: 573–576.

42. Hoult DI, Lauterbur PC (1979) The sensitivity of the zeugmatographic experiment involving human subjects. J Magn Reson 34: 425–433.

43. Bruner P, Ernst RR (1979) Sensitivity and performance time in NMR imaging. J Magn Reson 33: 83–106.

44. Haase A, Frahm J, Matthaei D, Hanicke W, Merboldt K-D (1986) FLASH imaging. Rapid NMR imaging using low flip-angle pulses. J Magn Reson 67: 258–266.

45. Glover GH, Pelc NJ, Shimakawa A (1987) GRASS movie techniques for gated studies. Proceedings 1987 Topical Conference on Fast Magnetic Resonance Imaging Techniques. Case Western Reserve University, Cleveland, Ohio. May 15.

MR Angiographic Imaging

M. Kouwenhoven, C.J.G. Bakker, M.J. Hartkamp, and W.P.Th.M. Mali

In developing a scan protocol for magnetic resonance angiography (MRA), the physician should be aware of the host of possiblities offered by present-day MRA. It is the purpose of this chapter to provide a global survey of current techniques [1] and options, and to discuss their merits and limitations. The focus will not be on technical details, but more on the practical consequences of each particular technique on items such as contrast to noise as a function of velocity. Each of the basic techniques [2] is discussed (inflow or time of flight, and phase contrast angiography) as well as a wide range of additional techniques. No attempt is made to give a historical survey [3], and references are only mentioned as suggestion for further in-depth reading, but not as a complete list of original references. Promising techniques such as echo planar imaging (EPI) [4] and spiral imaging [5] are not discussed here, because their availability is currently limited. Conventional and blood pool MR contrast agents [6] are not discussed either. The reader should have a basic understanding of the underlying MR physics, such as the concepts of slice selection, saturation, relaxation times, phase, k-space, various imaging techniques such as spin echo and gradient field echo [7–9], and basic postprocessing techniques such as the maximum intensity projection (MIP) [10].

Basic Methods

Inflow Angiography

The basic concept of inflow (or time of flight, TOF) MR angiography [11] is twofold:
1. Saturation of stationary tissue (inside the imaging volume)
2. Enhanced signal from fully magnetized inflowing blood

Saturation of Stationary Tissue

For optimum display of the vessel tree, containing moving blood, all stationary tissue in the imaging volume is saturated by applying repeated radiofrequency (RF) pulses so that it will produce almost no signal. As shown in Fig. 1, saturation requires a very short repetition time (TR) between these RF pulses, which is most easily achieved with a gradient field echo sequence. Typically, a *TR* of 25–30 ms is used for conventional gradient field echo techniques. Also, gradient field echo techniques do not suffer from flow voids caused by washout between the excitation pulse and the refocussing pulse as in spin echo techniques (see „Black Blood Angiography", below).

Enhanced Signal from Inflowing Blood

If fully magnetized, fresh, unsaturated blood (blood which has not received any on-resonance RF pulses recently) flows into the clinical volume of interest, it can produce a strong MR signal when excited by an RF pulse (see Fig. 2). Thus, its signal will be strongly enhanced, compared to the stationary, saturated tissue.

The maximum inflow effect is obtained if the fresh inflowing blood receives only one RF pulse during its time in the imaging excitation volume. As soon as the blood receives more than one RF excitation pulse, the saturation effect starts to occur, similar to that of the background tissue. The blood will receive only one RF pulse, and hence show the maximal inflow effect, when the velocity v complies with the following condition:

$$v \geq \frac{\mathrm{d}}{\mathrm{TR}}, \qquad (1)$$

where v is velocity of the blood (the velocity component perpendicular to the imaging plane), *TR* is RF repetition time, and d is excitation thickness;

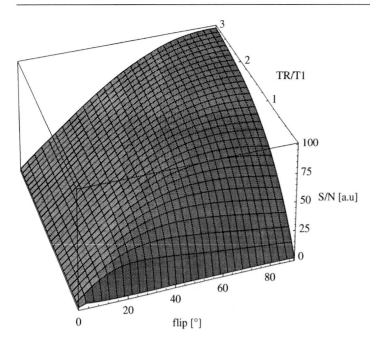

Fig. 1. Saturation of stationary tissue. Signal to noise (vertical axis, arbitrary units) vs. the flip angle and the *TR/T1* ratio. If *TR* is decreased, the spins in the tissue do not have time to fully relax, hence the signal decreases. In most MRA scans, the ratio *TR/T1* is very small (*TR* = ±25 ms, *T1* = 1000 ms, *TR/T1* = ±0.025) so that the signal from the tissue is effectively suppressed

depending on the technique used, this corresponds with:

2D: *d* = slice thickness
3D (single slab):   *d* = slab thickness
3D multiple slab: *d* = excitation thickness of
                                       every single slab

This condition applies to every pixel in those cases where the velocity varies over the vessel lumen (as in parabolic flow profiles, see Fig. 2). When flow is pulsatile, *v* does not simply represent the average velocity, but the condition in

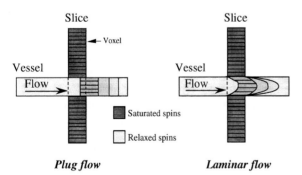

Fig. 2. Inflow or flow enhancement effect. The *left drawing* depicts plug flow, whereas the *right drawing* depicts laminar flow. The *dark shade* of the static excited slice represents its saturated spins: the inflowing spins are shown in a *brighter shade* to represent their relaxed state and hence their potential to give a large MR signal on the next RF excitation pulse

Eq. 1 should be evaluated for every point in time. The condition in Eq. 1 is met more easily if the flow is perpendicular to the imaging slice or slab. The following example illustrates the implications of this condition: with an average arterial flow rate of *v* = 50 cm/s and an average TR of about 25 ms it follows that the slice or slab thickness *d* should be *d* ≤ *v*. *TR* = 1.25 cm in order to obtain the maximal inflow effect. As is discussed later, it depends on the imaging technique used (2D or 3D) whether or not this condition is met. Important to note is that if *v* ≤ *d*/*TR*, flow enhancement still occurs, but it will be less pronounced. This depends strongly on the flip angle used as will be explained below (see Fig. 3). Several parameters can be controlled in order to comply with the condition in Eq. 1. Since the velocity of blood is difficult to control, the remaining parameters from Eq. 1 that are user defined are the repetition time *TR*, the excitation thickness *d*, and the excitation direction. Although not mentioned in Eq. 1, the RF excitation flip angle α plays an important role as will be explained below.

The *TR* is usually chosen as short as possible to obtain maximal background suppression, and also to shorten the total scanning time. In some special cases (e.g., very slow flow), the *TR* is increased in order to improve contrast between blood and static background tissues. The excitation thickness *d* depends on the type of imaging technique used (2D or 3D), and within that tech-

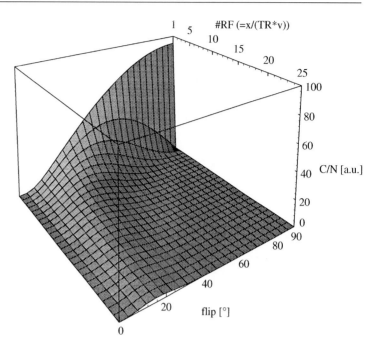

Fig. 3. Inflow MRA. Contrast to noise ratio (*C/N* vertical axis, in arbitrary units, a.u.) as a function of the flip angle and the number of received RF pulses (#RF). Notice that for a 90° excitation pulse, already at the second RF pulse there is no contrast left. This graph can be very helpful to optimize the flip angle if we know how many RF pulses the blood will receive between entering and leaving the excitation volume. The number of received RF pulses can be computed as #RF=$x/(TR.v)$, where x is the distance moved since entering the excitation volume. This graph could be understood more intuitively if we imagine the blood entering from behind, and rescale the #RF axis to distance x. (The numerical simulation to create this graph used a spoiled gradient field echo, a fixed *TR* of 30 ms, *T1* = 1000 ms. The *T1* of the flowing liquid and surrounding tissue are assumed to be equal)

nique on the selected slice (2D), total volume (3D), or slab (3D multi-slab) thickness. The excitation direction should preferably be chosen such that main flow direction is in the slice selection direction (perpendicular to the imaging plane).

An important parameter, especially in 3D MRA, is the RF excitation flip angle. Maximal inflow effect is always obtained if the condition in Eq. 1 is met, regardless of the flip angle used. However, if this condition is *not* met, the flip angle plays a critical role. Generally, the flip angle is taken as high as possible (leading to increased signal from fast-flowing blood, and better background suppression) without saturating the blood itself too much. For 2D methods, the above-mentioned condition is usually met, so that a large flip angle can be used, usually about 50–60°. (Although, in theory, 90° could be used, it is reduced to 50–60°, in order to prevent saturation of slow or in-plane flow, withhout significantly reducing the contrast to noise ratio). In 3D methods the condition in Eq. 1 is usually not met, because the volume or slab thickness is usually several centimeters [In 3D acquisitions, every RF pulse excites the entire 3D volume (single slab), or a large part of the 3D volume (multi-slab), instead of a single slice as in 2D.] The only way to avoid in and through plane saturation is to reduce the flip angle, usually to 15°–20° (see Fig. 3). Because in 3D multiple-slab

techniques (MOTSA, multi-chunk) the slab thickness is generally smaller than in single-slab techniques, the flip angle can be chosen a little larger, but usually no larger than 25°. Ghosting, a pulsatility artifact, is reduced when a smaller flip angle is used. Figure 3 shows the contrast to noise ratio (C/N) as a function of the flip angle and the number of RF pulses the inflowing blood has experienced. The C/N ratio is defined as the contrast between the tissues of interest divided by the noise:

$$\frac{C}{N} = \frac{S_{blood} - S_{background}}{N} \qquad (2)$$

Because the signal from the background ($S_{background}$) is usually very low, C/N≈S_{blood}/N. (Therefore, C/N and S/N are sometimes confused in MRA.) As clearly shown in Fig. 3, it takes more RF pulses to saturate the blood signal when smaller flip angles are used. If a vessel does not run straight through the volume of interest (perpendicular of the slice/volume), but follows an in-slice course instead, the blood in this vessel would become increasingly saturated, similar to the stationary tissue, and consequently be displayed with less contrast in an MR angiogram. As shown in Fig. 3, the number of RF pulses needed to saturate the blood completely depends heavily on the flip angle used. Vessels with very slow flow will hardly be displayed or not at all in the in-

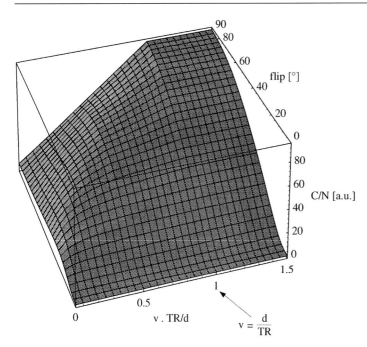

Fig. 4. Inflow singal (*C/N* vertical) vs. normalized velocity (*v. TR/d*) and flip angle for a 2D technique. Clearly, for a 90° flip angle, the signal decreases linearly when *v<d/TR* (*v.TR/d<1*). If the flip angle decreases, two effects are visible: (1) the overall signal decreases (for all velocities) and (2) the velocity threshold below which the inflow effect decreases markedly shifts from *v=d/TR* to lower velocities

flow MR angiogram. With the same repetition time TR, a thin imaging slice (2D) or volume (3D) will enable visualization of slower flow than is possible with a thicker slice/volume, since the distance the blood has to travel to cross the slice/volume is shorter for the thinner slice/volume. Figure 3 shows the effect of the flip angle and the number of RF pulses (received by the inflowing blood) on the contrast to noise ratio. It is also interesting to see the effect of flow velocity on blood signal for a 2D technique, given a certain slice thickness *d* and repetition time *TR*. This is shown in Fig. 4, where the contrast to noise ratio is displayed as a function of (normalized) velocity and flip angle. In summary, it can be stated that inflow (time of flight) MR angiography is concerned with the suppression of signal from stationary tissue and the enhancement of signal from flowing blood. The resulting difference in signal intensity between stationary tissue and flowing blood determines the contrast. Signal to noise ratio (of the stationary tissue) is subordinate in this respect.

Different Imaging Techniques: Multiple 2D, 3D, and 3D Multiple Slab

As explained above, the relationship between slice thickness and velocity of blood flow is an essential consideration in choosing a technique.

Multiple 2D. Perhaps the simplest technique is the 2D technique. In 2D inflow MR angiography, multiple 2D (M2D) slices are acquired. It is also referred to as sequential 2D imaging (S2D). The slices are acquired consecutively and individually reconstructed immediately after, or even during, the acquisition. After the acquisition and reconstruction of all slices, the slices are assembled into a single large volume on which a maximum intensity projection (MIP) in any direction can be performed. The slices usually overlap a little in order to avoid stepping artifacts on the MIP. M2D realizes a maximal inflow effect, because *d* (the slice thickness in 2D techniques) is small, typically several millimeters. A disadvantage of the 2D technique is its inherently low signal to noise ratio, which is partly compensated for by using a large flip angle. Of all the imaging techniques (3D, multi-slab, M2D), the 2D technique is most dependent on the direction of the flow; because of the large flip angle used (50°–60°), in-plane flow will be saturated rapidly. However, a high flip angle is needed in 2D MRA inflow techniques, in order to have an acceptable S/N ratio. Spatial presaturation (see additional techniques) is very effective with the M2D technique, because the presaturation slab moves with the slices („traveling" presaturation slab). The signal dependence on the velocity for a 2D technique is shown in Fig. 4.

3D. There are several differences between the 3D and the M2D techniques. Firstly, the slices are not acquired consecutively in 3D, but simultaneously; every RF pulse excites the entire volume. A 3D technique generally has a better signal to noise ratio (S/N) than a 2D technique, and is better suited to yield thin slices. Furthermore, since most 3D techniques use smaller voxels (compared with 2D), flow voids due to intravoxel dephasing will be reduced in 3D techniques. However, since the excitation volume is quite thick in 3D, the condition in Eq. 1 is usually not met, so that a smaller flip angle (typically 20°) should be used to maintain adequate contrast from blood (see Fig. 3).

The C/N ratio depends on the number of RF pulses the blood has received since entering the 3D imaging volume (see Fig. 3). Therefore, blood at the entrance side is usually brighter than at the exit side. Sometimes, this effect is reduced by varying the flip angle as a function of position (e.g. 15° at the entrance side and 25° at the exit side). This technique is referred to as TONE (Tilted Optimized Nonsaturating Excitation). Although the variation of the blood signal over the volume is reduced, a disadvantage of this method is that the background signal is no longer homogeneous, but now also varies over the volume.

3D Multiple Slab. In producing an MR angiogram of a relatively large volume of interest, a single 3D slab would result in an MR angiogram displaying only the larger vessels with relatively fast flowing blood. Smaller vessels can be visualized by dividing the single 3D slab into multiple 3D slabs [12, 13]. The multiple slab technique is also referred to as MOTSA (Multiple Overlapping Thin Slab Acquisition) or multi-chunk technique. The 3D multiple-slab technique is in fact a compromise between 3D and 2D imaging, with the advantages and disadvantages of both. Multiple-slab technique enables an imaging volume to be split into several subvolumes (slabs or chunks) of which each is imaged in 3D mode. In MRA, the slabs are imaged sequentially (in ascending or descending order), in order to optimize the inflow effect in each slab (although the slabs can also be imaged in an interleaved way, like the slices in multi-slice techniques). A disadvantage of the multiple-slab technique is the increase in scanning time due to the slab overlap. This overlap is necessary in order to compensate for the imperfect 3D slab selection profile. Another disadvantage of the multiple slab technique is a decrease in S/N ratio, proportional

to the slab volume. However, the decrease in S/N (of static tissues) is usually compensated for by the increase in C/N of the vessels. Each slab is acquired and reconstructed separately. After acquisition and reconstruction is completed, the separate 3D slabs are reassembled into a single volume. Although this technique can be used to enhance the inflow effect of smaller vessels, very small vessels with slow flow might still be missed. The choice of acquisition technique (3D, 3D multi-slab, or M2D) depends on the specific application.

In practice, for all three techniques only the (total) volume of interest is specified, as well as the number of slices or slabs, and their overlap.] The choice of technique really depends on the flow velocity, size, and tortuosity of the vessels to be visualized, as well as the total imaging volume to be covered. Although it is difficult to give general rules, the following guidelines may be helpful:

1. The 3D technique is preferred for larger vessels, or fast-flowing blood, and for higher resolution.
2. The 3D multiple-slab technique is preferred when a large volume is to be covered with a 3D technique, or if too much saturation occurs in a single-slab 3D technique.
3. The M2D technique is preferred for visualization of smaller vessels or slow flow, and for imaging of a large track of vessels, when high resolution is not required.

In order to get an impression of the consequences of the use of these techniques, they are compared for the same flow situation in Fig. 5.

Other Time of Flight Techniques. Blood „tagging" techniques using inversion pulses have been proposed [14–19] yielding good contrast angiograms using thick slices. „Outflow" techniques have also been proposed [20], where the signal from the stationary tissue as well as good contrast from the flowing blood is maintained. None of these techniques will be discussed here because their use is currently limited.

Phase Contrast Angiography

Phase contrast angiography (PCA) employs the phase shift of the MR signal induced by flowing spins to discriminate flowing blood from surrounding tissue [21, 22]. However, phase contrast techniques also rely on the refreshment of blood

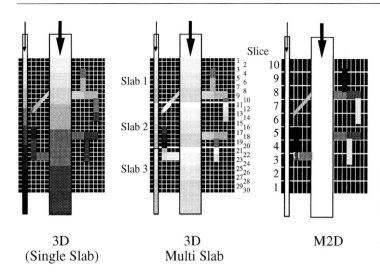

3D
(Single Slab)

3D
Multi Slab

M2D

Fig. 5. The MR contrast behavior of three inflow imaging techniques is shown for a large vessel with its branches, and for a smaller vessel (*left side*). The different effects of flow directions on the contrast are shown. (Drawing from an original idea by James Siebert.) Notice that in-plane flow is rapidly saturated with the M2D technique. Not drawn are the presaturation slabs, which are supposed to be present on the downstream side

in the imaging volume, although to a lesser extent than inflow techniques. Pulse sequences used in PCA are designed such that the phase shifts are proportional to the velocity of the flowing blood. With phase contrast methods, complete suppression of stationary tissue can be achieved by subtracting different acquisitions (as will be explained below), permitting depiction of very small vessels containing slowly flowing blood. Flexible adjustment of the velocity sensitivity (also called the PC-encoding velocity, denoted as V_{enc}) allows focussing on either fast flow or slow flow. Directional flow encoding can be selected in up to three orthogonal directions.

PCA can be used to obtain morphological and functional (quantitative flow, velocity) information, but we will treat quantitative flow techniques separately, although the acquisition technique for most quantitative flow measurements is almost identical. In fact, both functional and morphological information can be obtained from a single PC acquisition by performing different reconstructions. In principle (at least) four different types of reconstructions can be obtained from every single PCA acquisition:

1. One conventional "anatomical" magnitude image, containing only inflow (magnitude) effects, and no phase-based information (see Fig. 9).
2. One "magnitude of complex difference" image (here referred to as PCA/M) containing only qualitative flow information (see Fig. 7).
3. Up to three phase difference images (here referred to as PCA/P) each containing one velocity component, which together form the velocity vector (see Fig. 8).

4. One "speed" image containing the magnitude of the velocity vector, but no information about the direction of flow (see Fig. 8).

For the morphological vessel information, usually the magnitude of the complex (or vectorial) difference (see Fig. 6) is reconstructed for the following reasons:

1. A maximum intensity projection (MIP) should be applicable in order to reduce the reconstructed data set into one or several projections. On the PCA/M images, a MIP can be

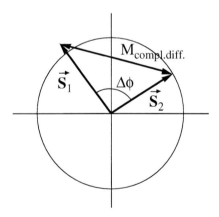

Fig. 6. Vector diagram of the phase difference $\Delta\phi$ and the magnitude of the complex or vectorial difference ($M_{compl.diff.}$). The two MR signal vectors $\mathbf{S}_1$ and $\mathbf{S}_2$ have a velocity-induced phase difference $\Delta\phi$. The magnitude of the complex difference is $M_{compl.diff.} = \mathbf{S}_1 - \mathbf{S}_2$. The magnitude (amplitude) of the signals $\mathbf{S}_1$ and $\mathbf{2}_2$ does not necessarily have to be equal, since this is also determined by the inflow effect. To appreciate the difference between phase difference and magnitude of complex difference, see also Fig. 10

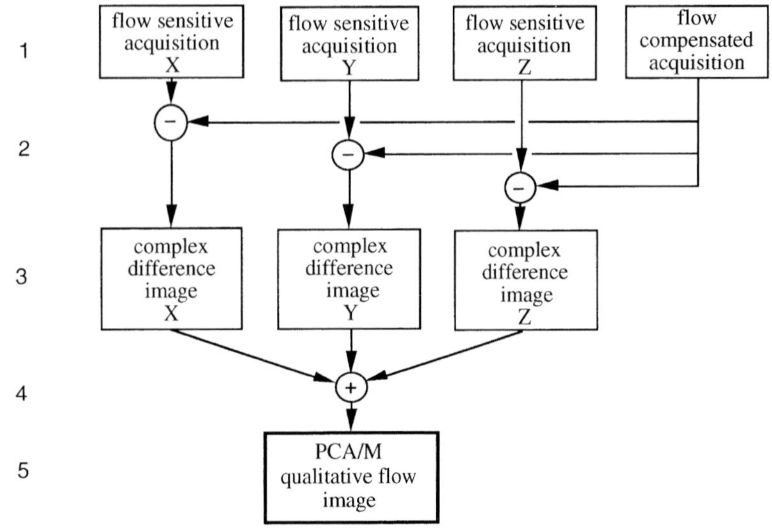

Fig. 7. Subtraction scheme for the PCA/M images (for the simple four-point method). The reconstructed complex data from the flow-compensated acquisition (*1*) is subtracted (*2*) from every flow-sensitized acquisition (*1*). From each set of complex difference data (*3*), the magnitude is computed. These magnitudes are compiled (*4*) to form one final PCA/M image (*5*). This image does contain qualitative flow information, but no quantitative velocity information

Fig. 8. Phase contrast angiography subtraction scheme for the phase difference images. Although the diagram looks similar to the one in Fig. 7, there are some essential differences. The reconstructed phase data from the flow-compensated acquisition (*1*) are subtracted (*2*) from the phase data from every flow-sensitized acquisition (*1*). This results in the phase difference images (*3*), each of which represents one orthogonal velocity component, which together form the velocity vector. In most cases these images are the final images, but in some cases the „speed" images are also computed (*4, 5*), *speed* = $\sqrt{v_x^2 + v_y^2 + v_z^2}$, which is simply the magnitude fo the velocity vector. It is very common for quantitative flow measurements to obtain only one velocity component

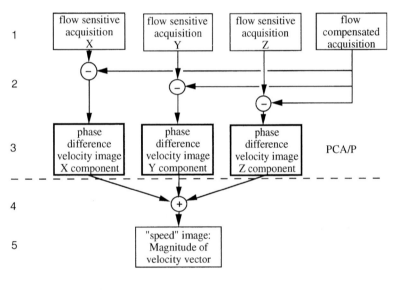

Fig. 9. Phase contrast angiography reconstruction scheme for the conventional „anatomical" modulus images. For every acquisition (*1*), the modulus images are reconstructed (*2, 3*), which are then added together (*4*) to obtain one averaged modulus image (*5*). These images contain no phase information (they are almost equivalent to normal flow-compensated gradient echo images)

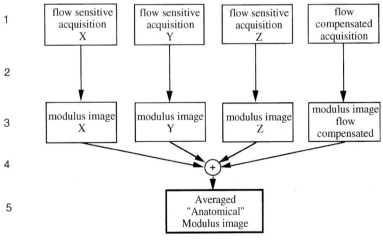

performed because the background has the lowest pixel value (close to zero). On the phase difference PCA/P images, a normal MIP is not useful, because the background does not have the lowest pixel values (backward flow generates negative pixel phase values, see Fig. 10).

A maximum absolute value projection [10] could eliminate this problem, but, as will be explained below, the noise in phase images can have a very large amplitude. The speed images also suffer from this large amplitude noise. Even though this noise can be filtered out in some cases by magnitude masking (see Fig. 16), the PCA/M images remain the preferred input for most projections.

2. PCA/M images are less sensitive to so-called phase wraps caused by phase aliasing. If the physical velocity exceeds the encoding velocity, a phase wrap will occur in the PCA/P image (see quantiative flow, and Figs. 10, 11). This property is generally exploited by setting the encoding velocity slightly *lower* than the highest expected physical velocity to be imaged if only the PCA/M images are required (as is often the case) (instead of setting it *higher* to avoid phase wraps as is necessary for the PCA/P phase difference images).

Phase is a fundamental property of all spins. Velocity-encoded images can be made because spins moving in the presence of a magnetic gradient field accumulate a flow-induced phase shift. This phase shift depends on the strength and duration of the gradients and on the velocity of the moving spins. Due to field inhomogeneities, the phase of the stationary tissue is not zero, and must be subtracted to make a PCA image. To accomplish this, a reference image can be used. The easiest reference image, used in the so-called simple four-point method, is a flow-compensated image (see additional techniques) where *all* (either stationary or flowing) spins have the same phase. More complicated schemes are commonly used [23] (Hadamard encoding) in which none of the acquisitions is flow compensated. To velocity encode an image, the amplitude of the dephasing and rephasing parts of a bipolar gradient (see Fig. 14) are adjusted such that if the physical velocity equals the chosen encoding velocity the phase shift will be $\pi = 180°$. All stationary spins will have the same phase as in the flow-compensated sequence, but the flowing spins are phase shifted by an amount dependent on their velocity.

An important aspect of PCA is that velocity encoding can only be performed in one direction at a time. This is different for inflow techniques, especially for 3D inflow techniques, which are sensitive to flow in every direction. In PCA, three velocity-encoded images are needed (each encoded in an orthogonal direction), plus one reference image, to get complete velicity information. This means a total of four images are needed to make one PCA image (see Figs. 7, 8). These four acquisitions are most commonly performed automatically, and are „invisible" to the user. Because four acquisitions are needed, PCA scans take longer than inflow or TOF MRA if the same spatial resolution is required. In practice, however, the superb background suppression of PCA facilitates a good compromise between resolution and scanning time. Moreover, PCA generally results in a good signal to noise ratio, because the four acquisitions are compiled into one single image (for the PCA/M image and for the conventional „anatomical" modulus image).

In special cases where the flow is known to be predominantly in only one or two (orthogonal) directions, it may suffice to only encode the acquisition for the anticipated flow directions, instead of for all three directions, thereby reducing scanning time.

Generally, the encoding velocity is equal for all encoded directions, but it is possible to make the encoding velocity direction dependent. This can sometimes be useful for better depiction of small branches of large vessels of which the flow is predominantly in one direction.

Background Suppression by Image Subtraction

The phase of the stationary tissue is the same in the flow-compensated and the flow-encoded sequence, but, due to field inhomogeneities, this phase is not zero. Stationary tissue signal is removed by subtracting the two images. The resulting image will only have flow information. If velocity encoding is done in all three orthogonal directions, three subtractions must be performed. The data can then be compiled to get one image with velocity information in all three directions. Diagrams of this process ore shown in Figs. 7–9.

Because the PCA/M images are both magnitude and phase dependent (magnitude of complex difference, see Fig. 6), the contrast is determined by the velocity of the spins, which determines the

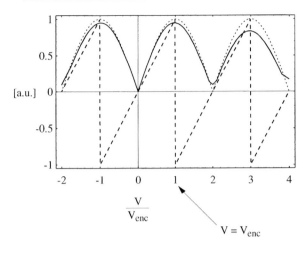

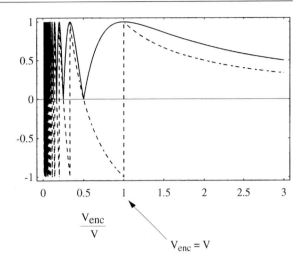

Fig. 10. The signal (vertical axis, arbitrary units) vs. velocity relation for phase difference images (PCA/P, *dashed line*) and the magnitude of the complex difference images (PCA/M, *solid line*) as a function of the flow velocity V (normalized with the encoding velocity V_{enc}). Notice that the phase difference images have a phase wrap at every odd multiple of $V = V_{enc}$, whereas the PCA/M images have their maxima at these points. The *thin dotted line* represents the theoretical curve for plug flow, but due to the spread of velocities within each voxel the minima are slightly elevated, whereas the maxima are slightly diminished. The inflow effects have not been taken into account for PCA/M in this graph. The signal vs. velocity relation of the „speed" images is equal to that of the phase difference images (*dashed line*), except that all negative values are converted to positive values

Fig. 11. The signal (vertical axis arbitrary units) vs. velocity relation for phase difference images (PCA/P, *dashed line*) and the magnitude of the complex difference images (PCA/M, *solid line*) as a function of the encoding velocity V_{enc} (normalized with the flow velocity, V). This graph contains the same information as the one in Fig. 10, but it can be helpful to show the effect of changing the encoding velocity when the flow velocity in the vessel of interest is known. The inflow effects have not been taken into account for PCA/M in this graph

phase difference, but also by the inflow (magnitude) effect. For this reason, the saturation effect will be less noticeable than inflow MRA, but will still be present. (If the magnitude is reduced, the magnitude of the complex difference will also be reduced.) One of the advantages of PCA is that the reconstructed data from each scan contain both the conventional („anatomical") magnitude images (see Fig. 9) and the complex difference magnitude (PCA/M, see Fig. 7) images for every slice. This allows good visualization of the vascular morphology (in the PCA/M images) in relation to the soft tissue (in the conventional magnitude images). Despite the short TR used, these „anatomical" magnitude images can still provide a relatively good S/N ratio in the static background tissues, because multiple acquisitions are averaged (see Fig. 9). Although not very common, because it generally requires a slightly different acquisition, the phase difference images (PCA/P) images which contain the quantitative informa-

tion, as well as the „speed" image, can also be reconstructed from the same (raw) data (see Fig. 8). This means that four different types of reconstructions can be obtained from the same PCA acquisition, each with relevant clinical information. Even though the velocity-induced phase shifts form the basis of PCA, the relation between the image contrast, the flow velocity, and the encoding velocity is not straightforward, as is shown in Figs. 10–13.

Different Imaging Techniques: 3D, 3D Multiple Slab, or 2D Single Slice

Although the available imaging techniques are the same as for inflow, the use of PCA has some typical consequences with respect to the imaging technique. However, they all share one important feature: if only the PCA/M images are reconstructed (and not the phase difference PCA/P im-

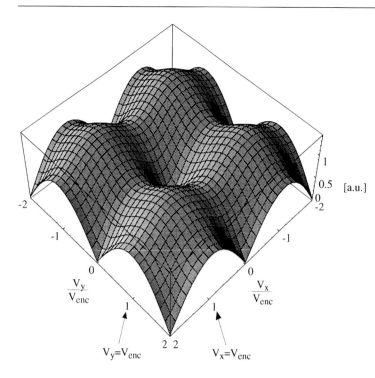

Fig. 12. The signal vs. velocity relation for the magnitude of the complex difference images (PCA/M) as a function of the flow velocities in *x*-direction V_x, and *y*-direction V_y (normalized with the encoding velocity V_{enc}). This graph is similar to the one in Fig. 10, but it shows the dependence on two velocity components in one graph. The inflow effects have not been taken into account for this graph

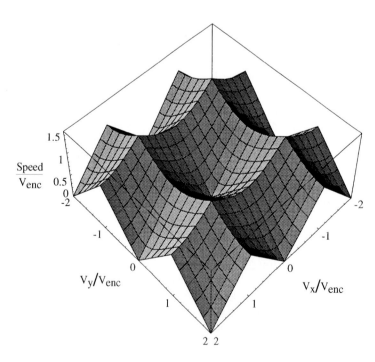

Fig. 13. The signal vs. velocity relation for the speed images, as a function of the flow velocities in *x*-direction V_x, and *y*-direction V_y (normalized with the encoding velocity V_{enc}). This graph shows the dependence on two velocity components in one graph. Speed $= \sqrt{v_x^2 + v_y^2 + v_z^2}$, v_z is assumed zero. The vertical speed axis is normalized with vene

ages), the encoding velocity V_{enc} is commonly chosen somewhat *lower* than the highest anticipated velocity (see Fig. 10) in order to increase the overall C/N ratio.

3D Phase Contrast Angiography

The 3D technique, as in 3D inflow, provides acquisition of multiple thin, contiguous slices with reduced intravoxel dephasing. This allows inspection of the vasculature from any projection angle with complete background suppression. Large volumes can be imaged (e.g., an entire brain). Even though saturation will occur, due to the excellent background suppression, there will be relatively good contrast even for the smaller vessels. The multiple-slab 3D technique can also be applied to PCA, but it is less commonly used than for inflow techniques. Similar to 3D inflow techniques, a small flip angle ($\pm 20°$) is used to avoid blood saturation.

2D Phase Contrast Angiography

Since background is suppressed very effectively in PCA, it is possible to image a very thick slice (several centimeters!) and still obtain a reasonable angiographic image. This would not be possible with conventional inflow techniques. Since a very thick slice can be used, it is most commonly used as a single-slice technique, which makes it a very fast technique. Due to its thick slice, the details of the smaller vessels can get lost, but this is usually outweighed by the advantage of its fast acquisition. Single thick-slice 2D PCA studies are often used as surveys for lengthier 3D scans. Single thick-slice 2D PCA also enables fast evaluation of the velocity sensitivity or encoding velocity. In combination with cardiac triggering, 2D cine PCA can be used to render a movie of flow at various phases of the cardiac cycle. Unlike 2D inflow techniques, a small flip angle ($\pm 20°$) is used to avoid blood saturation, because of the large slice thickness and in plane flow.

2D Cine Phase Contrast Angiography

Since the acquisition of a single thick PCA slice is very fast, and provides relatively good angiographic images, this technique is often combined with cardiac triggering (see additional techniques) to obtain temporal information, or with cardiac gating to reduce ghosting. Because in 2D PCA the slice is usually much thicker than the vessels, the image contrast gives only qualitative flow information (see Fig. 15a). For quantitative flow measurements, thinner slices are used, and another reconstruction is used (phase difference images PCA/P), where actual flow velocity values can be obtained.

Other Phase-Sensitive Techniques

Although PCA is the most commonly used phase-sensitive angiographic technique, other techniques, such as the dephase-rephase technique, are used as well. In this technique, two acquisitions are made, one is flow compensated and the other is not. In the non-flow-compensated acquisition, intravoxel phase dispersion will create deliberate flow voids in most parts of the vessel. The magnitude of both acquisitions is reconstructed and subtracted to obtain an image in which the background has been canceled [24]. This technique is sometimes also considered as a black blood technique.

Quantitative Flow

Magnetic resonance enables the noninvasive assessment of flow rates in blood vessels. Flow quantitation with MR uses the velocity-dependent phase shifts of flowing spins [25–27]. The quantitative flow feature permits the acquisition of a „flow image" from which the actual flow rates can be determined. In combination with cardiac triggering, flow rates can be determined at specified phases of the cardiac cycle. This enables the flow rates to be studied as a function of time. Quantitation of venous flow generally does not require cardiac triggering and is therefore very fast. Untriggered quantitation of arterial flow is not recommended unless the pulsatility index is very low [28]. An important feature of MR quantitative flow is that both the magnitude and direction of the flow can be determined in every pixel („backward" flow will induce a negative phase difference, see Fig. 10). From the same reconstructed phase difference image, both velocity (cm/s) and flux (or flow rate in cc/s or ml/s) can be obtained. In fact, the method employed for quantitative flow is very similar to that of PCA, with the difference that usually only one flow-sensitive direction is used (mostly perpendicular to the imaging plane), and that a higher encoding velocity is used to avoid phase wraps (see Fig. 10). In MR quantitative flow measurements, there is no arbitrary flow calibration factor. From physics it can be derived that for a bipolar gradient the velocity-induced phase shift Φ is linear with the velocity:

$$\Phi = v \, (\gamma \Delta A_g) \qquad (3)$$

where γ is the gyromagnetic ratio (a known constant), A_g the area of each gradient lobe, and Δ the time between the centers of the two gradient lobes, see Fig. 14. A_g and Δ depend on the user-defined velocity encoding. If the magnetic gradients are well controlled, as on modern MR machines, there is no need for any calibration. Sometimes, however, eddy currents can cause small phase offsets, which are automatically corrected for on some machines. Similar to normal imaging, at every pixel or voxel a value is obtained, Whereas in most MR images, the absolute pixel value does not have a clear meaning, in the case of quantitative flow, the pixel value represents the local velocity. This velocity value is a (weighted) average value, that is, it is proportional to the phase of the vector sum of the signal of all spins in a voxel. Because of this, partial volume effects can cause errors in the velocity measurements as shown in Fig. 15.

If velocity dispersion inside a voxel is large, the corresponding phase dispersion can cause the net signal to drop to zero, so that the magnitude of the signal becomes very small. However, in the phase difference image this will not show up as a signal void (pixel value zero), but will create a random, noise-determined phase value. In con-

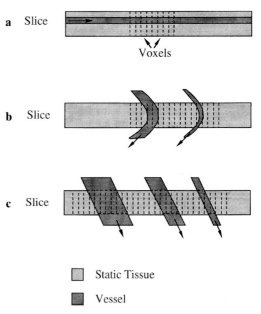

Fig. 15. Partial volume effects. For quantitative flow measurements this can affect the measured velocity value. *a*, in-plane flow; *b*, tortuous vessels; *c*, oblique flow. Whether or not the partial volume effects are significant depends on how small the vessel is compared with the voxel size (slice thickness)

trast to the regular magnitude images, where noise is usually hardly visible even in areas where the signal is very small or zero, the random phase noise is clearly visible in the phase (difference) images. This is due to the fact that, when the magnitude is extremely small, the phase is completely noise determined and hence random, meaning it can vary between maximum (π) and minimum ($-\pi$). In the phase image, this shows up as a „pepper and salt" like appearance of noise, clearly distinguishable from regions with normal signal. This same phenomenon also occurs for PCA, although it is never seen on the images, because usually only the complex difference magnitude and normal magnitude images are reconstructed. Mostly, the „pepper and salt" like noise occurs in regions with air (in lungs, and of course outside the patient). In many cases, magnitude masking can filter out the phase noise (after reconstruction) as shown in Fig. 16.

Quantitative flow is usually performed with a single thin 2D slice (3–10 mm), although it is also possible to combine it with 3D techniques, if very thin and/or multiple slices are needed. It is even possible to perform a 3D volume flow measurement in combination with cardiac (retrospective)

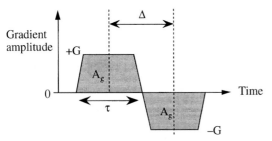

Fig. 14. Bipolar gradient. The velocity-induced phase shift of this gradient is proportional to $A_g \Delta = G \tau \Delta$, where A_g is the area under each gradient lobe and Δ the time interval between the centers of these lobes

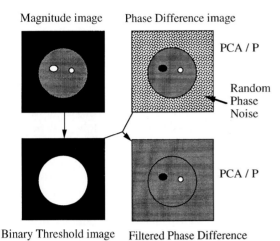

Magnitude image   Phase Difference image

PCA / P

Random
Phase
Noise

PCA / P

Binary Threshold image   Filtered Phase Difference

Fig. 16. Filter to remove the random phase noise from the phase difference (PCA/P) images by magnitude masking. All pixels for which the magnitude value is below a certain threshold are set to zero in the phase image

triggering to obtain both 3D spatial and temporal information, but this is not done very often due to the long scanning times. In 2D quantitative flow acquisition, the flow sensitivity is usually perpendicular to the imaging plane. The slice thus has to be planned perpendicular to the vessel of interest to avoid partial volume effects (see Fig. 15). The flip angle is usually between 25° and 50°, depending on the velocity and pulsatility of the flow (see Eq. 1). The encoding velocity V_{enc} has to be chosen somewhat *higher* than the maximum anticipated velocity to avoid phase wraps (see Fig. 10). Although several factors can affect the accuracy of the MR quantitative flow measurements [29, 30], many (mainly in vitro) verification studies have been performed [31–33], and it is rapidly gaining a reputation of being a reliable, accurate technique which does not depend strongly on the skill of the technician as in ultrasound.

Fourier Flow Imaging

The Fourier flow-imaging technique replaces the monopolar phase-encoding gradient commonly used for spatial encoding, by a bipolar velocity phase-encoding gradient. It is thus possible to obtain the spread of velocities within a voxel (instead of just one velocity value per voxel). For further reading on this subject we refer to the literature [34–37].

Black Blood Angiography

Flow distal to a stenosis is often disturbed (nonlaminar) or turbulent and leads to signal loss. This may result in an overestimation of the stenosis. This problem can be alleviated by the use of „black blood angiography." With this technique, blood signal is absent (black) and the vessel wall and potential plaques may be discriminated. Using spin echo sequences (with long echo time, TE) and presaturation on both sides of the imaging volume, the physician can assess vascular pathology with „black blood angiography" [38, 39]. The main motive to use spin echo techniques for black blood imaging is the spin washout in the time interval between the 90° excitation pulse and the (slice-selective) 180° refocussing pulse (see Fig. 17). If no presaturation is used, for a single-slice technique, the washout flow void will be complete when

$$v \geq \frac{2d}{TE} \qquad (4)$$

where d is the slice thickness, and *TE* is the echo time. From Eq.4 it is clear that a longer TE will decrease the velocity threshold for which a complete flow void will occur. For a multi-slice technique the relation becomes more complicated because signal might be (partially) refocussed in neighboring slices. Since a multi-slice sequence is

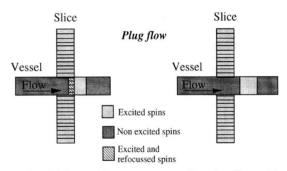

Fig. 17. Washout flow void for spin echo (single slice). The flow void can be partial (*left diagram*) or complete (*right diagram*). Both diagrams are drawn at the time of the 180° refocussing pulse (*t=TE/2*). If the 90° excitation and the 180° refocussing pulse are both slice selective (which is usually the case), spins which flow out of the slice during the time interval between the excitation and the refocussing pulse are not refocussed and hence do not contribute to the signal. The fresh spins which have entered the slice have not yet received a 90° excitation pulse and therefore cannot generate any signal after the 180° refocussing pulse

needed to cover a reasonable volume, this is one of the reasons why additional presaturation slabs are needed on one or both sides of the imaging volume. Often, also additional dephasing (spoiling) gradients are used in all three directions to dephase the remaining signal from slow flow. Very slow or recirculating flow might not be completely black, because it can recover from the presaturation, can be (partially) refocussed by the 180° pulses, and can be dephased insufficiently.

The above-mentioned dephase-rephase technique could also be considered as a black blood technique. Another black blood technique is a special type of turbo gradient field echo (see additonal techniques) where two inversion prepulses are used: the first of which is non-slice-selective and the second one is slice-selective [40]. The result is that blood outside the imaging volume is inverted, whereas the tissue in the selected volume remains unaffected. Proper choice of the inversion delay time between the two inversion pulses and the turbo imaging sequence (typically 600 ms) can null the signal from blood. In black blood techniques, a minimum intensity projection (mIP) has to be used instead of the more conventional maximum intensity projection (MIP), allowing processing images to be obtained with user-defined black blood MR angiography protocols. There are several potential problems with this technique, such as the fact that cortical bone and air in and outside the body will also be black, and thus shows up in the MIP. Therefore, the volume in which the projection is performed should be selected with care, and inspection of the original (or reformated) slices is recommended. Calcified plaques are also black in the images so that these lesions are not visible, which could potentially lead to an underestimation of the degree of the stenosis. Furthermore, with black blood angiography it is sometimes difficult to discriminate arteries and veins since the technique tends to make them both black.

Additional MRA Techniques

If all flow in the body were steady and laminar, and the vessels would not move, the above-mentioned techniques would be sufficient to image most vessels. However, most flow is pulsatile, and in some areas — mainly in or close to pathology — it may well be disturbed (nonlaminar) or even turbelent. Disturbed and/or turbulent flow causes intravoxel phase dispersion, which can be seen in MRA images as signal voids at places where disturbed or turbulent flow occurs. Such flow void artifacts can be reduced by choosing smaller voxel sizes and by reducing the gradient moments, resulting in shorter echo times (TE). Another way of reducing this type of flow void is to avoid peak systolic flow and acquire data only during diastole when the flow is much slower. The pulsatility of flow depends on whether it is venous or arterial. If the flow is arterial, in general, the closer it is to the heart, the more pulsatile it is. Motion of the vessels itself is another complicating factor; it can be due to pressure waves originating from the beating heart, motion due to breathing, or patient movement. In order to reduce breathing motion artifacts, several techniques have been developed such as breath-hold, respiratory triggering and gating, and the respiratory phase-encoding ordering [41, 42] (PEAR, ROPE, COPE). These techniques are not discussed here. All three factors (pulsatilitiy, nonlaminar flow, movement) create artifacts which can seriously affect the image qualitiy of MRA. A number of additional techniques have been developed which reduce or eliminate these artifacts. Other additional techniques mainly improve the contrast of the vessels, without specifically reducing any artifacts. Not all additional techniques can be combined with all basic methods, as wil be explained below. In many cases, more than one additional technique can be used simultaneously.

Cardiac Synchronization

Cardiac synchronization is used to reduce artifacts due to pulsatile flow and cardiac motion (ghosting). Besides artifact reduction, cardiac synchronization is used to obtain temporal information during the heart cycle. Several types of cardiac synchronization are used each with its specific applications. In the literature the terms cardiac triggering and cardiac gating are often confused. Although there is no clear consensus as to its definition, we define cardiac triggering as an acquisition mode in which many (typically 10–25) points in time (heart phases) are sampled, and cardiac gating as limiting the acquisition to a certain period (gate) in the cardiac cycle, the gate usually being of the order of several hundreds of milliseconds. Usually, with cardiac triggering only one phase-encoding gradient step (the same for all heart phases) is acquired per RR interval, whereas in gating several phase-endcoding gradient steps are acquired per gate. Recent developments have shown applications of a hybrid form of the two techniques [43–45], where temporal resolution is acquired with multiple phase-encoding gradient steps per RR interval. Also, retrospective gating can be considered as a form of triggering.

Cardiac Gating (Gated Sweep, Segmented k-Space)

Cardiac gating is an extension of the standard MRA methods, and can be used for both inflow and PCA. MR angiography of vessels with pulsating blood is frequently hampered by shift artifacts (ghosting) which could be interpreted as vessel anomalies; the signal is distributed into the phase-encoding direction, either as a diffuse bar, or as several discrete vessel „ghosts" (misregistered replicas), resulting in reduced signal intensity in the lumen of the vessel. Because of this, blood pulsation and retrograde flow can lead to signal intensity drops in (small) regions within the vessels, which could be misinterpreted as stenosis or thrombus. Cardiac gating suppresses these artifacts, as well as blurring due to movement of the vessels during the heart cycle [46].

By limiting the data acquisition to a specified heart phase interval (gate), determined by the user-defined gate delay and gate width (which can be in systole or diastole), excellent angiographic images with sharp vessel edges, improved contrast, and absence of pulsatility artifacts are obtained. Flow voids, which are frequently encountered in areas distal to stenosis, can sometimes be suppressed using diastolic gated acquisitions [47]; during diastole the flow is usually slower than during systole; consequently, the flow is less disturbed (or turbulent). Limiting the acquisition to diastole is only useful in those vessels where there is still significant flow in diastole, such as the carotid or renal arteries. However, since image acquisition is limited to a portion of the heart cycle only, scanning time is prolonged (inversely proportional to the gate width). When cardiac gating is combined with PCA (including quantitative flow), the different flow sensitivity directions can be interleaved within every gate (see below).

Cardiac gating can be performed in a steady state mode, where the RF pulses and gradients continue throughout the entire heart cycle, but the

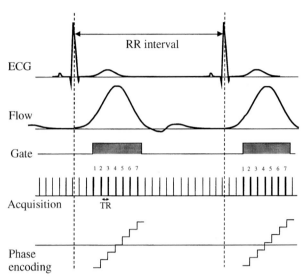

Fig. 18. Diagram of cardiac gating (gated sweep). A number of points are sampled in every gate (seven in this example), each with a different phase-encoding gradient value. The distance between the points is determined by the RF repetition time *TR*. If a steady state is maintained, the gradients and RF pulses continue outside the gate, but no data are acquired. In this example, the order of the phase-encoding steps within each gate is linear, but it is also possible to use a low-high (centric) phase-encoding order

acquisition of MR signal is limited to the selected gate (see Fig. 18). The cardiac gated technique is often referred to as a segmented k-space technique because the k-space is acquired in „segments" due to the fact that multiple phase-encoding steps are taken per heart beat. For the same reason it is also referred to as gated sweep technique (sweep through k-space). The cardiac gating technique can be combined with regular gradient field echo techniques, but also with turbo gradient field echo techniques, sometimes including magnetization preparation (inversion or saturation prepulses to suppress signal from static tussues). It is then frequently referred to as triggered turbo technique (Turbo Field Echo, TFE; Turbo FLASH, MP-RAGE, etc.)

Cardiac Triggering

Cardiac triggering can be used either to obtain temporal information about the flow or simply to suppress pulsation artifacts. Two main types of triggering exist: (conventional) prospective triggering and retrospective triggering (gating).

Prospective Triggering. This is the traditional type of cardiac triggering in which the acquisition is triggered by the ECG signal (R wave) (or by a peripheral pulse trigger). Every time a trigger signal is detected, the acquisition will sample data (multiple points in time or heart phases) during a predefined period, stops the acquisition, and waits for the next trigger signal. The predefined acquisition period should be shorter than the average heart beat interval. Due to the natural variation in the cardiac frequency, it is not possible to cover the complete heart cycle; the end-diastolic period is skipped (see Fig. 19) (unless the acquisition is extended to two or more RR intervals, which is not very common). Another drawback of this type of triggering is the so-called lightning artifact; due to the longer time interval between the RF pulses in the last and the next first sampled heart phase (compared with the interval between all other sampled heart phases), the tissues will give more signal in the first heart phase than in the other heart phases, due to the fact that they have more time to relax. When all the acquired heart phases are displayed in cinemode, this first heart phase will be brighter than all the others; hence the name lightning artifact.

Retrospective Triggering (Gating). The retrospective triggering technique is frequently referred to as retrospective gating [48], and is a powerful alternative for the conventional (prospective) triggering. The main difference with the prospective triggering is that the acquisition no longer waits for trigger signals, but steadily continues acquiring data, while the ECG signal is simultaneously recorded. Although other types of retrospective triggering exist, in the most common type, for every phase-encoding step, slightly more than one heart beat is sampled (default ±1.2 times the average RR interval). this ensures that even relatively long heart beats are fully covered (see Fig. 20). This retrospective oversampling factor is user defined and depends on the patient's heart beat variation. The reordering of the heart phases (for each phase-encoding profile, see Fig. 20) is most commonly performed "on the fly", during the scan, so that no additional reconstruction time is needed. The disadvantages of prospective triggering (lightning artifact, exemption of the end-diastole) are overcome with the retrospective triggering method. Moreover, the number of reconstructed heart phases can be selected relatively independent of the temporal re-

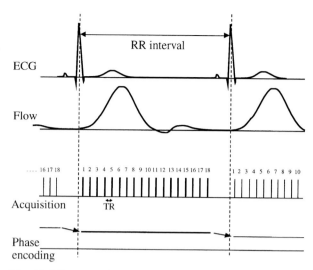

Fig. 19. Diagram of prospective triggering for a single-slice technique. The acquisition waits for the ECG trigger signal, and starts sampling a predefined number of points in time (1–18 in this example). The distance between these points is determined by the RF repetition time *TR*. Because of the natural variation in the heart beat frequency, the acquisition period has to be shorter than the average RR interval. Therefore, no information in end-diastole is obtained. All sampled points within each RR interval are acquired with the same phase-encoding gradient

solution of the acquisition as determined by the TR. In practice, however, the temporal resolution of the reconstructed heart phases is usually smaller than or equal to the temporal resolution of the scan. Thus, it is possible to reconstruct fewer heart phases than acquired to gain in signal to noise ratio. The technique is also referred to as retrospective gating because it is possible to select one or more (reconstruction) gates with arbitrary delay and width. Also, it is possible to use more than one heart beat (per phase-encoding step) in order to increase the temporal resolution of the scan. A practical disadvantage of retrospective triggering is that retrospective detection of ECG R-waves can be problematic. Because the acquisition no longer waits for an ECG signal, as in prospective triggering, but steadily goes on acquiring data, the ECG signal is continuously disturbed by the acquisition. For patients with a very weak ECG signal, it might not be possible to perform retrospective triggering, so that conventional (prospective) triggering has to be used.

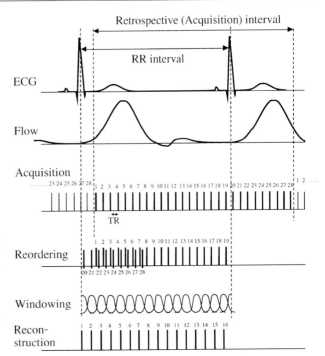

Fig. 20. Diagram of a common type of retrospective gating/triggering. The acquisition is not triggered to the ECG signal, but the ECG signal is recorded during acquisition. Because of this, the retrospective interval can start at any point in the heart cycle. In order to make sure that even long RR intervals are completely sampled, the retrospective acquisition period is longer than the average RR interval. During this period, multiple points in time are sampled (28 in this example), all with the same phase-encoding gradient value. The acquisition interval is determined by the RF repetition time *TR*. After, or during, the scan, the acquired samples are reordered such that all sampled points within one retrospective interval cover exactly one RR interval. The reconstruction sample interval can be chosen independently of the acquisition interval. In this example only 16 heart phases are reconstructed, while the acquisition would have allowed more. The windowing process takes care of the conversion from sampled points to reconstructed points; every reconstructed point is the result of a weighting of the acquired points, usually with a Gaussian-type filter

Cardiac Synchronization and Phase Contrast Techniques

When phase contrast techniques (including quantitative flow) are combined with cardiac synchronization (be it gating or triggering, prospective or retrospective) the flow-sensitive directions can either be acquired separately or interleaved. In the noninterleaved technique, every flow-sensitive direction needs one heart beat (in the case of only one encoding direction, two heart beats; in the case of all three directions, four heart beats.) The disadvantage of this noninterleaved method is that the scanning time is almost proportional to the number of flow-sensitive directions. The advantage is that a very high temporal resolution can be obtained. With the interleaved technique, all the flow-sensitive directions are measured within every heart beat. This has the advantage of reducing the total scanning time at the cost of reducing the maximal temporal resolution.

Intravoxel Dephasing (Flow Void) Reduction

Flow Compensation

Flow compensation is a technique where additional gradients are applied to compensate for the dephasing effect of the imaging gradients [49] (see Fig. 21). Compared with the situation where no flow compensation is used, the shortest possible TE will increase when flow compensation is switched on. Even though an increase in TE is generally not favored in MRA, application of flow compensation is mandatory in many cases for preserving the signal of flowing spins. Therefore, both for inflow and PCA, flow compensation is commonly applied. Misregistration artifacts which can occur with oblique (in-plane) flow are due to the difference in timing between the phase-encoding gradient and the readout gradient [50, 51]. This artifact can be reduced by flow compensation in the phase-encoding direction (shown in Fig. 21).

Partial Echo Sampling

Intravoxel dephasing flow voids are caused by a large variation of velocities within a voxel and by the presence of gradients. In order to reduce these intravoxel dephasing flow voids, the duration of the read-out gradients (including the flow-compensating gradients) can be reduced by partial echo sampling, where only the last part of the echo is sampled (see Fig. 22). This technique is also referred to as asymmetric echo sampling. As a consequence, the echo time TE is decreased,

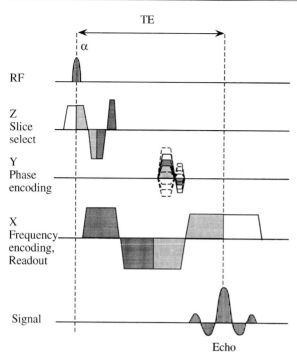

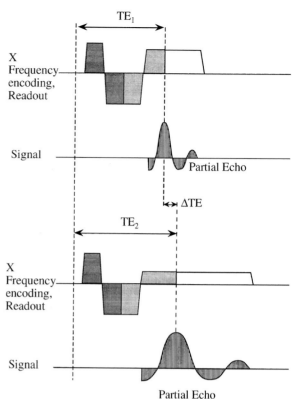

Fig. 21. Pulse sequence for a flow-compensated gradient echo. The *darker-shaded* gradient areas are the additional gradients needed for the flow compensation. They are added to the gradients which are necessary for imaging (*lighter-shaded* gradient areas)

Fig. 23. Readout gradient and data sampling for a flow-compensated gradient echo with partial echo sampling. Decreasing the ampliude of the readout gradient will decrease the sampling bandwidth, and hence increase the *S/N* ratio. In partial echo sampling this only slightly increases the echo time *TE* (the increase in *TE* would have been much larger when the full echo was sampled)

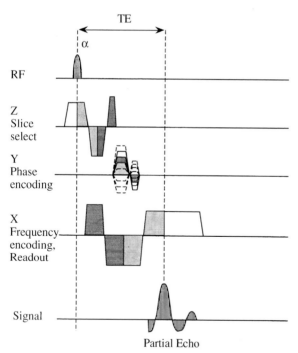

Fig. 22. Pulse sequence for a flow-compensated gradient echo with partial echo sampling. Because the first part of the echo is not sampled, the readout gradient is more compact, reducing the minimal echo time

and therefore also the TR, thus shortening the total acquisition time. The disadvantages of partial echo sampling are a decrease in S/N ratio, a slight loss of resolution in the readout direction, and the need for a phase correction on every sampled echo [52]. This phase correction is performed automatically, but it lengthens the reconstruction time. Partial echo sampling is commonly used both for inflow MRA and for PCA. However, for quantitative flow it is generally not recommended, because here the phase difference images are reconstructed, which are slightly affected by the phase correction. Partial echo sampling is often used in combination with the shortest possible TE. In order to obtain a large increase in S/N ratio, it can be worthwhile to decrease the acquisition bandwidth (see Fig. 23). This can be done either by manually decreasing the bandwith (which results in an increased TE) or by increasing the (shortest) TE (by only 1 or 2 ms) on machines with an automatic bandwidth optimization. This is a very effective way to improve the S/N ratio without losing diagnostic image quality (unless severely disturbed flow is anticipated).

Contrast Enhancement Techniques: Prepulses

Presaturation

In many cases, discrimination between arterial and venous flow is desirable. In MR angiography this can be achieved by suppressing signal from either arterial or venous flow. Suppression is achieved by positioning a thick (usually 5–10 cm) presaturation slab adjacent to the volume of interest. Within this slab, saturation (pre)pulses are applied, so that the magnetization is destroyed. Blood flowing from this presaturation slab into the imaging volume will produce negligible signal (at least for the first hundred milliseconds after leaving the presaturation volume). Presaturation is very effective with inflow MRA, because both presaturation and inflow depend mainly on T1 (magnitude) effects. Application of presaturation in combination with PCA is possible, but the presaturation will be less effective in suppressing the blood signal, because the signal in PCA images is a mixture of magnitude and phase (difference) effects, the latter of which is not affected by presaturation. For the multiple 2D single-slice technique (M2D), the one-sided presaturation slab moves with the position of the slice being imaged in order to provide effective suppression of arterial or venous flow („traveling" presaturation slab). If presaturation is combined with the 3D multiple-slab technique, the presaturation slab does move with the imaging slab; the gap between the presaturation slab and the current imaging slab remains constant.

Fat Suppression

Inflow MRA is frequently hampered by high fat signal, possibly obscuring small vessels with low contrast in the maximum intensity projection (MIP). In PCA *all* static background tissues, including fat, are effectively suppressed, which is the reason that fat suppression techniques are mainly used for inflow techniques. Several fat suppression techniques have been developed, which either use the fact that the resonance frequency of fat is slightly different from that of water, or the fact that the T1 of fat is shorter than the T1 of any other tissue. A popular T1 based fat suppression method is STIR (short inversion time recovery). In MRA, this is not used very often, because the inversion pulse needed also affects the blood signal. An easy and frequently applied technique is a simple method where the echo time TE is chosen such that the water and fat signal are out of phase, and thus cancel each other if a voxel contains both water and fat. For machines operating at field strengths of 0.5 T this occurs at odd multiples of TE = 6,9 ms, at field strengths of 1 T at odd multiples of TE = 4.6 ms, and for field strengths of 1.5 T at odd multiples of TE = 2.3 ms. For MRA, practical values are TE = 6.9 ms for both 0.5 T and 1.5 T, and TE = 4.6 ms for 1.0 T. This technique results only in a reduction (not a complete suppression) of the fat signal, and is only effective for voxels which contain both fat and water. Another method, chemical shift presaturation fat suppression (SPIR, FATSAT), uses a saturation prepulse applied at fat resonance. This method is sensitive to field inhomogeneities, because it should selectively saturate fat, without saturating water, the resonance frequency of which is very close to that of fat. Because this technique increases the repetition time TR in normal inflow sequences, its use is mainly limited to cases where the TR has to be long anyway (e.g., for imaging of venous flow) and to turbo inflow squences (see below), where it does not affect the TR, because it acts as a prepulse. Often, it is also possible to exclude fat from the MIP, simply by performing a „target" MIP where only a part of the acquired volume (without fat) is used for the projection.

Magnetization Transfer

Magnetization transfer (MT) prepulses manipulate contrast by reducing the signal from certain tissues such as brain, liver, and muscle [53]. Other tissues like fat and CSF are hardly affected by MT. MTC (MT contrast) is created by RF prepulses which saturate the „bound water pool" (protons in macromolecules with an extremely short T2) without saturating the „free water pool" (relatively free protons with a „normal" T2). Due to cross-relaxation between the „free water pool" and the „bound water pool" a new equilibrium is created, in which the tissue of interest (which is part of the free proton pool) has less available longitudinal magnetization and also a shorter T1. The magnetization of the „bound pool" can either be destroyed by frequency selective off-resonance pulses (see Fig. 24) or by binomial pulses on-resonance (121, 1331). In inflow MRA the main goal of MT is suppression of the static background to increase the contrast between blood and static tissues. This will increase the small vessel conspicuity. Because the background suppression in PCA is excellent, MT is not clinically used for PCA, but only for inflow MRA. MT has been successfully applied to inflow MRA in the brain [54, 55]. Both on-resonance and off-resonance MTC RF pulses are successful in suppressing the signal of the static brain tissue by about 40 % maximally. Moreover, it has been shown in vitro that *nonflowing* blood also shows an MTC signal reduction of about 20 %. MTC signal reduction of *flowing* blood depends on the MTC technique being used, but will be between 0 % and 20 %. Thus, MTC results in a gain of between 20 % and 40 % in blood contrast. Similar to inflow enhancement for normal excitation RF pulses, the (unwanted) reduction of the blood signal due to MTC RF pulses depends on the number of MTC pulses it has received, and on the MTC RF frequency characteristics. In general, off-resonance MTC pulses affect the blood signal less than on-resonance (binomial) MTC pulses. This can be explained by the fact that the *transparent* bandwidth of on-resonance MTC pulses (usually about 800 Hz,

depending on the MTC pulse length) is limited by the RF transmit power and Specific Absorption Rate (SAR) limits. With off-resonance MTC pulses it is easier to limit the *excitation* bandwidth by using a shaped RF pulse and making the RF pulse relatively long. For MRA, usually the off-resonance MT prepulses are used, typically with a duration of 10–15 ms and with a frequency offset of about 1 kHz. The RF power of these pulses should be very large, typically equivalent to a flip angle of about 500°–1000°. Because of the length of this MT prepulse, the minimal TR is increased, typically to 40–45 ms (and with it the total scanning time). Because the fat signal is hardly suppressed by the MT pulses, not only the contrast between blood and MT-sensitive tissues increases by MT, but also the contrast between fat and these tissues. This sometimes makes it difficult to appreciate the gain in blood contrast by MT.

Turbo Techniques

The main features of turbo gradient field echo techniques [56, 57] as far as inflow angiography is concerned are its for extremely short repetition times TR and the use of magnetization preparation prepulses (inversion or saturation) for superior static background tissue suppression. Skillful application of these prepulses can reduce the background tissue signal intensity to an absolute minimum (see Fig. 25). This permits the appreciation of small vessels with slow flow. To ensure complete effectiveness of the prepulses, each series of phase-encoding steps is split up into a user-definable number of scan segments or „shots" (segmented k-space). The order of the phase-encoding steps within every shot can be either low-high (centric) or linear. In this way optimal contrast between vessels and stationary tissue in turbo inflow angiography is realized. Multiple shots can be combined with cardiac triggering/gating in order to freeze motion due to cardiac pulsations. The combination of segmented turbo inflow and cardiac triggering/gating makes the inflow technique a powerful method for the study of pulsating blood vessels (all major arteries).

In the literature, turbo techniques are referred to as Turbo Field Echo (TFE), Turbo FLASH (Fast Low Angle SHot), MP-RAGE (Magnetization Prepared-Rapid Acquisition Gradient Echo), etc. Most often, in MRA, the turbo sequence is performed with an inversion prepulse, in combina-

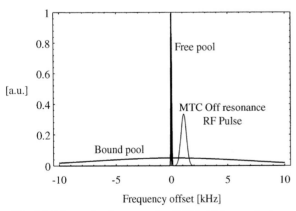

Fig. 24. Magnetization transfer (MT). This graph demonstrates the narrow resonance spectrum of the free water pool, and the broad resonance spectrum of the bound water pool (due to its very short *T2*) An off-resonance RF pulse is also shown, used to generate the magnetization transfer contrast (MTC). These off-resonance pulses only excite the (invisible) bound water pool and have only an indirect effect on the free water pool

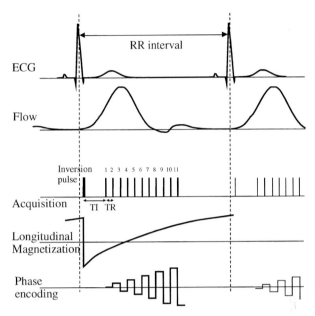

Fig. 25. Turbo sequence. A slice-selective inversion pulse inverts the longitudinal magnetization of the imaging volume. During the inversion delay time *TI*, fresh blood flows in, and the static spins recover from the inversion. The phase-encoding order is centric (low-high) in this example in order to sample the center of k-space at the beginning of the „shot" when the longitudinal magnetization (of the static background) is close to zero. Since the center of k-space determines most of the global contrast, in this way the static background is effectively suppressed

tion with cardiac triggering, as shown in Fig. 25. At every detected R wave, after a user-defined trigger delay, a slice-selective inversion prepulse is applied, inverting all spins inside the imaging volume (including blood). During the following user-defined inversion delay time TI, fresh blood will flow into the imaging volume, and the inverted blood will flow out. Furthermore, the longitudinal magnetization of the static tissue, which has been inverted, will relax to its original state, crossing zero at some point in time. When the blood inside the imaging volume has been refreshed sufficiently, and the longitudinal magnetization of the static tissue is close to zero, a number of profiles with different phase-encoding steps are acquired in one shot. The order of the phase-encoding steps is usually low-high (centric) so that the low phase-encoding steps (the center of k-space) which determine the main contrast in the image are acquired at the beginning of the shot, when longitudinal magnetization of the static background tissue is close to zero. In this way, the signal from the background is very effectively suppressed. One problem with this type of technique is that not all tissues can be „nulled" at the same time, depending on the TI. Generally fat, having a short TI, is the most problematic. To alleviate this problem, turbo techniques can also be combined with fat saturation as has been recently described [58]. Similar to the gated sweep technique, the turbo sequence acquisition can be limited to systole, when the flow is maximal, or to diastole, where the flow is slower and hence less disturbed. Limiting the acquisition to diastole is only useful in those vessels where there is significant flow in diastole, such as the carotid or renal arteries.

The cardiac gated sweep technique and the triggered turbo sequences are similar in the way they acquire the k-space in segments. The difference between the two techniques is that in turbo techniques no steady state is maintained, and that gated sweep technique does not feature any prepulses other than presaturation prepulses. If presaturation is used, in the turbo sequence the presaturation pulse is applied only once per shot, whereas in the gated sweep technique it is applied every TR. Turbo techniques can also be combined with phase contrast techniques, although in PCA no inversion or saturation prepulses are used, but only presaturation prepulses (outside the imaging volume) to discriminate between venous and arterial flow.

Appendix A

Phase Effects

The motion-induced phase shift ϕ of the MR signal depends on the spin displacement function $\mathbf{x}(t)$ and on the gradient function $\mathbf{G}(t)$. (a bold notation is used to denote vectors). We assume that the main static perfectly homogeneous field $\mathbf{B}_0$ is in the z direction, and that the static field contains a small constant inhomogeneity $\mathbf{b}_0(\mathbf{x})$. The gradient vector function $\mathbf{G}(t)$ can be expressed as $\mathbf{G}(t) = \nabla B_z(\mathbf{x},t)$, and its corresponding magnetic field as $B_{Gz}(\mathbf{x},t) = \mathbf{G}(t) \cdot \mathbf{x}$. Because the magnetic gradients are assumed to be linear, $\mathbf{G}(t)$ does not depend on $\mathbf{x}$. For simplicity, we consider only the gradient fields in the main field direction, so that $\mathbf{G}(t)$ is written as a vector instead of a tensor. The local field strength B_z as experienced by a moving isochromatic spin group with coordinates $\mathbf{x}(t)$ can thus be written as

$$B_z(\mathbf{x}(t)) = B_{0z} + b_{0z}(\mathbf{x}(t)) + \mathbf{G}(t) \cdot \mathbf{x}(t) \quad \text{(A1)}$$

Using the resonant condition

$$\omega(\mathbf{x},t) = \gamma \cdot B_z(\mathbf{x},t) \quad \text{(A2)}$$

where γ is the magnetogyric ratio, the phase ϕ of the MR signal (after demodulation with the Larmor frequency $\omega_0 = \gamma \cdot B_{0z}$) from an excited isochromatic spin group at $\mathbf{x}(t)$ can be expressed as

$$\phi = \phi(\text{TE}) - \phi(0) = \int_0^{\text{TE}} \omega(\mathbf{x}(t)) - \omega_0 \, dt =$$
$$\gamma \int_0^{\text{TE}} b_{0z}(\mathbf{x}(t)) + \mathbf{G}(t) \cdot \mathbf{x}(t) \, dt$$
$$\text{(A3)}$$

where t=0 is defined as the center of the RF excitation pulse (we neglect the effects due to the (relatively long) duration of the RF pulse) and t=TE as the center of the formed echo. Furthermore, any displacement function $\mathbf{x}(t)t$ that is continuously differentiable around an arbitrary time expansion point $t=t_{\text{exp}}$ can be written as a Taylor expansion series around t_{exp}. If, for convenience, we write the nth derivative of position $\mathbf{x}$ at time t_{exp} as

$$\mathbf{x}^{[n]}(t_{\text{exp}}) \equiv \frac{d^n \mathbf{x}(t_{\text{exp}})}{dt^n}, \text{ we can write } \mathbf{x}(t) \text{ as}$$

$$\mathbf{x}(t) = \sum_{n=0}^{\infty} \frac{1}{n!} \mathbf{x}^{[n]}(t_{\text{exp}}) \cdot (t - t_{\text{exp}})^n$$
$$= \mathbf{x}(t_{\text{exp}}) + \mathbf{v}(t_{\text{exp}}) \cdot (t - t_{\text{exp}}) + \frac{1}{2}\mathbf{a}(t_{\text{exp}}) \cdot$$
$$(t - t_{\text{exp}})^2 + \frac{1}{6}\mathbf{j}(t_{\text{exp}}) \cdot (t - t_{\text{exp}})^3 + \dots \quad \text{(A4)}$$

In practice, only a limited number of derivatives are used in order to describe the motion function $\mathbf{x}(t)$. The phase sensitivity to the nth derivative of position $\mathbf{x}^{[n]}(t_{\text{exp}})$ is determined by the nth gradient moment $\mathbf{M}_n$:

$$\mathbf{M}_n(t_{\text{exp}}) \equiv \frac{\gamma}{n!} \int_0^{\text{TE}} \mathbf{G}(t) \cdot (t - t_{\text{exp}})^n dt$$
$$(\text{SI unit}: \text{rad.s}^n/\text{m}) \quad \text{(A5)}$$

Notice that due to our unconventional Taylor expansion (Eq. A4), the integration limits (0-TE) do not change when t_{exp} is changed. This is impor-

tant, because it means that changing t_{exp} does not imply a shift in „observer" time scale; the timing is always determined by the gradient $\mathbf{G}(t)$.

For convenience, we denote the first four sensitivities as $\mathbf{M}_x \equiv \mathbf{M}_0$, $\mathbf{M}_v \equiv \mathbf{M}_1$, $\mathbf{M}_a \equiv \mathbf{M}_2$, $\mathbf{M}_j \equiv \mathbf{M}_3$, and the phase shift due to the field inhomogeneity as $\phi_{\text{inh}} = \gamma_0 \int_0^{\text{TE}} b_{0z}(\mathbf{x}(t)) dt$. If we now substitute Eqs. A4 and A5 in Eq. A3 we get

$$\phi = \phi_{\text{inh}} + \sum_{n=0}^{\infty} \mathbf{x}^{[n]}(t_{\text{exp}}) \cdot \mathbf{M}_n(t_{\text{exp}}) \quad \text{(A6a)}$$

$$\phi = \phi_{\text{inh}} + \mathbf{x}(t_{\text{exp}}) \cdot \mathbf{M}_x + \mathbf{v}(t_{\text{exp}}) \cdot \mathbf{M}_v(t_{\text{exp}}) +$$
$$\mathbf{a}(t_{\text{exp}}) \cdot \mathbf{M}_a(t_{\text{exp}}) + \mathbf{j}(t_{\text{exp}}) \cdot \mathbf{M}_j(t_{\text{exp}}) + \dots \quad \text{(A6b)}$$

For most flow velocity measurements, a phase difference technique is used in order to eliminate the phase contribution ϕ_{inh} of the field inhomogeneity $\mathbf{b}_0(\mathbf{x})$. Two acquisitions are made with gradient functions $\mathbf{G}_1(t)$ and $\mathbf{G}_2(t)$, which have different flow sensitivities, such that the gradient difference function $\Delta\mathbf{G}(t) = \mathbf{G}_1(t) - \mathbf{G}_2(t)$ is bipolar. Finally, the reconstructed pixel phases ϕ_1 and ϕ_2 are subtracted. According to Eq. A3, the net phase shift $\Delta\phi = \phi_1 - \phi_2$ of a phase difference technique using two gradient functions $\mathbf{G}(t)$ and $\mathbf{G}_2(t)$ can be written as

$$\Delta\phi = \gamma \int_0^{\text{TE}} \Delta\mathbf{G}(t) \cdot \mathbf{x}(t) \, dt \quad \text{(A7)}$$

The inhomogeneity term in Eq. A/3, $\phi_{\text{inh}} = \gamma \int_0^{\text{TE}} b_{0z}(\mathbf{x}(t)) dt$, is eliminated, because it is the same for both acquisitions. (Eddy currents can induce other phase shifts which will not completely cancal after subtraction, but they are neglected here.) For flow measurements, the gradient difference function $\Delta\mathbf{G}(t)$ is usually designed to be a (more or less odd) bipolar gradient sequence. From Eqs A7, A5, and A6, the net phase sensitivity can be written as

$$\Delta\mathbf{M}_n(t_{\text{exp}}) = \frac{\gamma}{n!} \int_0^{\text{TE}} \Delta\mathbf{G}(t) \cdot (t - t_{\text{exp}})^n dt$$
$$= \mathbf{M}_{n1}(t_{\text{exp}}) - \mathbf{M}_{n2}(t_{\text{exp}}) \quad \text{(A8)}$$

Since $\Delta\mathbf{M}_x = \mathbf{O}$, we can rewrite Eq. A6 as

$$\Delta\phi = \mathbf{v}(t_{\text{exp}}) \cdot \Delta\mathbf{M}_v + \mathbf{a}(t_{\text{exp}}) \cdot \Delta\mathbf{M}_a(t_{\text{exp}})$$
$$+ \mathbf{j}(t_{\text{exp}}) \cdot \Delta\mathbf{M}_j(t_{\text{exp}}) + \dots \quad \text{(A9)}$$

Appendix B

Table B1. Survey of relative advantages and disadvantages of MRA techniques [59]

Technique	Advantages	Disadvantages
Inflow general	Reprojection and subvolumes possible Presaturation works well	Thrombus may simulate flow Tortuous vessels give less contrast than vessels which go straight through the slice/volume
M2D inflow	Contrast very dependent on flow direction (due to large flip angle) Sensitive to slow flow (maximum inflow effect) Reasonable scanning times (for small volumes) No saturation effects for flow perpendicular to imaging plane	Low spatial resolution (thick slices) Large voxels, more intravoxel dephasing Motion artifacts (stripe artifacts) Insensitive to in-plane flow (saturation effects) Longer *TE* than 3D techniques Relatively poor *S/N* Scanning time increases with length of vessel track
3D inflow (single slab)	Sensitive to flow in all directions (small flip angle) Short scanning times High spatial resolution Very short *TE* Good *S/N* ratio Small voxels Less dephasing (due to smaller voxels and shorter *TE*)	Insensitive to slow flow Field distortion artifacts (air-bone) Limited track of vessels (saturation) Sensitive to motion (blurring and ghosting, swallowing) Less static background suppression than with 2D (due to smaller flip angle)
3D inflow (multi-slab MOTSA multi-chunk)	See 3D inflow single slab Larger track of vessels possible More sensitive to slow flow Better static background suppression when larger flip angle is used	Less *S/N* for smaller slabs Field distortion artifacts (air-bone) Sensitive to motion (blurring and ghosting, swallowing) Longer scanning time than with single slab due to slab overlap Residual Venetian blind artifacts
MTC prepulse (inflow techniques)	Additional suppression of several tissues, including brain, muscle, liver	Longer *TR*; longer scanning time Higher *SAR* (more W/kg) Not always possible to avoid reduction of blood signal
Prepulses (turbo inflow techniques)	Additional suppression background tissue	Sometimes reduction of blood signal caused by prepulse
PCA general	Variable velocity encoding, allowing depiction of slow and fast flow Excellent background suppression Minimized saturation effects, large track of vessels Differentiation between flowing and stationary blood (hemorrhage) Directional flow images possible	Long *TE* (more turbulence effects) Presaturation works less effective, only for small track of vessel
2D PCA	Short scanning time Thick slice possible (several cm) Can be used as survey No MIP necessary (single thick slice)	No reprojection images Large voxel size (thick slice) Low *C/N* (partial volume) Signal loss with overlapping vessels (due to large slice thickness)
2D cine PCA	Time resolution Hemodynamic flow information	See 2D PCA Needs cardiac triggering, longer scanning times

Table B1. (continued)

Technique	Advantages	Disadvantages
3D PCA	Small voxels (less intravoxel dephasing) Preprojection and subvolumes possible	Long acquisition time Motion sensitive Field distortion artifacts (air-bone)
QF general	Variable velocity encoding, allowing measurement of slow and fast flow Quantitative (velocity cm/s and or flux cc/s, stroke volume) Through-plane and/or in-plane measurement	
2D QF	Short scan times	Relatively thick slice (usually 5–10 mm)
3D QF	Flow information in multiple slices Thin slices, smaller voxels, so less intravoxel dephasing	Longer scanning times (proportional to number of slices)
Cine QF (2D and 3D)	Time resolution Hemodynamic flow information	Needs cardiac triggering
Cardiac gating (gated sweep segmented k-space) Inflow+PCA	Less blurring due to movement of the vessel caused by pulsatility of the blood Reduction of ghosting Diastolic gating: slower flow, less flow voids in stenosis, increased specificity Systolic gating: higher flow: more signal, more flow voids in stenosis: increased sensitivity	Longer scanning time (compared with no gating)

PCA: phase contrast angiography; QF: quantitative flow.

References

1. Siebert JE, Pernicone JR, Potchen EJ (1992) Physical principles and application of MRA. Seminars in Ultrasound, CT and MRI 13: 227–245
2. Masaryk TJ, Lewin JS, Laub G (1991) Magnetic resonance angiography. In: Stark DD, Bradley WG (eds) Magnetic resonance imaging Mosby, St Louis, pp 299–334
3. Crooks LE, Haacke EM (1993) Historical overview of MR angiography. In: Potchen EJ, Haacke EM, Siebert JE, Gottschalk A (eds) Magnetic resonance angiography, concepts & applications. Mosby, St. Louis, pp 3–8
4. Cohen MS (1993) Echo planar flow imaging. In: Magnetic resonance angiography, concepts & applications. Potchen EJ, Haacke EM, Siebert JE, Gottschalk A (eds) Mosby, St. Louis pp 297–304
5. Jackson JI, Nishimura DG, Macovski A (1992) Twisting radial lines with application to robust magnetic resonance imaging of irregual flow. Magn Reson Med 25: 128–139
6. Marchal G, Bosmans H, McLachlan SJ (1993) Magnetopharmaceuticals as contrast agents. In: Potchen EJ, Haacke EM, Siebert JE, Gottschalk A (eds), Magnetic resonance angiography, concepts & applications. Mosby St. Louis, pp 305–322
7. van der Meulen P, Groen JP, Cuppen JJM (1985) Very fast MR imaging by field echoes and small angle excitation. Magn Reson Imaging 3: 297–299
8. Wehrli FW, Haacke EM (1993) Principles of MR imaging. In: Potchen EJ, Haacke EM, Siebert JE, Gottschalk A (eds) Magnetic resonance angiography, concepts & applications. Mosby, St. Louis, pp 9–34
9. van der Meulen P, Groen JP, Tinus AMC, Bruntink G (1988) Fast field echo imaging: an overview and contrast calculations. Magn Reson Imaging 6: 355–368
10. Siebert JE, Rosenbaum TL (1993) Image presentation and postprocessing. In: Potchen EJ, Haacke EM, Siebert JE, Gottschalk A (eds) Magnetic resonance angiography, concepts & applications. Mosby, St. Louis, pp 220–245
11. Keller PJ, Saloner D (1993) Time of flight flow imaging. In: Potchen EJ, Haacke EM, Siebert JE, Gottschalk A (eds) Magnetic resonance angiography, concepts & applications. Mosby, St. Louis, pp 146–159
12. Parker DL, Yuan C, Blatter DD (1991) MR angiography by multiple thin slab 3D acquisition. Magn Reson Med 17: 434–451
13. Blatter DD, Parker DL, Robinson R (1991) Cerebral MR angiography with multiple overlapping thin slab acquisition. Radiology 179: 805–811

14. Edelman RR, Siewert B, Adamis M, et al. (1994) Signal targeting with alternating radiofrequency (STAR) sequences: application to MR angiography. Magn Reson Med 31: 233–238
15. Nishimura DG, Macovski A, Pauly JM, Conolly SM (1987) MR angiography by selective inversion recovery. Magn Reson Med 4: 193–202
16. Nishimura DG, Macovski A, Jackson JI et al. (1988) Magnetic resonance angiography by selective inversion recovery using a compact gradient echo sequence. Magn Reson Med 8: 96–103
17. Dixon WT, Du LN, Gado M et al. (1986) Projection angiograms of blood labeled by adiabatic fast passage. Magn Reson Med 3: 454
18. Sardashti M, Schwartzberg DG, Stomp G, Dixon WT (1990) Spin-labeling angiography of the carotids by presaturation and simplified adiabatic inversion. Magn Reson Med 15: 192–200
19. Dixon WT, Sardashti M, Castillo M, Stomp G (1991) Multiple inversion recovery reduces static tissue signal in angiograms. Magn Reson Med 18: 257–268
20. Doyle M, Mulligan A, Matsuda T, Pohost GM (1992) Outflow refreshment angiography: bright blood, bright tissue technique. Magn Reson Imaging 10: 887–892
21. Dumoulin CL, Souza SP, Pelc N (1993) Phase sensitive flow imaging. In: Potchen EJ, Haacke EM, Siebert JE, Gottschalk A (eds) Magnetic resonance angiography, concepts & applications. Mosby, St. Louis, pp 173–186
22. Dumoulin CL, Souza SP, Walker MF, Wagle W (1989) Three-dimensional phase contrast angiography. Magn Reson Med 9: 139–149
23. Pelc NJ, Bernstein MA, Shimakawa A, et al. (1991) Encoding strategies for three-directional phase-contrast MR imaging of flow. J Magn reson Imaging 1: 405–413
24. Axel L, Morton D (1987) MR flow imaging of motion by velocity-compensated/uncompensated difference images. J Comput Assist Tomogr 11: 31
25. van Dijk P (1984) Direct cardiac NMR imaging of heart wall and blood flow velocity. J Comput Assist Tomogr 8: 429–436
26. Bryant DJ, Payne JA, Firmin DN, Longmore DB (1984) Measurement of flow with NMR imaging using a gradient pulse and phase difference technique. J Comput Assist Tomogr 8: 588–593
27. Firmin DN, Dumoulin CL, Mohiaddin RH (1993) Quantitative flow imaging. In: Potchen EJ, Haacke EM, Siebert JE, Gottschalk A (eds) Magnetic resonance angiography, concepts & applications. Mosby, St. Louis, pp 187–219
28. Hofman MBM, Kouwenhoven M, Sprenger M, van Rossum AC et al. (1993) Nontriggered magnetic resonance velocity measurement of the time-average of pulsatile velocity. Magn Reson Med 29: 648–655
29. Buonocore MH, Bogren H (1992) Factors influencing the accuracy and precision of velocity-encoded phase imaging. Magn Reson Med 26: 141–154
30. Wolf RL, Ehman RL, Riederer J, Rossman PJ (1993) Analysis of systematic and random error in MR volumetric flow measurements. Magn Reson Med 30: 82–91
31. Nordell B, Stahlberg F, Ericsson A, Ranta C (1988) A rotating phantom for the study of flow effects in MR imaging. Magn Reson Imaging 6: 695–705
32. Meier D, Maier S, Bösinger P (1988) Quantitative flow measure ments on phantoms and blood vessels with NMR. Magn. Reson. Med 8: 25–34
33. Ku DN, Biancheri CL, Pettigrew RI, Peifer JW, Markou CP, Engels H (1990) Evaluation of magnetic resonance velocimetry for steady flow. ASME J Biomechanical Engineering 112: 464–472
34. Moran PR (1982) A flow velocity zeugmatographic interlace for NMR imaging in humans. Magn Reson Imaging 1: 197–203
35. Wendt RE, Wong WF (1992) Nuclear magnetic resonance velocity spectra of pulsatile flow in a rigid tube. Magn Reson Med 27: 214–255
36. Feinberg DA, Crooks LE, Sheldon P, et al. (1985) Magnetic resonance imaging and velocity vector components of fluid flow. Magn Reson Med 2: 555–566
37. Hennig J, Mueri M, Brunner P, Friedburg H (1986) Quantitative flow measurement with the fast Fourier flow technique. Radiology 161: 717–720
38. Edelman RR, Mattle HP, Wallner B et al. (1990) Extracranial carotid arteries. evaluation of „black blood" MR angiography. Radiology 177: 45–50
39. Lin W, Haacke EM, Edelman RE (1993) Black blood imaging. In: Potchen EJ, Haacke EM, Siebert JE, Gottschalk A (eds) Magnetic resonance angiography, concepts & applications. Mosby, St. Louis, pp 160–172
40. Edelman RR, Chien D, Kim D (1991) Fast selective black blood imaging. Radiology 181: 655–660
41. Haacke EM, Patrick JL (1986) Reducing motion artifacts in two dimensional Fourier transform imaging. Magn Reson Imaging 4: 359–376
42. Bailes DR, Gilderdale DJ, Bydder GM et al. (1985) Respiratory ordered phase encoding (ROPE): a method for reducing respiratory motion artifacts. J Comput Assist Tomogr 9: 835–838
43. Frederickson JO, Pelc JN (1994) Time-resolved MR imaging by automated data segmentation. J Mang Reson Imag 4: 189–196
44. Keegan J, Firmin D, Gatehouse P, Longmore D (1994) The application of breath hold velocity mapping techniques to the measurement of coronary artery blood flow velocity: phantom data and initial in vivo results. Magn Reson Med 31: 526–536
45. Buonocore M, Gao L (1994) Experimental study of the effects of „fractional" gating on flow measurements. Magn Reson Med 31: 429–436
46. de Graaf RG, Groen JP (1992) MR Angiography with pulsatile flow. Magn Res Imaging 10: 25–34
47. Saloner D, Selby K, Anderson CM (1994) MRA Studies of arterial stenosis: improvements by diastolic gating. Magn Reson Med 31: 196–203
48. Lenz GW, Haacke EM, White RD (1989) Retrospective cardiac gating: a review of technical aspects and future directions. Magn Reson Imaging 7: 445–455
49. Duerk JL, Wendt RE III (1993) Motion artifacts and motion compensation. In: Potchen EJ, Haacke EM, Siebert JE, Gottschalk A (eds) Magnetic resonance angiography, concepts & applications. Mosby, St. Louis, pp 80–133

50. Moran PR, Nalcioglu O. Juh SC (1987) Oblique vascular displacement flow artifacts in conventional MRI sequences. Magn Reson Imaging 5: 34–35

51. Frank LA, Crawley AP, Buxton RB (1992) Elimination of oblique flow artifacts in magnetic resonance imaging. Magn Reson Med 25: 299–307

52. McGibney G, Smith MR, Nichols ST, Crawley A (1993) Quantitative evaluation of several partial fourier reconstruction algorithms used in MRI. Magn Reson Med 30: 51–59

52. Flamig DP, Pierce WB, Harms SE, Griffey RH (1992) Magnetization transfer contrast in fat-suppressed steady-state three-dimensional MR images. Magn Reson Med 26: 122–131

54. Edelman RE, Sungkee SA, Chien D et al. (1992) Improved time-of-flight MR angiography of the brain with magnetization transfer contrast. Radiology 25: 372–399

55. Pike GB, Hu BS, Glover GH, Enzmann DR (1992) Magnetization transfer time-of-flight magnetic resonance angiography. Magn Reson Med 25: 372–379

56. van Vaals JJ, Groen JP, van Yperen GH (1991) Recent progress in fast MR imaging. Medica Mundi 36: 152–167

57. Haase A (1990) Snapshot FLASH MRI. Applications to T1, T2 and chemical-shift imaging. Magn Reson Med 13: 77–89

58. Li D, Haacke EM, Mugler JP, Berr S, et al. (1994) Three-dimensional time-of-flight MR angiography using selective inversion recovery RAGE with fat saturation and ECG-triggering: application to renal arteries. Magn Reson Med 31: 414–422

59. Huston J, Ehman RL (1993) Comparison of time-of-flight and phase-contrast MR neuroangiographic techniques. Radiographics 13: 5–19

Cerebrovascular MR Imaging

J. Hennig and K. U. Wentz

This chapter presents an introduction to applications of cerebrovascular magnetic resonance angiography (MRA). The emphasis is placed on outlining experimental possibilities (and pitfalls) of angiographic techniques with a view to the clinical relevance of the respective examinations.

The quality of MR angiograms has improved continuously since the first demonstration of images from human vessels at the fourth annual meeting of the Society of Magnetic Resonance in Medicine in 1985 [1, 2]. Although the large number of presentations on MRA are not adequately reflected in the number of day-to-day applications of these techniques in clinical routine, MRA can still be said to have changed the outlook of diagnostic MR imaging especially for examinations of cervical and cerebral vessels.

Methodological Aspects

The basic techniques in use today were introduced during the first years of its development. They are described by Crooks and Hylton and Kouwenhoven et al. (this volume) and are therefore discussed only briefly here, with special emphasis on the problems and possibilities of their application to the cerebrovascular system.

Time-of-flight (TOF) techniques can be performed either as sequential two-dimensional single-slice experiments for vessels with slow flow or directly by three-dimensional data acquisition for high flow [3–7]. Both use gradient-echo imaging sequences with short recovery times. For two-dimensional acquisition high flip angles are commonly used. This leads to very low signal for stationary matter while the signal from blood flowing through the imaged slice appears bright due to an exchange of unsaturated spins. Three-dimensional angiograms can then be produced by maximum-intensity projections (MIP) through a stack of such images [8–10]. A problem with TOF methods lies in the fact that total cancelation of stationary tissue cannot be achieved, which always leads to problems in detecting very small vessels with low velocity. This has led to techniques for further reducing stationary signals using additional radiofrequency (RF) pulses either for additonal saturation of spins within the same slice [11, 12] or for signal attenuation via magnetization transfer suppression [13].

An additional problem arises when a fresh thrombus is submitted to TOF angiography. The short T_1 of such a clot leads to a bright signal in spite of zero flow. This is demonstrated in Fig. 1, which shows a two-dimensional TOF image from a patient with a thrombus in the left transverse sinus. The thrombus appears as bright as the signal of flowing blood in the controlateral vessel. The lack of blood flow is demonstrated by a fast Fourier flow [14] image (Fig. 1, bottom).

The relative signal enhancement of flowing blood versus stationary matter decreases when the flowing spins remain in the imaged slice longer than the repetition time of the experiment. The flowing spins are then also saturated, and their signal amplitude is reduced. This is the case when the flow velocities are low, slice thickness is large, or with in-plane flow. Consequently visualization of extremely thin vessels requires the use of very thin slices of 1 mm or less. For the acquisition of angiograms of small vessels with slow flow this effect leads to long overall acquisition times due to the necessity of acquiring a large number of thin slices. One way of reducing acquisition time is to use a limited number of phase-encoding steps. In the limiting case this leads to acquiring only a single projection per slice, a technique that has been presented as line-scan angiography. The reduced spatial resolution in the phase-encoding direction allows, of course, the reconstruction of an angiogramm only in the direction of the phase-encoding gradient. The lower overall signal-to-noise ratio also leads to problems in the detection of smaller vessels. This limited sensitivity of line-scan angiography has hitherto prohibited the clinical use of this method for the examination of cerebral and cranial vessels.

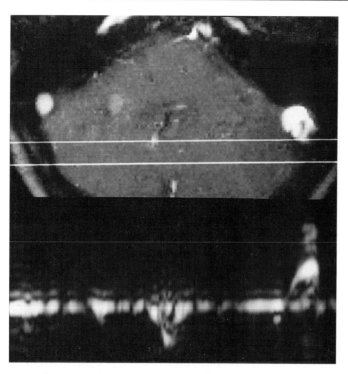

Fig. 1. Enlarged section of a transversal two-dimensional TOF image in a patient with suspected thrombosis of the right lateral sinus (TR = 50 ms, TE = 8 ms, flip angle 60°). *Below,* a fast Fourier flow image displaying flow through a coronal plane located in the position of the *horizontal bars* (*above*). The downward flow in the sagittal sinus is demonstrated as the flow parabola in the center of the image and flow through the left sinus transversus (*arrows, right*), whereas no flow is seen in the right sinus (*arrows, left*). This demonstrates that the bright signal in the TOF image is due to the short T1 of the thrombus and not to inflow. (J. Hennig, D. Ott, Radiological Clinic, University Freiburg, 2T Bruker S 200F)

A second variant of TOF methods uses the excitation of one or several thicker slabs with three-dimensional phase encoding directly to produce a three-dimensional angiogram [15–17]. This technique typically uses lower flip angles and longer repetition times to reduce the saturation of flowing spins. Even then vessels often appear brighter and larger on the side on which blood enters the slab. This effect can be reduced by the TONE method [18], which uses a trapezoidal pulse shape that leads to an effective lower flip angle at the entry side. Figure 2 compares a conventional TOF angiogram (Fig. 2a) to an image acquired with a TONE pulse (Fig. 2b). The latter better delineates vessels downstream from the entry side in the imaged volume. A problem with TONE pulses is the rather complicated dependence of the signal intensity on blood velocity, the dwell time of blood in the volume under examination, and the spatially variable flip angle of the RF pulses. This is illustrated in Fig. 3a, where the gradient of the flip angle is chosen so that the vessels on the entry side appear darker than those further downstream, as compared with a homogeneous flip angle as shown in Fig. 3b.

The suppression of signals from stationary tissue is somewhat better in two-dimensional TOF methods due to the possibility of using large flip angles. For optimum resolution of the final three-dimensional angiogram in the direction of the slice-selection gradient the three-dimensional acquisition, however, does offer the advantage of a continuous representation of the total volume. This avoids the typical "pearl chain" artifact of angiograms reconstructed from two-dimensional slices, which occurs when the spacing of successive slices is too large, or if the signal from the vessel varies between slices due to arterial pulsatility (Fig. 4).

The second effect used to produce MR angiograms also relies on flow velocity namely on the velocity-dependent dephasing of spins flowing along a magnetic field gradient. When two experiments with opposed phase sensitization are performed, an angiogram can be produced by substraction of the two datasets [19–24]. An intrinsic advantage of this method is the perfect cancelation of stationary spins with the possibility of detecting even small vessels (Fig. 5). A disadvantage is the long acquisition time (two to six times that of TOF with identical parameters), especially when flow sensitization is performed in all three directions. In addition, maximum signal intensity is achieved only for those spins whose velocity leads to exact opposition of the signal phases. Spins with lower or higher velocity yield

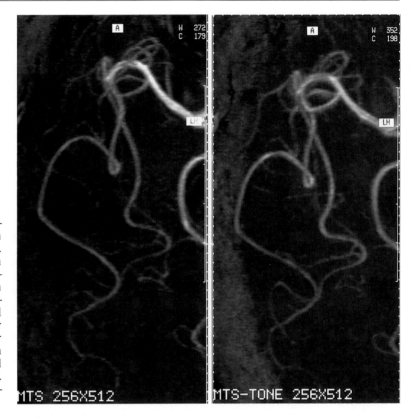

Fig. 2. Comparison of two high-resolution TOF techniques, both using magnetic transfer supresion. *Right*, a rising flip angle between entrance and exit slice of the three-dimensional volume (TONE). In this healthy volunteer the peripheral branches of the middle cerebral artery (*below*) have slightly better flow signal when magnetic transfer suppression with TONE excitation is used compared to conventional TOF angiogram (*left*) (K. U. Wentz, EFMT, Bochum 1.5 T, Magnetom SP 63)

less signal. This problem is especially awkward for those spins which lead to 360° dephasing. These signals cancel one another just as signal from stationary tissue. Phase-substraction angiograms are therefore optimal only for a given flow velocity. Knowledge of the expected velocities is therefore required before performing such an experiment. A problem of phase-substraction methods is of course the require-

ment of perfect reproducibility of the experiment. This has vastly improved with state-of-the-art gradient systems using actively shielded gradients. The nonreproducibility due to patient movement can be minimized by interleaving the various subtraction steps.

A possibility in all angiographic techniques is the supression of signal from parts of the vessel by introducing appropriate saturation pulses. The ad-

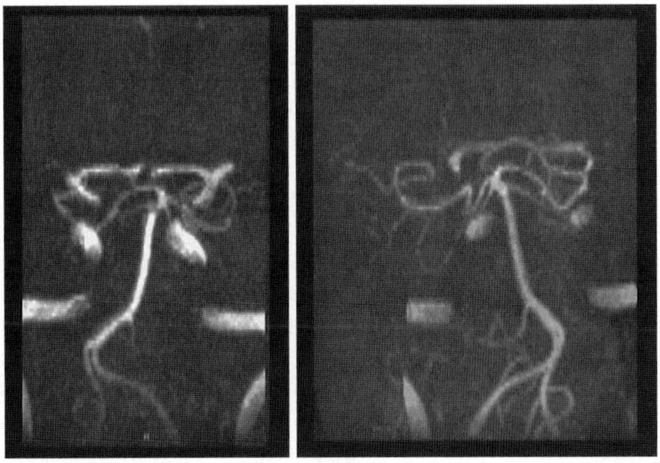

Fig. 3. Comparison of a three-dimensional TOF angiogram of a healthy volunteer with (**a**) and without (**b**) TONE pulse. The TONE MRA gives higher signal in the distal part of the vessels

a   b

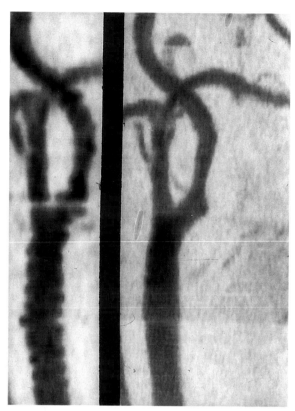

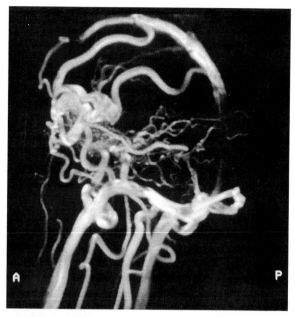

Fig. 5. Phase-contrast angiogram of the head of a patient with a large AV malformation. Acquisition time 15 min. (0.5 T, Gyroscan T5-II, Dr. Keller, University Bonn)

Fig. 4. Angiogram of the carotis bifurcation using a sequential two-dimensional TOF technique (*left*) and a three-dimensional acquisition in three slabs (*right*). Due to the pulsatility of flow with concurrent variation of the signal intensity and to the size and location of the arteries, the vessels in the two-dimensional acquisition show a typical "pearl chain" appearance (G. Bongartz, Radiological Clinic, University Münster, 1.5 T, Magnetom SP 63)

dition of saturation slabs caudal to the imaged volume leads to the supression of arterial blood in cerebrospinal examinations and thus to the generation of venograms. Arteriograms can be produced by adding saturation slabs craniad to the imaged volume. In addition, signal from single vessels can be saturated. This allows for the so-called selective angiography [25]. The main application is in the examination of cross-flow profiles in patients with carotid occlusion. In addition, the flow dynamics in arteriovenous (AV) malformations can be studies (Fig. 6).

The two basic mechanism for MRA suffer from some common problems. The most important of these is the dependence of MRA signal on blood flow. The appearance of the signal is determined principally by the local blood flow properties, which are hard to predict especially in patholo-

gical vessel conditions. Turbulence leads to intravoxel dephasing with subsequent loss of signal amplitude. The inability to display areas of turbulent flow is especially disturbing in the assessment of stenoses. Turbulence caused by the stenosis causes signal obliteration downstream from the lesion [26, 27]. The stenosis is therefore overestimated and appears to be extended into the downstream part of the vessel.

A further problem relates to the observation of pulsatile flow. The changes in the flow velocity in arteries over the cardiac cycle lead to a peroidic signal variation in TOF examinations and to a variation in the flow-dependent phase in phase-subtraction angiography. Both effects cause the appearance of pulsatility ghosts of arteries displaced in the phase-encoding direction of the image. Several possibilities exist to minimize these artifacts. The simplest approach is to use signal averaging, which leads to coherent signal enhancement of the true signal while the artifacts add up incoherently, their relative signal amplitude is therefore reduced. The strong disadvantage of this approach is in considerably prolonging the examination time.

In TOF methods flow-compensated gradients can be used to reduce the dephasing of spins [28]. Since flow compensation always requires longer

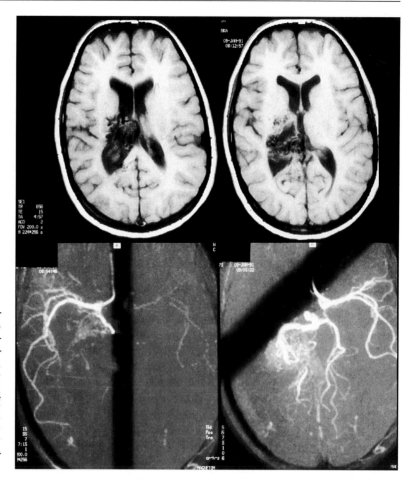

Fig. 6. Transverse T1-weighted images (*above*) and MR angiograms of a patient with an AV malformation. Selective MRA with saturation of the right internal carotid artery demonstrates blood supply mainly by the posterior cerebral artery. Flow signal suppression of the basilar artery shows additional supply via small branches of the posterior communicating artery (K. U. Wentz, EFMT, 1.5 T, Magnetom SP 63)

echo times, with subsequent signal loss due to T_2^* effects, normally only first-order flow compensation is used. This works especially well for moderate signal variations, where the first-order approximation appears sufficient.

For fast velocity changes and high velocity gradients the use of very short echo times is often superior to flow compensation. With the fast and strong gradients available today, echo times shorter than 7 ms can be easily achieved which lead to very few or no artifacts even for the observation of strongly pulsatile vessels such as the carotid arteries. For three-dimensional examinations (both TOF and phase-substraction techniques) the echo times can be made even shorter due to the thicker slices used here [10, 29].

Further advances in MRA use larger image matrices to improve spatial resolution. This leads to better demonstration of smaller voxels by reduction of the partial volume effect from surrounding tissue. Since the signal loss depends on the velocity dispersion inside each voxel, an improved re-

solution using smaller voxels automatically improves the signal quality of larger vessels as well. The reduced sensitivity of high-resolution angiograms to space-dependent changes in the velocity pattern leads to a more continuous representation of even smaller vessels and thus reduces the danger of false-positive diagnosis of stenoses.

Higher resolution also affords a better distinction between small vessel loops and aneurysms. As shown in Fig. 7, a suspected aneurysm is easily demonstrated to be a small loop in the high-resolution angiogram. State-of-the-art angiograms with image matrix sizes up to 1024 × 1024 are displayed in Figs. 7–9. A certain disadvantage of high-resolution scans lies in the fact that the higher spatial resolution is achieved only by using longer echo times. For high-flow turbulence this may lead to increased flow void in spite of the smaller voxel size.

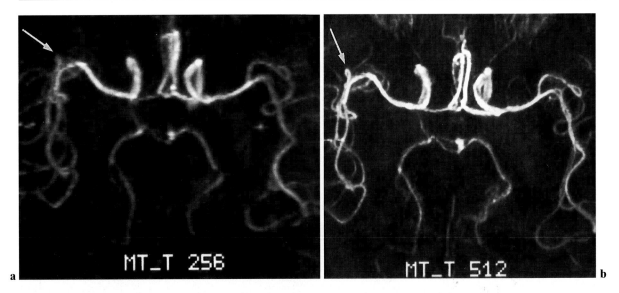

Fig. 7a,b. MRA demonstrating the circle of Willis and the left and right median arteries of a normal volunteer with magnetization transfer suppression acquired with 256×256 (**a**) and 512×512 (**b**) in-plane resolution. The vessel loop clearly demonstrated in the high-resolution image (*arrow*) might easily be misread as a small aneurysm in the lower-resolution scan. (G. Bongartz, Radiological Clinic, University Münster, 1.5 T, Magnetom SP 63)

Applications

Conventional X-ray angiography provides excellent angiograms with high spatial and temporal resolution. However, it has several drawbacks which make the search for alternative approaches such as MRA extremely attractive. These include the following: (a) While the insertion of the needle or catheter can be regarded as a low-risk procedure from a clinical point of view, it is nevertheless an invasive procedure which is not automatically well-tolerated by all patients and requires a higher degree of justification than a noninvasive image acquisition. (b) There is a risk of adverse reactions related to the use of contrast agents, which can be particularly troubling in severely ill patients. (c) The multiple exposure to X-rays is certainly the most severe drawback of conventional angiography. Due to these drawbacks its application is restricted to cases in which the clinical situation strictly requires such an examination.

Compared to MRA it must also be kept in mind that the basic physical effect used to visualize the vascular lumen is fundamentally different. Whereas X-ray methods use the filling of the vessel lumen with contrast agent to visualize the vascular structure, MRA relies on the flow properties of blood. This leads to different modes of operations for the two modalities. Contrast-enhanced MRA can be used by nonselective venous injection of gadolinium compounds for special applications such as the visualization of small vessels, the search for the nidus of AV malformations, and the demonstration of a recanalized sinus thrombosis. Selective injection of contrast agents typical for X-ray angiography has hitherto not been introduced into MRA. Although techniques to allow tracking of catheters by MRA have recently been demonstrated, there have as yet been no demonstrations of clinical applications of such devices. The possibility of conducting a selective catheter MRA is currently prohibited by the size and limited access of the MR magnet. Future developments of "open magnet" designs will demonstrate whether catheter angiography by MRA can find a place in interventional neuroradiology. Although the possibility of selectively visualizing vessels by injecting MR contrast agents (e. g., Gd-DTPA) via catheter has been demonstrated for vessels in the abdomen, it remains to be seen whether such a procedure will find sufficient acceptance to warrant the increased costs and effort. A disadvantage of catheter MRA is certainly the fact that it at least partially eliminates the noninvasive nature of the technique. The advantages of eliminating prolonged X-ray exposure,

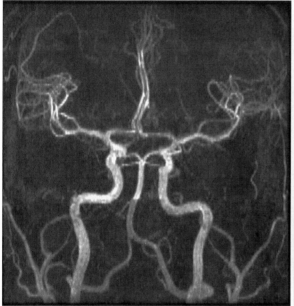 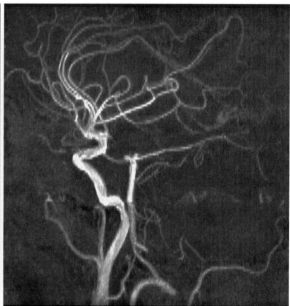

a   b

Fig. 8a, b. Triple-slab acquisition with an anterior projection of all intracranial arteries (**a**) and a lateral projection of the right carotid territory and the posterior circulation (**b**) (K. U. Wentz, EFMT, Bochum, 1.5 T, Magnetom SP 63)

however, remain. Selective catheter angiography currently remains a domain of X-ray techniques. The most significant clinical application of MRA today is in ruling out macroangiopathy due to atherosclerosis, especially in combination with Doppler ultrasound. Additional applications include the analysis of AV malformations, thrombosis, and subclinical aneurysms. The current state of the art is described in below.

Arteriovenous Malformations

A distinct advantage of MRA in the diagnosis of AV malformations is its ability to depict the morphological changes in the surrounding anatomical structures in one examination session. Displacement of brain tissue, formation of edema, compression of ventricles, and acute hemorrhage can easily be detected.

Examples of MR angiograms of AV malformations are presented in Figs. 4, 6, and 10. Although the angiogram does not give direct information about the supplying and draining vessels, this information can in most cases be achieved by selec-

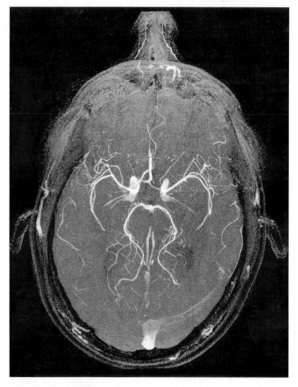

Fig. 9. Three-dimensional TOF MRA of a healthy volunteer, 512×512 acquisition matrix interpolated to a 1024×1024 display matrix. (1.5 T, Gyroscan ACS-II, Philips Medical Systems)

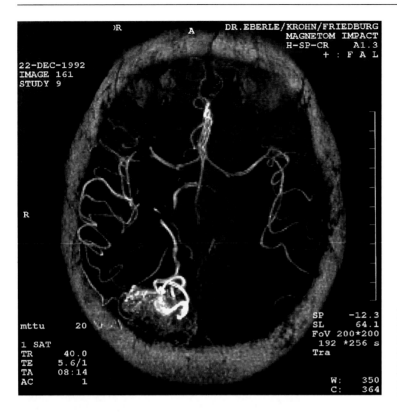

Fig. 10. AV malformation after intracerebral occipital bleeding. The arterial supply is demonstrated via the right a cerebri posterior. Venous drainage proceeds to the sagittal superior sinus (H. Friedburg, Karlsruhe, 1 T, Magnetom Impact)

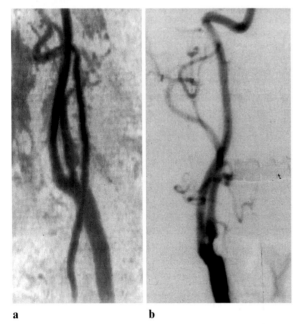

a   b

Fig. 11 a, b. Carotid stenosis demonstrated by MRA (**a**) and DSA (**b**). The MR image was acquired using three-dimensional TOF with 128 partitions and a TONE pulse. (G. Bongartz, Radiological Clinic, University Münster, 1.5 T, Magnetom SP 63)

tive MRA using saturation slices covering potential candidates, as shown in Fig. 6. MRA thus helps not only in the diagnosis but also in selecting candidates for surgical treatment, radiotherapy, and/or embolotherapy. It therefore serves as a helpful preangiographic procedure.

Stenoses and Vascular Occlusions

The possibility of detecting stenoses is demonstrated in Figs. 11 and 12, showing stenosis and occlusion of the carotid artery [10, 16, 29]. Digital subtraction angiography (DSA; Fig. 11b) demonstrates the competetive quality and diagnostic validity of MRA using state-of-the-art equipment and methodology. In evaluating MR angiograms it must be kept in mind that the turbulent flow around stenosis may lead to various degrees of cancelation of signals; this depends strongly on the MRA technique. Although the inherent overestimation of the degree of the stenosis can be reduced by increasing the spatial resolution and by shortening the echo times, stenoses are still likely to be overestimated. In extreme cases a false-

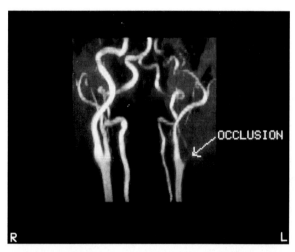

Fig. 12. Occlusion of the left carotid artery demonstrated by three-dimensional TOF MRA. (0.5 T, Gyroscan T5-II, Dr. Keller, University Bonn)

positive diagnosis may be made in regions of vascular obstructions with highly turbulent flow. The fact that atherosclerotic plaques tend to form at regions of unstable flow such as vessel bifurcations increases the tendency to false-positive findings. Furthermore, a reduction in signal intensity, with subsequent erroneous diagnosis of stenosis, is also possible in regions in which strong susceptibility effects lead to signal dephasing. This may be the case at the base of the skull. For very narrow passage through the bone the

Fig. 13. Patient with a stenosis of the left median arter (*arrow*). The stenosis was confirmed by Doppler ultrasound. (G. Bongartz, Radiological Clinic, University Münster, 1.5 T, Magnetom SP 63)

concurrent signal loss is easily mistaken as a stenosis.

The detection of intracranial stenosis requires optimized techniques, first, to obtain a good representation of the particular vessel under study and, second, to reliably define any lack of signal as a stenosis. This requires motion-compensated, short echo time and high-resolution TOF or phase-substraction techniques. Figure 13 demonstrates the visualization of a stenosis of the left median artery by MRA. Flow turbulence is also a severe problem in the diagnose of intracranial stenoses. The problem is somewhat less than in the carotid arteries due to the lesser pulsatility of arterial flow in the intracranial vessels.

Figure 14 demonstrates of the occlusion of a small vessel as visualized by MRA. The T2-weighted image (Fig. 14a) reveals a small area of infarction as a consequence of an occlusion of vertebral occlusion (Fig. 14b).

Currently MRA appears to be diagnostic only when the findings are negative, e.g., no vascular pathology is discerned. When vascular pathology is demonstrated by MRA, other methods, such as Doppler ultrasound or X-ray angiography, are needed to confirm the diagnosis. Future improvements to make MRA a more reliable diagnostic tool will depend on improvement in its image resolution and a further reduction in echo times.

The detection of total vessel occlusion is somewhat more reliable when proper techniques are used. This is especially true when MRA reveals vessels of similar size and blood velocities near a missing vessel.

Care must be taken with pseudo-occlusions in three-dimensional MRA. In patients with ischemic infarcts in whom the three-dimensional

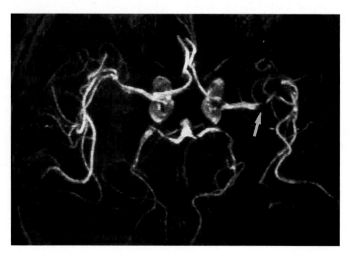

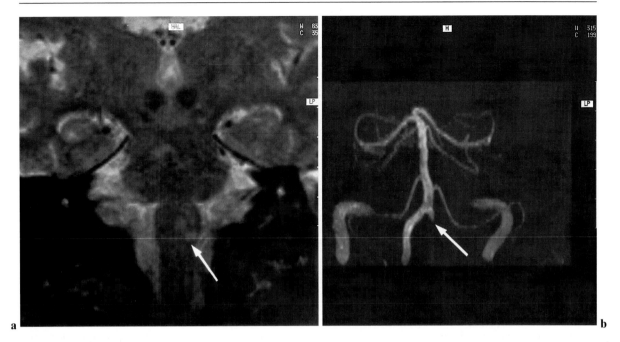

a   b

Fig. 14 a, b. A 68-year-old man with hemiparesis on the right and left paresis of the tongue (ipsilateral lesion of the hypoglossal nerve). T2-weighted imaging demonstrates left anterior infarction of the subpontine medulla (**a,** *arrow*) which is due to vertebral occlusion as demonstrated by MRA (**b,** *arrow*). Lacunar lesion of the pons. (K. U. Wentz, EFMT, Bochum, 1.5 T, Magnetom SP 63)

This requires TOF MRA in three planes. Note, for example, the missing part of the vessel in the phase-contrast angiogram in Fig. 15, in which the flow is in the craniocaudal direction. The benefit of MRA for the diagnosis lies in the fact that conventional MR images taken within the same examination period can be used not only to produce

angiogram does not show the pertinent vessel two-dimensional TOF MRA or flow quantitation should be used to distinguish true occlusion from apparent (pseudo-)occlusion.

MRA can also be used as a quantitative tool for flow measurements via phase mapping or, better, Fourier flow techniques. Whether such techniques can improve the diagnostics of stenosis remains to be determined.

Thrombosis

Figures 15 and 16 demonstrate the ability to detect thrombosis of the sagittal sinus by MRA. Although susceptibility artifacts from the skull bones may obstruct visualization of the sinus, this problem can be overcome by sufficiently shortenning echo times. In demonstrating the sagittal sinus in its full length the changing direction of flow must be taken into account.

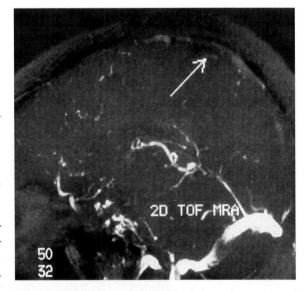

Fig. 15. Thrombosis of the sagittal sinus demonstrated by two-dimensional TOF MRA. (G. Bongartz, Radiological Clinic, University Münster, 1.5 T, Magnetom SP 63)

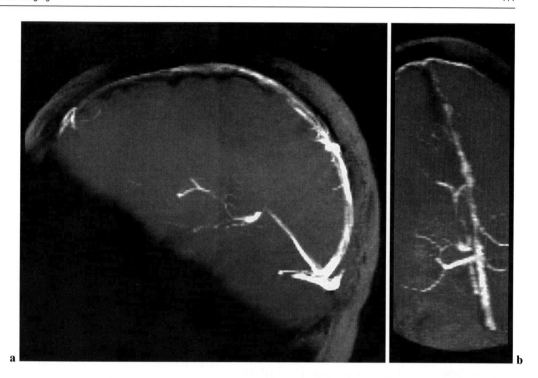

a   b

Fig. 16a, b. Patient after recanalization of a thrombus in the sagittal sinus. The two-dimensional TOF MRA in sagittal (**a**) and transverse (**b**) views demonstrates patency of the vessel and an irregular shape of the lumen as a consequence of incomplete recanalization. (H. Friedburg, Karlsruhe, 1 T, Magnetom Impact)

images of the thrombus itself but also from any parenchymal changes accompanying the vascular pathology.

Aneurysms

MRA has been proposed as an efficient screening method for chronic and subclinical aneurysms down to a diameter of about 3 mm [30]. It must be pointed out, however, that this is true only for high-resolution MRA. Otherwise, as has been pointed out above, small vascular loops are easily mistaken as aneurysms (Fig. 17). The screening of large groups in the general population, such as the members of families with high incidence of aneurysms and other risk groups using high-resolution MRA would be possible, however, only at considerable cost.

The MRA demonstration of a larger aneurysm before and after embolization is demonstrated in Fig. 17. The highly turbulent flow in and around such aneurysms normally does not allow the outlining of its full lumen. However, the information provided by MRA is sufficient to localize the embolization material. Especially for follow-up examinations the MRA technique therefore offers the opportunity to perform frequent control examinations, avoiding repetitive X-ray examinations.

In acute cases of suspected rupture of an aneurysm with subarachnoidal bleeding MRA should not be used due to its low sensitivity in detecting acute hemorrhage. Patients with suspected hemorrhage should be examined by conventional angiography.

Conclusions

With state-of-the-art equipment and methodology MRA has reached a stage of considerable refinement. Distinct advantages of the MRA approach include its possibility to perform repetitive examinations and the possibility of combining angiography with high-resolution and high-contrast imaging of brain parenchyma in a single examination.

MRA serves as a useful preangiographic procedure. After clinical examination and Doppler ultrasound patients from the groups discussed above should be referred to MRA. This specifical-

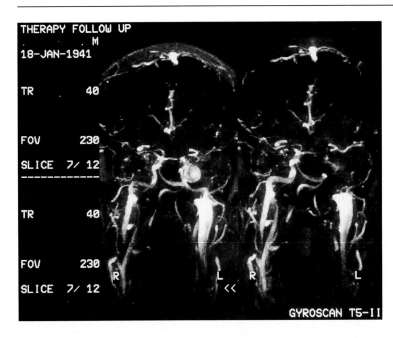

Fig. 17. Follow-up of a patient with a cerebral aneurysm before (*left*) and after (*right*) balloon embolization. (0.5 T, Gyroscan T5-II, Dr. Keller, University Bonn)

ly excludes indications for direct DSA, such as the examination of tumor vascularization and suspected intracranial hemorrhage.

The first MRA examination should be a high-resolution, multislab, three-dimensional TOF scan with magnetization transfer. If this reveals no pathology, and extracranial ultrasound is negative, vascular pathology can be excluded, without further examinations such as DSA. With positive finding in the initial MRA for reliable definition of vascular pathology such as occlusion versus pseudo-occlusion, stenosis of uncertain degree, and AV malformation, more specific MRA sequences should be obtained, such as three-dimensional FISP with minimum echo time, two-dimensional TOF, selective MRA, and black blood MRA, depending on the specific pathology. DSA should be performed only if MRA does not provide definite diagnosis, and therapeutic consequences are to be expected. In more than 50 % of cases with suspected vascular pathology on the basis of clinical examination and Doppler ultrasound MRA can establish the diagnosis, and X-ray angiography can be avoided.

It should, however, be emphasized that MRA today is far from being a push-button method. Whereas a negative diagnosis can be ascertained reliably using the procedures described above, to define an existing pathology considerable skill, experience as well as utilization of standard techniques such as ultrasound and radiography are required.

References

1. Wedeen VJ, Rosen BR, Buxton R, Edelman RR, Meuli R, Brady TJ (1985) MRI angiography and flow volume quantitation. Proc. IVth Ann. Meeting SMRM, London, p. 618.
2. Müri M, Juretschke HP, Bösch C, Hennig J, Brunner P (1985) The examination of the vascular system by methods of MR imaging. Proc. IVth Ann. Meeting SMRM, London, p. 589.
3. Singer JR, Crooks LE (1983) Nuclear magnetic resonance blood flow measurements in the human brain. Science 221: 654–656.
4. Wehrli FW, MacFall JR, Axel L, Shutts D, Glover GH, Herfkens RJ (1984) Approaches to in-plane and out-of-plane flow imaging.
5. Bradley WG, Waluch V (1985) Blood flow: magnetic resonance imaging. Radiology 154: 443.
6. Wehrli FW, Shimakawa A, Gullberg GT, MacFall JR (1986) Time-of-flight MR flow imaging: selective saturation recovery with gradient refocussing. Radiology 160: 781–785.
7. Dixon WT, Du LN, Gado M et al. (1986) Projection angiograms of blood labeled by adiabatic fast passage. Magn. Reson. Med. 3: 454.
8. Gullberg GT, Wehrli FW, Shimakawa A et al. (1987) MR vascular imaging with fast gradient refocusing pulse sequence and reformatted images from transaxial sections. Radiology 165: 241.
9. Edelman RR, Wentz KU, Mattle H et al. (1989) Projection arteriography and venography: initial clinical results with MR. Radiology 172: 351.
10. Keller PJ, Drayer BP, Fram EK et al. (1989) MR angiography with two-dimensional acquisition and three-dimensional display. Radiology 173: 527.
11. Wehrli FW, Shimakawa A, MacFall JR et al. (1985) MR imaging of venous and arterial flow by a selective saturation – recovery spin echo (SSRSE)

method (1985). J. Comput. Assist. Tomogr. 9: 537–545.

12. Hennig J, Mueri M, Friedburg H, Brunner P (1987) MR imaging of flow using the steady state selective saturation method. J. Comp. Assist. Tomogr. 11: 872.

13. Pike GB, Hu BS, Glover GH, Enzmann DR (1992) Magnetization transfer contrast enhanced time-of-flight angiography. Proc. XIth Ann. Meeting SMRM, Berlin, p. 218.

14. Hennig J, Mueri M, Brunner P, Friedburg H (1988) Quantitative flow measurement with the fast Fourier flow technique. Radiology 166: 237–240.

15. Laub G, Kaiser W (1988) MR angiography with gradient motion refocusing. J. Comput. Assist. Tomogr. 12: 377.

16. Masaryk TJ, Modic MT, Ruggieri PM et al. (1989) Three-dimensional (volume) gradient-echo imaging of the carotid bifurcation: preliminary clinical experience. Radiology 171: 793.

17. Ruggieri PM, Laub G, Masryk TJ et al. (1989) Intracranial circulation: pulse sequence considerations in three-dimensional (volume) MR angiography. Radiology 171: 785.

18. Purdy D, Cadena G, Laub G (1992) The design of variable tip angle slab selection (TONE) pulses for improved 3-D MR angiography. Proc. XIth Ann. Meeting SMRM, Berlin, p. 882.

19. Macovsky A (1982) Selective projection imaging: applications to radiology and NMR. IEEE Trans. Med. Imaging 1: 42.

20. Moran PR (1982) A flow velocity zeugmatographic interlace for NMR imaging in humans (1982). Magn. Reson. Imaging 1: 197.

21. Dumoulin CL, Hart HR (1986) MR angiography. Proc. Vth Ann. Meeting SMRM, Montreal, p. 1095.

22. Dumoulin CL, Hart HR (1986) Magnetic resonance angiography. Radiology 161: 717.

23. Alfidi RJ, Masaryk TJ, Haacke EM et al. (1987) MR angiography of peripheral, carotid and coronary arteries. AJR 149: 1097.

24. Axel L, Morton D (1986) A method for imaging blood vessels by phase compensated/uncompensated difference images. Magn. Reson. Imaging 4: 153.

25. Mattle HP, Wentz KU (1992) Selective magnetic resonance angiography of the head. Cardiovasc. Intervent. Radiol. 15: 65–70.

26. Evans AJ, Blinder RA, Herfkens RJ et al. (1988) Effects of turbulence on signal intensity in gradient echo images. Invest. Radiol. 23: 512.

27. Podolak MJ, Hedlund LW, Evans AJ et al. (1989) Evaluation of flow through simulated vascular stenoses with gradient echo magnetic resonance imaging. Invest Radiol. 24: 184.

28. Pattany PM, Marino R, McNally JM (1986) Velocity and acceleration desensitization in 2DFT MR imaging. Magn. Reson. Imaging 4: 154.

29. Masaryk TJ, Modic MT, Ross JS (1989) Three dimensional (volume) gradient-echo imaging of the carotid bifurcation: preliminary clinical experience. Radiology 171: 801.

30. Ross KS, Masaryk TJ, Modic MT et al. (1990) Intracranial aneurysms: evaluation by MR angiography. Am. J. Neuroadiol 11: 449.

Coronary MR Imaging

M.B. Scheidegger and P. Boesiger

Introduction

X-Ray contrast angiography represents the gold standard for the diagnosis of coronary artery disease (CAD), and images of the coronary arteries of adequate quality for interventional requirements are produced only with this modality. However, this technique is invasive requiring catheterization, it is expensive, and it carries a small risk. Therefore, it is less well suited for repeated follow-up examinations. For these applications a noninvasive assessment of coronary artery disease would be highly desirable.

Magnetic resonance angiography (MRA) has been developed and applied for imaging of the carotid arteries, the intracranial arteries, the peripheral vessels, and the large vessels in the thorax and abdomen. More recently the major proximal segments of the coronary arteries have been successfully visualized. However, mainly due to breathing artifacts, heart motion, and insufficient spatial resolution of cardiac magnetic resonance images, progress in that field has been been slow. In the early attempts conventional magnetic resonance (MR) techniques were used to visualize the proximal segments of the epicardial coronary arteries, although the image quality was extremely variable, and very often unpredictable [1, 2].

Recent advances in MRA technology have helped to improve image quality. The use of respiration gating and breat-holding (BH) together with rapid image acquisition techniques considerably reduce the respiratory motional artifacts in high-resolution cardiac imaging. Several authors have recently reported preliminary data on successful imaging of the coronary arteries in volunteers and in patients with CAD [3–12]. This chapter provides a brief overview of the present state of coronary MRA.

Methods

Magnetic Resonance Imaging Methods for Coronary Artery Angiography

Since the precise control of respiratory motion is crucial in coronary artery MRA, methods can be classified according to the approach to the solution of this problem. A single MR image can be acquired (1) in a single heart beat, (2) in a single breath-hold, or (3) over multiple breath-hold periods or breathing cycles.

Image Acquisition in a Single Heart Beat

Only with echo-planar image (EPI) acquisition techniques and the use of a special gradient system is it currently possible to acquire one single MR slice image in as little as 50 ms. Poncelet et al. [13] used EPI to measure coronary blood flow velocities. However, the spatial resolution of approximately 2–4 mm was similar to the diameter of the examined vessels and was thus insufficient to accurately distinguish normal from stenotic segments. Extensive improvements in image resolution are needed to use EPI techniques for coronary artery MRA.

Image Acquisition in a Single Breath-Hold Period

Edelman et al. [3, 4, 7] and Macovski et al. [5, 6] developed approaches with breath-holding where patients have to hold their breath for 12–25 s. During this interval one single-slice image of approximately 4 mm thickness with an in-plane resolution of about 1.5 mm^2 is acquired. In ref. [7] a segmented k-space fast-field echo sequence is used. Eight to ten phase-encoding profiles are measured in a time interval of approximately 100–120 ms during diastole. Repetitive breath-hold periods are necessary to complete the acqui-

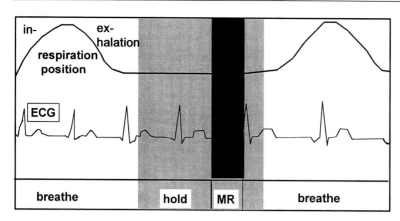

Fig. 1. Breathing scheme for the "multiple-slice, multiple-breath-hold" technique. The inspiration level is shown by the *solid line (top of figure)*. Breathing is close to normal with a short inspiration/expiration sequence followed by approximately 2 s of breathing arrest after full exhalation (*area with gray overlay*). The MR signals are acquired during one diastole (*dark overlay*). Approximately 170 such cycles are needed for the acquisition of an MR coronary angiogram

sition of a full MR image data set. Artifact-free high-quality images are obtained, and with suitable slice orientation the number of slices or breath-hold periods, respectively, can be kept to a minimum. These are nevertheless long apnea phases for cardiac patients, and one problem is that it is difficult to reproduce precisely the inspiration level and thus the slice position.

Image Acquisition over Multiple Respiratory Cycles, or Multiple Short Breath-Hold Periods

The breath-hold periods can be shortened if MR signals for a single slice are acquired over multiple breath-hold periods. Such a breathing scheme is sketched in Fig. 1. The solid line depicts the inspiration level. Breathing is close to normal with just a slightly prolonged exhalation phase. During the 2–2.5 s apnea at the end of exhalation, one or two cardiac cycles can be used for MR data acquisition. Synchronization with the data acquisition is either done by the patient, waiting until the MR acquisition with its gradient noise is over, or by accurate respiratory motion detection devices, such as a pneumatic chest belt.

Conventional MR equipment and sequences rather than ultrafast imaging can be used with such breathing schemes. The scheme is ideally suited for the multiple-slice acquisition technique. MR signals of one phase-encoding step are obtained within one diastole. The first slice is acquired during early diastole in the apex of the heart. The slice „moves up" in a linear sequence during diastole, towards the base of the heart, until, at end diastole, the last slice within the ascending aorta is imaged. To enhance the contrast between coronaries and surrounding tissue, slices overlap

each other, causing a partial saturation of the overlapping portions of the slices [14]. With a slice acquisition interval of 17 ms, 30–60 slices are acquired with a slice thickness of 3.5 mm and an overlap of 1.5 mm. The MR signal of myocardium thus stems from an only 2-mm-thin slice, whereas signals from blood in the coronary arteries flowing in the opposite direction of the slice movement originate from a 3.5-mm-thick portion due to inflow. Signals from blood moving parallel to the slice movement direction are suppressed to a certain extent. First-order flow compensation is applied, resulting in an echo time of 7.5 ms, the imaged area is 170×250 mm, and the in-plane resolution is 1 mm^2. All our examinations have been performed on a commercial 1.5-T whole body Philips Gyroscan ACS-II MR scanner with no modifications. A special heart quadrature surface coil is used, and the patients are placed in the prone position. The image volume of 80–120 mm thickness is positioned to cover as much as possible of the proximal coronary arteries; in most cases the whole heart is covered.

Approximately 170 such inspire-expire-wait cycles are needed for one full data set corresponding to the acquisition of 170 phase-encoding steps, resulting in an acquisition time of 9–13 min. The total examination time is approximately ½ h. Data for each slice are acquired at a different time in diastole, but data for every single slice image are acquired always at the same time point within diastole, so that periodic heart motion does not blur the individual images.

The proximal parts of the coronary arteries are largely embedded in fat; therefore, good fat suppression is a key point in coronary artery MRA to enhance local image contrast, and to avoid chemical shift artifacts. In the multiple-slice sequence fat suppression is achieved by highly selective saturation pulses on the fat resonance. Since these pulses last 15 ms, only one fat suppression pulse is applied every 100 ms with a pulse angle of 105°. A fat suppression ratio above 7.5 is achieved.

Display of Coronary Angiograms

The multiple-breath-hold multiple-slice technique with its overlapping slice sequence generates a rather low image contrast between the coronary arteries and the myocardial tissue. The tiny coronary arteries cannot be viewed after application of the Maximum Intensity Projection algorithm [15], since they are covered within the large bright areas of chamber blood. A quick visual impression of the coronary arteries is best obtained by looking at the cine movie across all slices. A semiautomatic segmentation of the coronary arteries is performed on a computer workstation. A „seed" is put into the orifices of both the left and right coronary arteries, and then the algorithm tries to track the vessels in consecutive slices. At vessel branches and at sites of severe stenoses, operator input is required. Normal right coronary arteries consistently exhibit sufficient local image contrast to be traced automatically. The left main, the left anterior descending, and circumflex coronary arteries require some user interaction. The segmented arteries together with a short piece of the ascending aorta are then reconstructed and displayed with a 3D presentation package on the same workstation. The reconstructed vessels can be rotated into any desired view.

Validation with Contrast Angiography

For the validation of the MRA procedure an X-ray contrast angiogram is obtained in all cases during the interventions with percutaneous transluminal coronary angioplasty (PTCA). Vessel diameter measured with MRA and digitized films from computerized contrast angiography [16] have been compared for validation of the MRA procedure with the multiple-short breath-hold technique. Three to five diameter measurements per patient have been carried out including the proximal right [$n=13$], the proximal left (left main, left circumflex, left anterior descending ($n=28$), and the distal right coronary artery

($n=3$). In total, 44 vessel segments were evaluated, and side branches or bifurcations served as landmarks. After manual segmentation coronary diameter was determined over a length of approximately 5 mm from single MR images using a specially designed computer program. For each site ten measurements were performed, and the results were averaged. Only nonstenotic segments were measured, since the vessel diameter within stenotic lesions could not be determined accurately by MR due to signal loss at these locations. A good correlation ($r=0.76$, $p<0.001$) with an intercept of 0.8 mm and a slope of 0.71 was observed. Accuracy (mean difference) was 0.19 mm, and precision (standard deviation of mean difference) 0.39 mm. With the exception of one uncooperative patient, all patient examinations were evaluated. There seems to be a slight overestimation of coronary artery diameter by MRA mainly at the smaller diameters, which is probably due to image blurring (motion artifacts) and/or partial volume effects.

Clinical Applications

Patients with known coronary artery disease have been imaged, usually 1 day before PTCA, to evaluate whether the stenotic lesion could be identified with the MR procedure. Another MR examination was performed 1–8 days after the intervention [11]. Figure 2 shows a representative series of MR slice images of the right coronary artery from the ostium to the middle segment of the vessel. Data are taken from a patient with a severe lesion in the proximal left anterior descending coronary artery, and an unobstructed right coronary artery.

A representative example of a patient with a severe stenosis in the proximal left anterior descending coronary artery is shown in Fig. 3, with 3D reconstructions from the MR data sets acquired 1 day before and 1 day after PTCA. The stenotic lesion is seen as a short interruption of the artery due to signal loss (arrow in the left-hand image) which has completely disappeared in the right-hand image. One to four follow-up examinations are performed in these patients, normally 3, 6 and 12 months after PTCA, for the detection of restenosis. So far, in one patient a restenosis was found and the vessel was redilated.

In an ongoing study, the stenotic lesion, or the patency of the vessel in the follow-up examination,

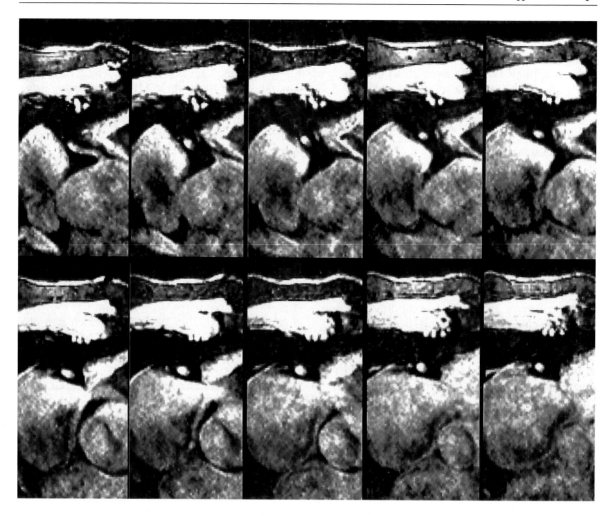

Fig. 2. Zoomed MR images of the right coronary artery: A sequence of 10 out of 48 acquired images is presented, covering the ostium and the proximal course of the right coronary artery. The suppression of fat signals avoids fat shift artifacts and results in a high local image contrast between the coronary artery and the surrounding fat tissue

was correctly classified with MRA in 25 of 30 vessels, in 83% of the examined cases therefore. Nondiagnostic images were obtained in 15% of the examinations. One patient did not understand the breathing pattern and was incooperative.

Manning et al. [3] reported a sensitivity of 97% and a specificity of 70% for the MR technique for correctly classifying patients as having or not having serious coronary artery disease. Pennell et al. [12] found similar results in a smaller number of patients.

Perspectives

Several recent studies [3, 4, 11, 12] have shown that, using available MRA technology, in a majority of patients reasonable quality coronary angiograms can be obtained. The right coronary artery can be most consistently visualized due to its proximity to the chest wall and to the applied surface coil. The results are less optimal for the left anterior descending coronary artery, and even less so for the circumflex artery largely due to the greater distance between the circumflex artery and the surface coil. In addition the larger motional excursion of the anterolateral and inferior segments of the heart at the basal level is detrimental.

The image quality now appears to be sufficiently reproducible over repeated examinations of the same patient in follow-up examinations. However, a constant, high image quality is still not

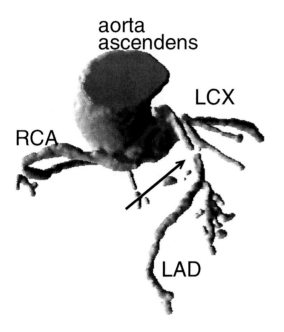
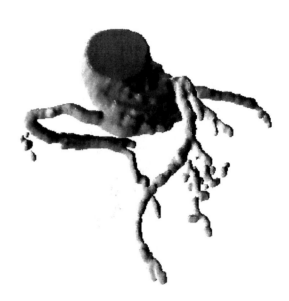

Fig. 3. Three-dimensional reconstruction of the coronary vessels of a 53-year-old patient with a severe lesion of the left anterior descending coronary artery. The image on the left of the figure is acquired 1 day before treatment of the lesion with PTCA. The lesion is rendered as a short interruption due to signal loss within the stenosis. The image on the right is acquired 1 day after the intervention. The dilated vessel segment can be identified as open. In further follow-up examinations up to 1 year after the treatment no restenosis was observed

achieved in all patient examinations and a considerable patient-to-patient variation of the MR image quality remains. This could be attributed to either heart rate variations and/or breathing artifacts, and appears to be the main challenge in a further development of MRA of the coronary arteries.

Using surface coils, at present an in-plane image resolution of 1×1 mm with 2- to 3-mm-thick slices can be obtained. This spatial resolution is sufficient to image the proximal segments of the main coronary arteries. It is also sufficient to distinguish between a completely normal vessel and a severe proximal lesion. High-grade stenoses often exhibit considerable signal loss within and a few millimeters downstream of the constriction. The image resolution is, however, not sufficient to visualize the more distal segments or smaller side branches, and it is also not sufficient for detection of mild stenoses with less than 50% reduction in cross-sectional vessel area. An improved spatial resolution will be necessary to visualize the distal segments of the coronary arteries.

The segmentation of the coronary vessels is possible only semiautomatically, and is therefore associated with a considerable observer dependence. Nevertheless, 3D reconstructions help to find potential lesions quickly. Final assessment of the stenotic region is always done on the basis of the unprocessed MR images. A fully automated vessel segmentation would solve this problem, but the local image contrast would have to be improved considerably. Such an improvement is expected to result from the application of intravascular contrast agents, which should be available in a few years. Intravascular contrast agents which selectively lower the longitudinal relaxation time T_1 of blood within the vasculature could improve the signal-to-noise ratio, or, in a trade-off, the image resolution could be enhanced.

The long-term goal is the noninvasive primary diagnosis of coronary artery disease in patients at high risk. For this task, the MRA technology must be improved to eliminate the combined cardiac and respiratory motion artifacts while bringing the spatial image resolution down to the submillimeter range.

References

1. Paulin S, von Schulthess GK, Fossel E, Krayenbuehl HP (1987) MR imaging of the aortic root and proximal coronary arteries. Am J Roentgenol 148: 665–670
2. Underwood SR (1991) Imaging of acquired heart disease. In: Underwood SR, Firmin DN (eds) Magnetic resonance for the cardiovascular system. Blackwell, London, pp 41–67
3. Manning WJ, Li W, Edelman RR (1993) A preliminary report comparing magnetic resonance coronary angiography with conventional angiography. N Engl J Med 328: 828–832
4. Manning WJ, Li W, Boyle NG, Edelman RR (1993) Fat-suppressed breath-hold magnetic resonance coronary angiography. Circulation 87: 94–104
5. Meyer CH, Hu BS, Nishimura DG, Macovski A (1992) Fast spiral coronary artery imaging. Magn Reson Med 28: 202–213
6. Sang SJ, Hu BS, Macovski A, Nishimura DG (1991) Coronary angiography using fast selective inversion recovery. Magn Reson Med 18: 417–423
7. Edelman RR, Manning WJ, Burstein D, Paulin S (1991) Coronary arteries: breath-hold MR angiography. Radiology 181: 641–643
8. Li D, Paschal CB, Haacke EM, Adler LP (1993) Coronary arteries: three-dimensional MR imaging with fat saturation and magnetization transfer contrast. Radiology 187: 401–406
9. Doyle M, Scheidegger MB, Pohost GM (1993) Coronary artery imaging in multiple 1-sec breath holds. Magn Reson Imag 11: 3–6
10. Cho ZH, Mun CW, Friedenberg RM (1992) NMR angiography of coronary vessels with 2-D planar image scanning. Magn Reson Med 20: 134–143
11. Scheidegger MB, Vassalli G, Hess OM, Boesiger P (1993) Magnetic resonance coronary arteriography before and after PTCA. In: Proceedings of the 12th annual meeting, Society of Magnetic Resonance in Medicine, Location p 563 Berkeley, 1993
12. Pennell DJ, Keegan J, Firmin DN, Gatehouse PD, Underwood SR, Longmore DB (1993) Magnetic resonance imaging of coronary arteries: technique and preliminary results. Br Heart J 70: 315–326
13. Poncelet BP, Weiskoff RM, Wedeen VJ, Brady TJ, Kantor H (1993) Time of flight quantification of coronary flow with echo-planar MRI. Magn Reson Med 30: 447–457
14. Matsuda T, Doyle M, Pohost GM (1992) Slice thickness reduction by partial overlapping presaturation. Magn Reson Med 24: 358–363
15. Rossnick S, Kennedy D, Laub G (1986) Three dimensional display of blood vessels in MRI. In: Proceedings of the IEEE computers in cardiology conference. IEEE, Piscataway, pp 193–196
16. Buechi M, Hess OM, Kirkeeide RL, et al: (1990) Validation of a new automatic system for biplane quantitative coronary arteriography. Int J Card Imaging 5: 93–103

Peripheral Vascular MR Imaging

M. J. Hartkamp, C. J. G. Bakker, M. Kouwenhoven, and W. P. Th. M. Mali

Introduction

The primary aim of vascular investigation of the lower extremities is to determine the level, extent, and severity of peripheral vascular disease, in order to select an appropriate therapeutic approach. Specifically, essential requirements are determination of focal or diffuse disease, evaluation of the severity of stenotic disease and the length of the diseased segment, identification of the level of reconstitution distal to an occlusion, and imaging of patent target vessels for bypass grafting. Until recently, angiography and color Doppler were the main techniques used to provide this information. The conventional angiogram has been the mainstay of visualization for many decades. During the past 5 years conventional film screen angiography has been complemented by digital subtraction angiography (DSA), leading to improved contrast resolution, faster film handling, and increased scope for interventions. The main disadvantages of the technique are its invasiveness (albeit minimal), use of contrast agents with the inherent risk of complications (renal dysfunction, puncture site trauma), two-dimensional (2D) display, limited physiological information, frequently required overnight hospital stays, and relatively high cost.

Color Doppler investigation has developed into an important diagnostic tool during the past 5 years, and is used to determine the severity and extent of the disease. It is noninvasive, provides both qualitative (presence or absence of lesions) and quantitative information (peak systolic velocities), and can cover the extent of a limb in 20 min. Disadvantages of color Dopper include the relatively high degree of operator dependency, and lack of an angiogram-type display. Furthermore, in some patients, the iliac arteries and the femoropopliteal regions are sometimes difficult to investigate, and experience with Doppler of the infrapopliteal vessels is limited. The considerable disadvantages of conventional techniques, such as the invasiveness of angiography and the operator dependency of color Doppler, have instigated the development and improvement of magnetic resonance angiography (MRA). Currently, the main clinical role of MRA is to investigate the infrapopliteal vessels as potential targets for bypass surgery, and to substitute for conventional angiography in cases wherever conventional angiography is contraindicated. Over the past 10 years MRA has grown from an experimental investigative tool into a method that can be used for clinical practice. Technical developments such as the introduction of gradient-recalled echo, reduced echo time, segmented k-space, cardiac triggering, and fat suppression prepulses have resulted in MRA acquisitions that can be performed within reasonable scanning time (<30 min), with improved image quality, providing both morphological and quantitative information. Flow quantification is now possible on most (upgraded) magnetic resonance imaging (MRI) systems, thus providing a more complete evaluation during a single examination. The main advantages of MRA are its noninvasive character, high sensitivity [1–7], multiple projection post-processing potential, and the virtue of combining morphological and quantitative analysis in a single examination.

This chapter provides a general survey of published clinical experience to date, clinical indications based on our own experience, and suggestions for acquisition protocols. Essential MRA techniques, concepts, and artifacts relevant to peripheral vasculature are also discussed. Various pulse sequences are discussed in greater detail in the chapter on MRA techniques.

Clinical Approach: Diagnostic Techniques and the Role of MRA

The past 10 years have seen considerable changes in the diagnosis and therapy of patients with peripheral vascular disease. Stenotic disease and occlusions are the main problem in the category of patients with peripheral vascular disease (excluding the abdominal aorta). Classification of patients into categories with respect to their clinical presentation was formerly based on the Fontaine classification, which has since been complemented by the SVS/ISCVS[1] categories (Table 1) [8, 9]. The SVS/ISCVS classification is based on both clinical symptoms and objective criteria such as ankle pressure and the treadmill test. Whether treatment is necessary or not depends on the patient's classification combined with the patient's particular history. If the desired treatment consists of medication or exercise, no further diagnostic workup is generally required. However, if surgery or an endovascular procedure is considered, further diagnostic evaluation is necessary to determine the precise location and extent of the lesion. This can be done by conventional angiography, color Doppler, and MRA.

Doppler is increasingly applied as the initial investigation to determine whether patients have localized disease (stenosis and occlusions up to 10 cm) which is treatable with percutaneous transluminal angioplasty (PTA), or whether generalized disease is present requiring surgery. Thus

[1] Society for Vascular Surgery (SVS) and International Society for Cardiovascular Surgery (ISCVS).

selection of patients for PTA is effected on the basis of color Doppler, and the site of a lesion determines whether an antegrade or retrograde puncture is performed. During the PTA session, the lesion is angiographically confirmed prior to the dilatation procedure. In those cases in which surgical intervention is planned, an angiogram is performed to visualize distal runoff vessels, enabling the surgeon to select the best site for a distal anastomosis of the bypass. Color Doppler has been used sparingly for this purpose, due to operator dependency and the long examination time required to investigate the subtrifurcation vessels. It is especially in this region that MRA can provide important morphological and functional information.

Treatment considerations differ according to the various vascular regions. Stenoses and occlusions in the iliac region are mainly treated by endovascular techniques. The combination of color Doppler and endovascular treatment seems to be quite adequate in the majority of patients. Endovascular pressure measurements remain the gold standard for the definitive assessment of iliac artery stenoses. In the femoropopliteal region color Doppler is frequently used to assess the extent of the lesion. It is critical to determine whether the popliteal artery is patent above the knee, and whether the trifurcation is functional. If so, a femoropopliteal bypass is feasible. If disease is located distal to the trifurcation, or when disease is of a more generalized nature, the angiogram should be performed.

Thus, presently, the role of MRA is generally limited to the following three instances: (1) in cases where conventional angiography fails to identify

Table 1. SVS/ISCVS Classification of Ischemic Limb Disease

Grade	Rutherford category	Clinical description	Fontaine classification	Suggested treatment
0	0	Asymptomatic	I	None
I	1	Mild claudication	II	Vascular intervention/reconstruction
	2	Moderate claudication		Vascular intervention/reconstruction
	3	Severe claudication		Vascular intervention/reconstruction
II	4	Ischemic rest pain	III	Vascular intervention/reconstruction
III	5	Minor/focal gangrene, ulcera, diffuse ischemia	IV	Vascular intervention/reconstruction/ excision
	6	Major gangrene, extending above metatarsals, foot not salvageable		Vascular intervention/reconstruction/ excision/amputation

suitable (distal) runoff vessels for bypass surgery; (2) substitution for conventional angiography in patients at risk for contrast-related complications such as contrast allergy or renal impairment; and (3) in cases of increased risk of embolic complications due to invasive procedures. The value of MRA as a noninvasive follow-up technique after interventions has yet to be established.

Clinical Use of MRA and Experience

Results of Clinical Trials

Reviewing the current literature, it is concluded that only few systematic studies have been performed which address the value of MRA for peripheral arterial vascular disease evaluation. Most have concentrated on the lower extremity vessels, and can be classified as evaluations of morphological features (which focus on detection of stenoses, occlusions, and/or detection of distal reconstitution of vessels), or as MR flow quantitation studies.

An initial study by Mulligan et al. [10] concluded that color Doppler ultrasound correlated better with X-ray angiography (XRA) as a standard of reference for lower extremity vascular disease than MRA did. At the time Mulligan et al. used a considerably longer minimal echo time than current protocols, which can account for their unfavorable results, since longer echo times allow for increased intravoxel phase dispersion, resulting in signal loss. Yucel et al. [1–3, 11] investigated the value of MRA for morphological features, with XRA as the main standard of reference, and found an accuracy of 94 % for identification and gradation of diseased segments, and a sensitivity of 100 % for the identification of aneurysms and detection of distal patent tibial vessels as is seen in Table 2. Other studies performed by the same group yielded similar results (see Table 2) with sensitivity and specificity of MRA within the 88 % – 100 % range for stenosis and occlusion detection and classification [1–3, 11, 12]. A 2D time of flight (TOF) technique was used, which is known to overestimate the degree of stenosis in comparison to XRA, especially apparent on maximum intensity projections (MIPs), although inspection of the axial slices allows improved accuracy in grading. Surprisingly, 2D TOF has also been reported to systematically underestimate stenoses [6, 13]. Owen et al. [4–7, 14, 15] extended their trials to

include evaluation of the clinical implications of MRA, by comparing the interventional plans based on MRA with those based on XRA findings, in addition to evaluation of morphological MRA features. Their most important conclusion was the striking superiority of MRA in detection of patent distal target vessels for bypass grafting: MRA detected 24 % [5] and 48 % [4] more patent distal vessel segments in total, of which there were 13 % [5] and 24 % [4] more popliteal segments, and 49 % [5] and 62 % [4] more tibial segments (see also Table 2). The clinical implications were such that the identification by MRA of X-ray angiographically occult distal vessels obviated intraoperative exploration (to avoid amputation), saving operating time, and preventing multiple incisions on the patient. It is important to note that DSA was only used in 11 patients [5] and 3 patients [4] in these studies, which raises the question whether DSA should not have been used in all patients in whom XRA failed to detect distal target vessels, since intraarterial DSA has been demonstrated to be more sensitive for distal vessel visualization [16–18]. (Smith et al. included 50 patients [16] and Kaufman et al. 133 patients [17] in their studies comparing intraarterial DSA with conventional film screen angiography.) Results of trials comparing intraarterial DSA and MRA should be available in the near future [19], to ensure that MRA is compared with the fairest possible standard of reference with regard to distal vessel visualization. Furthermore, it should be pointed out that neither Owen et al. [4–7, 13–15] nor Yucel et al. [1–3, 11] incorporated cardiac synchronization or integrated prepulses in the MRA imaging protocols used in their clinical trials as listed in Table 2.

Little has been published about the controversy [1, 6, 13] concerning grading of stenoses with MRA in peripheral vessels. Most authors claim that the severity of a stenosis can be approximated by the existence and length of a poststenotic signal void [1, 2]; however, no attempts have been made to standardize grading by visual features on MR angiograms, due to the complexity of the phenomenon. Spielmann et al. [20] describe the existence of poststenotic jets in MRI, producing signal voids dependent on flow velocity rather than the degree of stenosis, and in which imaging parameters proved to be critical. Since imaging parameters are far from standardized in various MRA applications, it seems that stenosis grading will remain controversial. One must keep in mind that grading is only of relative importance

Table 2. Results of clinical trials

Ref.	No. of pts., limbs	Vascular trajectory	No. of segments	Clinical presentation	Standard of reference (gold standard)	Classification of disease	Results	Accuracy	Sensitivity	Specificity
1	19 pts., 29 limbs	Iliac Femoropopliteal Tibial		12 ASOD 4 grafts 4 aneurysms	XRA in 21 limbs Surgery in only 5 limbs US Doppler in 1 limbs	A. Iliac/femorals/grafts: 100% stenosis >75% stenosis 50–75% stenosis <50% stenosis B. Tibial: patent or occluded C. Aneurysms	A. ASOD/grafts: MRA/gold standard 16/16 3/5 3/4 – B. All patent detected by MRA C. All 5 detected by MRA	A. 94% B. 100% C. 100%		
2	25 pts.	Aorta Iliacs Femorals Popliteal a.	206	ASOD	XRA	100% stenosis[1] 70–99% stenosis[2] 50–69% stenosis[3] <50% stenosis[4]	84% of segments correctly classified Level of distal reconstruction correct in 29/32 vessels		100%[1] 90%[1+2] 92%[1+2+3]	98%[1] 97%[1+2] 88%[1+2+3]
3	24 pts.	Iliacs Femorals Popliteal a. Infrapopliteal a.	175	PAOD	XRA	Normal or stenosis <50% diseased	Discrepancies in 8.3% of limbs Iliacs[1] OA: 94%/κ: 0.88 Common femoral[2] OA: 97%/κ: 0.93 All segments[3] OA: 98%/κ: 0.96		100%[1] 100%[2] 100%[3]	92%[1] 96%[2] 97%[3]
4	23 pts., 25 limbs	Popliteal a. to pedal arch	350	PAOD	Intraoperative XRA Postinterventional XRA Intraoperative exploration DSA in 3 patients	Patent or occluded	Discrepancies in 72% of limbs Discrepancies in 22% of segments All due to superior detection of distal runoffs by MRA		Detection of distal runoffs: 100%	
5	51 pts., 55 limbs	Popliteal a. to pedal arch	1540	PAOD	Intraoperative XRA Postinterventional XRA Intraoperative exploration DSA in 11 patients	Patent or occluded	Discrepancies in 48% of limbs All due to superior detection of distal runoffs by MRA 4/11 DSA pts.: superior detection of runoffs by MRA		Detection of distal runoffs: 100%	
7	51 pts. 22 pts. Total: 73	Popliteal a. to pedal arch Aorta to prox. femoral a.	1007	Symptomatic peripheral vascular disease	Intraoperative XRA Postinterventional XRA Intraoperative exploration	Normal Stenotic Diseased Occluded	Clinically relevant discrepancies in 16% of pts. Discrepancies in 12% of segments 82% of discrepancies due to superior detection of runoffs by MRA		Detection of distal runoffs: 100%	

pts., patients; ASOD, atherosclerotic occlusive disease; PAOD, peripheral arterial occlusive disease; XRA, X-ray angiography; DSA, digital subtraction angiography; OA, observer agreement; κ, kappa, kappa's measure of agreement beyond chance.

in peripheral vascular disease, since management is determined predominantly by the longitudinal extent of diseased segments. Hemodynamic evaluation of the severity of stenoses is perhaps superior in this respect.

Validity studies concerning hemodynamic assessment of lower extremity vascular disease with quantitative 2D cine phase contrast (PC) MRA [21–24] are limited to three small-scale studies performed on healthy subjects. Caputo et al. [22] demonstrated the feasibility of applying velocity-encoded 2D cine PC MRA as a tool for hemodynamic assessment by comparison with color Doppler in ten healthy subjects. Likewise, Meyer et al. [24] concluded that MR phase-encoded flow velocity measurements are useful for physiological studies of peripheral vascular dynamics before and after exercise in their study on eight healthy individuals. Dousset et al. [25] studied the popliteal arteries in 11 healthy subjects with an MR Fourier flow-encoding technique, with temporal resolution. They concluded that MR imaging can provide detailed hemodynamic information, including intraluminal velocity distribution, and can thus allow quantitation of true flow rates. However, systematic clinical trials on patients with peripheral vascular disease have yet to be performed to determine the definite role of MR flow quantitation in this area.

It is necessary to stimulate the use of MRA, and to gain confidence with its use on the part of vascular surgeons. Evaluation of MRA in other clinical applications such as aneurysms, preoperative tumor evaluation, follow-up after interventional procedures, and venography is scarce.

Clinical Experience

Our own experience with three different 2D TOF MRA protocols is in general agreement with other published material [19]. We used the Gated Sweep 2D Inflow (Inflow = TOF), standard ungated 2D Inflow, and Turbo Inflow protocols supplied with the Philips Gyroscan T5 II 0.5-T MR system and obtained the best imaging results with the Turbo Inflow method, also known as the Magnetization Prepared Turbo Field Echo[2] (MP-TFE) technique [26]. Basically, MP-TFE is a 2D TOF technique combined with cardiac gating, an in-

tegrated inversion prepulse (180° prepulse) for improved background suppression, and segmented k-space acquisition for scanning-time reduction, resulting in good-quality MR angiograms acquired within reasonable scanning time (<30 min scanning time from the adductor canal to the foot, approx. 45 min including time needed for repositioning of the coil). The Gated Sweep protocol proved to be time consuming, although imaging results were good. The standard 2D Inflow protocol resulted in moderate image quality since ghosting was not compensated for by cardiac synchronization, and a relatively high signal from bone marrow fat compromised vessel identification on MIPs. Turbo Inflow, on the other hand, was faster than the standard 2D Inflow method, and produced images with no pulsatility artifacts, and improved quality MIPs due to augmented (bone marrow) fat suppression. Our initial clinical experience with the 2D cine PC quantitation methods has also been encouraging. Indeed, the combination of 2D TFE MRA of the subtrifurcation vessels (for example, a single acquisition with an extremity coil) for morphological evaluation with subsequent hemodynamic assessment of the identified vessels using 2D cine PC, seems to be most promising.

Clinical Trial

We have investigated a total of 30 patients, to date, with peripheral vascular disease of the lower extremity referred to the Radiology Department's angiography unit for either preoperative diagnostic contrast angiography for bypass intervention, or for PTA. Each patient was imaged with one of the three MRA TOF protocols as mentioned above, and subsequent intra-arterial DSA was performed within 24 h of the MRA, in order to compare MRA with intra-arterial DSA as the standard of reference. The results of this trial were not available at the time this chapter was written, but should be available in early 1995 [19]. The following sections on suggested protocols and common artifacts are based on our experience gained during the course of the trial. To illustrate the clinical potential of MRA a short account of two cases investigated at our hospital is given below. Case 1 is an example of MRA's superior sensitivity to patent distal vessels. In case 2, the MR angiogram identified a patent posterior tibial artery suitable for reconstructive surgery in a

---

[2] Turbo Field Echo (Philips) is turbo gradient echo, synonymous for turbo-FLASH and RAGE.

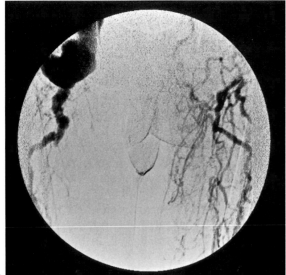

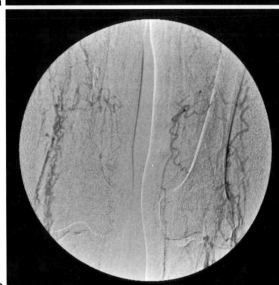

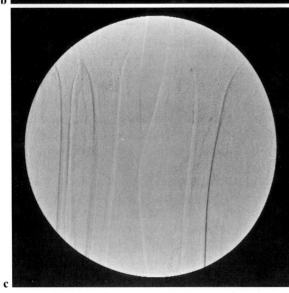

a

b

c

patient with a previous history of severe (non-ionic) contrast hypersensitivity. This obviated the need for intraoperative exploration and multiple incisions.

Case 1. A 71-year-old male patient with a previous history of extensive vascular disease (angina pectoris, hypercholesterolemia, aneurysmectomy of the right common femoral artery, and four coronary bypass grafts) was admitted to hospital with symptoms of lower extremity ischemia: claudication in both legs, and rest pain in the right foot. Clinical assessment concluded hypertension, grade I – category 2 ischemic disease of the left leg (see Table 1 for grading features), and grade II – category 4 ischemic disease of the right leg. No peripheral pulses were found upon palpation. Intra-arterial DSA revealed a stenosis of the abdominal aorta, with an aneurysm continuing into both common iliac arteries. Flow in the left external iliac artery was compromised. Moreover both superficial femoral arteries were occluded with very faint reconstitution of the popliteal arteries via collaterals. No distal vessels were identified below the popliteal artery despite state-of-the-art intra-arterial DSA, shown in Fig. 1. MRA was performed shortly afterwards and demonstrated flow in both anterior tibial arteries as shown in Fig. 2, enabling appropriate intervention to be performed, resulting in a successful femoroanterior tibial Varivas bypass of the right leg. An aortabifemoral (bifurcation) prosthesis was also positioned. It was concluded that the trifurcation and distal vessels could not be identified by intra-arterial DSA due to stagnation of contrast in multiple proximal aneurysms and dilution of contrast in extensive collateral networks.

Case 2. A 72-year-old female patient suffering from advanced diabetes mellitus type II, nephropathy, peripheral atherosclerotic occlusive disease, duodenal ulcera, steatosis hepatis, obesity, hypertension, venous engorgement of the lower extremities, and generalized osteoarthrosis was admitted to hospital with symptoms of grade III – category 5 ischemia of the right foot. Her medical history also noted a right-sided femoropopliteal

Fig. 1 a–c. Intra-arterial DSA study of the patient in case 1 (see text). This patient demonstrates multiple aneurysms proximally; despite using state of-the-art DSA technique, distal vessels in the calf were not visualized

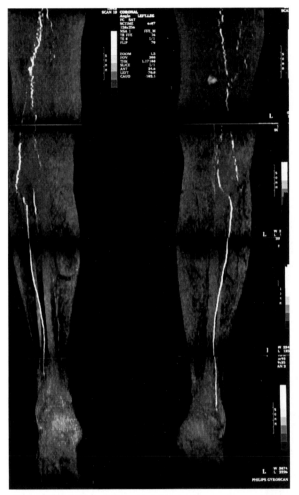

Fig. 2. MRA of both lower extremities of the same patient as demonstrated in Fig. 1 (case 1 in text). Anteroposterior MIPs are shown, acquired at four different stations and compiled to show the entire length in a continuous fashion. Both anterior tibial vessels are shown clearly by the MP-TFE technique (see text), which demonstrates superior sensitivity of MRA for distal vessel visualization compared with intra-arterial DSA (Fig. 1). (Soft tissue borders of the first and second acquisition stations do not coincide due to pressure applied to the skin by the extremity (knee) coil at the level of the first acquisition)

bypass, amputation of the second through fourth digits of the right foot, and severe contrast hypersensitivity. Upon admission the bypass was at risk, and an MRA of the subtrifurcation vessels demonstrated slow flow in the posterior tibial artery only (Fig. 3). On the basis of the MRA findings a femoroposterior tibial bypass was performed, which initially functioned successfully. Within 1 week the bypass was occluded, and subsequent

thrombectomy was performed. In conclusion, unfortunately amputation of the lower leg was inevitable.

Protocols

Acquisition Considerations

It is helpful to consider the advantages and disadvantages of 2D time of flight (TOF) (also known as Inflow MRA) and 2D cine PC techniques when deciding which technique to use. Three-dimensional acquisitions are most impractical and are therefore unpopular for the lower extremities due to the very long scanning times required for the large fields of view concerned.

2D Time of Flight

The advantages of 2D TOF are its sensitivity to a wide range of velocities, including slow flow, acquisition of multiple slices, allowing postprocessing resulting in projections from a multitude of angles, faint residual background signal providing anatomical landmarks, and selectivity for caudally (arterial) or cranially (venous) directed flow determined by postitioning of the presaturation slab. A frequently recurring question on behalf of clinicians concerns the lower threshold of flow sensitivity of a particular acquisition. The sensitivity to (slow) flow of 2D TOF pulse sequences is dependent on the time interval TR used, and the slice thickness; maximal inflow enhancement (signal) is achieved if all spins within a slice of a selected thickness are completely replenished between two RF excitations (time interval TR). This is achieved when the flow velocity (v) equals or exceeds δ/TR (δ = slice thickness). For signal detection, a certain fraction of $v = \delta/TR$ or greater will suffice. Any flow in the appropriate direction with a velocity of δ/TR will certainly be detected by the acquisition concerned, and flow with a lower velocity might be detected; however, this is dependent on other scanning and flow parameters (see also chapter on MRA techniques). In general, 2D TOF provides excellent morphological information because it is extremely sensitive to detection of stenoses, occlusions, and reconstituted distal vessels [1-7, 11, 14, 15], thus providing a "road map" of the arterial tree for global (morphological) evaluation. Several disadvan-

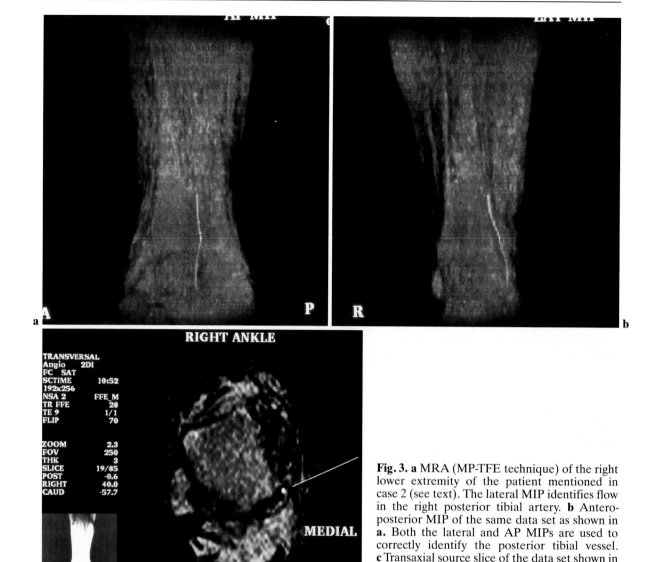

Fig. 3. a MRA (MP-TFE technique) of the right lower extremity of the patient mentioned in case 2 (see text). The lateral MIP identifies flow in the right posterior tibial artery. **b** Antero-posterior MIP of the same data set as shown in **a.** Both the lateral and AP MIPs are used to correctly identify the posterior tibial vessel. **c** Transaxial source slice of the data set shown in **a** and **b,** which identifies the medially located posterior tibial artery at the level of the ankle

tages of 2D TOF are the time requirements to image large fields of view such as an entire lower extremity, although the application of k-space segmentation (TFE, see protocol section below) has effected substantial reductions in imaging time. Other disadvantages include overestimation of stenosis due to intravoxel phase dispersion, and insensitivity to retrograde flow when applying selective MRA or venography. Slice orientation selection, which is invariably transverse in the lower extremities, is suboptimal for certain regions such as tortuous iliac arteries or the anterior tibial artery origin (see "In-Plane Flow Saturation" below).

2D Phase Contrast

Two-dimensional PC MRA provides direct projections: a single thick slice acquisition results in a single projection. Unlike 2D TOF, 2D PC employs arbitrary slice orientation with respect the vessel, since PC is sensitive to all motion relative to the flow encoding gradient(s). 2D PC is not hampered by time considerations associated with the large extent (of vessels) to be imaged, since the vessels can be imaged with coronal or sagittal acquisitions accommodating their longitudinal course, in contrast to 2D TOF where slices are

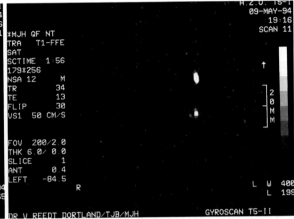

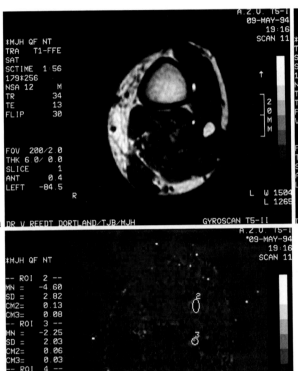

Fig. 4a–c. Untriggered 2D PC quantitative flow study of the left calf in a patient with lower extremity vascular disease. The anterior tibial and peroneal arteries are identified. **a** FFE-M image (Fast Field Echo = gradient echo-Modulus = magnitude image) demonstrates the anatomy. **b** PCA-M image of the same slice as in **a** (Phase Contrast Angio-Modulus = angiographic image) demonstrates blood flow in the anterior tibial and peroneal artery. **c** PCA-P image of the same slice as in **a** and **b** (Phase Contrast Angio-Phase = phase-type image) demonstrates the quantitative information needed to calculate flow, which is performed by applying an ROI to the target vessels. The ROI calculations in the right margin indicate the average flow velocity *(MN)* in cm/s, and the luminal area *(CM2)* in cm^2. Multiplication of the MN with CM2 yields the average volume flow in ml/s

acquired perpendicular to the vessels. Background signal is eliminated by subtraction in PC MRA, rendering improved vessel visualization in projections of small caliber or slow flow vessels, such as in the foot. Selection of the velocity sensitivity may require (time-consuming) velocity sampling, since velocities in diseased arteries are unpredictable: they are increased at stenoses and decreased distal to stenoses. Other disadvantages of PC include motion artifacts due to bowel gas overlying the iliac arteries, and the availability of a single projection plane only. Complementary 2D PC acquisitions are required, for instance coronal and sagittal, to achieve the depth information necessary to accurately locate vessels.

Two-dimensional PC produces anatomical images (magnitude images) (FFE-M[3]) and angiogram-type images (PCA-M[4]), and can also be used to produce phase-type images (PCA-P[5]), in which only vague anatomical outlines remain, and signal intensity conveys quantitative information, in order to calculate flow velocities and flow volumes. Figures 4 and 5 show the corresponding image types of a 2D PC acquisition. These different image types can be produced whether or not cardiac synchronization is used.

Usually, cardiac synchronization is used for 2D PC studies of the lower extremities, which reduces pulsatility artifacts such as ghosting (although this also applies to the 2D TFE TOF protocol) and provides temporal resolution during the cardiac cycle providing a multiphase acquisition is performed. Lanzer et al. [27] demonstrated improved PC angiography in the aortoiliac and femoropopliteal vessels when using the Rapid Sequential Excitation (RSE) angiographic pulse sequence, resulting in improved vessel contrast due to reduction of flow-related phase shift subtrac-

---

[3] FFE-M, Fast Field Echo-Modulus images: magnitude (anatomical) images of the PC data set.

[4] PCA-M, Phase Contrast Angio-Modulus images: angiographic images after background subtraction of the PC data set.

---

[5] PCA-P, Phase Contrast Angio-Phase images: quantitative phase images of the PC data set. See also Figs. 4 and 5.

tion errors, and reduced motion-related subtraction errors (of motion other than blood flow). In the RSE mode, the flow-compensated and flow-sensitive profiles are acquired in a favorable "back to back" temporal order with respect to triggering.

The subsequent phases of the cardiac cycle are usually displayed in consecutive temporal order, known as cine mode. Such acquisitions are therefore known as 2D cine PC. A single slice is thus imaged a number of times, depending on the number of phases selected within a heart-beat period, and each phase image then represents a sequential section of the cardiac cycle.

If phase-type images are intended for quantification of flow, the acquisition is usually performed in a single-slice, multiphase mode (cardiac triggered) with the slice oriented perpendicular to the vessel of interest. Perpendicularity ensures that only one flow-encoding direction is necessary to detect the main flow component, and also enables accurate calculation of the luminal area to be carried out. Cardiac-triggered quantitative 2D cine PC enables pulsatility measurements and velocity waveform analysis for hemodynamic evaluation to be performed.

Velocity quantitation is an inherent advantage of PC techniques, since the phase shift measured, which also determines signal intensity, is directly proportional to the velocity of the moving spins ($\Delta \Phi = \gamma m v$; $\Delta \Phi$ = phase shift; γ = gyromagnetic ratio, m = gradient moment difference between the two acquisitions; and v = velocity [22]). Volumetric flowrate is equal to the average spatial velocity of a vessel multiplied by the cross-sectional luminal area of the vessel; thus calculation of flow volumes (ml/s) is also a PC feature.

Clinical Applications and Protocols

Clinical applications of peripheral vascular MRA are as follows:

1. Evaluation of peripheral arterial disease
2. Target vessel identification for bypass surgery
3. Aneurysm detection
4. Follow-up after interventional procedures
5. Venography

Our experience indicates that the 2D TFE TOF protocol (Table 3) provides good image quality within reasonable scanning times: a presaturation pulse is used to reduce stationary tissue signal,

Table 3. 2D TFE TOF protocol

Scan time	5:40 (min:s)
Scan technique	TFE[a]
Scan mode	Multiple 2D
TR	13 ms
TE	6 ms
Flip angle	70°
TFE prepulse	180° (inversion)
Prepulse delay (TI)	250 ms[b]
Coil	Knee/extremity
No. of slices	65
Slice thickness	4 mm
Slice overlap	−1 mm
FOV	200
Rectangular FOV	50%
Slice order	Ascending
NSA	1
Matrix	128 × 256
Cardiac triggering	Yes
Presaturation slab	Parallel/caudal
Slab thickness	100 mm
Slab gap	5 mm

[a] TFE, turbo field echo = RF-spoiled turbo gradient echo (turbo FLASH = RAGE).
[b] variable

Table 4. 2D cine PC flow quantification protocol, cardiac gated

Scan time	4:02 (min:s)
Scan technique	FFE[a]
Scan mode	2D
TR	34
TE	13
Flip angle	30
Angiography mode	Phase contrast
PC velocity	50–100 cm/s[b]
PC flow direction	Superior-inferior
Coil	Knee/extremity
No. of slices	1
Slice thickness	6 mm
FOV	200 mm
Rectangular FOV	80%
NSA	1
Matrix	180 × 256
Cardiac synchronization	Retrospective
Retrospective period	1.2 beats
No. of heart phases	15–25
Presaturation slab[c]	Parallel/caudal
Slab thickness	50 mm
Slab gap	5 mm

[a] FFE, fast field echo = gradient echo.
[b] PC velocity: for the femoral arteries 100 cm/s is recommended, for the popliteal and distal arteries 50–100 cm/s is recommended.
[c] The presaturation slab can be used to suppress the infrapopliteal veins.

and k-space segmentation is applied for faster acquisitions. (The reader is referred to the chapter on MRA techniques for a detailed explanation of the pulse sequences.) Our standard protocols are listed in Tables 3 and 4, with adaptations provided in the text, where necessary, pertaining to the following four vascular regions: iliac and common femoral vessels, superficial and deep femoral vessels, the popliteal and infrapopliteal trajectory, and vessels of the foot. Obviously, these are suggestions only, based on our experience, as well as on literature reviews as indicated. Clearly, due to the flexibility of MRA, other acquisition techniques may prove to be at least as good as those suggested here.

Evaluation of Peripheral Vascular Disease

Initial localization and determination of focal or diffuse disease in order to select subjects for PTA or bypass surgery can be done noninvasively by performing a morphological evaluation combined with hemodynamic assessment with MRA. Initial "road mapping" of the lower extremity arterial tree is complicated by the large extent of the vessels concerned, and therefore usually performed in a multistation mode.

Iliac Vessels

To date most protocols have employed 2D TOF for the iliac arteries. The 2D TFE TOF protocol is suggested, the relatively large caliber of the vessels allowing use of the body coil, a slice thickness of 3–5 mm, and a field of view of 32 cm.

PC is perhaps a good alternative suited to the oblique course of (tortuous) iliac vessels; indeed it is advantageous to apply an additional flow-encoding gradient (besides the standard superior-inferior flow-encoding gradient) in the left-right direction with the PC technique for the iliacs. If software allows, different velocity sensitivities could be applied for each of the two gradients for an optimal signal in the respective flow directions.

Femoral Vessels, Popliteal and Infrapopliteal Trajectory, and Pedal Vessels

Two-dimensional TFE TOF is our method of choice for morphological examination of this region, since TOF has been shown to be extremely sensitive in detecting stenoses, occlusions, and reconstituted distal vessels [1–7, 11, 14, 15], and allows exact localization of the identified vessels and collaterals relative to the stationary tissue outlines as defined on axial source slices, with additional spatial referencing by MIPs from varying angles. Previous studies have illustrated the advantage of multiple projections in this region [4]. In imaging the femoral vessels, the vessel caliber is such that the body coil can be used, with a 3- to 5-mm slice thickness, and a field of view (FOV) of 25 cm. In the popliteal and infrapopliteal arteries, an extremity coil is used for improved resolution, with an effective slice thickness of 3 mm (4 mm with 1 mm overlap) and a FOV of 20 cm. The coil is usually repositioned four times to image the popliteal artery to the pedal arch. Markers attached to the skin surface perpendicular to the longitudinal axis of the leg can be used to indicate the point of overlap between consecutive acquisitions on a survey image.

After initial localization of the vascular lesions, which can be overestimated with 2D TOF, an accurate noninvasive hemodynamic assessment of the stenoses can be made with quantitative 2D cine PC. A transversely orientated single-slice, multiphase acquisition (see Table 4) is positioned first above and then below the lesion. Depending on the subject's heart rate, the number of cardiac phases is selected, and a velocity sensitivity of 50–100 cm/s is used to prevent aliasing (phase wrap). Measurements can be performed on the vessel of interest by selecting a region of interest (ROI) corresponding to the lumen of the vessel on the anatomical images (magnitude images) as is shown in Figs. 4 and 5, and applying an identical ROI to the corresponding phase images. The spatial mean velocity of the selected ROI for each phase is determined, and plotted along the y coordinates of a graph, with the phase number along the x-axis to yield a velocity waveform. Hemodynamically significant lesions have monophasic waveforms, and the pulsatility index can be calculated as shown in Eq. 1 [22], which has been shown to correlate well with the pulsatility index as determined by Doppler ultrasound [22]. Peak systolic velocity can also be determined, by cast-

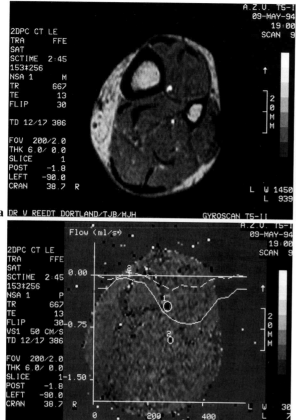

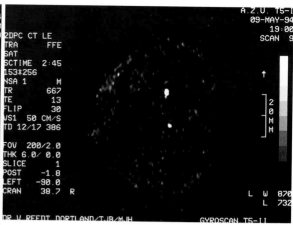

Fig. 5a–c. Cardiac Gated 2D cine PC Quantitative Flow study of the left calf in a patient with lower extremity vascular disease. Only 1 phase of the 17 is shown here. **a** FFE-M image (see Fig. 4) identifies the anterior tibial and peroneal arteries. **b** PCA-M image of the same slice as in **a**. **c** PCA-P image of the same slice as in **a** and **b,** with the flow curve superimposed, demonstrating the flow variations measured during the cardiac cycle (*y*-axis, ml/s; *x*-axis, time during the cardiac cycle in ms)

ing a line profile through the vessel lumen on the peak systolic phase image, and determining the range of intensity-linked velocities along the projected line.

$$PI = ((PSFV) - (PDRV))/MCCV \qquad (1)$$

where PI is pulsatility index, PSFV is peak systolic forward velocity, PDRV is peak diastolic reverse velocity, and MCCV is mean cardiac cycle velocity.

Multiplication of the area of the ROI (vessel lumen) with the mean spatial velocity (in cm/s) yields the volume flow (in ml/s) through the vessel concerned.

Thus both morphological and hemodynamic features of the diseased vessels can be determined noninvasively in order to select an appropriate intervention in a single MR examination.

Target Vessel Identification for Bypass Surgery

The 2D TFE TOF protocol with the aforementioned adaptations (above) is also our method of choice for the detection of target vessels for bypass surgery.

Pedal Vessels

For pedal vessels with very slow flow a 2D cine PC study with a low velocity sensitivity may be useful for improved visualization of the smaller caliber vessels due to selectable sensitivity to very slow flow and elimination of background signal by subtraction [28]. Two or more projections, i.e., coronal and sagittal projections, should be acquired for accurate localization of the vessels.

Aneurysms

Both techniques (2D TOF and 2D PC) have been tested for aneurysm imaging [28]. If slow flow is predicted, 2D cine PC is perhaps preferable since 2D TOF tends to saturate slow flow, especially if turbulent.

Conventional contrast angiography and MRA depict intraluminal flow in a similar manner; thus complementary SE MR imaging should be performed to assess the presence of intraluminal thrombus. In preparation of surgical correction by bypass grafting, the inflow and outflow vessels can be assessed by the protocols suggested above.

Preoperative Tumor Evaluation

Experience in this area is limited. Swan et al. [29] suggest a technique to combine SE MR images with 2D cine PC images to produce combined angiographic-stationary tissue (CAST) images. A cardiac-triggered, 2D PC MRA acquisition is performed of the region under investigation, and the resulting study is combined with an SE MRI image of the same anatomical region. The pixels of the MRA image are weighted to prevent obscuring the MRA signal by the higher total signal of the SE image. The technique was successfully applied for preoperative evaluation of limb salvage [29].

Follow-up After Interventional Procedures

With regard to follow-up, it might be rewarding to use surgical ligatures instead of clips in anticipation of the future role of MRA. The advantages of using a noninvasive technique such as MRA are especially clear in the follow-up setting. We suggest the protocols as described above for "road mapping" and, if necessary, 2D cine PC for supplemental hemodynamic evaluation.

Venography

Spritzer et al. [30] report that 2D TOF is very sensitive for venography from the level of the popliteal vein upward. MR venography of veins of the calf is less successful, basically because venous flow is slower at this level, and intermittent, coinciding with intermittent muscular contractions.

According to the same author, MR venography is the only reliable investigative tool for identification of deep venous thrombosis in pelvic veins.

Iliac Veins

Two-dimensional TOF is suggested with a 5 mm slice thickness, 5 mm interslice gap, 128 × 256 matrix, and a FOV at the pelvis depending on the patient's size (40-28 cm), which is decreased as one moves distally from the pelvis. In the pelvis, the body coil is used, with four excitations [30].

Veins of the Thigh

In the thigh the body coil is used, and the number of excitations is reduced to two [30].

Veins of the Calves

For the calves, the extremity coil is suggested, with a 256 × 256 matrix, a rectangular FOV of 20–30 cm, and one excitation. Supplemental SE images (and phase contrast) are suggested in order to identify thrombus [30].

Common Artifacts

An important prerequisite for the successful application of MRA in the clinical setting is familiarity with the artifacts associated with the MRA technique (and how to approach them). In the next section a review of 2D TOF and 2D PC artifacts is given, as well as how they can be recognized, and suggestions to overcome them. Common artifacts are: (1) in-plane flow saturation, (2) movement artifacts, (3) saturation of cranially directed retrograde flow (in TOF only), (4) black band artifact (in TOF only), (5) ghosting, (6) metallic clip artifact, and (7) poststenotic signal void. Phase contrast MRA, enabling velocity and flow quantification to be carried out, uses different imaging techniques, with specific difficulties such as: (1) phase aliasing artifact (phase wrap) and (2) sensitivity to ROI selection for quantitative measurement purposes.

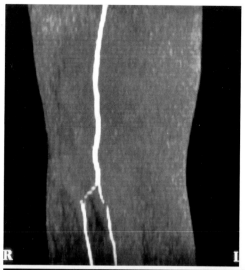

Fig. 6. a Anteposterior MIP of a 2D TOF acquisition of the lower extremity, demonstrating in-plane flow saturation, resulting in diminished signal intensity, at the origin of the anterior tibial artery. **a** Inspection of the subsequent transaxial source slices of the corresponding MIP in **b–e** reveals adequate flow in the aforementioned anterior tibial artery origin

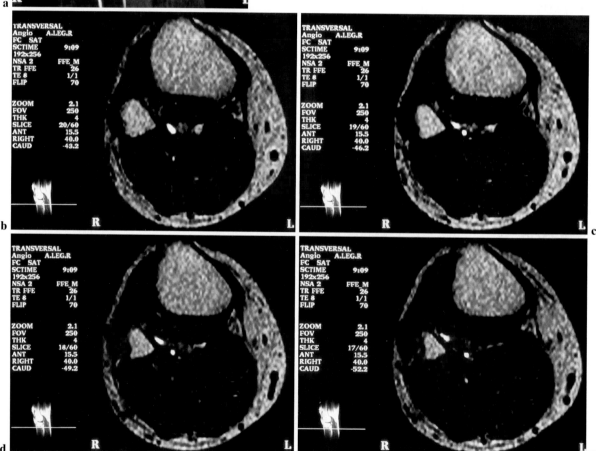

In-Plane Flow Saturation

The MR signal of blood flowing within the plane of acquisition diminishes due to repetitive exposure to excitation pulses (with relatively large flip angles) within the slice (saturation). With 2D TOF of the lower extremities, this occurs mostly with any flow perpendicular to the longitudinal axis of the lower extremity. This is especially evident at the external iliac arteries and the origin of the anterior tibial artery, shown in Fig. 6a. These vessel portions have an oblique course; therefore the spins of flowing blood are more often exposed to repetitive RF pulses in the imaging plane than those of blood flowing perpendicular to the imaging plane. Signal is diminished in oblique vessels, which is exaggerated on the MIPs, and can be misinterpreted as stenosis by the inexperienced eye. It is important that the axial slices are consulted to differentiate between in-plane flow artifact and veritable stenosis, since the axial slices will demonstrate sufficient signal in the case of artifact as is shown in Fig. 6b–e. In-plane flow saturation becomes more severe as the vessel portion courses increasingly in-plane. Moreover, since the MIP is based on multiple 2D slices, vessels that course obliquely will be displayed with a "stepping artifact" to a greater or lesser degree, as is shown in Fig. 6a, depending on the quality of the MIP and slice thickness.

Movement Artifact

Less commonly, movement artifact is seen especially in patients with rest pain (or tissue necrosis) causing restlessness of the lower extremity during the examination. Figure 7 demonstrates movement artifacts on the MIP, which result from dis-

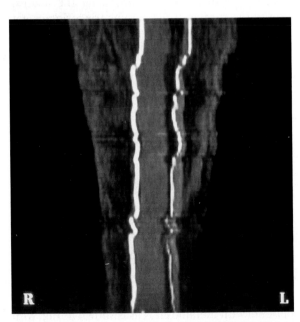

Fig. 7. Anteroposterior MIP of a 2D MP-TFE TOF data set of the lower extremity demonstrating movement artifact: inspection of the skin contours at the corresponding levels confirms movement. Lesions may be overlooked by misinterpretation as movement artifact, and therefore inspection of the axial slices is necessary

placement of the individual source slices with respect to each other. This is rarely misinterpreted as stenosis; however, in some instances stenoses could be missed on these MIPs. Inspection of the skin contours on the MIP will confirm movement artifact, and consultation of the axial source slices is important in these cases for reliable interpretation of the vessel lumen. In the group of patients with grade II and III (SVS/ISCVS) ischemic disease, intramuscular administration of 10 mg morphine prior to examination can be very helpful to prevent movement during the MRA acquisition.

Retrograde Flow

A disturbing artifact is the saturation of cranially directed arterial flow due to the venous presaturation pulse, which occurs with retrograde flow in vascular segments fed by collaterals or grafts. Figure 8 shows an intra-arterial DSA and an MRA of the same peripheral vascular trajectory in a patient, the DSA study demonstrating flow in the popliteal artery (supplied by an end-to-side bypass vessel), which is not visualized on the MR angiogram. In this case it is concluded that cranially directed retrograde flow exists in the popliteal artery. Any cranially directed flow is saturated by the traveling presaturation pulse positioned caudally to the imaging slice in order to saturate venous flow. The incidence of this artifact is reported to be very low: Owen et al. [7] report nonvisualization of retrograde flow in only 1 out of 1007 segments (73 patients); in our study it occurred in 1 out of 30 patients.

Black Bands

An extremely rare artifact in clinical practice is the black band (also known as horizontal stripe) artifact. This is caused when there is a moderate to strong retrograde flow phase in subjects with triphasic flow. During the retrograde flow phase, spins that have been saturated by the venous presaturation pulse slab can flow cranially into the imaging slice, and cause signal void since their magnetization has been presaturated. This artifact is encountered in the experimental setting when healthy individuals with strong triphasic flow patterns are subjected to 2D TOF acquisitions using the traveling venous presaturation slab. It is rare in patients with peripheral vascular disease be-

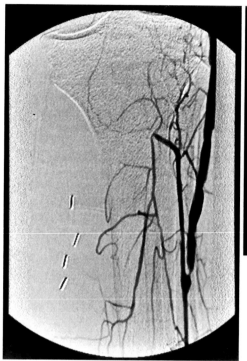
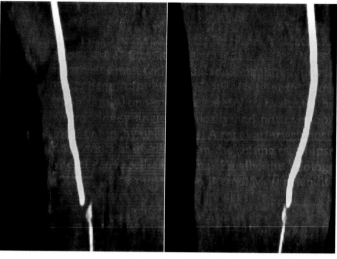

Fig. 8. a Intra-arterial DSA of a patient demonstrating flow in a femoroanterior tibial bypass graft and in the anterior tibial artery. A stenosis of the distal anastomosis is also noted. **b** lateral and AP MIPs of a 2D TOF MRA examination of the same patient acquired within 24 h of the DSA shown in **a**. Although the bypass is visualized clearly, the MR angiogram fails to visualize flow in the proximal part of the anterior tibial artery, hence it is concluded that flow in the proximal portion of the anterior tibial artery is retrograde (directed cranially). Retrograde flow is saturated by the traveling venous presaturation pulse. The stenotic distal anastomosis shows a short signal void on the lateral MIP

cause their flow patterns are most often biphasic due to proximal stenoses and loss of elasticity of the vessel walls. The artifact can be overcome by increasing the gap between the presaturation slab and the imaging slice ("slab gap").

Ghosting

Ghosting is an MRA term used to describe misregistered replicas of flow signal along the phase-encoding axis. Figure 9 demonstrates artifactual replicas ("ghosts") of the original vessel image. Ghosting occurs with pulsatile flow: pulsatile flow causes variations in signal amplitude between the subsequent phase-encoding steps, producing replicas in the phase-encoding direction. Ghosting is usually reduced by synchronizing the acquisition to the cardiac cycle: cardiac triggering or gating. We found ghosting to occur in 42% of our patients imaged with a 2D TOF protocol without cardiac synchronization, in contrast to none in the group imaged with the cardiac gated 2D TFE TOF protocol.

Metallic Clips

This artifact belongs to the group of susceptibility artifacts. Metallic clips, reminiscent of previous bypass or other interventional operations, may cause signal dropout or lead to image distortion in the same way as they do in regular MR imaging. The presence of metallic clips in the lower extremities does not necessarily exclude the patient from peripheral MRA, although most intracranial clips do. We have performed successful MRA in patients with metallic clips as is shown in Fig. 8. It is recommended that an MRA be performed in these cases and the result judged for interpretability rather than to exclude these patients from the outset. The use of a mid- or lowfield strength MR system will reduce clip artifacts.

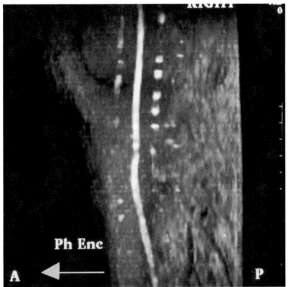

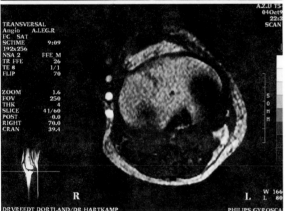

Fig. 9. a Lateral MIP of a 2D TOF MRA examination of the lower extremity at the level of the knee, using an untriggered TOF technique. Ghosting artifact is demonstrated in a bypass graft with pulsatile flow. The *arrow* indicates the phase-encoding *(Ph Enc)* direction of the acquisition. **b** Transaxial source slice of the same data set as in **a**. Ghost vessels are imaged along the phase-encoding axis of the slice

Poststenotic Signal Void

Poststenotic signal void has been reported on MIPs [1–3] although other authors claim that MRA systematically overestimates stenosis based on inspection of the transaxial slices [6, 13]. It is well known that TOF MRA of the carotid arteries is associated with overestimation of stenoses. Our experience demonstrates the tendency of stenoses to produce short signal voids on MIPs of MR angiograms in incomplete occlusions as diagnosed

by intra-arterial DSA. Complete occlusions are depicted as longer segments of signal void, in which signal is regained after reconstitution of flow in the vessel concerned.

Aliasing (Phase Wrap)

An essential artifact encountered only in PC MRA is aliasing: diminished signal intensity which occurs when the velocity of flow supersedes the selected velocity sensitivity, even causing severe signal reduction when flow velocity becomes an even multiple of the selected velocity. PC-phase images as produced by flow quantification pulse sequences are also influenced by aliasing.

Region of Interest Management

To calculate flow curves and mean velocity on phase reconstructions of the PC study, an ROI is drawn to include the slowest flow adjacent to the vessel wall, and thus the ROI should coincide with the inner border of the vessel lumen as is shown in Figs. 4 and 5. (To measure the *range* of velocity inside the vessel, a line profile can be drawn along its orthogonal section.) Volume flow measurements are performed by choosing a similar ROI around the vessel lumen; however, slightly larger ROIs will not influence the measurements to the same degree as with velocity flow measurements, since inclusion of pixels displaying stationary tissue will be cancelled by their zero velocity in volume flow calculations. Especially mean velocity measurement is extremely sensitive to small variations of ROI selection. It is best to perform the ROI on zoomed images.

Maximum Intensity Projection

In general, stenotic vessel segments have a lower signal intensity and are easily lost on the MIP due to superimposition of structures with a (slightly) higher signal intensity. Therefore, a stenosis often appears more severe on a MIP. After locating a stenosis on the MIP, overestimation of the stenosis is best avoided by determining the degree of stenosis on the transaxial (source) slices.

Future Developments and Perspective

Full realization of the clinical potential of MRA requires continuing clinical studies and further improvements with regard to the efficiency of the technique, spatial and contrast resolution, suppression of artifacts, processing, and display. Current research extends to all these areas and will be briefly summarized below.

Efficiency. At present, an MRA examination of the peripheral arteries usually requires repositioning of (different) coils, which is time-consuming and tedious. The development of dedicated, extended extremity coils and the construction of coils that operate in synergy will definitely lead to more efficient use. A revolutionary development which is expected to improve the efficiency and efficacy of MRA is the implementation of ultra-fast imaging techniques, such as echo-planar imaging (EPI), GRASE (a combination of turbo-spin echo and echo-planar imaging), and spiral imaging (including 2D EPI PC) [31]. Even real-time interactive MR flow imaging seems to be feasible. Such fast angiography and flow quantification techniques are expected to be particularly effective in the evaluation of peripheral vascular disease.

Resolution. The spatial resolution of MRA is still inferior to that of conventional angiography. However, the gap is being narrowed by hardware and software modifications which permit thinner slices, smaller fields of view, and larger matrices. With respect to contrast resolution, the peripheral vessels constitute a difficult area, due to the slow average velocity of blood flow, in particular below the popliteal trifurcation and distal to hemodynamically significant lesions. Contrast in TOF angiograms of the peripheral arteries is further compromised by the relatively bright signal of bone marrow and subcutaneous fat, although integration of dedicated prepulses in current pulse sequences has achieved substantial improvements in this respect. Marked improvements in vessel conspicuity have recently been made by gating the acquisition to the period of maximum systolic flow and by the application of fat suppression techniques. Slow flow is easily saturated, alleviation of which has been demonstrated by using relaxation agents which reside intravascularly for several hours, exhibiting only little leakage to soft tissues. These blood-pool agents, such as albumin-gadolinium diethylene triamine penta-acetic acid (albumin-DTPA), have not yet been approved for human use. Clearly, the option of selective presaturation of venous flow is eliminated after administration of contrast material.

Alternatively, slow flow can be dealt with by application of PC angiography. PC methods provide flow-related images of the vascular system and permit quantitative measurements of velocity and volume flow rates. Unfortunately, the pulsatility of blood flow complicates the selection of an optimal velocity sensitivity to provide good image quality and avoid aliasing artifacts. For 2D PC, promising results have been obtained with an ECG-gated cine acquisition in which the velocity sensitivity is adapted for each phase in the cardiac cycle. Optimization of 3D PC is currently pursued by selecting independent velocity for each flow-encoding direction.

Artifacts. Reduction of flow misregistration artifacts and reduction of flow-related signal losses are currently under study with application of stronger, faster, and thus more compact gradients. Such gradients allow shorter echo times and smaller fields of view and are expected to overcome the tendency of MRA to overestimate lesions and, consequently, improve the utility of MRA for evaluating stenotic disease. Although partial echo sampling is already common practice, development of algorithms that compensate for lost data is still continuing.

Postprocessing and Display. Maximum intensity projection (MIP) constitutes the most widely employed method by which an angiogram-type display is derived from the source data. Apart from the fact that MIP introduces disturbing artifacts and is only applicable if blood provides the highest signal (or the lowest signal, as is the case in black blood MRA), MIP does not attempt to differentiate vessel and background but simply looks for the highest signal intensities in a chosen projection direction. Current research – which is not specific to peripheral MRA – is directed at vessel-tracking techniques (segmentation) which attempt to discriminate between vessels and background tissues by applying segmentation and connectivity algorithms. These methods preserve depth information and allow 3D rendering of vascular structures.

This short survey of current developments merely indicates some areas of interest in peripheral

MRA, and the next few years should be decisive as to the ultimate role of MRA in the assessment of peripheral vascular disease.

References

1. Yucel EK, Dumoulin CL, Waltman AC (1992) MR angiography of lower-extremity arterial disease: preliminary experience. J Magn Reson Imaging 2: 303–309
2. Yucel EK, Kaufman JA, Geller SC, Waltman AC (1993) Atherosclerotic occlusive disease of the lower extremity: prospective evaluation with two-dimensional time-of-flight MR angiography [see comments]. Radiology 187: 637–641. Comment in: Radiology (1993) 187: 615–617
3. Cambria RP, Yucel EK, Brewster DC, L'Italien G, Gertler JP, La Muraglia GM, Kaufman JA, Waltman AC, Abbott WM (1993) The potential for lower extremity revascularization without contrast arteriography: experience with magnetic resonance angiography. J Vasc Surg 17: 1050–1057
4. Owen RS, Carpenter JP, Baum RA, Perloff LJ, Cope C (1992) Magnetic resonance imaging of angiographically occult runoff vessels in peripheral arterial occlusive disease [see comments]. N Engl J Med 326: 1577–1581. Comment in: N Engl J Med (1992) 326: 1624–1626; comment in: N Engl J Med (1992) 327: 1319–1320
5. Carpenter JP, Owen RS, Baum RA, Cope C, Barker CF, Berkowitz HD, Golden MA, Perloff LJ (1992) Magnetic resonance angiography of peripheral runoff vesseles [see comments]. J Vasc Surg 16: 8007–815. Comment in: J Vasc Surg (1993) 17: 1136–1137
6. Schnall MD, Holland GA, Baum RA, Cope C, Schiebler ML, Carpenter JP (1993) MR angiography of the peripheral vasculature. Radiographics 13: 920–930
7. Owen RS, Baum RA, Carpenter JP, Holland GA, Cope C (1993) Symptomatic peripheral vascular disease: selection of imaging parameters and clinical evaluation with MRA. Radiology 187: 627–635
8. Rutherford RB, Flanigan DP, Gupta SK (1986) Suggested standards for reports dealing with lower extremity ischaemia. J Vasc Surgery 4: 80–94
9. Rutherford RB, Becker GJ (1991) Standards for evaluating and reporting the results of surgical and percutaneous therapy for peripheral arterial disease. Radiology 181: 277–281
10. Mulligan, SA, Matsuda TM, Lanzer P, et al. (1991) Peripheral arterial occlusive disease: prospective comparison of MR angiography and color duplex US with conventional angiography. Radiology 178: 695–700
11. Yucel EK (1992) Magnetic resonance angiography of the lower extremity and renal arteries. Semin Ultrasound CT MR 13: 291–302
12. Steinberg FL, Yucel EK, Dumoulin CL, Souza SP (1990) Peripheral vascular and abdominal applications of MR flow imaging techniques. Magn Reson Med 14: 315–320
13. Owen RS, Baum RA, Carpenter JR, et al. (1992) Identification and quantification of peripheral vascular stenoses with MR angiography (Abstr.). Radiology 185: 277
14. Schiebler ML, Listerud J, Holland G, Owen R, Baum R, Kressel HY (1992) Magnetic resonance angiography of the pelvis and lower extremities. Works in progress. Invest Radiol 1 [Suppl 2]: S90–S96
15. Hertz SM, Baum RA, Owen RS, Holland GA, Logan DR, Carpenter JP (1993) Comparison of magnetic resonance angiography and contrast arteriography in peripheral arterial stenosis. Am J Surg 166: 112–116
16. Smith TP, Cragg AH, Berbaum KS, Nakagawa N (1992) Comparison of the efficacy of digital subtraction and film-screen angiography of the lower limb: prospective study in 50 patients. AJR 158: 431–436
17. Kaufman SL, Chang R, Kadir S, Mitchell S, White RI Jr (1984) Intraarterial digital subtraction angiography in diagnostic arteriography. Radiology 151: 323–327
18. Darcy MD (1991) Lower extremity arteriography: current approach and techniques. Radiology 178: 615–621
19. Hartkamp MJ, et al. (1994) Peripheral vascular disease evaluation with MRA. (Unpublished data) University Hospital Utrecht, Utrecht, The Netherlands
20. Speilmann RP, Schneider O, Thiele F, Heller M, Bücheler E (1991) Appearance of poststenotic jets in MRI: dependence on flow velocity and on Imaging parameters. Magn Res Imaging 9: 67–72
21. Girmin G, Nayler GL, Kilner PJ, Longmore DB (1990) The application of phase shifts in NMR for flow measurement. Magn Reson Med 14: 230–241
22. Caputo GR, Masui T, Gooding GAW, Chang J-M, Higgins CB (1992) Popliteal and tibioperoneal arteries: feasibility of two-dimensional time-of-flight MR angiography and phase velocity mapping. Radiology 182: 387–392
23. Caputo GR, Higgings CB (1992) Magnetic resonance angiography and measurement of blood flow in the peripheral vessels. Invest Radiol [Suppl] 27: S97–S101
24. Meyer RA, Foley JM, Harkema SJ, Sierra A, Potchen EJ (1993) Magnetic resonance measurement of blood flow in peripheral vessels after acute exercise. Magn Res Imagi 11: 1085–1092
25. Dousset V, Wehrli FW, Louie A, Listerud J (1991) Popliteal artery hemodynamics: MR imaging-US correlation. Radiology 179: 437–441
26. Yucel EK, Gillams AR, Silver MS, McCall P, Carter AP (1993) MR angiography of iliac vessels: quantitative comparison of three inflow techniques. SMRM Abstracts, p 185. Vol 1 Book of Abstracts of the 12 Annual Scientific Meeting of the Society of Magnetic Resonance in Med, NY
27. Lanzer P, Bohning D, Groen J, Gross G, Nanda N, Pohost G (1990) Aortoiliac and femoropopliteal phase-based NMR angiography: a comparison between FLAG and RSE. Magn Reson Med 15: 372–385

28. Steinberg FL (1994) Peripheral MRA ready for wide clinical use. Diagnostic imaging Winter: 32–38
29. Swan JS, Weber DM, Korosec FR, Grist TM, Heiner JP (1993) Technical note: combined MRI and MRA for limb salvage planning. J Comput Assist Tomogr 17: 339–342
30. Spritzer, CE (1993) Venography of the extremities and pelvis. MRI Clinics of North America December 1993: 239–251
31. Debaten JF (1994) Abstract no. 44 (p 51), Abstract no. 341 (p 367), Abstract no. 392 (p 420). In: Book of Abstracts of the 11th Meeting of the ESMRMB. European Society for Magnetic Resonance in Medicine and Biology

Section II
Computed Tomography

Computed Tomographic Angiography

M. S. van Leeuwen, L. J. Polman, J. Noordzij, and B. Velthuis

Introduction

Computed tomographic angiography (CTA) is a vascular imaging technique based on the rapid acquisition of volumetric CT data during the bolus phase of intravenously administered contrast [1–3]. CTA is a recent diagnostic technique and is still under development. Only preliminary studies on its diagnostic value have been performed. In this chapter the technique is described and the clinical experience of various research groups with a number of specific CTA applications is discussed. The latest generation of CT scanners are equiped with slip-ring current and data transfer. This makes it possible to rotate the assembly of X-ray tube and X-ray detectors continuously. During this continuous rotation the patient can be moved at a constant speed through the plane of the X-ray tube and detectors. The simultaneous linear movement of the patient and continuous rotation of the X-ray tube creates a helical path of the X-ray beam relative to the patient's longitudinal axis. From the continuous, helical data acquisition, axial CT slices can be reconstructed at any desired location along the longitudinal axis of the examined volume. Overlapping slices can be reconstructed with no additional radiation to the patient, improving anatomic resolution in the longitudinal direction and enabling image reconstructions to be performed in any desired plane [4, 5]. The quality of these reconstructions is markedly improved from conventional CT due to the continuous helical data acquisition. In conventional CT, data acquisition and subsequent table transport takes 6–12 s for each slice. With helical CT a full rotation usually takes 1 s and, depending on the capacity of the X-ray tube, up to 50 rotations can be acquired in one scan. Therefore, the time needed to image a large number of overlapping slices is dramatically reduced. Vascular detail is optimized because the entire volume of interest is scanned at peak vascular enhancement during a single breath-hold.

Methods

In order to comprehend the diagnostic scope and technical limitations of CTA, basic knowledge is required of the technical parameters inherent in helical data acquisition, and of different means of image display.

Data Acquisition

As in conventional CT, image quality depends on the combination of contrast and spatial resolution [6, 7]. Contrast and spatial resolution in the transverse plane is defined by the X-ray contrast between anatomic structures, the diameter of the volume of interest, or field of view (FOV), and the reconstruction filter used. Data acquisition during peak vascular enhancement will result in optimal contrast between vascular lumina and surroundings. Consequently, intravenous contrast is administered with a mechanical injector at a high injection rate, and the delay between start of injection and image acquisition is adjusted to the region under study. The size of the FOV is minimized to include only the region of interest, thus further optimizing in-plane resolution. The reconstruction filter is adjusted to optimize the balance between signal-to-noise ratio and in-plane resolution. Spatial resolution along the longitudinal or Z-axis is limited by the slice thickness, but can be improved by using overlapping reconstructions. Slice thickness itself is the end product of the collimation size, the table speed, and the reconstruction algorithm used to reconstruct axial slices from the helical data.

In any CTA application, helical scanning and contrast parameters have to be adjusted to the anatomy under investigation. For instance, if a large volume has to be investigated, as in CTA of aortic disease, a large number of rotations are required. If aortic dissection is suspected, the entire thoracoabdominal aorta can be imaged in one acquisition if 10 mm/s table speed and 10-mm slice collimation are chosen. Resolution on the Z-axis will be poor due to volume averaging in thick slices. However, in-plane resolution is not influenced by slice thickness, and intimal tears can be depicted accurately along their entire length. Conversely, if the abdominal aorta is investigated for aneurysmal disease, the presence and location of accessory renal arteries must be assessed. A total of 40–50 rotations with a table speed of 5 mm/s and a collimation of 5 mm will cover the entire abdominal aorta and still yield sufficient resolution on the Z-axis. In order not to exceed 150 ml of contrast an injection rate of 2–2.5 ml/s, with a scan delay of 30 s, will provide a high intravascular contrast level during the entire acquisition.

If CTA is optimized for detection and grading of stenoses in the renal arteries, which are usually located in the transverse plane, resolution on the Z-axis should be as high as possible and collimation and table speed should preferably be kept at or below 3 mm and 3 mm/s respectively. To optimize spatial resolution intense vascular enhancement at the level of the renal arteries is required. This can be achieved by measuring the transit time between peripheral injection and peak enhancement at the level of the renal arteries after injection of a small amount of contrast. Thus, the scan delay is optimized and the injection rate can be set at 3–5 ml/s to provide maximum contrast and spatial resolution at the desired anatomic level.

Although the compromise between imaged volume and resolution on the Z-axis applies to all CTA applications, differences in CT scanners exist. The total amount of rotations with sufficient X-ray power varies between 24 and 50 in one acquisition. Consequently, the scanner with the maximal amount of rotations will be able to image a longer anatomic region with comparable resolution in the Z-axis, or an equal anatomic volume with improved resolution along the Z-axis. At our institute we use a spiral CT scanner (SR 7000, Philips Medical Systems, Best) capable of 50 consecutive rotations with a rotation time of 1 s. A tube voltage of 120 kV and a tube current of 250 mAs is possible, which is relatively high for spiral CT and provides a good signal-to-noise ratio.

To compensate for the limitation in the amount of rotations, a table speed in excess of the collimation can be chosen. For instance, if table speed is increased from 5 to 10 mm/s without an increase in collimation, a twofold increase in imaged volume is achieved. However, the resolution along the Z-axis will be significantly lower, due to increased volume averaging.

Image Display

Due to the continuous helical data acquisition, overlapping axial slices can be reconstructed at any desired location along the Z-axis. To minimize partial volume averaging, the distance between the center of the reconstructed slices (reconstruction index) should be approximately half the collimation and table speed [7]. Thus, an acquisition with 5 mm collimation and 5 mm/s table speed should be reconstructed with a reconstruction index of 2 or 3 mm, whereas an acquisition with 10 mm collimation and 10 mm/s table speed should be reconstructed with a reconstruction index of 5 mm.

The reconstructed, overlapping, axial slices can be displayed on film, comparable to conventional CT. However, interpreting vascular anatomy on a series of cross-sectional images on a light box is cumbersome and prone to inaccuracies. The overall geometry of the investigated vascular region is difficult to perceive due to the obliquity and tortuosity of the vascular structures relative to the axial slices. For the same reason, detection and grading of stenoses on the axial slices alone can be difficult. To overcome these limitations different postprocessing procedures can be performed on the CT operator console or alternatively, off-line, on a dedicated workstation [8].

Cine Display

The entire stack of overlapping axial slices can be loaded into image memory, and can be subsequently displayed in interactive cine mode. Perception of vascular anatomy is more intuitive, and the time needed to examine a large stack of slices is markedly reduced. By tracking the vascular structures in the craniocaudal direction of the data set, focal abnormalities can be searched for, and the optimal level for assessment of disease severity is easily found.

Multiplanar Reformatting

The stack of overlapping axial slices can be reconstructed along any desired plane by using a multiplanar reformatting (MPR) algorithm. Coronal and sagittal reformations are valuable in displaying longitudinal vascular structures such as the aorta. More recent algorithms allow curved and curved-oblique reformations. Using these algorithms, reformatting along the tortuous course of a vessel results in display of the full extent of the vessel in a single image.

Although informative, some limitations are inherent to MPR. Spatial resolution of the reformations is a resultant of in-plane resolution in the axial slices and longitudinal resolution, defined by collimation, table speed, and reconstruction index. Because in-plane resolution is markedly superior to longitudinal resolution, definition of vascular detail will be low if the course of the vessel deviates significantly from the longitudinal axis. Also, if MPR is used for grading of stenoses, off-axis reformations will result in overestimation of stenoses, while eccentric stenoses can be underestimated by inappropriately chosen reformation planes.

Maximum Intensity Projection

With a maximum intensity projection algorithm (MIP), angiogram-type display is achieved. The entire stack of transverse images is loaded into computer memory and a set of parallel mathematical rays traverses the data volume. Every ray identifies the voxel with the highest CT density (HU or Houndsfield Unit) along its path and displays it on a projection plane perpendicular to the rays. Because a single MIP lacks depth, a cine loop can be created, built up of multiple projections with increasing serial angulation. The resulting display is comparable to that of conventional angiography, but allows an infinite number of projections. In order to be displayed, the vessel of interest should have the highest number of HUs along the path of the imaginary projection rays. Consequently, bone or densely enhanced veins can obscure arterial lumina. To solve this problem, bone or veins can be removed from the axial slices by manual or semiautomatic editing.

The use of MIP to display CTA data has advantages and disadvantages. MIP provides an efficient means of conveying a survey of the anatomic data because all the vascular structures with sufficient density are displayed in the projections. Another advantage of MIP is its relative insensitivity to partial volume averaging.

If a vessel follows a tortuous course, its transverse segments will suffer significantly from volume averaging due to relatively low resolution along the Z-axis. The HU values in such transverse segments will represent a mixture of luminal contrast and a significant portion of surrounding soft tissue and fat. Conversely, longitudinally oriented segments of the vessel will suffer less from volume averaging, and the HU values will represent luminal contrast, with only a small fraction of surrounding soft tissue and fat. As a result, HU values, equivalent to CT density, can vary greatly among different vessels filled with the same concentration of contrast, depending on their relative size and orientation with respect to the transverse plane. Consequently, MIPs display a tortuous vessel with varying densities, higher in its vertical segments and lower in its horizontal segments. Interpretation of MIPs of medium-sized and large arteries is not affected by this phenomenon, because the difference in density is not interpreted as a difference in luminal diameter. Only in transverse vessels with a diameter significantly smaller than the collimation and table speed, volume averaging may result in poor or nonvisualization of these vessels on MIP.

A limitation inherent in MIP is the need to remove overlying structures with densities equal to or higher than the vessels of interest. This editing process is time consuming and may result in partial loss of anatomic information.

Shaded Surface Display

Shaded surface display (SSD) is a surface-rendering algorithm, which results in three-dimensional renderings of the surfaces of the structures of interest. In contrast to MIP, an HU threshold is chosen, dividing the continuous scale of HUs in a binary data set of values above and below the threshold. All voxels with densities below the threshold will be excluded from the reconstruction, and all voxels with densities above the threshold will be included.

Similar to MIPs, SSDs vividly display the vascular anatomy in a single image. However, apparent vessel size is strongly dependent on the chosen threshold, creating a significant subjective element in the procedure. Due to volume averaging, vertical segments of a vessel will be displayed wider than horizontal parts. Also, since all anatomic structures with a density above the threshold will be included in the SSD, plaque calcification can be displayed as part of the vessel lumen, resulting in underestimation of stenoses. Manual editing of the axial slices can prevent the inclusion of calcified plaque in the lumen, but such editing is time consuming and adds another subjective element to the resultant surface renderings.

Conclusions

Cine display and MPR are efficient means of presenting the information contained in the axial slices. MIP and SSD are postprocessing algorithms which require operator time and input, and result in overall images of vascular anatomy. An important difference between SSDs and MIPs is that in the latter no threshold is used; all pixels are shown with a density according to their original HU value. Conversely, in SSD, HU values are reduced to a binary data set in which each pixel either belongs to the volume of interest or is excluded.

Clinical Applications

CT Angiography in Carotid Artery Disease

Diagnostic Issues

Atherosclerotic carotid artery changes are a major cause of intracranial thromboembolic disease. Detection and quantification of carotid artery disease has gained renewed clinical interest due to the striking sixfold stroke reduction after endarterectomy in comparison with medical treatment alone in patients, with a diameter reduction of 70 % – 99 %, as reported in the interim results of the NASCET and ECST studies [9, 10]. The demonstrated beneficial effects of carotid surgery in patients with severe stenoses calls for a vascular imaging technique which is accurate in identifying patients with severe stenoses, and carries minimal risk to the patient.

The standard of reference in grading severity of carotid stenoses is selective angiography. However, this invasive technique carries a risk of permanent neurologic damage, ranging from 0.09 %

as reported in a nonselected group of patients with cerebral angiography, to 4 % as reported in patients with atherosclerotic carotid disease, in whom a stenosis above 30 % was suspected on the basis of color Doppler ultrasound examination [11, 12]. Furthermore, a selective carotid angiogram costs between US $3000 and $6000, leading to an estimated annual total in the range of US $500 million dollars for the United States health care system (D.E. Strandness, personal communication).

The risk of serious complications and the high cost of carotid angiography have stimulated the development of noninvasive techniques for carotid disease evaluation. Noninvasive carotid imaging will have to answer three questions successfully in order to replace selective angiography: (1) does it identify patients with 70 % – 99 % stenoses accurately, (2) does it distinguish complete occlusion from severe stenosis, and (3) does it demonstrate tandem lesions in the carotid circulation? [13].

Ad (1) High sensitivity is required to identify all patients who may benefit from carotid endarterectomy. High specificity is required to prevent exposure of patients with minimal or moderate stenoses to the risk of surgery, for whom benefit from endarterectomy has not yet been proven (in the NASCET study perioperative morbidity in the surgical group was 5.5 % compared with 3.3 % in the same time interval in the medical group) [9].

Ad (3) The therapeutic implications of coexisting severe stenoses in the intracranial carotid circulation are a controversial matter. Some argue that in the presence of such stenoses surgery should not be performed, while others have not been able to demonstrate disadvantageous outcomes in these patients [13, 14]. The need to demonstrate tandem lesions is to be approached in the context of a low prevalence of such disease; in the NASCET study only 7 of 659 patients with severe carotid stenoses demonstrated significant intracranial vascular disease: 4 severe stenoses and 3 aneurysms [9].

Acquisition Technique

Atherosclerotic disease of the carotid arteries is invariably located at the level of the carotid bifurcation and in the proximal internal carotid artery. Disease can be limited to a short segment, and in the presence of more extensive disease the point of maximum stenosis may be short. The existence of a predeliction site of disease allows for a standardized acquisition protocol, whereas detection of short stenoses requires thin slices.

In our hospital the following acquisition technique is used: a lateral scout view identifies the lower border of the sixth cervical vertebral body. From this level upward 50 consecutive rotations are acquired; collimation, 3 mm; table speed, 3 mm/s; reconstruction index, 2 mm, 120 kVp, 250 mAs; FOV, 160 mm; matrix, 512. Contrast injection: 150 ml nonionic contrast (300 mg I/ml), injected at 2.5 ml/s; scanning is started after a delay of 25 s. In order to prevent motion artifacts, patients are instructed to breathe quietly and to avoid swallowing. With this protocol a craniocaudal distance of 15 cm is covered, and a survey of the carotid bifurcation and the larger part of the extracranial internal carotid is obtained (Fig. 1). We have recently started experimenting with 1.5 mm collimation, 1.5 mm/s table speed, and a reconstruction index of 1 mm. This technique provides improved depiction of short stenoses; however, a distance of only 7.5 cm can be covered, visualizing only the carotid bifurcation and the most proximal part of the internal carotid.

Display

The reconstructed axial slices can be studied on film on a light box or viewed in interactive cine mode on a workstation, the latter being more efficient, allowing for rapid identification of the carotid bifurcation and the region of maximum luminal reduction. MPRs can be created, preferably along the course of the internal carotid. Alternatively, the axial slices can be postprocessed on- or off-line to generate MIPs or SSDs. Both techniques generate a survey of the carotid circulation in one image, which can be rotated to demonstrate the most severe luminal reduction.

With all techniques difficulties are experienced in assessing the severity of stenoses (Fig. 1). The axial slices are difficult to read if the stenotic carotid segment is oblique with respect to the transverse plane. Also, the window width and window level of the images will affect the diameter of the apparent lumen. MPR along the course of the carotid is very sensitive to proper placement of the reformatting plane, which may result in over- or underestimation of stenoses. MIP readily differentiates calcified plaque from luminal contrast.

However, calcified plaque at the site of maximum narrowing may obscure the lumen, preventing accurate assessment of the luminal diameter. The results of SSD rely heavily on the selected threshold value. If too low a threshold is chosen, stenosis will be underestimated, and vice versa. Also, if a single threshold value is used instead of a threshold range, calcified plaque is included in the lumen and stenosis is underestimated. Calcified plaque can be manually removed to improve MIP and SSD reconstructions, but such removal is time consuming and, to some extent, operator dependent.

Clinical Results

The first reported studies on CTA of the carotids differ in their methods and conclusion. In two separate studies [15, 16] SSD was used to grade carotid stenosis into four categories: mild, moderate, severe, and occluded. Consensus readings of SSDs and angiograms demonstrated an overall agreement of 92 % and 82 %, respectively; and no readings differed by more than one category. Schwartz et al. used the attenuation value of the lumen at the level of maximum stenosis to define the threshold, while Dillon et al. derived a threshold by comparing the luminal density of a normal region with the HU value of the sternocleidomastoid muscle, representing the density of unenhanced vessel wall. In a third study, Marks et al. performed MIPs and angiograms on 28 carotids and found overall agreement in grading of stenoses of 89 % [17]. All three studies concluded that CTA is a promising noninvasive technique for detecting and grading carotid stenoses.

In contrast to these studies, Castillo reported agreement of only 50 % in a study comparing MIPs with angiograms in ten patients [18]. However, his technique was limited by a collimation of 5 mm, a table speed of 5 mm/s, and a very short scan delay of 10 s.

Recently, 5 observers compared interactive cine mode, MIP, and SSD with the same CTA acquisitions (3 mm slice thickness) with selective angiograms in 49 carotids (Polman, unpublished data). Interactive cine mode demonstrated the best overall performance as measured by receiver operating characteristic (ROC) analysis (AUC, 0.82), but also the lowest interobserver agreement (K, 0.62), demonstrating a substantial learning curve. Very short stenoses were consis-

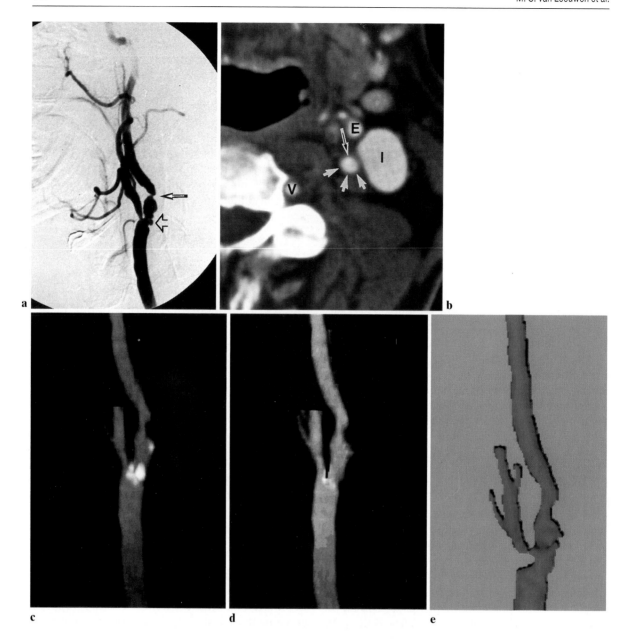

Fig. 1 a–l. Selective carotid angiogram and CTA with 3 mm and 1.5 mm collimation in a patient with severe stenosis in the left internal carotid artery. **a** Angiogram demonstrates ulcerated plaque in the bifurcation *(open arrow)*, stenosis of the external carotid, and, more distally, severe stenosis in the internal carotid *(black and white arrow)*. **b** Three-millimeter section of the stenosis in the internal carotid. Averaging due to 3 mm collimation results in a summation of stenosis *(black and white arrow)* and distal wider lumen *(short arrows); E,* external carotid; *I,* jugular vein; *V,* vertebral artery. **c** MIP demonstrates circumferential calcification at the level of the bifurcation, preventing accurate assessment of the lumen. **d** After removal of calcification by manual editing, the lumen is better visualized. On MIP, the stenosis in the internal carotid is underestimated due to averaging. **e** SSD also underestimates the stenosis due to averaging. No image of the 3-mm data demonstrates the ulcer.

Two weeks later, the same patient underwent CTA with 1.5 mm collimation, 1.5 mm/s table speed, and 1 mm re-

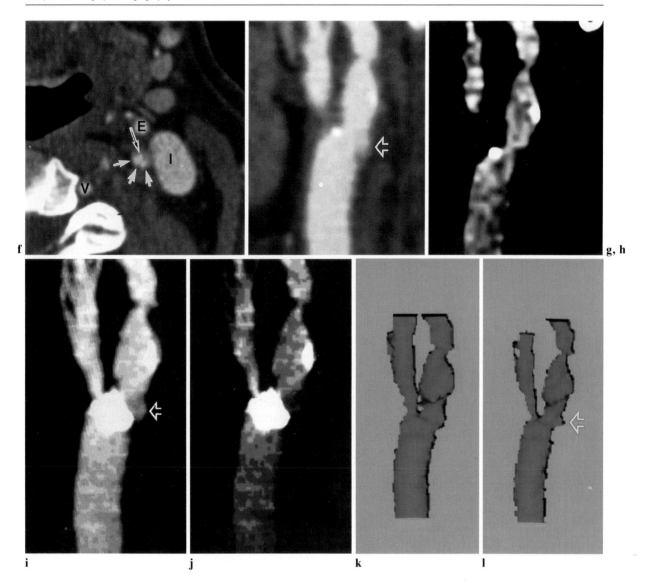

f

g, h

i   j   k   l

construction index. **f** Axial slice demonstrates severe stenosis *(black and white arrow)* and part of distal, poststenotic internal carotid *(short arrows)* in one image (cf. Fig. 1 b). **g** Curved sagittal MPR of the carotid bifurcation demonstrates the stenosis and suggests the ulcer *(open arrow)*. **g, h** The severity of stenosis on MPR is affected by the window width and window level, the narrow window **(h)** demonstrating the severity of stenosis more realistically. **i, j** Unedited MIP of the 1.5-mm slices is affected by window width and level in the same manner as MPR. The ulcer is best depicted on the wide window setting **(i)**, whereas the severity of the stenosis is best depicted on the narrow window setting **(j)**. **k, l** Two SSDs, one with a low **(k)** and one with a higher threshold **(l)**. The calcification at the bifurcation was removed by manual editing. A higher threshold results in a more severe stenosis. Note that the ulcer *(open arrow)* is best depicted on the high-threshold SSD

tently underestimated by one category with all three display techniques. These results have prompted us to explore the use of 1.5 mm collimation and 1.5 mm/s table speed to minimize volume averaging in short stenoses, and to further optimize the use of the interactive cine mode.

Circle of Willis CTA

Diagnostic Issues

In 75% of patients with subarachnoid hemorrhage (SAH), a ruptured saccular aneurysm is the cause of bleeding. The disease carries a poor prognosis with a mortality rate of around 50%, half of which die within the first 24 h [19, 20]. A high morbidity characterizes the surviving patients, with only 26% – 58% achieving good recovery [19–21]. The leading causes of death and disability, besides the direct effects of the initial hemorrhage, are vasospasm and rebleeding.

Vasospasm occurs in up to 50% of patients [22]. The incidence of vasospasm increases daily in the first 7 days with a maximum in the 4- to 14-day period [21, 22]. However, only minimal vasospasm or none is seen on initial angiography in more than 90% of patients during the first 4 days [21].

Rebleeding occurs in 22% of patients, 70% of which occurs during the first 6 h, and 88% within 24 h [19]. Rebleeding is associated with a very high mortality (75%) compared with those that do not rebleed (39%). According to Inagawa et al. [19], rebleeding is not related to age or sex of patients, shape or size of aneurysm, or even blood pressure on admission. Angiography increases the risk of rebleeding, especially in the first 6 h [19].

Early surgery (0–3 days), prior to the peak period of vasospasm, will reduce the risk of rebleeding and permit more aggressive treatment of vasospasm with hypertensive and hypervolemic therapy [19, 23]. However, in a large, nonrandomized study early surgery lowered the rate of rebleeding but did not prevent vasospasm [23]. No distinct difference in overall outcome of early surgery (0–3 days) compared with delayed surgery (11–14 days) was found. Only in the intermediate period was the outcome worse. Patients who were alert on admission had the most favorable outcome with early surgery. A smaller, randomized study also showed no significant difference between early and late surgery [24]. Early

surgery will become more advantageous if the management of vasospasm becomes more effective. Also, "very early surgery", i.e., within hours after admission, can potentially prevent the large amount of rebleeding which occurs in the first 6 h.

Angiography is still the method of choice for detecting aneurysms. The goals of the examination are: identification of the ruptured aneurysm, location of the neck and parent artery, identification of multiple aneurysms, detection of vasospasm, and assessment of the patency of the circle of Willis. Angiography identifies an aneurysm in approximately 85% of patients [20]. A false-negative angiogram can be due to vasospasm and should be repeated in 1–2 weeks. The majority (78%) of aneurysms are small (<12 mm) [21]. Up to 25% of patients demonstrate multiple aneurysms; therefore three- to four-vessel angiography is needed. Most aneurysms arise from the anterior communicating artery, the internal carotid artery, and the middle cerebral artery. In 4% – 10% a vertebrobasilar aneurysm is present.

Computed tomography angiography offers the possibility of a quick and noninvasive examination. Ideally, it should provide an expedient diagnosis, obviating the need for angiography in selected patients, subsequently making earlier surgery possible. Probably, CTA cannot reliably identify vasospasm, however, spasm is absent or only minimally present in 90% of patients in the first few days.

Acquisition Technique

The vessels which constitute the circle of Willis are small, more or less parallel to the scanning plane, and located close to the bony structures of the skull base and sella turcica. In addition, the size of aneurysms is often in the millimeter range. Therefore, maximal spatial resolution is required and thin slices and optimal contrast enhancement are essential.

We use the following protocol in patients with SAH: a lateral scout identifies the dorsum sellae. The circle of Willis is presumed to be located 0.5 cm above the dorsum sellae. A scan plan is set to include the region 3 cm below to 3 cm above the presumed level of the circle of Willis: technique, 40 rotations; collimation, 1.5 mm; table speed, 1.5 mm/s; reconstruction index, 1 mm, 140 kVp, 125 mAs; FOV, 160 mm; matrix, 512. Contrast injection is 180 ml nonionic contrast (300 mg I/ml), injected at 4 ml/s; scanning is started after a delay of 25 s. Patients are instructed to breathe calmly and to avoid swallowing.

Display

The axial slices can be viewed on film, or interactively in cine mode. On the axial slices, identification of the vascular segments is difficult, and cine mode is helpful. Also, differentiation between small vessels, very tortuous vessels, and small aneurysms may be difficult.

A survey of the willisian circulation can be created with MIP or SSD (Fig. 2). The varying obliquity of the vessels in and around the circle will result in different appearances on the MIP and SSD images. On MIP in-plane vessels are less sharply delineated and of lesser density than longitudinally oriented vessels. Also, due to the principle of MIP, wider vessels with resulting high density will obscure thinner vessels with resulting lower density. Superpositioning of surrounding bony structures is to be remedied by manual or semiautomatic editing. SSD images will overestimate the vessel diameter in vertical parts, and simulate spasm due to diminished diameter in the horizontal parts. Adjacent vessels may seem to fuse due to partial volume effects.

Clinical Results

Few studies have described CT as a diagnostic technique for identification of cerebral aneurysms. In 1987, before the introduction of helical CT, Schmid et al. described a study of 102 consecutive patients, with suspected aneurysm of the cerebral arteries [25]. After a noncontrast CT of the skull, 12–20 1.5-mm slices were taken during administration of 100 ml contrast. MPR was used to create sagittal and coronal reconstructions of a possible aneurysm. With this technique the authors were able to visualize 71/76 (93.4%) aneurysms prospectively and 74/76 (97.4%) retrospectively. In three patients an aneurysm was falsely suspected.

Recently, Aoki et al. used helical CT (1.5 mm collimation and 1.5 mm/s table speed) in 15 patients with clinically suspected cerebral aneurysms [26]. Using a threshold of 100 HUs, SSDs were constructed, without deleting bone. With this tech-

nique they were able to detect all (15/15) aneurysms and demonstrate their necks and the parent arteries. In one patient an aneurysm was falsely suspected, at a location where angiography demonstrated a small, tortuous vessel.

Napel et al. [1] used MIP to visualize CTA data from the circle of Willis. They used semiautomatic bone removal and were able to consistently visualize the intracranial part of the internal carotid, including its intracavernous course and the cerebral arteries, beyond the A1 and M1 segments. They argued that MIP is superior to SSD in circle of Willis visualization since it is less susceptible to the effects of volume averaging.

The studies cited agree that CTA of the circle of Willis can be used for early diagnosis and location of cerebral aneurysms in patients with SAH. Schmid et al. described three conditions where CTA alone is sufficient for preoperative evaluation: (1) adequate identification of the aneurysm, parent vessel, and complete circle of Willis; (2) identification of a temporal hematoma around an aneurysm in the middle cerebral artery in deteriorating patients; and (3) detection of an aneurysm of the posterior communicating artery in patients with oculomotor nerve palsy [25].

With the current helical scanners and the variety of postprocessing algorithms available, it can be expected that, in the near future, a substantial percentage of patients with SAH can be operated upon as soon as CTA, performed on admission, has demonstrated sufficient anatomic information.

CT Angiography in Pulmonary Embolism

Diagnostic Issues

Pulmonary embolism (PE) is a common disease entity with an estimated incidence in, for example, the United States of 630000 cases annually [27]. It is lethal in 30% of untreated patients. Administration of adequate anticoagulant therapy can lower the mortality rate to 8%. However, the estimated complication risk of such therapy totals 32%, 13% being severe bleedings [28]. Consequently, a sensitive and a specific diagnostic test for the detection of PE is needed.

In patients with clinically suspected PE, ventilation/perfusion (V/Q) scanning is often used as the screening test. The sensitivity of the perfusion scan is 98% in the detection of PE. Specificity is less: in high-probability V/Q scans, PE is found in

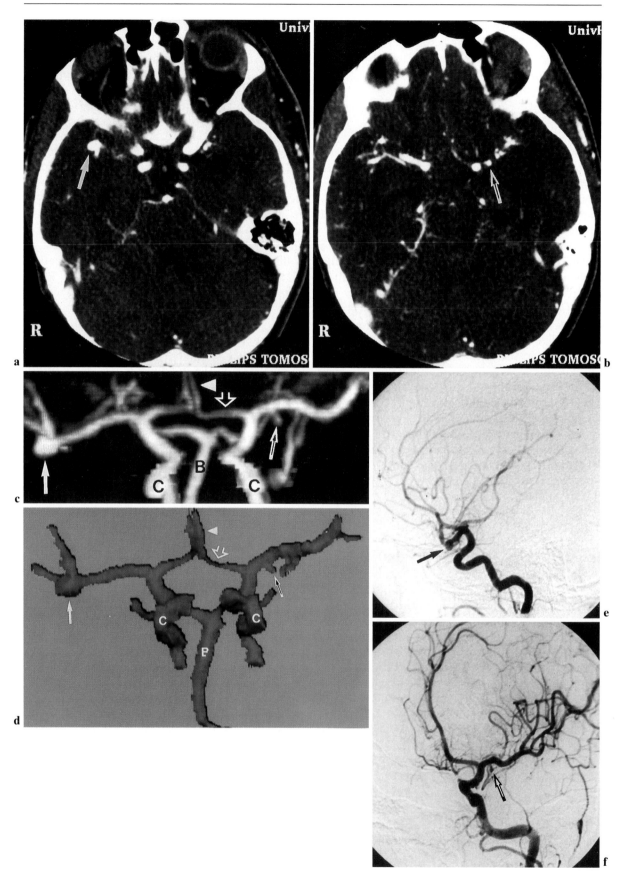

only 88%, and in indeterminate V/Q scans the prevalence of PE is reported to be 33% [29]. Therefore, pulmonary angiography is often needed to confirm PE in the large group of patients with indeterminate V/Q scans. Pulmonary angiography is reliable in detecting emboli in segmental, lobar, and main pulmonary arteries. However, it is an expensive and invasive test with 2.7% morbidity and 0.2% mortality [30].

The rapid acquisition of helical CT enables direct, noninvasive visualization of pulmonary emboli. Clinical studies indicate that helical CT may be an ideal tool in the diagnosis of PE, preventing the need for V/Q scans and largely replacing pulmonary angiography.

Acquisition and Display Technique

The central part of the pulmonary arterial system is located below the level of the aortic arch and above the domes of the diaphragm. In most patients this region can be covered with 24–30 rotations with the following technique: collimation, 5 mm; table speed, 5 mm/s; reconstruction index, 3 mm. Scans are made during breath-hold, or shallow respiration. To prevent streak artifacts a contrast agent with a concentration of 12% iodide can be used, totaling 120 ml, administered at an injection rate of 7 ml/s [31]. In patients with possible pulmonary hypertension or right ventricular failure a contrast agent with a concentration of

◀ **Fig. 2 a–f.** CTA and selective angiography in a patient with suspected aneurysm. **a, b** On the axial slices a large aneurysm *(white arrow)* at the end of the right M1 segment is demonstrated. The left M1 segment demonstrates a small, caudally directed aneurysm *(black and white arrow)*. **c, d** MIP **(c)** and SSD **(d)** of the willisian circulation. On the axial slices bone was removed by manual editing. The threshold for SSD was adjusted to demonstrate the circle of Willis optimally. Both aneurysms *(arrows)* are displayed clearly on the MIP and SSD images. Note how partial volume averaging affects the MIP and SSD display of the anterior cerebral arteries. The horizontal A1 segments *(open arrow)* are affected by volume averaging due to their relatively small diameter compared with the 1.5 mm slice thickness. As a result, the A1 segments are depicted less brightly on MIP, and of a smaller diameter on SSD, compared to the vertical A2 segments *(arrowhead)*. The closely adjacent, vertical A2 segments appear to be fused on SSD due to in-plane volume averaging, but are clearly separated on MIP. **e, f** Selective right and left carotid angiogram demonstrates the aneurysms *(arrows)*, which were both successfully clipped

30% iodide can be used, totaling 90 ml, injected at a rate of 5 ml/s. Scanning is started 10 s after the beginning of contrast administration.

The overlapping axial slices are best visualized in interactive cine mode. To date, postprocessing algorithms seem to offer no advantage over axial slices.

Clinical Results

Several studies have described the CT appearance of PE [32–41]. However, only recently have attempts been made to define the role of CT in patients with suspected PE, as reported in two studies [31, 42].

Remy-Jardin evaluated 42 patients suspected of PE with contrast-enhanced helical scanning and selective pulmonary angiography [31]. Detection of central PE included analysis of the main, lobar, and segmental pulmonary arteries. Partial filling defects, complete filling defects, and the "railway track" sign (thromboembolic masses surrounded by contrast) were recorded. Overall quality of vascular opacification was insufficient in one case (2%) and good or excellent in 98%. Twenty-two pulmonary arteries in six patients were not interpretable due to their oblique ($n = 19$) or parallel course ($n = 3$) relative to the scan plane. Central pulmonary thromboembolism was excluded in 23 patients with helical CT, which was confirmed by pulmonary angiography. In 19 patients, CT demonstrated pulmonary embolism which was confirmed angiographically in 18 patients. In the only false-positive CT, angiography demonstrated asymmetry in pulmonary vascular opacification due to increased pulmonary arterial resistance on the left side in a trauma patient with ipsilateral pleural effusion and parenchymal consolidation.

Teigen et al. reported 86 patients studied with electronic beam CT [42]. Of all the anatomic zones, visualization was considered adequate in 96%. Among the 86 patients, CT was considered positive for PE in 39 and negative in 47 patients. Pulmonary angiography, V/Q scintigraphy, and surgical or autopsy findings were used as a reference standard. Sensitivity and specificity were not established; yet the authors felt that electron beam CT has the potential to become a primary non-invasive examination for PE.

Precise knowledge of the anatomy of the bronchovascular system is necessary for proper interpretation of CT studies of pulmonary vessels. The presence of intersegmental lymph nodes and apparent filling defects in small pulmonary veins in the upper lobes may mimic the appearance of segmental arterial emboli. Perivascular edema can be misinterpreted as chronic embolic material. Imaging of vessels parallel to the scan plane is problematic due to volume averaging.

It seems logical that CTA might supplant V/Q scintigraphy as the screening tool of choice in suspected pulmonary embolism. Furthermore, CTA seems an attractive imaging technique for follow-up of patients with central thromboembolism after anticoagulant or lytic therapy. An important advantage of CTA is that other intrathoracic pathology is accurately depicted on CT.

However, large prospective studies, focussing on patient outcome, are needed to reduce the need for V/Q scanning and pulmonary angiography in patients with clinically suspected PE.

CT Angiography in Aortic Disease

Diagnostic Issues

Suspected aneurysmal disease or aortic dissection are the most frequent indication for aortic imaging. The length and maximal width of the luminal and thrombotic part of the aortic aneurysm and the relationship to renal and visceral arteries constitute the key concern for the surgeon. Furthermore, elongation of the aorta and iliacal vessels, location and extent of mural thrombus, calcification, and coexisting periaortic pathology can influence surgical planning.

In aortic dissections the precise extent of the dissecting hematoma needs to be assessed. The primary laceration is frequently located in the ascending aorta or at the junction of the aortic arch and descending aorta. From the site of primary laceration, the false lumen can extend distally over a varying distance; retrograde extension of the false passage is usually limited. Extension of the dissection into aortic side branches, with possible impairment of blood flow, rupture into the pericardial sac, and aortic insufficiency are the major sequelae of dissection.

Angiography is often used to evaluate aortic disease. Disadvantages are the examination time, relatively high cost, and invasiveness of the procedure, with the risk of complications. The number of possible projections is limited and periaortic pathology is not visualized.

Already, CTA has proved to be very useful in the visualization of the thoracic and abdominal aorta. It is a rapid, minimally invasive diagnostic test, which can be performed as an outpatient procedure and can demonstrate the vast majority of anatomic information needed for patient management (Fig. 3).

Acquisition Technique

The scanning parameters used for CTA of the aorta are defined by the length of the region of interest. In thoracic scans a collimation of 10 mm and a table speed of 10 mm/s is used with a reconstruction index of 5 mm. If only the ascending aorta, the aortic arch, and the proximal part of the descending aorta need to be visualized, a slice thickness of 5 mm with a reconstruction index of 2 mm is used. Abdominal scans are performed with a slice thickness of 5 mm and a reconstruction index of 2 mm and the FOV is adjusted to include the aneurysm and the kidneys. In all three acquisitions 140 ml of a nonionic contrast agent is injected at a rate of 2 ml/s. Scanning is started 20–30 s after the beginning of contrast injection, depending on whether the thoracic or abdominal aorta is examined. Patients are instructed to hyperventilate before, and hold their breath during, the acquisition.

One of the issues in CTA of the aorta is the timing of the contrast bolus throughout the entire scanning period. Some institutes assess the individual circulation time with a continuous scan at a single level after infusion of a small amount of contrast (± 20 m) at a flow rate of 3 ml/s. The elapsed time till peak enhancement is measured and the individual scan delay is adjusted accordingly. However, with the protocol used at our institute with a fixed 20- or 30-s scan delay, the thoracic and abdominal aorta and surrounding pathology are well opacified in the vast majority of patients.

Display

Images can be reviewed on a workstation in cine mode, which demonstrates best the advantages of volumetric scanning. The whole extent of the thoracic and abdominal aorta can be displayed smoothly, and aortic branches are easily tracked. In this way most anatomic and pathologic find-

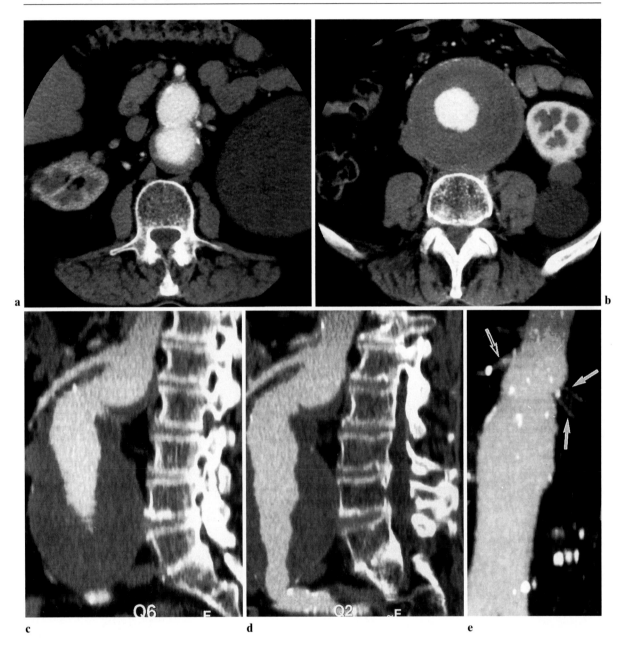

Fig. 3 a–e. Preoperative CTA in a patient with abdominal aneurysm. **a, b** Axial slices at the cranial end and at the level of the largest transverse diameter. **c, d** Sagittal and curved sagittal MPR. The curved reformat is made along the center of the aortic lumen, which is marked on the orthogonal MPRs. The advantage of curved MPR is that it can display the full extent of the aneurysm in one image. **e** MIP is not very useful in aneurysms. Thrombus is not visualized and the origin of the aortic branches is often superimposed on the aortic lumen (*white arrows,* branches of left renal artery; *black and white arrow,* right renal artery). **f–i** Different SSDs of the aneurysm

ings, such as extension of the aneurysm, relation to renal arteries, and size of mural thrombus, can be demonstrated. In the presence of dissection, intimal flaps and true and false lumina are displayed well.

Multiplanar reformats with orthogonal and curved reconstructions are of good quality due to the overlapping slices. A curved reconstruction demonstrates a survey of the extent of the aneurysm or dissection, and the relative position of mural thrombus, calcifications, and intimal flaps.

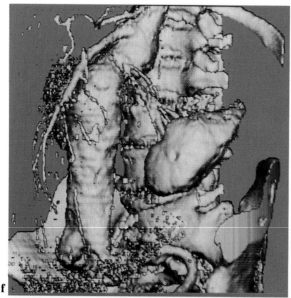

f

Fig. 3. f Left anterior oblique (LAO) projection. If no editing is performed, thrombus is not visualized and structures with equal or higher density, like bone and kidney, are all displayed. **g–i** Anteroposterior, LAO, and left lateral projection. After editing, thrombus *(yellow)* and lumen *(red)* can be individually displayed without surrounding structures, allowing assessment of the origins of the right *(black and white arrow)* and left *(white arrows)* renal arteries relative to the thrombus and the luminal dilatation. Note the elongation of the iliac arteries

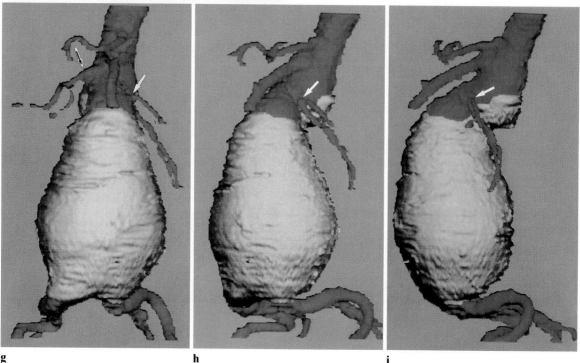

g   h   i

Three-dimensional renderings, such as SSD or MIP, provide the surgeon with anatomic information in a single image, which is important for pre-operative planning. SSDs demonstrate the opacified aorta and its branches together with bony structures, such as spine and pelvis. Because the threshold is selected by the operator, loss of information is possible. The density of mural thrombus is almost equal to that of soft tissue, which makes automatic reconstruction impossible. To obtain images with mural thrombus in relation to aortic lumen and aortic branches manual editing is necessary, which is time consuming.

In MIP no threshold is used, and lumen and calcifications are easily distinguished. Like SSDs, MIPs require suppression of bony structures and manual editing is needed to remove them.

Clinical Results

CT angiography of the aorta can be performed in an outpatient setting, and is less invasive, less costly, much quicker, and often more informative in comparison to conventional angiography. Rubin et al. [2] mentioned consistent imaging of second-to-fourth order aortic branches and good correlation with conventional angiography. All the major aortic branches were clearly demonstrated, except in-plane vessels with severe stenosis.

Costello et al. [43] examined 19 patients with suspected abdominal aneurysmal disease and demonstrated aortic aneurysms in 16 cases. Angiography was available in seven patients, in whom the extent of the aneurysm and the number and location of renal arteries were confirmed. Differential opacification of true and false lumens were also well displayed with CTA, although only a small amount of contrast was used prior to a 24-s thoracic scan [44].

Balm et al. [45] mentioned MPR as a valuable tool for evaluating the craniocaudal appearance of aortic pathology. In complex cases such as supra- and juxtarenal aneurysms, recurrent aneurysms, dissections, and anatomic variants, SSDs were more useful.

At our institute CTA has become the examination of choice for abdominal aneurysms and thoracoabdominal dissections. Contrary to conventional angiography, CTA demonstrates mural thrombus, aortic calcifications, and additional abnormalitie such as perianeurysmal fibrosis and hematomas. In most cases two-dimensional viewing functions, i.e., cine mode and MPR, are sufficient to obtain the anatomic information the surgeon needs for preoperative evaluation.

CTA provides all the information needed for minimal invasive aneurysmal repair by means of a percutaneously inserted endovascular prosthesis. Accurate measurements of the aortic aneurysm, necessary for a made-to-measure endovascular prosthesis, can be made with a curved multiplanar reformat based on a line positioned centrally in the aorta. Reconstructions parallel and perpendicular to this curve provide projections which best demonstrate the true diameter and length of the aneurysm. SSDs are used in case of elongation of the aorta and iliacs and to visualize the extent of luminal dilatation in relation to mural thrombus and aortic branches.

CT Angiography in Renal Artery Stenosis

Diagnostic Issues

Renal artery stenosis (RAS) is a potentially curable cause of hypertension, with a prevalence of less than 5 % in patients with arterial hypertension. Stenoses in excess of 50 % are considered hemodynamically significant. Due to the large number of patients with hypertension and the small percentage of patients with RAS, a heavy burden is placed on diagnostic workup. A high sensitivity is required to find and subsequently treat all the patients with RAS, and a relatively high specificity is needed to prevent unnecessary invasive procedures in the large group of patients with hypertension. Angiography is not suited as a screening procedure due to its invasiveness and cost. Less invasive procedures such as duplex Doppler and magnetic resonance (MR) angiography have not reached the required high sensitivity and specificity as yet. Captopril renography is a good screening test for RAS, but does not provide anatomic information.

Preliminary studies indicate that CTA of the renal arteries may be sufficiently accurate in the detection and grading of RAS to be used as a screening procedure.

Acquisition Technique

The relatively small size, transverse course, variable craniocaudal location, and frequent plurality of renal arteries require an optimal scanning technique [46].

The location and number of renal arteries can be appreciated on a noncontrast scan from the level of Th12 downward. Subsequent optimal contrast enhancement requires assessment of the individual transit time at the level of the renal arteries. Galanski et al. report that the measured time from the start of the test injection to peak enhancement should be increased by 5 s to allow for the longer injection time needed for the larger contrast volume. The actual CTA acquisition is started at the origin of the superior mesenteric artery. Between 100 and 150 ml nonionic contrast (300 mg I/ml) is injected at 3–5 ml/s. Patients with a body weight above 60 kg receive 150 ml at 3.5 ml/s, and 2.5 ml/kg contrast is given to patients of less than 60 kg body wt. In young patients with a transit time below 15 s, injection rate is increased to 5 ml/s to compensate for the increased dilution caused by their higher cardiac output.

Collimation and table speed are kept as low as possible to minimize partial volume averaging. Galanski et al. report good results with a standard 2-mm slice thickness and a reconstruction index of 1 mm. This can be increased to 3 mm slice thickness and a reconstruction index of 2 mm in obese patients and in patients in whom a larger craniocaudal distance has to be scanned because of suspected accessory renal arteries on the non-contrast scan.

Display

Interactive cine mode of the axial slices, MPR, SSD, and MIP can all be used to view the volumetric data (Fig. 4). MPR is most informative if a curved reconstruction is made along the often tortuous course of the renal artery. The highest spatial resolution is the in-plane resolution of the axial slices. Consequently, luminal diameter is best judged on these images. However, if the course of the vessel at the point of stenosis is oblique with respect to the scan plane, interpretation is difficult and curved MPR, MIP, or SSD may be useful.

If SSD is used, a threshold has to be chosen, which best fits the individual enhancement level. Due to partial volume effects, small calcifications may be erroneously represented as part of the lumen, leading to underestimation of stenosis. In MIPs, bone has to be removed by manual editing. The enhancing aortic lumen or calcified plaque in aortic plaque may be superimposed on the origins of renal arteries, precluding accurate assessment of luminal diameter.

Clinical Results

Galanski et al. prospectively examined 22 patients with suspected renovascular hypertension with CTA and intraarterial digital subtraction angiography (DSA) [46]. Postprocessing was performed to create MPRs, MIPs, and SSDs. Renal arteries were examined on the axial slices, MPRs, MIPs, and SSDs and each renal artery was graded 0–4: 0, no stenosis; 1, mild stenosis (<50 %); 2, moderate stenosis (50 % – 75 %); 3, severe stenosis (76 % – 99 %); and 4, occlusion.

Contrast enhancement was good or excellent in 19/22 patients. In 5 patients 11 accessory arteries

were present on DSA and all were detected on CTA. Twenty-two arteries in 15 patients demonstrated RAS or occlusion of a renal artery on DSA, and all were correctly detected and localized with CTA. In 4/22 stenoses a difference in CTA and DSA grading of stenosis occurred. Two stenoses were underestimated (grade 2 on CTA, grade 3 on DSA), one case of fibromuscular hyperplasia was overestimated (grade 3 on CTA, grade 2 on DSA), and one short occlusion with well-developed collateral circulation was graded as grade 3 stenosis.

The authors report that the axial slices are the most important display mode. In 15 of 22 patients the axial slices alone were conclusive. The combination of interactive cine display and curved MPR yielded almost the same results as all four viewing modalities combined. Only one grade 2 ostial stenosis was underestimated as grade 1 and correctly diagnosed as grade 2 with MIP.

The quality of MIP images depended on vessel enhancement, size, course with respect to the scan plane, and differentiation of renal arteries from overlying enhancing veins. In four patients renal arteries were inadequately displayed due to insufficient contrast, and in six patients renal veins prevented accurate assessment of the renal artery. Although grading of stenoses was less accurate than the axial slices in combination with MPR, the authors use MIP as the optimal presentation to document the anatomic findings. Also, MIP may be helpful in the detection and grading of ostial stenoses.

Fig. 4 a–b. Angiography and CTA of the renal arteries ▶ in a patient with hypertension. **a** Aortogram in deep inspiration demonstrates stenoses in both right renal arteries *(arrows)* and a normal left renal artery *(L)*. **b–e** Axial slices at the level of the origins of the renal arteries. **b** Origin of the left renal artery *(arrowhead)* is oblique relative to the scan plane, and therefore difficult to assess on one slice. **c** Cranial right renal artery demonstrates a very narrow lumen *(black and white arrow)* shortly after its origin. **c** Two millimeters below **d** the lumen widens again *(black and white arrow)*, distal to a small calcification. **e** The tortuous caudal right renal artery demonstrates a stenosis at its origin *(white arrow)* due to mural thrombus in the aorta. **f, g** Curved coronal MPR through the right cranial and left renal arteries. In **f** the reformatting plane is in the middle of the vessels, whereas **g** demonstrates a curved reformat 1 mm anterior to **f**. Note how the origin of the left renal artery seems stenosed on the off-axis reformat *(open arrow)*. *Black and white arrow,* stenosis in cranial right renal artery

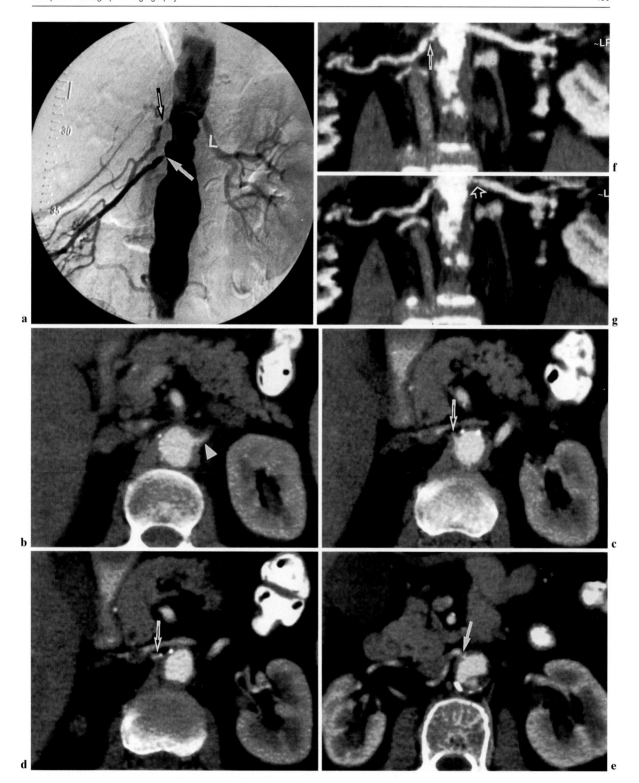

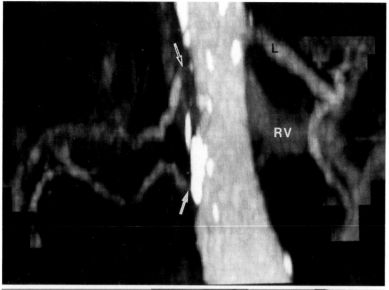

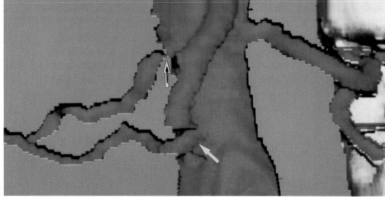

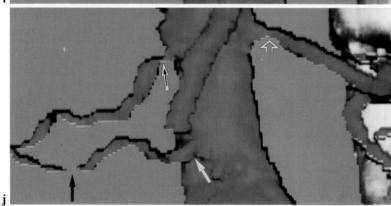

Fig. 4. h MIP demonstrates a normal left renal artery *(L)*, severe stenosis in the cranial right renal artery *(black and white arrow)*, and calcified aortic plaque superimposed on the origin of the caudal right renal artery *(white arrow)*. Due to volume averaging horizontal parts of the right renal arteries are presented in a darker gray than the oblique and vertical parts. *RV,* left renal vein. **i, j,** SSD with a lower **(i)** and a higher **(j)** threshold. Note that a higher threshold results in a stenosis in the left renal artery *(open arrow)* and a pseudo-occlusion *(black arrow)*, due to volume averaging, in a horizontal part of the caudal right renal artery. Compare with Fig. 4 h. The stenosis at the origin of the caudal right renal artery *(white arrow)* is not apparent on the SSDs

Shaded surface display was only useful in one patient with a kidney transplant and a tortuous renal artery. In most patients the diagnostic value was limited due to merging of lumen and classification, and due to the consistent overestimation of severe stenoses as pseudo-occlusions. Consequently, two short occlusions with good collateral circulation could not be differentiated from the pseudo-occlusion appearance of severe stenoses. The authors conclude that CTA of the renal arteries is an excellent technique for the detection, localization, and grading of renal artery stenoses. Rubin et al. described 31 patients with suspected RAS, examined with CTA and angiography [47].

The authors compared SSD and MIP with conventional angiography as the standard of reference. The authors did not grade the stenoses on the axial images. Sensitivity for detecting stenoses >70 % stenosis was 92 % for MIP and 59 % for SSD. Accuracy of stenosis grading was 80 % for MIP and 55 % for SSD.

The lower performance of CTA than in the study of Galanski et al. can be explained by the omission of the axial images and MPRs for grading, and by differences in acquisition technique. In Rubin's study, collimation was always 3 mm and table speed varied between 3 and 6 mm. Consequently, the acquisition technique is more prone to volume averaging compared with the 2–3 mm collimation and 2–3 mm table speed as used by Galanski et al.

Conclusions

Preliminary studies on the diagnostic value of CTA in a number of applications demonstrate good results for the evaluation of aortic disease, pulmonary embolism, and renal artery stenosis. Additionally, CTA seems promising for grading of carotid stenosis and detection of intracerebral aneurysms.

The reported studies stress the need for optimal technique in data acquisition and image display. Technical developments in helical CT will provide more flexibility in scanning parameters, allowing the acquisition of more and thinner slices in one acquisition to overcome the problems of limited scan length and volume averaging. The actual data acquisition often takes no more than a few minutes. However, several applications are time intensive due to off-line postprocessing. Developments in postprocessing algorithms will result in quicker and more automatic image processing, which is essential for the introduction of these techniques on a larger scale.

The appearance and severity of vascular pathology is dependent on the display technique used. Research is needed to define the optimal display method for each application. The current trend favors the use of nonprocessed axial slices and curved MPR for detection and grading of disease. SSD and MIP are mainly used for survey.

In each developing application, the potential role of CTA must be considered; is it meant to be a screening procedure or a confirmatory test? As soon as acquisition and display techniques are op-timized for a specific application, prospective studies will have to examine diagnostic accuracy. Thus, CTA can find its proper place among the other vascular imaging techniques.

References

1. Napel S, Marks MP, Rubin GD, Dake MD, et al. (1992) CT Angiography with spiral CT and maximum intensity projection. Radiology 185: 607–610
2. Rubin GD, Dake MD, Napel SA, McDonnel CH, Jeffrey RB Jr (1993) Three-dimensional spiral CT angiography of the abdomen: initial clinical experience. Radiology 186: 147–152
3. Dillon EH, van Leeuwen MS, Fernandez MA, Mali WPTM (1993) Spiral CT angiography. AJR 160: 1273–1278
4. Kalender WA, Seissler W, Klotz E, Vock P (1990) Spiral volumetric CT with single-breath-hold technique, continuous transport, and continuous scanner rotation. Radiology 176: 181–183
5. Crawford CR, King KF (1990) Computed tomography scanning with simultaneous patient translation. Med Phys 17: 967–982
6. Barnes JE (1992) Characteristics and control of contrast in CT. RadioGraphics 12: 825–837
7. Polacin A, Kalender WA, Marchal G (1992) Evaluation of section sensitivity profiles and image noise in spiral CT. Radiology 185: 29–35
8. Vahlensieck M, Lang Ph, Chan WP, Grampp S, Genant HK (1992) Three-dimensional reconstruction, part I: applications and techniques. Eur Radiol 2: 503–507
9. NASCET Collaborators (1991) Beneficial effect of carotid endarterectomy in symptomatic patients with high-grade carotid stenosis. N Engl J Med 325: 445–453
10. ECST Collaborators (1991) MRC European Carotid Surgery Trial: interim results for symptomatic patients with severe (70–99 %) or with mild (0–29 %) carotid stenosis. Lancet 337: 1235–1243
11. Grzyska U, Freitag J, Zeumer H (1990) Selective cerebral intraarterial DSA. Neuroradiology 32: 296–299
12. Davies KN, Humphrey PR (1993) Complications of cerebral angiography in patients with symptomatic carotid territory ischaemia screened by carotid ultrasound. J Neurol Neurosurg Psychiatry 56: 967–972
13. Masaryk TJ, Obuchowski N (1993) Noninvasive carotid imaging: caveat emptor. Radiology 186: 325–328
14. Schuler JJ, Flanigan DP, Lim LT, Keifer T, et al. (1982) The effect of carotid siphon stenosis on stroke rate, death, and relief of symptoms following elective carotid endarterectomy. Surgery 92: 1058–1067
15. Schwartz RB, Jones KM, Chernoff DM, Mukherji SK, et al. (1992) Common carotid artery bifurcation: evaluation with spiral CT. Radiology 185: 513–519

16. Dillon EH, van Leeuwen MS, Fernandez MA, Eikelboom BC, Mali WPTM (1993) CT angiography: application to the evaluation of carotid artery stenosis. Radiology 189: 211–219
17. Marks MP, Napel S, Jordan JE, Enzmann DR (1993) Diagnosis of carotid artery disease: preliminary experience with maximum-intensity-projection spiral CT angiography. AJR 160: 1267–1271
18. Castillo M (1993) Diagnosis of disease of the common carotid artery bifurcation: CT angiography vs catheter angiography. AJR 161: 395–398
19. Inagawa T, Kamiya K, Ogasawara H, Yano T (1987) Rebleeding of ruptured intracranial aneurysms in the acute stage. Surg Neurol 28: 93–99
20. Van Gijn J (1992) Subarachnoid haemorrhage. Lancet 339: 653–655
21. Kassell NF, Torner JC, Haley EC Jr, Jane JA, et al. (1990) The International Cooperative Study on the Timing of Aneurysm Surgery, part 1: overall management results. J Neurosurg 73: 18–36
22. Hijdra A, Braakman R, Van Gijn J, Vermeulen M, Van Crevel H (1987) Aneurysmal subarachnoid hemorrhage. Complications and outcome in a hospital population. Stroke 18: 1061–1067
23. Kassel NF, Torner JC, Jane JA, Haley EC Jr, Adams HP (1990) The international cooperative study on the timing of aneurysm surgery, part 2: surgical results. J Neurosurg 73: 37–47
24. Öhman J, Heiskanen O (1989) Timing of operation for ruptured supratentorial aneurysms: a prospective randomized study. J Neurosurg 70: 55–60
25. Schmid UD, Steiger HJ, Huber P (1987) Accuracy of high resolution computed tomography in direct diagnosis of cerebral aneurysms. Neuroradiology 29: 152–159
26. Aoki S, Sasaki Y, Machida T, Ohkubo T, et al. (1992) Cerebral aneurysms: detection and delineation using 3-D-CT angiography. AJNR 13: 1115–1120
27. Dalen JE, Alpert JS (1975) Natural history of pulmonary embolism. Prog Cardiovasc Dis 17: 259–270
28. Mant MJ, Thong KL, Birtwhistle RV, O'Brien BD, et al. (1977) Haemorrhagic complications of heparin therapy. Lancet I: 1133–1135
29. PIOPED Investigators (1990) Value of the ventilation/perfusion scan in acute pulmonary embolism. Results of the prospective investigation of pulmonary embolism diagnosis (PIOPED). JAMA 263: 2753–2759
30. Mills SR, Jackson DC, Older RA, Heaston DK, Moore AV (1980) The incidence, etiologies, and avoidance of complications of pulmonary angiography in a large series. Radiology 136: 295–299
31. Remy-Jardin M, Remy J, Wattinne L, Giraud F (1992) Central pulmonary thromboembolism: diagnosis with spiral volumetric CT with the single-breath-hold technique; comparison with pulmonary angiography. Radiology 185: 381–387

32. Sinner WN (1978) Computed tomographic patterns of pulmonary thromboembolism and infarction. J Comput Assist Tomogr 2: 395–399
33. Godwin JD, Webb WR, Gamsu G, Ovenfors C-O (1980) Computed tomography of pulmonary embolism. AJR 135: 691–695
34. DCarlo LA Jr, Schiller NB, Herfkens RL, Brundage BH, Lipton MJ (1982) Noninvasive detection of proximal pulmonary artery thrombosis by two-dimensional echocardiography and computerized tomography. Am Heart J 104: 879–881
35. Breatnach E, Stanley RJ (1984) CT diagnosis of segmental pulmonary artery embolus. J Comput Assist Tomogr 8: 762–764
36. Chintapalli K, Thorsen K, Olson DL, Goodman LR, Gurney J (1988) Computed tomography of pulmonary thromboembolism and infarction. J Comput Assist Tomogr 12: 533–559
37. Kälebo P, Wallin J (1989) Computed tomography in massive pulmonary embolism. Acta Radiol [Diag] (Stockh) 30: 105–107
38. Ren H, Kuhlman JE, Hruban RH, Fishman EK, et al. (1990) CT of inflation-fixed lungs: wedge-shaped density and vascular sign in the diagnosis of infarction. J Comput Assist Tomogr 14: 82–86
39. Erol C, Candan I (1993) Non-invasive methods in the diagnosis of chronic major-vessel thromboembolic pulmonary hypertension. Eur Heart J 14: 1004–1005
40. Verschakelen JA, Vanwijck E, Bogaert J, Baert AL (1993) Detection of unsuspected central pulmonary embolism with conventional contrast-enhanced CT. Radiology 188: 847–850
41. Tardivon AA, Musset D, Maitre S, Brenot F, et al. (1993) Role of CT in chronic pulmonary embolism: comparison with pulmonary angiography. J Comput Assist Tomogr 17: 345–351
42. Teigen CL, Maus TP, Sheedy PF II, Johnson CM, Stanson AW, Welch TJ (1993) Pulmonary embolism: diagnosis with electron-beam CT. Radiology 188: 839–845
43. Costello P, Gaa J (1993) Spiral CT angiography of the abdominal aorta and its branches. Eur Radiol 3: 359–365
44. Costello P, Dupuy DE, Ecker CP, Tello R (1992) Spiral CT of the thorax with reduced volume of contrast material: a comparative Study. Radiology 183: 663–666
45. Balm R, Eikelboom BC, van Leeuwen MS, Noordzij J Spiral CT-Angiography of the Aorta Eur J Vasc Surg (1994) 8, 544–551
46. Galanski M, Prokop M, Chavan A, Schaefer CM, et al. (1993) Renal arterial stenoses: spiral CT angiography. Radiology 189: 185–192
47. Rubin GD, Dake MD, Napel S, Jeffrey RB Jr, et al. (1994) Spiral CT of renal artery stenosis: comparison of three-dimensional rendering of techniques. Radiology 190: 181–189

Section III
Intravascular Ultrasound

Coronary Intravascular Ultrasonography

D. Hausmann. P. J. Fitzgerald, and P. G. Yock

Introduction

Intravascular ultrasound is a promising new technique that provides tomographic, cross-sectional images of the vessel lumen and wall *in vivo*. The development of intravascular ultrasound started in the early 1970s when Bom and coworkers [1] designed a phased-array device with 32 elements mounted on a 9-F catheter tip; this system provided two-dimensional, real-time ultrasound images. The increasing use of percutaneous balloon angioplasty and the development of other interventional devices in the 1980s renewed the interest in intravascular ultrasound imaging [2]. During the past 5 years various catheter designs have been developed and are now commercially available. The experience from several centers using intravascular ultrasound indicates that this technique may have some advantages over other modalities currently used for coronary imaging. *Fiberoptic angioscopy* provides an excellent image of wall surface structures such as intima flaps, dissections, plaque ruptures, and thrombus. However, angioscopy does not allow imaging of structures beyond the vessel wall surface and requires continuous flushing to obtain a blood-free view. *Contrast angiography* gives an image of the silhouette of the vessel lumen and thereby an excellent overview of epicardial vessels. However, this technique is limited by the fact that plaque growth does not necessarily lead to luminal narrowing. Furthermore, coronary atherosclerosis is often diffuse, plaque is located eccentrically in the vessel, and the vessel lumen is often elliptical. Angiography therefore only indirectly reflects the amount of the atherosclerotic plaque and, of course, offers effectively no information about the compositon of the plaque. In this context, the advantages and disadvantages of *intracoronary ultrasound* are addressed in this chapter. Following a description of the technical background and imaging procedure, the potential clinical applications of this technique are discussed.

Technical Background

The currently available intravascular ultrasound systems are based on two different catheter designs using either mechanical or phased-array transducers (Fig. 1). *Mechanical* systems are single imaging element devices that either have a rotating mirror that directs the ultrasound beam to the transducer or a rotating transducer. This allows circumferential scanning of the ultrasound beam and acquisition of a two-dimensional image. Rotation is provided by a flexible cable traveling through the catheter and connected to an external motor drive. In *solid-state* systems multiple elements are located in a cylindric array at the tip of the catheter and are activated in sequences to produce a two-dimensional image. The solid-state approach has the advantages that no parts in the catheter are moving; mechanical systems provide a better image quality, due to better dynamic range and higher resolution.

Spatial image resolution is a direct function of frequency, i.e., higher frequencies yield better resolution. However, the depth of the ultrasound field also depends on the transducer frequency, so that in practice transducers of 20- to 30-MHz are used for coronary imaging whereas 10- to 20-MHz transducers are appropriate for peripheral arteries. The outer diameter of the coronary ultrasound catheters currently ranges between 2.9 and 5.5 F. In solid-state systems the guide wire runs coaxially through the catheter shaft, and therefore no wire artifact appears on the image. Mechanical catheters are usually delivered with a wire running along the transducer ("rapid exchange" modus).

The resolution of the system is a major factor for the image quality. Resolution is defined as the minimal distance between two points that can be discriminated, and this is influenced by the catheter aperture as well as the transducer frequency. Axial resolution of the system is always better than lateral resolution; thus structures aligned on a

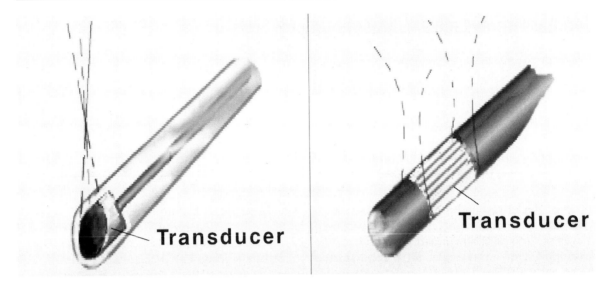

Transducer

Fig. 1. Different designs of intravascular ultrasound catheters. *Left*, mechanical intravascular ultrasound system with rotating transducer; *Right*, solid-state device with multiple elements placed circumferentially around the catheter

Fig. 2. Three-dimensional reconstruction of intracoronary ultrasound images. Standard cross-sectional images are acquired during slow pullback of the ultrasound catheter. The figure shows the same reconstructed segment in different oblique views, and the eccentric accumulation of the plaque can easily be seen (*arrow*)

radial beam from the transducer can be discriminated with greater accuracy than structures positioned in the lateral direction. Practically speaking, eccentric placement of the ultrasound catheter in the vessel significantly degrades image quality due to geometric distortion of vascular morphology. For solid-state systems at 20 MHz axial resolution in the near field is 0.15 mm and lateral resolution is 0.4 mm; out-of-plane resolution ("slice-thickness" of the image) is reported to be approximately 1 mm [3]. Mechanical systems at 20 MHz provide axial resolution of 0.28 mm, lateral resolution of 0.55 mm, and out-of-plane resolution of nearly 2 mm [3].

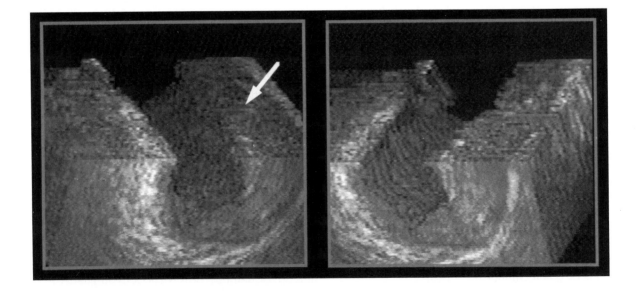

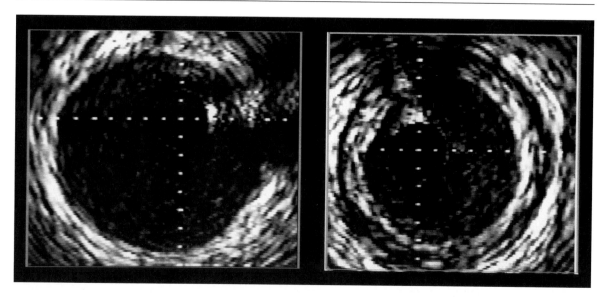

Fig. 3. Intracoronary ultrasound imaging. *Left*, normal intravascular ultrasound image of the left anterior descending coronary artery; the layers of the vessel wall cannot be discriminated; *Right*, concentric intimal thickening of the left anterior descending artery in a patient 1 year after heart transplantation

In addition to the conventional two-dimensional display of ultrasound images, three-dimensional reconstructions have recently been introduced (Fig. 2). For this purpose ultrasound images are acquired during a timed pullback of the ultrasound catheter through a vessel segment; a pullback speed of 0.5–1.0 mm/s is provided by a motor-driven device. The ultrasound cross-section acquired during the pullback are processed by computer and reconstructed to a visual display. These displays allow different operator-controlled views of the imaged segment. Three-dimensional reconstruction of ultrasound images may improve the assessment of structures in which cross-sectional *and* longitudinal perspectives are useful, such as dissections or deposits of calcium.

Interpretation of Intracoronary Ultrasound Images

Images obtained by intravascular ultrasound are a combination of the underlying vessel morphology and artifacts caused by the imaging technique; understanding both parts and their interaction is fundamental for correct interpretation of normal and abnormal ultrasound images.

Image of Normal Coronary Arteries

The center of the intravascular ultrasound image is a black hole produced by the imaging element itself. The surrounding lumen of the vessel shows a weak, speckled echo pattern caused by reflection of the ultrasound beam at red blood cells. The intensity of the blood backscatter increases with the ultrasound frequency used. Furthermore, backscatter is influenced by blood flow velocities, with blood backscatter being highest in areas of low flow velocity [4]. Depending on the type of ultrasound equipment used, the image in a small arc of the circumference is significantly attenuated by an artifact of the catheter strut and by the guide wire running along the imaging element. The basis for the ability of intravascular ultrasound to discriminate between different layers of the coronary vessel wall is their difference in acoustic properties at 20–30 MHz. The media of coronary arteries (muscular type) contains only small amounts of elastin and collagen; this contributes to the relatively echolucent appearance of the media as compared to the adventitia and intima. On the ultrasound scan the media therefore appears as a dark band. Only these different characteristics of the vessel wall layers allow identification of the outer border of atherosclerotic plaque [5]. The internal elastic lamina is a highly reflective structure; it may even cause a "blooming" effect, with overrepresentation of the internal elastic lamina on the ultrasound scan. Since the truly "normal" intima consists only of a single cell

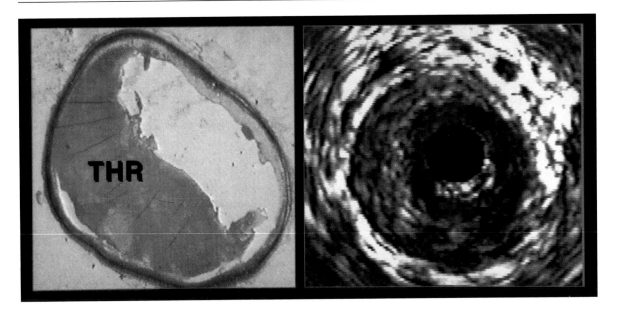

Fig. 4. *In vivo* intravascular ultrasound image of a large thrombus (*THR*) in a rabbit aorta (*right*) and the corresponding histologic specimen. Discrimination between thrombus and soft plaque by intravascular ultrasound imaging may be difficult

layer and is usually too thin to be delineated, the first inner layer of the vessel wall on an ultrasound image at 20–30 MHz is the internal elastic lamina. Thickening of the intima begins at birth and can be detected by histology [6] or intravascular ultrasound [7] even in healthy young adults. Intima thickness in early childhood is approximately 50 μm and increases to 200–250 μm at the age of 40 years. Whether intimal thickening per se represents a pathologic process therefore remains unclear. For clinical routine it appears appropriate to consider a coronary vessel wall as "normal" when no three-layer appearance is present, or the layer of the intima/internal elastic lamina is represented by only a thin line of < 200 μm [8]. An example of a normal coronary artery vessel wall without three-layer appearance is shown in Fig. 3.

Image of Atherosclerotic Coronary Arteries

Atherosclerosis of the coronary artery vessel wall leads to thickening of the intima layer and, in the presence of advanced disease, thinning of the media. The media, which is the major component of

the normal vessel wall, is substantially attenuated in areas of overlying plaque, probably because of primary atrophy or as a result of intravasation of the plaque [9–11]. Intravascular ultrasound studies with histologic validation have shown that media thickness in the absence of atherosclerotic lesions is approximately 0.6 mm, decreasing to 0.1 mm in the area of advanced plaque [10]. Since detection of the outer border of the atherosclerotic plaque relies on identification of echolucent media, moving the ultrasound proximal and distal into areas of less media attenuation may be useful in cases with advanced plaque and no clear media layer.

A major advantage of intravascular ultrasound imaging compared to other imaging techniques is its ability to differentiate plaque composition; this provides important information regarding the natural history of the disease as well as the response of the plaque to interventions. According to studies comparing in vitro ultrasound images of human atherosclerotic vessels and the corresponding histologic specimens, accurate differentiation between soft, fibrous, and calcified plaque is possible [12, 13]. Calcified plaques are brightly reflective on the ultrasound scan and show a drop-out of the image peripherally to the calcium deposit. As a result, visualization of vessel wall structures, in particular the outer border of the plaque, in this area is complicated. Fibrous plaques also show a bright echo on the ultrasound image but usually cause no intense shadowing; however, depending on transducer characteristics, thick layers of fibrous plaque may also lead to drop-out. Soft plaque is less reflective and causes no shadowing of peripheral structures. Localized lipid deposits, often occurring within fibrous tissue, are also hypoechoic structures and in favorable cases can be detected by ultrasound imaging [13]. A major limitation of currently available intravascular ultrasound imaging systems is their difficulty in differentiating thrombotic material in the vessel lumen from soft tissue or from areas of low blood flow velocity [14]. One characteristic feature of fresh thrombus is the "scintillating" appearance; however, organized thrombus may appear very similar to soft plaque. Figure 4 shows the *in vivo* ultrasound image of a thrombus in a rabbit aorta subsequently confirmed by histology; from the ultrasound image it is difficult to differentiate thrombus from soft plaque. Differentiation of thrombus and lipid-rich plaque is a strength of angioscopy because of the high image resolution and color capabilities. Tissue characterization during intravascular ultrasound may be helpful in discriminating plaque types and thrombotic material. This approach is based on analysis of the backscattered ultrasound signal, which reveals greater information than the image presentation alone. Fitzgerald et al. [15] have shown that thrombus and soft plaque reveal different radiofrequency signals, and that this method may improve the recognition of different tissue types.

Besides the qualitative assessment of plaque composition, intracoronary ultrasound has the advantage of allowing cross-sectional two-dimensional measurements of the vessel lumen and wall dimensions. Compared to histology this technique has been shown to provide reliable measurements of lumen area and diameter [12, 13, 16–19] as well as wall thickness of arteries [12, 13, 16, 17]. Intracoronary ultrasound has also been shown to give quantitative information of the luminal dimensions that correlates well with angiographic data [20–23]; however, following mechanical intracoronary interventions, correlation between the techniques is weak, probably because of the complex and irregular contour of the lumen post-intervention [19, 24].

Pitfalls in Image Interpretation

Eccentric and nonorthogonal placement of the ultrasound catheter in the vessel lumen causes image distortion [25]. Figure 5 illustrates ultrasound images obtained from incorrect catheter placement.

In mechanical transducer, air bubbles in the catheter housing may significantly attenuate image quality. Thorough flushing before and, if necessary, during placement of the catheter in the vessel is mandatory.

Calcium deposits in the plaque cause shadowing of underlying structures; these drop-outs must be differentiated from other phenomena such as air bubbles in the imaging catheter.

Blood backscatter intensity increases in areas of low blood flow velocity [4], such as dissections, when blood flow is reduced from occlusion of tight lesions by the ultrasound catheter itself. In these cases lumen and vessel wall structures can show similar acoustic properties, and delineation of the vessel wall can be difficult. Intracoronary injection of echogenic agents can increase the blood backscatter intensity allowing correct delineation of the vessel wall surface [26].

Differentiation of thrombus from soft plaque using the conventional 20- to 30-MHz ultrasound technique can sometimes cause problems.

Since intravascular ultrasound imaging provides a cross-sectional view of the vessel wall, the longitudinal orientation in the vessel can be difficult. For longitudinal orientation the typical appearance of branches should be used, and the direction of the catheter movement during imaging should be recorded on video tape. Finally, the positon of the ultrasound catheter in the vessel should be documented by fluoroscopy.

In mechanical catheters failure to achieve a precise rotation can result in nonuniform rotational distortion of the ultrasound image.

Imaging Procedure

Initialization and Imaging

The imaging procedure depends to some degree on the type of ultrasound equipment used. In mechanical catheters air must be removed from the space between the imaging element and the surrounding sheath by flushing. The ultrasound catheter must be connected to the ultrasound scanner; in mechanical systems the catheter is at the same time connected to the motor drive which rotates the mirror or imaging element. For placement of the ultrasound catheter a guiding catheter is placed into the coronary ostium, and a guide-

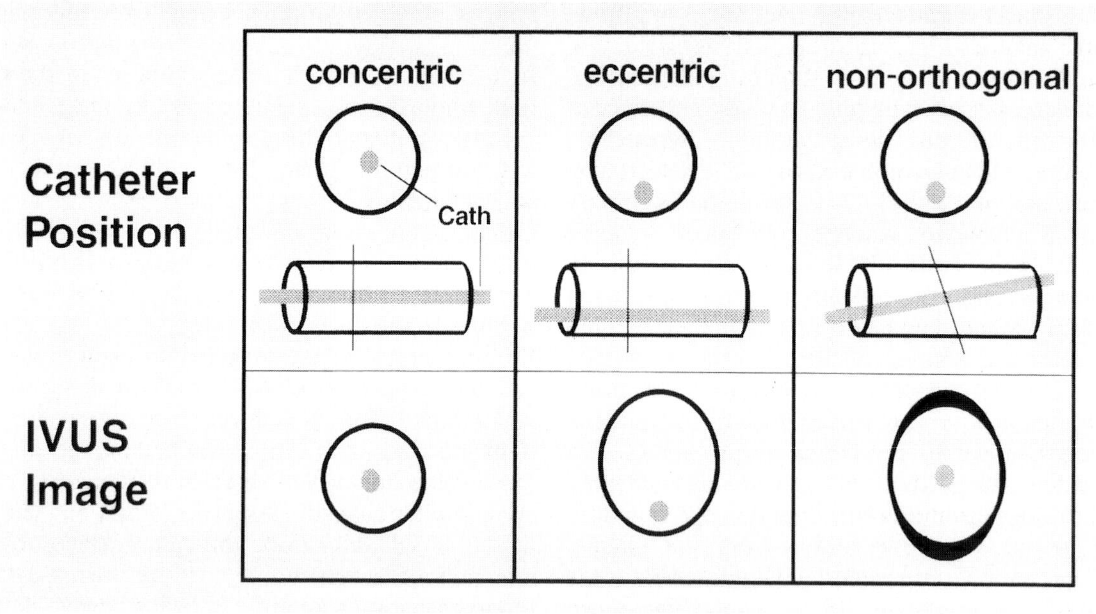

Fig. 5. Importance of catheter placement in the vessel. Orthogonal placement of the ultrasound catheter in the center of the lumen provides accurate ultrasound images; eccentric and nonorthogonal placements of the catheter cause distortion of the ultrasound image

wire is advanced into the target vessel using standard techniques. The size of the guiding catheter depends on the outer diameter of the ultrasound catheter; the size of the guide wire is usually 0.014 in. An additional dose of heparin should be given to prevent thrombus formation. In some centers intracoronary or sublingual nitroglycerin is given routinely before the procedure to prevent spasm during catheter placement. The ultrasound imaging catheter is then advanced over the wire into the vessel. As soon as the ultrasound catheter leaves the tip of the guiding catheter, the settings for gain, compression, and reject should be adjusted meticulously until an ultrasound image with optimal dynamic range is obtained. The ultrasound image should allow reliable differentiation between the different layers of the vessel wall; in the near field the time-gain control should be reduced to deemphasize the blood backscatter, and in the far field the gain should be gradually increased. If no optimal image can be obtained, the catheter should not be advanced further into the coronary vessels because of the potential risk of catheter passage without obtaining adequate information from the study. When an optimal image is obtained, the ultrasound catheter can be advanced further into the target segment under careful fluoroscopic guidance. Recordings on video tape are made for off-line analysis. Calibration markers are superimposed on the image for diameter and area measurements. For longitudinal orientation of the catheter position, branch points should be identified on the ultrasound image and the position should be documented using fluoroscopy with and without contrast injection.

Technical Problems and Potential Complications

Since ultrasound catheters are stiff in the region of the imaging element, advancing the catheter to the target segment can be a problem when curved segments must be crossed. Although smaller catheter designs are now available, it can also be difficult to cross very tight lesions, especially those with superficial calcium deposits. Crossing tight lesions with the ultrasound catheter may cause a certain amount of "dottering" effect (mechanical expansion). Furthermore, imaging of the distal portion of coronary vessels is limited by the size of the imaging catheter. Another technical problem can be that despite intensive flushing before insertion of the ultrasound catheter, the intravascular image can still be impaired by air bubbles. Potential complications of intracoronary ultrasound imaging are spasm, thrombus formation, occlusion, and dissection of the vessel; in addition, placement of the ultrasound catheter into tight lesions can cause reversible myocardial ischemia. Conclusive data on the overall incidence of complications of the ultrasound procedure are currently not available, and complications are reported only in studies with small numbers of patients (<60). In these studies vessel spasm occurred in 0% [16, 27] to 14% [23, 28, 29] of the cases. In a preliminary report of Erbel et al. [30] 11/218 (5%) of intracoronary ultrasound studies could not be completed due to technical or patient-related complications. A multicenter, "multicatheter" registry on acute complications of intracoronary ultrasound has recently been established by our group. Ultrasound procedures performed in transplant patients and in patients with native coronary disease with and without intervention are included from nearly 30 centers; the initial data will be available in 1995. Whether manipulation of the ultrasound catheter in the coronary vessels may cause chronic injury resulting in acceleration of the progression of atherosclerosis and/or changes in endothelial function remains uncertain at this point.

Clinical Applications

The introduction of intravascular ultrasound and the ability to obtain cross-sectional images of the vessel lumen and wall in vivo have renewed the interest in morphologic studies of coronary atherosclerosis. Using this technology new insights into the natural history of coronary artery disease regarding regression of coronary atherosclerosis, prognosis of "unstable" plaque, vasculopathy after heart transplantation, as well as the use of new interventional devices can be obtained.

Natural History of Caronary Artery Disease

Soon after the introduction of coronary angiography the limitations of this technique for assessment of the true anatomic amount of atherosclerosis became clear [31, 32]. Compared to the histologic specimens, premortem [33–38] and postmortem angiography [31, 32, 40] only poorly reflects the true amount of atherosclerotic plaque. Angiography visualizes the silhouette of the vessel lumen rather than the plaque itself; this fundamental problem remains even with further refinement of angiographic techniques (multiple orthogonal views, quantitative angiography, videodensitometry, digital subtraction technique). Potential explanation for the discrepancies between angiography and the true anatomic amount of atherosclerosis are the following: (a) The media is substantially attenuated in advanced coronary atherosclerosis; this may partially compensate for lumen reduction during plaque growth [9–11]. (b) Angiographic detection and quantification of lumen narrowing is based on comparison of a "lesion" to a reference segment that is considered as normal. However, histologic [36] and epicardial echocardiographic studies [41] have clearly shown that coronary arteries are often diffusely diseased. This may lead to an angiographic appearance without localized narrowings or to considerable underestimation of the atherosclerotic plaque by angiography. (c) The lumen shape of atherosclerotic coronary vesels is often elliptical or D-shaped [33, 42] or located eccentrically in the vessel [33, 40]; this also causes problems in the angiographic assessment of these lesions. (d) Compensatory mechanisms during plaque development cause coronary artery enlargement in relation to plaque growth; luminal narrowing may be delayed until the plaque occupies approximately 30%–40% of the potential vessel lumen [43–46]. Stiel et al. [46] have applied this concept to the angiographic assessment of coronary atherosclerosis; they showed that compensatory enlargement accounts for angiographic underestimation of mild stenosis whereas underestimation of high-grade stenosis is based mainly on enlargement of the reference segment erroneously considered to be normal by angiography. Compensatory enlargement of coronary arteries has also been shown by intravascular ultrasound [47, 48] and is believed to be more pronounced in soft plaque whereas calcified plaque might prevent then compensatory mechanisms [49]. With regard to intracoronary catheter-based interventions, plaque accumulation up to 30%–40% of the potential vessel lumen in the reference segment that is considered to be normal indicates that the "desirable" lumen in the target lesion may be grossly underestimated by angiography [50].

During the past 5–10 years it has become clear that regression and/or retardation of progression of coronary atherosclerosis in humans is possible [51–56], especially when intensive lipid-lowering therapy is initiated. In contrast to angiography, intravascular ultrasound visualizes the entire cross-section of the plaque rather than only the lumen narrowed by the plaque. In light of the described limitations of angiography, especially for detection of early atherosclerotic changes, intravascular ultrasound might become a useful complementary tool for further regression studies. Preliminary studies in animals have shown that changes in atherosclerotic plaque burden can be accurately tracked by intravascular ultrasound [57].

The impact of plaque compositon on the natural course of coronary artery disease has gained increasing interest in recent years [58, 59]. After slow growth over a long time period the atherosclerotic plaque can progress abruptly to high-grade stenosis or occlusion causing acute clinical events of coronary heart disease. This acute aggravation is usually caused by plaque disruption, hemorrhage, and thrombus formation [58, 59]. This concept explains the high incidence of mild or moderate lesions found before acute myocardial infarction [60, 61] or after thrombolytic therapy of acute mayocardial infarction [62]. Plaques with lipid deposition and a thin fibrous cap are at particular risk for rupture due to mechanical instability [63]; in contrast, calcified or fibrous lesions with low lipid content seem to be more stable. Stabilization of these plaques by depletion of lipid pools might also account for the discrepancies between the relatively small improvement in lumen stenosis compared to the much higher reduction in coronary events during lipid-lowering therapy [52]. Initial observations indicate that intravascular ultrasound might be a useful tool for identification of these moderate though potentially unstable lesions [24, 64].

Intravascular ultrasound has an advantage over angiography in being able to image the correct geometry of the plaque and the lumen. Angiography often underestimates the eccentricity of lesions [65]; even in high-grade lesions the plaque may be located eccentrically in the vessel [33, 40]. However, the eccentricity of the lesion and the amount of residual normal wall segment might have important implications for the planning of catheter-based intracoronary interventions, for example, atherectomy directed to maximal bulk of the plaque or reducing recoil during balloon angioplasty. The extent of the disease-free wall can also be determined by intravascular ultrasound; since normal vessel wall indicates preserved media and smooth muscle function, this is important for understanding the effect of vasodilatatory drugs in atherosclerotic vessels [40, 66]. Different lumen shapes (circle, ellipse, D-shaped, star-shaped, cresentic) can easily be distinguished by intravascular ultrasound; all noncircular shapes can cause under- and overestimation when cross-sectional area is determined by angiography [42].

Transplant Vasculopathy

Coronary transplant vasculopathy is the major cause of death in patients after heart transplantation who survive at least 1 year [67]. The principal cause of transplant vasculopathy appears to be immune-mediated damage of the coronary endothelium. Five years after the transplantation, approximately 50 % of patients have coronary artery disease that is detectable by angiography. However, fibrous thickening of the intima is present as early as 1 month after transplantation; after 1 year the majority of patients have moderate or severe intimal thickening [68]. Besides fibrous intima thickening, atherosclerotic plaque similar to that of nontransplant atherosclerosis can be detected in some patients [69]. Due to the diffuse nature of transplant vasculopathy and the concentric pattern of intimal thickening, angiography is normal in most cases despite significant intima disease [68, 69]. A typical intravascular ultrasound image of the proximal left anterior descending artery in a patient 1 year after transplantation is shown in Fig. 3. Due to the limitations of angiography intravascular ultrasound has been used to detect vasculopathy in an earlier stage of the disease than angiography. Compensatory enlargement of the vessel comparable to that observed in nontransplant atherosclerosis may account for the absence of luminal narrowing on angiography [70].

In addition to morphologic abnormalities, transplant vasculopathy is associated with changes in vasoreactivity. Intravascular ultrasound offers a useful tool to study coronary reactivity and morphologic changes simultaneously in these patients. It has been shown that vascular smooth muscle relaxation is impaired in these patients during rejection [71] or in the presence of advanced initial thickening [72]. Yeung et al. [73] have shown that endothelial function can be evaluated by acetylcholine testing during intravascular ultrasound in these patients. These authors found that endothelial dysfunction occurs early in the course of the disease and may be present even before intimal thickening.

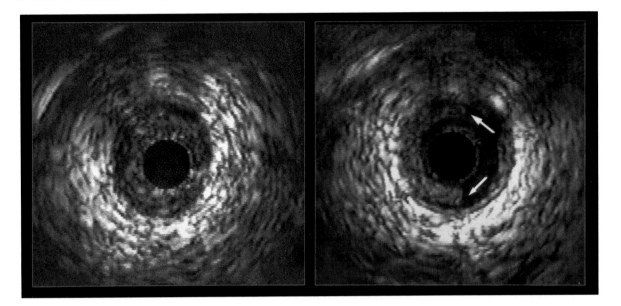

Fig. 6. Intravascular ultrasound imaging before and after balloon angioplasty. *Left*, concentric soft plaque before angioplasty; *Right*, after angioplasty, intravascular ultrasound visualizes the expanded lumen and the dissections of the vessel wall (*arrows*)

Catheter-Based Intracoronary Interventions

Balloon Angioplasty

Intravascular ultrasound provides the ability to study the relative contributions of different mechanisms of lumen gain during angioplasty, such as plaque compression and tearing, dissection, and stretching of the normal wall [74–76] (Fig. 6). Intravascular ultrasound imaging has confirmed pathology studies showing that the amount of tearing caused by balloon inflation is greater than that shown by contrast angiography [19, 28]. In one study dissections were detected in 50%–70% by ultrasound scanning compared to only 20%–40% by contrast angiography [50]. Depth and extent of dissection after inflation are detected by intravascular ultrasound in favorable cases; this technique is able to identify whether a dissection of only the intima layers had occurred or the dissection extents into deeper layers. This is of potentially major clinical importance since involvement of deep structures has been shown to provoke more restenosis after balloon angioplasty [77].

Besides assessment of dissections *after* angioplasty, intravascular ultrasound has the potential to predict the location of the dissection based on preinterventional plaque characteristics. Two sites in the plaque are predisposed to dissection. First, differences in the distensibility are especially high at the edge of an eccentric plaque (between plaque and normal wall segment). At this site, the normal wall is stretched away during inflation and the angulation between the normal wall segment, and the plaque creates a dissection plane. Second, the interface between localized calcium deposits and surrounding softer tissue is predisposed to tearing during inflation because stress is highest at these points [78]. For detection of localized calcium deposits ultrasound scanning is far more sensitive than fluoroscopy [28, 79]; in addition, the exact location of the calcium deposits in the plaque can be assessed by intravascular ultrasound but not with fluoroscopy.

Intravascular ultrasound is also able to demonstrate the extent of elastic recoil. Initial data suggest that recoil is greatest in lesions without clear evidence of tearing in the region of the plaque [65]. After balloon inflation the residual lumen of the lesions can be defined exactly by ultrasound measurements in order to decide whether additional balloon inflations are required, and which balloon size is preferable. As pointed out, angiographic comparison to a normal reference segment does not reveal the true potential vessel size; intravascular ultrasound may thereby help to better identify the "desirable" vessel lumen and the final size of the balloon used.

Recently, combined angioplasty/imaging devices have been developed. A design using a multiple-

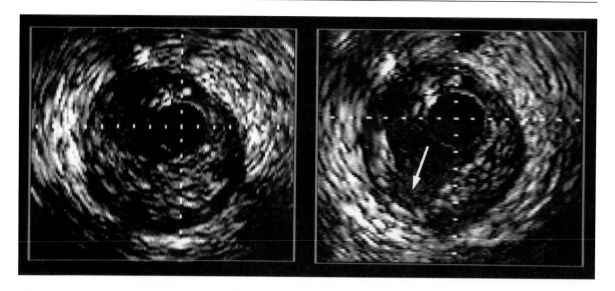

Fig. 7. Intravascular ultrasound imaging before and after directional atherectomy. *Left*, eccentric soft plaque before atherectomy; *Right*, intravascular ultrasound shows the site of the atherectomy cuts (*arrow*)

element device combined with an angioplasty balloon has been reported [80]. In this prototype the imaging element is mounted directly behind the balloon. In a multicenter experience using a combined device decisions in approximately one-third of all interventions were changed by the information provided by the imaging data [81]. Another design has been reported with a mechanical device mounted at the same level as the balloon, allowing for simultaneous imaging during balloon inflation [82].

Directional Atherectomy

Since intravascular ultrasound is able to image the atherosclerotic plaque, and the primary goal of directional coronary atherectomy (DCA) is plaque removal, this technique appears ideal for evaluation of morphology before and after DCA. Due to compensatory dilation of the vessel at the site of plaque growth, major parts of the plaque are usually located outside the vessel contour that is defined by the angiographically normal reference segment. Furthermore, angiographically normal reference segments are nearly always diseased, with up to 30%–40% of the potential vessel area covered by plaque. Using inravascular

ultrasound it has been shown that excellent angiographic results after atherectomy still have a large amount of residual plaque [83]. Studies using intravascular ultrasound have also confirmed previous angiographic observations that "dottering" the lesions is a significant contribution of the actual lumen gain after DCA, accounting for up to 50% of the lumen gain [83].

Ultrasound scanning can accurately show the depth and location of the cuts (Fig. 7). The extent of this injury may be important for the degree of restenosis after the interventions. During angiographically guided directional atherectomy one-half of interventions show cuts that extend into the media, and that one-third of the cuts even reach the adventitia. The direction of the DCA device into the area of maximal plaque my be clinically important, especially when highly eccentric lesions are treated. Intravascular ultrasound is currently the only technique that can provide rotational orientation. For this purpose a branch near the target lesion should be identified by ultrasound and the angle to the area of the deepest extent of the plaque measured. The DCA device can then be inserted, and by using the branches on angiography as reference points it can be directed to the maximal plaque accumulation [84].

Other important factors for the results of atherectomy are the extent and location of calcium [85]. Prior angiographic studies have suggested that atherectomy should not be performed in highly calcified lesions. However, angiography or fluoroscopy grossly underestimate the extent of calcium [28, 79], and assessment of the location

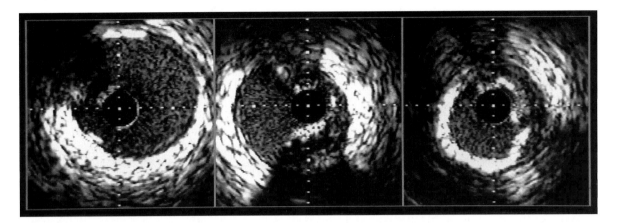

Fig. 8. Intravascular ultrasound imaging of a plaque with superficial calcification in the left main coronary artery. *Left*, normal ultrasound image in the proximal portion of the vessel. *Middle*, plaque with superficial calcium (causing shadowing in the far field) in the middle portion of the vessel; *Right*, intravascular ultrasound imaging shows a ring of superficial calcium surrounding the vessel lumen in the distal portion of the left main coronary artery

(deep or superficial) of the calcium deposits in the plaque is nearly impossible. It has been shown that only 50 % of the tissue can be retrieved by atherectomy if superficial calcium is present on the ultrasound scan as compared to plaques with no or only deep calcium [85]. When a complete ring of calcium is present, tissue retrieval is minimal (Fig. 8).

Combined devices with atherectomy and imaging capabilities have also been developed in recent years [83]. One prototype catheter has been tested in vitro and in animal experiments. An image out of the open housing is provided, so that the target lesion can be evaluated before cutting. Initial results suggest that medial injury can be reduced by this device. A commercially available combined atherectomy/imaging device is currently entering clinical testing.

Rotational Atherectomy

Rotational atherectomy is a relatively efficient approach for removing plaque tissue in lesions with superficial calcium. Intravascular ultrasound has demonstrated that in approximately 75 % of patients referred for balloon angioplasty the target lesions shows significant calcification, either deep or superficial in the plaque. In 50 % of the pa-

tients at least two quadrants of the circumference are covered by calcium [79]. These lesions appear ideal for rotational atherectomy. In soft plaque, however, the postinterventional lumen is not ideally round and is smaller than the largest burr used. This may be due to a combination of less effective plaque ablation and more spasm of the vessel. The extent of superficial calcium can be significantly reduced by rotational atherectomy as shown by intravascular ultrasound; further treatment of these lesions by other devices is then possible [86].

Stents

Due to the metal struts intravascular ultrasound imaging provides an excellent view of intracoronary stents. The various stent designs have different aspects during intravascular ultrasound as described in detail elsewhere [87]. Three-dimensional reconstruction of ultrasound images may be particularly useful for stents. In lesions considered for stenting intravascular ultrasound can provide important information about the underlying composition and the shape of the lesion and the extent and depth of any dissection. Preliminary observations indicate that cases with severe dissection after angioplasty, in which differentiation between dissection and true lumen may be difficult, ultrasound can correctly identify the dissection and allow successful stent placement [89]. Intravascular ultrasound provides good visualization of the stent/vessel size matching and immediate quantitative assessment of the effects of stent placement [88]. Imcomplete expansion of stents may be associated with a higher risk for thrombosis because more metal surface is exposed to blood, and local flow disturbances are more likely. Finally, restenosis can also be easily defined using intravascular ultrasound since the metal struts provide an ideal reference marker for the original lumen border.

Summary and Future Directions

Intravascular ultrasound is a new technique that provides tomographic, cross-sectional images of the vessel lumen and wall *in vivo*. For imaging of coronary arteries mechanical or solid-state transducers with frequencies of 20–30 MHz are used; the catheter size currently ranges between 2.9 and 5.5 F. Discrimination between different layers of the coronary vessel wall by ultrasound is based on their different acoustic properties at 20–30 MHz. The media has an echolucent appearance compared to adventitia and intima; in contrast, the internal elastic lamina is a highly reflective structure. Soft, fibrous, and calcified plaques can be differentiated by their typical pattern on the ultrasound scan. Intravascular ultrasound provides an image of the plaque whereas contrast angiography shows a lumenogram of the vessel. Since early atherosclerosis does not result in luminal narrowing, these changes can be detected only by techniques that visualize the plaque directly. Intravascular ultrasound may therefore be helpful for detection of early transplant vasculopathy; furthermore, changes in plaque burden during regression studies may also be better detected than by contrast angiography. Intravascular ultrasound imaging is increasingly used for the guidance of catheter-based intracoronary interventions. It allows detection of vessel wall dissections, identification of calcified or eccentric plaque accumulation, and exact measurement of luminal dimensions before and after the procedure.

Future developments in intravascular ultrasound are expected to include the combination of imaging and therapeutic devices. Combined angioplasty/imaging and atherectomy/imaging devices are currently undergoing experimental testing; guide wires with imaging capabilities have also been developed recently. Future improvements in imaging technology will include the refinement of three-dimensional reconstruction of ultrasound scans and possibly the introduction of forward viewing systems. Tissue characterization may be helpful to better discriminate different plaque types and will potentially provide prognostic infor-

mation on plaque stability. However, the general acceptance of intravascular ultrasound will probably depend on its relevance for therapeutic device selection, particularly for choosing among the second generation catheters; in this respect, the impact of plaque calcification on device performance appears to be the most important factor.

References

1. Bom N, Lancee CT, van Egmond FC: An ultrasonic intracardiac scanner. Ultrasonics 1972; 72–76
2. Yock PG, Johnson EL, Linker DT: Intravascular ultrasound: development and clinical potential. Am J Card Imag 1988; 2: 185–193
3. Benkeser PJ, Churchwell AL, Lee C, Abouelnasr DM: Resolution limitations in intravascular ultrasound imaging. J Am Soc Echocardiogr 1993; 6: 158–165
4. Yamada EG, Fitzgerald PJ, Sudhir K, Hargrave VK, Yock PG: Intravascular ultrasound imaging of blood: the effect of hematocrit and flow on backscatter. J Am Soc Echo 1992; 5: 385–392
5. Yock PG, Linker DT, Angelsen BAJ: Two-dimensional intravascular ultrasound: technical development and initial clinical experience. J Am Soc Echo 1989; 2: 296–304
6. Enos WF, Holmers RH, Beyer J: Coronary disease among united states soldiers killed in action in korea. Preliminary report. JAMA 1986; 256: 2859–2862
7. St. Goar FG, Pinto FJ, Alderman EL, Fitzgerald PJ, Stinson EB, Billingham ME, Popp RL: Detection of caronary atherosclerosis in young adult hearts using intravascular ultrasound. Circulation 1992; 86: 756–763
8. Fitzgerald PJ, Goar FG, Connolly RJ, Pinto FJ, Billingham ME, Popp RL, Yock PG: Intravascular ultrasound imaging of coronary arteries. Is three layers the norm. Circulation 1992; 86: 154–158
9. Crawford T, Levene CI: Medial thinning in atheroma. J Pathold 1953; 66: 19–23.
10. Gussenhoven EJ, Frietman P, The SHK, van Suylen RJ, van Egmond FC, Lancee CT, van Urk H, Roelandt JRTC, Stijnen T, Bom N: Assessment of medial thinning in atherosclerosis by intravascular ultrasound. Am J Cardiol 1991; 68: 1625–1632
11. Isner JM, Donaldson RF, Fortin AH, Tischler A, Clarke RH: Attenuation of the media of coronary arteries in advanced athersclerosis. Am J Cardiol 1986; 58: 937–939
12. Potkin BN, Bartorelli AL, Gessert JM, Neville RF, Almagor Y, Roberts WC, Leon MB: Coronary artery imaging with intravascular high-frequency ultrasound. Circulation 1990; 81: 1575–1585
13. Gussenhoven EJ, Essed CE, Lance CT, Mastik F, Frietman P, van Egmond FC, Reiber J, Bosch H, van Urk H, Roelandt J, Bom N: Arterial wall characteristics determind by intravascular ultrasound imaging: an in vitro study. J Am Coll Cardiol 1989; 14: 947–952

14. Pandian NG, Kreis A, Brockway B: Detection of intraarterial thrombus by intravascular high frequence two-dimensional ultrasound imaging in vitro and in vivo studies. Am J Cardiol 1990; 65: 1280–1283

15. Fitzgerald PJ, Connolly AL, Watkins RD, et al: Distinction between soft plaque and thrombus by intravascular tissue characterization (Abstract). J Am Coll Cardiol 1991; 17: 111A

16. Hodgson JM, Graham SP, Savakus AD, Dame SG, Stephens DN, Dhillon PS, Brands D, Sheehan H, Eberle MJ: Clinical percutaneous imaging of coronary anatomy using an over-the-wire ultrasound catheter system. Int J Card Imag 1989; 4: 187–193

17. Pandian NG, Kreis A, Brockway B, Isner JM, Sacharoff A, Boleza E, Caro R, Muller D: Ultrasound angioscopy: real-time, two-dimensional, intraluminal ultrasound imaging of blood vessels. Am J Cardiol 1988; 62: 493–494

18. Nishimura RA, Edwards WD, Warnes CA, Reeder GS, Holmes DR, Tajik AJ, Yock PG: Intravascular ultrasound imaging: in vitro validation and pathologic correlation. J Am Coll Cardiol 1990; 16: 145–154

19. Tobis JM, Mallery JA, Gessert J, Griffith J, Mahon D, Bessen M, Moriuchi M, McLeay L, McRae J, Henry WL: Intravascular ultrasound cross-sectional arterial imaging before and after balloon angioplasty in vitro. Circulation 1989; 80: 873–882

20. St. Goar FG, Pinto FJ, Alderman EL, Fitzgerald PJ, Stadius ML, Popp RL: Intravascular ultrasound imaging of angiographically normal coronary arteries: An in vivo comparion with quantitative angiography. J Am Coll Cardiol 1991; 18: 952–958

21. Davidson CJ, Sheikh KH, Harrison JK, Himmelstein SI, Leithe ME, Kisslo KB, Bashore TM: Intravascular ultrasonography versus digital subtraction angiography: a human in vivo comparison of vessel size and morphology. J Am Coll Cardiol 1990; 16: 633–636

22. Nissen SE, Grines CL, Gurley JC, Sublett K, Haynie D, Diaz C, Booth DC, DeMaria AN: Application of a new phased-array ultrasound imaging catheter in the assessment of vascular dimensions: in vivo comparison to cineangiography. Circulation 1990; 81: 660–666

23. Nissen SE, Gurley JC, Grines CL, Booth DC, McClure R, Berk M, Fischer C, DeMaria AN: Intravascular ultrasound assessment of lumen size and wall morphology in normal subjects and patients with coronary artery disease. Circulation 1991; 84: 1087–1099

24. Hodgson JM, Reddy KG, Suneja R, Nair RN, Lesnefsky EJ, Sheehan HM: Intracoronary ultrasound imaging: correlation of plaque morphology with angiography, clinical syndrome and procedural results in patients undergoing coronary angioplasty. J Am Coll Cardiol 1993; 21: 35–44

25. DiMario C, Madretsma S, Linker D, The SHK, Bom N, Serruys PW, Gussenhoven EJ, Roelandt JR: The angle of incidence of the ultrasonic beam: a critical factor for the image quality in intravascular ultrasonography. Am Heart J 1993; 125: 442–448

26. Hausmann D, Fitzgerald PJ, Yock PG, Daniel WG: Intravaskulärer Kontrast-Ultraschall: eine neue Methode zur Erkennung komplexer Wandstrukturen. Z Kariol 1993; 82: 111 (Abstract)

27. Violaris AG, Linnemeier TJ, Campbell S, Rothbaum DA, Cumberland DC: Intravascular ultrasound imaging combined with coronary angioplasty. Lancet 1992; 339: 1571–1572

28. Honye J, Mahon DJ, Jain A, White CJ, Ramee SR, Wallis JB, Al-Zarka A, Tobis JM: Morphological effects of coronary balloon angioplasty in vivo assessed by intravascular ultrasound imaging. Circulation 1992; 85: 1012–1025

29. Tobis JM, Mallery J, Mahon D, Lehmann K, Zalesky P, Griffith J, Gessert J, Moriuchi M, McRae M, Dwyer ML, Greep N, Henry WL: Intravascular ultrasound imaging of human coronary arteries in vivo: Analysis of tissue characterization with comparison to in vitro histological specimens. Circulation 1991; 83: 913–926

30. Erbel R, Ge J, Gerber T, Görge G, Rupprecht HJ, Meyer J: Safety and limitations of intravascular ultrasound: experience with 325 consecutive procedures. Circulation 1992; 86 (Suppl I): I–195. (Abstract)

31. Eusterman JH, Achor RWP, Kincaid OW, Brown AL: Atherosclerotic disease of the coronary arteries. A pathologic-radiologic correlative study. Circulation 1962; 26: 1288–1295

32. Gray CR, Hoffmann HA, Hammond WS, Miller KL, Oseasohn RO: Correlation of arteriography and pathologic findings in the coronary arteria in man. Circulation 1962; 26: 494–499

33. Vlodaver Z, Frech R, Van Tassel RA, Edwards JE: Correlation of the antemortem coronary arteriogram and the postmortem specimen. Circulation 1973; 47: 162–169

34. Grondin CM, Dyrda I, Pasternac A, Campeau L, Bourassa MG, Lesperance J: Discrepancies between cineangiographic and postmortem findings in patients with coronary artery disease and recent myocardial revascularization. Circulation 1974; 49: 703–708

35. Isner JM, Kishel J, Kent KM, Ronan JA, Ross AM, Roberts WC: Accuracy of angiographic determination of left main coronary arterial narrowing. Angiographic-histologic correlative analysis in 28 patients. Circulation 1981; 63: 1056–1064

36. Arnett EN, Isner JM, Redwood DR, Kent KM, Baker WP, Ackerstein H, Roberts WC: Coronary artery narrowing in coronary heart disease: comparison of cineangiographic and necropsy findings. Ann Int Med 1979; 91: 350–356

37. Kemp HG, Evans H, Elliott WC, Gorlin R: Diagnostic accuracy of selective coronary cinearteriography. Circulation 1967; 36: 526–533

38. Schwartz JN, Kong Y, Hackel DB, Bartel AG: Comparison of angiographic and postmortem findings in patients with coronary artery disease. Am J Cardiol 1975; 36: 174–178

39. Hutchins GM, Bulkley BH, Ridolfi RL, Griffith LSC, Lohr FT, Piasio MA: Correlation of coronary arteriograms and left ventriculograms with postmortem studies. Circulation 1977; 56: 32–37

40. Freudenberg H, Lichtlen PR: Das normale Wandsegment bei Koronarstenosen — eine postmortale Studie. (The normal wall segment in coronary stenoses — a postmortal study). Z Kardiol 1981; 70: 863–869

41. McPherson DD, Hiratzka LF, Lamberth WC, Brandt B, Hunt M, Kieso RA, Marcus ML, Kerber RE: Delineation of the extent of coronary atherosclerosis by high-frequency epicardial echocardiography. N Engl J Med 1987; 316: 304–309

42. Thomas AC, Davies MJ, Dilly S, Dilly N, Franc F: Potential errors in the estimation of coronary arterial stenosis from clinical arteriography with reference to the shape of the coronary arterial lumen. Br Heart J 1986; 55: 129–139

43. Glagov S, Weisenberg E, Zarins CK, Stankunavicius R, Kolettis GJ: Compensatory enlargement of human atherosclerotic coronary arteries. N Engl J Med 1987; 316: 1371–1375

44. Zarins CK, Weisenberg E, Kolettis G, Stankunavicius R, Glagov S: Differential enlargement of artery segments in response to enlarging atherosclerotic plaques. J Vasc Surg 1988; 7: 386–394

45. McPherson DD, Sirna SJ, Hiratzka LF, Thorpe L, Armstrong ML, Marcus ML, Kerber RE: Coronary arterial remodeling studied by high-frequency epicardial echocardigraphy: an early compensatory mechanism in patients with obstructive coronary atherosclerosis. J Am Coll Cardiol 1991; 17: 79–86

46. Stiels GM, Stiel LSG, Schofer J, Donath K, Mathey DG: Impact of compensatory enlargement of atherosclerotic coronary arteries on angiographic assessment of coronary artery disease. Circulation 1989; 80: 1603–1609

47. Hermiller JB, Tenaglia AN, Kisslo KB, Phillips HR, Bashore TM, Stack RS, Davidson CJ: In vivo validation of compensatory enlargement of atherosclerotic coronary arteries. Am J Cardiol 1993; 71: 665–668

48. Nissen SE, Booth DC, Gurley JC, Bates M, Yamagishi M, Fischer C, DeMaria AN. Coronary remodelling in CAD: intravascular ultrasound evidence of vessel expansion. Circulation 1991; 86 (Suppl II); II–437. (Abstract)

49. Mintz GS, Bonner RF, Bouek PC, Kent KM, Pichard AD, Satler LF, Leon MB: Lesion composition determines compensatory vessel wall responces and plaques and plaque accumulation in native coronary artery stenoses: an intravascular ultrasound study. J Am Coll Cardiol; 1993: 326A (Abstract)

50. The GUIDE Trial Investigators (1993) Discrepancies between angiographic and intravascular ultrasound appearance of coronary lesions undergoing Intervention. A report of phase I of the „GUIDE" trial. J Am Coll Cardiol 21; 118A. (Abstract)

51. Kane JP, Malloy MJ, Ports TA, Phillips NR, Diehl JC, Havel RJ: Regression of coronary athersoclerosis during treatment of familial hypercholesterolemia with combined drug regimens. JAMA 1990; 264: 3007–3012

52. Brown G, albers JJ, Fisher LD, Schaefer SM, Lin JT, Kaplan C, Zhao XQ, Bisson BD, Fitzpatrick VF, Dodge HT: Regression of coronary artery disease as a result of intensive lipid-lowering therapy

in men with high levels of apolipoprotein B. N Engl J Med 1990; 323: 1289–1298

53. Cashin-Hemphill L, Mack WJ, Pogoda JM, Sanmarco ME, Azen SP, Blankenhorn DH: Beneficial effects of colestipol-niacin on coronary atherosclerosis. A 4-year follow-up. JAMA 1990; 264: 3013–3017

54. Blankenhorn DH, Kramsch DM: Reversal of artherosis and sclerosis. The two components of atherosclerosis. Circulation 1989; 79: 1–7

55. Lichtlen PR, Hugenholtz PG, Rafflenbeul W, Hecker H, Jost S, Deckers JW: Retardation of angiographic progression of coronary artery disease by nifedipine. The Lancet 1990; 335: 1109–1113

56. Ornish D, Brown SE, Scherwitz LW, Billings JH, Armstrong WT, Ports TA, McLanahan SM, Gould KL: Can lifestyle changes reverse coronary heart disease? The Lancet 1990; 336: 129–133

57. Gupta M, Connolly AJ, Zhu BQ, Sievers RE, Sudhir K, Sun YP, Parmley WW, Fitzgerald PJ, Yock PG: Quantitative analysis of progression of atherosclerosis by intravascular ultrasound: validation in a rabbit model. Circulation 1992; 86 (Suppl. I): I–518.

58. Davies MJ, Thomas AC; Plaque fissuring — the cause of acute myoacardial infarction, sudden ischaemic death, and crescendo angina. Br Heart J 1985; 53: 363–373

59. Ambrose JA, Winter SL, Stern A, Eng A, Teichholz LE, Gorlin R, Fuster V: Angiographic morphology and the pathogenesis of unstable angina pectoris. J Am Coll Cardiol 1985; 5: 609–616

60. Little WC, Constantinescu M, Applegate RJ, Kutcher MA, Burows MT, Kahl FR, Santamore WP: Can coronary angiography predict the site of a subsesquent myocardial infarction in patients with mild-to-moderate coronary artery disease. Circulation 1988; 78: 1157–1166

61. Lichtlen PR, Nikutta P, Jost S, Deckers JW, Wiese B, Rafflenbeul W: Anatomical progresson of coronary artery disease in humans as seen by prospective, repeated, quantitated coronary angiography. Relation to clinical events and risk factors. Circulation 1992; 86: 828–838

62. Brown BG, Gallery CA, Badger RS, Kennedy JW, Mathey D, Bolson EL, Dodge HT: Incomplete lysis of thrombus in the moderate underlying atherosclerotic lesin during intracoronary infusion of streptokinase for acute myocaridal infarction: quantitative angiographic observations. Circulation 1986; 73: 653–661

63. Loree HM, Kamm RD, Stringfellow RG, Lee RT: Effects of fibrous cap thickness on peak circumferential stress in model atherosclerotic vessels. Circ Res 1992; 71: 850–858

64. Nissen SE, Gurley JC, Booth DC, Berk MR, Yamagishi M, Fischer C, DiMaria AN. Differences in intravascular ultrasound plaque morphology in stable and unstable patients. Circulation 1991; 84 (Suppl. II): II–436

65. The GUIDE Trail Investigators (1992) Lumen enlargement following angioplasty is related to plaque characteristics. A report from the GUIDE Trial. Circulation 86 (Suppl. I): I–531

66. Saner HE, Gobel FL, Salomonowitz E, Erlien DA, Edwards JE: The disease-free wall in coronary atherosclerosis: its relation to degree of obstruction. J Am Coll Cardiol 1985; 6: 1096–1099

67. Schroeder JS, Gao S, Hunt SA, Stinson EB: Accelerated graft coronary artery disease: diagnosis and prevention. J Heart Lung Transplant 1992; 11: 258–266

68. St.Goar FG, Pinto FJ, Alderman EL, Valantine HA, Schroeder JS, Gao ZS, Stinson EB, Popp RL: Intracoronary ultrasound in cardiac transplant recipients: in vivo evidence of "angiographically silent" intimal thickening. Circulation 1992; 85: 979–987

69. Ventura HO, Ramee SR, Ashit J, White CJ, Collins TJ, Mesa JE, Murgo JP: Coronary artery imaging with intravascular ultrasound in patients following cardiac transplantation. Transplantation 1992; 53: 216–219

70. Jaski BE, Skowronski EW, Stewart JB, Gordon JB, Smith SC: Detection of fatal coronary arteriopathy in a heart-transplant recipient by intravascular ultrasonography. N Engl J Med 1991; 325: 358–359

71. Pinto FJ, St. Goar FG, Fischell TA, Stadius ML, Valantine HA, Alderman EL, Popp RL: Nitroglycerin-induced coronary vasodilation in cardiac transplant recipients. Evaluation with in vivo intracoronary ultrasound. Circulation 1992; 85: 69–77

72. Hausmann D, Mügge A, Fitzgerald PJ, Yock PG, Daniel WG: Nitroglycerin-induced coronary vasodilation in heart transplant patients is impaired by intimal thickening. J Am Coll Cardiol 1993: 21 (Abstract Suppl.): 334A (Abstract)

73. Yeung AC, Anderson T, Meredith I, Uehata A, Ryan TJ, Selwyn AP, Mudge GH, Ganz P: Endothelial dysfunetion in the development and detection of transplant coronary artery disease. J Heart Lung Transplant 1992; S69–S73

74. Tenaglia AN, Buller CE, Kisslo KB, Stack RS, Davidson CJ: Mechanisms of balloon angioplasty and directional coronary atherectomy as assessed by intracoronary ultrasound. J Am Coll Cardiol 1992; 20: 685–691

75. Potkin BN, Keren G, Mintz GS, Duek PC, Pichard AD, Satler LF, Kent KM, Leon M: Arterial responses to balloon coronary angioplasty: an intravascular ultrasound study. J Am Coll Cardiol 1992; 20: 942–951

76. Losordo DW, Rosenfield K, Pieczek A, Baker K, Harding M, Isner JM: How does angioplasty work? Serial analysis of human iliac arteries using intravascular ultrasound. Circulation 1992; 86: 1845–1858

77. Forrester JS, Fisbein M, Helfant R, Fagin J: A paradigm for restenosis based on cell biology: clues for the development of new preventive therapies. J Am Coll Cardiol 1991; 17: 758–769

78. Fitzgerald PJ, Ports TA, Yock PG: Contribution of localized calcium deposits to dissection after angioplasty: An observational study using intravascular ultrasound. Circulation 1992; 86:64–70

79. Mintz GS, Douek P, Pichard AD, Kent KM, Satler LF, Popma JJ, Leon MB: Target lesion calcification in coronary artery disease: an intravascular ultrasound study. J Am Coll Cardiol 1992; 20: 1149–1155

80. Hodgson JM, Cacchione JG, Berry J, et al. Combined intracoronary ultrasound imaging and angioplasty catheter: initial in-vivo studies. Circulation 1990; 82 (Suppl III): III–676.

81. Caccione JG, Reddy K, Richards F, Sheehan H, Hodgson JM: Combined intravascular ultrasound/angioplasty balloon catheter: initial use during PTCA. Cathet Cardiovasc Diagn 1991; 24: 99–101

82. Isner JM, Rosenfield K, Losordo DW, Rose L, Langevin RE, Razvi S, Kosowsky BD: Combination balloon-ultrasound imaging catheter for percutaneous transluminal angioplasty. Validation of imaging, analysis of recoil, and identification of plaque fracture. Circulation 1991; 84: 739–754

83. Yock PG, Fitzgerald PJ, Sykes C, et al.: Morphologic features of successful coronary atherectomy determined by intravascular ultrasound imaging. Circulation 1990; 82 (Suppl. III): III–676

84. Kimura BJ, Fitzgerald PJ, Sudhir K, Amidon TM, Strunk BL, Yock PG: Guidance of directed coronary atherectomy by intracoronary ultrasound imaging. Am Heart J 1992; 124: 1365–1369

85. Fitzgerald PJ, Muhlberger VA, Moes NY et al: Calcium location within plaque as a predictor of atherectomy tissue retrieval: an intravascular ultrasound study. Circulation 1992; 86 (Suppl. I): I–516 (Abstract)

86. Mintz GS, Pichard AD, Popma JJ, Kent KM, Satler LF, Leon MB: Preliminary experience with adjunct directional coronary atherectomy after high-speed rotational atherectomy in the treatment of calcific coronary artery disease. Am J Cardiol 1993; 71: 799–804

87. Slepian MJ: Application of intraluminal ultrasound imaging to vascular stenting. Int J Card Imag 1991; 6: 285–311

88. Cavaye DM, Tabbara MR, Kopchok GE, Termin P, White RA: Intraluminal ultrasound assessment of vascular stent deployment. Ann Vasc Surg 1991; 5: 241–246

89. Schryver TE, Popma JJ, Kent KM, Leon MB, Eldredge S, Mintz GS: Use of intracoronary ultrasound identify the "true" coronary lumen in chronic coronary dissection treated with intracoronary stenting. Am J Cardiol 1992; 69: 1107–1108

Peripheral Intravascular Ultrasonography

E. J. Gussenhoven, A. van der Lugt, S. H. K. The, W. Li, F. C. van Egmond, H. Pieterman, and H. van Urk

Introduction

In recent years the development of percutaneous endovascular interventions has prompted research on new intravascular diagnostic devices; of these, intravascular ultrasound is a promising tool. Since this technique provides histologic like high resolution cross-sectional images of the artery, it is especially useful to describe morphologic characteristics of the vessel wall in conjunction with interventional techniques [1–6].

In vitro studies demonstrated that intravascular ultrasound can distinguish the elastic from the muscular type of arteries [1]. In elastic arteries (e. g., carotid artery) the elastin fibers present in the tunica media are responsible for a homogeneously bright arterial wall. In muscular arteries (e. g., coronary and iliofemoral arteries) the smooth muscle cells present in the tunica media result in the typical three-layered appearance of the arterial wall. In the presence of an arteriosclerotic lesion it has been found that basically three types of lesions can be distinguished: (a) lesions that are echographically "soft" correspond to fibromuscular and/or fibrous lesions, (b) those that are echographically "hard" with ultrasonic shadowing beyond the lesion correspond to calcified atherosclerotic lesions, and (c) a distinct hypoechoic region inside an echographically "soft" lesion generally indicates a large lipid deposit. In addition, quantitative validation studies have shown that intravascular ultrasound measurements correlate closely with histologic data [1, 4].

Since the histopathologic and quantitative validation of intravascular ultrasound has been established in vitro, the precise role of this technique in the clinical setting is being determined in ongoing studies. It is realistic to say that only if intravascular ultrasound provides important data that affect clinical decisions or prognoses, is this new diagnostic technique here to stay. The major goals in the treatment of vascular obstructive disease are improving the primary and long-term success rate of interventions, reducing the restenosis rate, and reducing complications. The use of intravascular ultrasound may contribute to these goals. Initially it may help to improve the definitions of in vivo vascular pathology before and after (endo)vascular interventions. Later it may provide useful information for better selecting patients for specific and/or additional treatment modalities such as balloon angioplasty, atherectomy, stenting, or a primary bypass operation and in this way improve the overall results of therapy.

This chapter provides a brief overview of the intravascular ultrasound methodology currently employed in our Departments of Radiology and Vascular Surgery, summarizes the current clinical applications and results in peripheral arterial disease, and compares intravascular ultrasound and angiography.

Methods

Intravascular Ultrasound Investigation

The present intravascular ultrasound systems used in peripheral arteries fall into two categories: electronic and mechanical systems. The catheter of the phased-array device contains multiple (32 or 64) small acoustic elements which are positioned cylindrically around the catheter tip. By introducing electronically switched time delays subgroups of elements may together form an echo image. Conversely, mechanical devices are based either on the rotating mirror principle or on the rotation of the ultrasound element itself. Both phased-array and mechanical systems operate at either 20 or 30 MHz.

The Departments of Radiology and Vascular Surgery at Erasmus University Hospital Rotterdam use a mechanical 30-MHz imaging system (Du-MED, Rotterdam, The Netherlands). The transducer is mounted on a 4.1-F catheter and rotates up to 16 images per second [7]. Axial

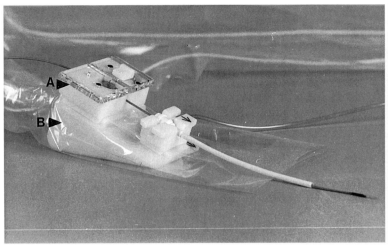 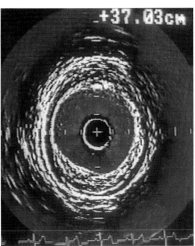

Fig. 1. *Left,* displacement sensing device showing the sensing unit (*A*) attached to the registration (*B*). For clinical studies the ultrasound catheter is advanced via the sensing unit and sheath into the vessel. *Right,* the position of the ultrasound catheter tip in relation to the radiopaque ruler (37.03 cm) is documented instantaneously on the videoscreen. The soft eccentric lesion (*6 o'clock*) results in an area obstruction of 30 %. Note medial thinning beyond the lesion. +, Catheter; calibration, 1 mm

resolution of the system is 80 μm, and lateral resolution is greater than 225 μm at a depth of 1 mm. The resulting images are displayed on a monitor via a videoscanned memory and stored on a VHS system. The ultrasound catheter is sterilized with ethylene oxide. A radiopaque ruler is used to match angiographic and ultrasound data. The presence and location of obstructive lesions are first assessed routinely by single-plane angiography using a 7-F sheath placed into the common femoral artery. The ultrasound catheter is advanced over a guide wire (monorail system) to the level of the obstruction and if possible beyond the obstructive lesion. Under fluoroscopic control a series of cross-sections are then recorded during pull-back of the catheter. When a stenosis is present, recordings are made at 5- or 10-mm intervals. At each level the catheter is kept in position long enough for recording. To eliminate the effects of echogenic blood saline can be injected via the side port of the sheath; this procedure facilitates off-line analysis of the still frames. After intervention (e.g., balloon angioplasty, bypass surgery) a repeat angiogram is made, followed by a second examination by intravascular ultrasound.

To document the position of the ultrasound catheter tip within the artery real-time cineangiography or fluoroscopy can be combined instantaneously with ultrasound imaging using split-screen videotaping. Documentation of the position of the ultrasound catheter tip compared with the radiopaque ruler facilitates comparison of the ultrasound data before and after intervention and comparison of these results with the angiographic records [7, 8]. Secondly, a displacement sensing device can be used providing instantaneous online orientation of the location from which the ultrasound images were derived within the vascular tree, with known interslice distance (Fig. 1) [9, 10].

Definition and Terminology

– Muscular artery: recognized by three contiguous layers encircling the lumen: the hypoechoic media seen between the inner echodense layer (intima and internal elastic lamina) and outer echodense layer (external elastic lamina and adventitia; Fig. 2)
– Vein: echographically recognized by a homogeneous vessel wall (Fig. 2)
– ePTFE (Gore-tex) prosthesis: seen as a highly reflective echo structure (Fig. 2)
– Soft lesion: recognized as having a homogeneous echo structure without shadowing (Fig. 3)
– Hard lesion: recognized by the presence of a bright echo structure casting peripheral shadowing (Fig. 3)

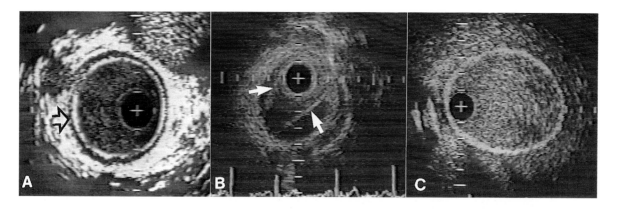

Fig. 2. Intravascular ultrasound cross-sections showing the characteristics of a muscular artery (**A**), a vein together with valves (**B**, *arrows*), and a Gore-tex prosthesis (**C**). Note that the hypoechoic media (*open arrow*), typical for a muscular artery, is seen amidst internal elastic lamina/intima and adventitia. +, Catheter; calibration, 1 mm

– Fresh thrombus: recognized as a soft lesion having a homogeneous echo structure
– Organized thrombus: seen as a soft lesion having a homogeneous echo structure
– Concentric lesion: defined as a lesion distributed along the entire circumference of the vessel wall in a cross-section (Fig. 4)
– Eccentric lesion: defined as a lesion involving one part of the circumference of the vessel wall in a cross-section, leaving the remaining part disease free (Figs. 1, 3)
– Dissection: defined as the presence of a separation of the lesion from the underlying arterial wall (Fig. 4)
– Plaque rupture: identified as an interruption in the lesion (intimal) surface (Fig. 4)
– Internal elastic lamina rupture: defined as an interruption in the internal elastic lamina (Fig. 4).

Quantitative Analysis

To understand the ultimate effect of an intervention the corresponding ultrasound images before and following intervention can be analyzed with a digital videoanalyzer as described previously. Briefly, the commercially available analysis system is developed on an IBM PC/AT (IBM, Boca Raton, USA) equipped with a frame-grabber and PC mouse device. Each image reproduced on the analyzer videoscreen can be contour traced (Fig. 5). To facil-

itate the quantitative analysis, real-time images can be replayed on a separate videomonitor. The following parameters can be analyzed [11, 12]:
– Free lumen area (mm^2): defined as the area encompassed by the inner boundary of the intimal surface (characterized also by the presence of blood flow)
– Media-bounded area (mm^2): defined as the native vessel area bounded by the hypoechoic medial layer

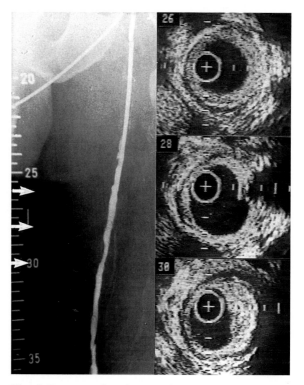

Fig. 3. Intravascular ultrasound cross-sections and corresponding angiogram with radiopaque ruler showing difference in a soft lesion (*level 26*) and hard lesions (*levels 28, 30*). +, Catheter; calibration 1 mm. (From [8])

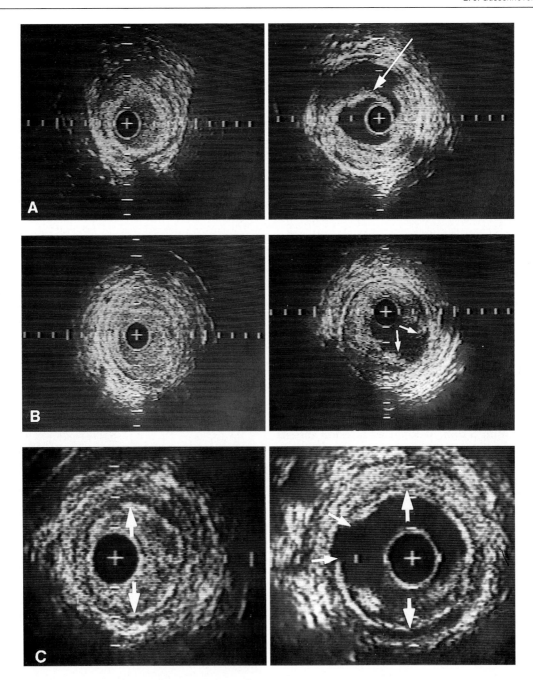

Fig. 4 A–C. Corresponding intravascular ultrasound cross-sections obtained prior to (*left panels*) and following (*right panels*) balloon angioplasty, showing three basic anatomic features that may occur as result of a balloon angioplasty. **A** Dissection (*arrow*). **B** Plaque rupture (*arrows*). **C** Internal elastic lamina rupture (*arrows at 9 o'clock*). Note the increase in media-bounded area (*vertical areas*). Before intervention an eccentric soft lesion was present in **A**; in **B, C** a concentric soft lesion was involved. + Catheter; calibration, 1 mm

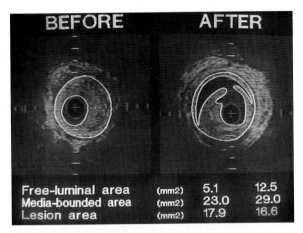

Fig. 5. Intravascular ultrasound cross-sections of the superficial femoral artery showing the traced contours of the free lumen and media-bounded lumen area. The region enclosed by the two contours is the lesion area. The quantitative results obtained before and after balloon angioplasty are provided. +, Catheter; calibration, 1 mm. (From [8])

– Lesion area (mm²): calculated as the difference between media-bounded area and free lumen area

In those instances where partial drop-out of echoes from the luminal contour (for free lumen area) or medial layer (for media-bounded area) were noted, the contours were estimated by means of continuity from adjacent sections.

Results

Intravascular Ultrasound and Balloon Angioplasty

Comparison of corresponding intravascular ultrasound images prior to and following balloon angioplasty confirmed for the first time unequivocally that luminal enlargement by balloon angioplasty is produced primarily by overstretching the arterial wall with the lesion volume remaining practically constant (Figs. 4–6). The increase in free lumen area was generally associated with an increase in media-bounded area and a decrease in medial thickness (median media thickness from 0.6 mm to 0.3 mm) [8]. In addition, it was observed that the increased free lumen area was unrelated to the type of lesion (hard or soft). Overstretching was almost always accompanied by a dissection and a plaque rupture and sometimes by an internal elastic lamina rupture (Figs. 4, 5). With respect to the internal elastic lamina rupture it was found that the original diameter of the vessel was relatively small in relation to the balloon size. It was also observed that soft lesions were more frequently associated with dissection and plaque rupture than were hard lesions (56% versus 28%, respectively). In some instances partial or complete disappearance of the lesion suggested dislodging and embolization of the lesion as an additional effect of balloon angioplasty (see also Figs. 4c, 6).

Fig. 6. Comparison of free lumen, media-bounded and lesion areas before and after balloon angioplasty in a total of 106 ultrasonic cross-sections. Each pair of cross-sections obtained before and after intervention is interconnected. Note the increase in free lumen and media-bounded area, whereas lesion area remains practically unchanged. In some cases partial or total disappearance of the lesion occurs

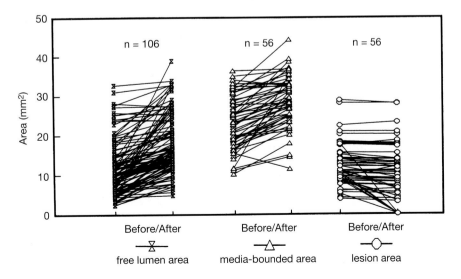

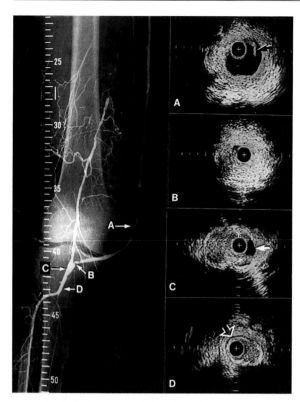

Fig. 7. *Left,* angiogram with corresponding intravascular cross-sections (*A–D*) immediately following bypass surgery (vein graft). The ultimate result judged from angiogram was ambiguous. *Right,* intravascular ultrasound images (*A–D*) corresponding to positions indicated on the angiogram. Intravascular ultrasound evidenced an obstructive lesion proximal to (*B*) and at the anastomotic site. *A Black arrow,* valve remnants. *C Arrow* points to the narrow free lumen area. *D Open arrow,* media of the popliteal artery. +, Catheter; calibration, 1 mm

Intravascular Ultrasound and Bypass Anastomosis

Intravascular ultrasound has been used to assess the effectiveness of bypass anastomosis using either ePTFE Gore-tex (Gore, Flagstaff, USA) or saphenous vein bypass [13]. It became evident that adequate anastomoses can be distinguished from obstructive anastomoses that require immediate reintervention (Fig. 7). In addition, it was found that the ultrasound data can solve ambiguous angiographic results. For instance, following saphenous bypass surgery the angiogram revealed an ambiguous obstruction proximal to the anastomosis. Using intravascular ultrasound an external compression was clearly visualized. Subsequent to tendon cleavage intravascular ultrasound and angiography revealed normal findings.

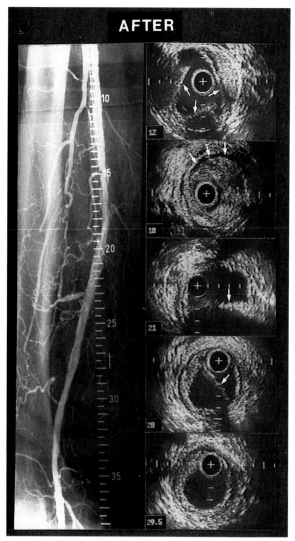

Fig. 8. Angiographic and intravascular ultrasound cross-sections obtained from the superficial femoral artery following balloon angioplasty. The ultrasound images best elucidated the variability in anatomy. A dissection was seen both angiographically and by ultrasound at levels 12, 18, 21, and 28. The degree of stenosis was less than 50 % at level 12.5 with both techniques. At level 18 angiography judged the stenosis less than 50 %; however, ultrasound revealed 50 %–90 % stenosis (75 %). The lesion is seen dissected from the arterial wall (*arrows*). The dissection seen at level 21 resulted in a large dropout of echoes beyond the dissection. At this level no semiquantitative analysis could be made. At level 29.5 a normal vessel was seen. +, Catheter; calibration, 1 mm

Intravascular Ultrasound and Angiography

By comparing angiography and intravascular ultrasound in peripheral arteries a good correlation was found for the recognition of eccentric or

Table 1. Results of the percentage area obstruction assessed semiquantitatively by visual inspection and quantitatively using a computer-aided analysis system

		Percentage area obstruction		
Semiquantitative analysis	Normal	$<50\%$	$50\%-90\%$	$>90\%$
Quantitative analysis	$18.0\% \pm 10.5\%$	$43.2\% \pm 7.1\%$	$65.1 \pm 8.0\%$	$83.0\% \pm 9.1\%$

concentric lesions prior to intervention and the extent of dissections seen following intervention [14, 15] (Fig. 8). Plaque rupture and particularly internal elastic lamina rupture were uniquely documented by intravascular ultrasound. Comparison of the semiquantitative analysis of the degree of luminal narrowing (normal, $<50\%$, $50\%-90\%$, $>90\%$ stenosis) from angiograms (diameter stenosis) and corresponding intravascular ultrasound cross-sections (area stenosis) showed that the two techniques agreed in 75%. In 25%, however, the degree of stenosis was judged more severe on ultrasound (Fig. 8). One reason why contrast angiography may overestimate the true lumen diameter during projection imaging is that from a mathematical point of view a 50% diameter stenosis is equivalent to a 75% area stenosis; the ultrasonic grade therefore appears more severe than the angiographic grade. Another reason for this discrepancy is the fact that angiography uses the alleged normal vessel segment as reference. In contrast, intravascular ultrasound uses the arterial media as reference to quantify the degree of area obstruction (Fig. 5). Furthermore, it was found that the degree of stenosis assessed by visual inspection of the intravascular ultrasound cross-sections corresponds well with the quantitative analysis (Table 1) using a digital videoanalyzer. This suggests that intravascular ultrasound may serve as an on-line decision-making device prior to and following intervention (Fig. 7). It is important to mention that quantitative analysis of the ultrasonic images that were initially judged semiquantitatively by visual inspection as normal revealed a mean area obstruction of 18% (Table 1). This underlines the fact that angiographic reference segments may indeed not be as "normal" as alleged. The significance of the stenosis seen echographically immediately following intervention is underlined by the observation that five of the eight patients in whom intravascular ultrasound evidenced a residual stenosis of $50\%-90\%$ required a reintervention.

Discussion

Intravascular ultrasound appears to have several advantages over angiography. The technique provides both qualitative and quantitative information about the vessel wall and atherosclerotic lesions that cannot be obtained by any other method in comparable details and accuracy [7, 8, 13–19]. Before intervention the nature of an obstruction may be elucidated, and heavily calcified lesions can be distinguished from soft lesions. These morphologic features provide clues for the selection of patients for various treatment modalities [13, 19, 20]. In our hands, planned interventions have not been performed on the basis of morphologic data provided laser angioplasty was not used in the presence of concentric calcified obstructive lesion but rather bypass surgery. Similarly, atherectomy is not applied in the presence of superficial calcified lesions; however, when calcification is deep inside a lesion, atherectomy may be performed successfully.

Furthermore, the ultrasound technique provides a better understanding of the pathophysiologic effects of balloon angioplasty. The increase in free lumen area seen echographically following balloon angioplasty is based on stretching of the media-bounded area while the plaque area remains practically unchanged [8]. Whether a more complete debulking of the lesion should be performed as accomplished, for example, by atherectomy remains to be determined. The clinical implications of the intravascular ultrasonographic finding that soft lesions are more frequently associated with dissection and/or plaque rupture than hard lesions remain to be determined.

It has been found that angiography may underestimate the degree of stenosis seen before and after intervention [14, 15, 20, 21]. This is of paramount importance, particularly in the light of increasing the primary success of intervention. Similarly, unexpected stenosis detected by intravascular ultrasound distal to obstructive lesions following intervention has led to additional surgical intervention. We experienced that five of the eight patients in whom intravascular ultrasound evidenced a 50%–90% area stenosis following balloon angioplasty required reintervention (three patients within 2 weeks and two within 6 months). At present our reseach seeks to define the point within the range of 50%–90% area stenosis and in the free lumen area that determines the necessity for additional revascularization.

Similarly as angiography may overestimate the arterial lumen, the inappropriate internal elastic lumina and media rupture seen on intravascular ultrasound following balloon angioplasty may sometimes be avoided by proper balloon sizing. Balloon size estimates based on angiographic images often results in oversizing; this difficulty is avoided when intravascular ultrasound is used [15, 22]. In addition, intravascular ultrasound has been shown to have an impact on the interpretation of ambiguous angiographic findings [13, 23], and at the same time may prevent complications.

The role of intravascular ultrasound in evaluating the primary success of the intervention, evaluating restenosis, and selecting optimal treatment for individual lesions is evolving; additional balloon angioplasties have been performed based on intravascular ultrasound criteria [24, 25]. In other instances the ultrasound information has led to modification of the angioplasty procedure [20]. Detection of plaque rupture and dissection can be used to monitor the proper and selective placement of stents: selective positioning of short stents at the entry and/or reentry of a dissection may be of value in the effort to reduce the restenosis phenomenon.

From our clinical experience to date we conclude that intravascular ultrasound enables us to extend our knowledge and understanding of the ultimate result of vascular intervention.

Randomized studies are required to determine the specific variables that are predictive of early and late success after balloon angioplasty.

References

1. Gussenhoven EJ, Essed CE, Lancée CT, Mastik F, Frietman P, van Egmond FC, Reiber J, Bosch H, van Urk H, Roelandt J, Bom N (1989) Arterial wall characteristics determined by intravascular ultrasound imaging: and in vitro study. J Am Coll Cardiol; 14: 947–952.

2. Gussenhoven WJ, Essed CE, Frietman P, Mastik F, Lancée C, Slager C, Serruys P, Gerritsen P, Pieterman H, Bom N (1989) Intravascular echographic assessment of vessel wall characteristics: a correlation with histology. Int J Card Imaging; 4: 105–116.

3. Nishimura RA, Edwards WD, Warnes CA, Reeder GS, Holmes DR, Tajik AJ, Yock PG (1990) Intravascular ultrasound imaging: in vitro validation and pathologic correlation. J Am Coll Cardiol; 16: 145–154.

4. Tobis JM, Mallery JA, Gessert J, Griffith J, Mahon D, Bessen M, Moriuchi M, McLeavy L, McRae M, Henry WL (1989) Intravascular ultrasound cross-sectional arterial imaging before and after balloon angioplasty in vitro. Circulation; 80: 873–882.

5. Gussenhoven EJ, Frietman PAV, The SHK, van Suylen RJ, van Egmond FC, Lancée CT, van Urk H, Roelandt JRTC, Stijnen T, Bom N (1991) Assessment of medial thinning in atherosclerosis by intravascular ultrasound. Am J Cardiol; 68: 1625–1632.

6. Lockwood GR, Ryan LK, Gotlieb AI, Lonn E, Hunt JW, Liu P, Foster FS (1992) In vitro high resolution intravascular imaging in muscular and elastic arteries. J Am Coll Cardiol; 20: 153–160.

7. Gussenhoven EJ, Lugt vd A, The SHK, de Feyter P, Serruys PWE, Suylen v RJ, Lancée CT, van Urk H, Pieterman H (1993) Similarities and differences between coronary and iliofemoral arteries related to intravascular ultrasound. Intravascular ultrasound. Eds. Roelandt, Gussenhoven, Bom; Kluwer Academic Press, 1993 pp 45–62.

8. The SHK, Gussenhoven EJ, Zhong Y, Li W, van Egmond F, Pieterman H, van Urk H, Gerritsen GP, Borst C, Wilson RA, Bom N (1992) The effect of balloon angioplasty on the femoral artery evaluated with intravascular ultrasound imaging. Circulation; 86: 483–493.

9. Gussenhoven EJ, Li W, Lugt vd A, Strijen v MJL, Stigter CMM, The SHK, van Egmond F, Mali WPTM, Bom N (1993) Accurate displacement sensing device provides reproducible intravascular ultrasound images. J Am Coll Cardiol; 21: 119 A.

10. Gussenhoven EJ, Strijen v MJL, Lugt vd A, Li W, The SHK, Egmond FC, Honkoop J, Peters RJG, de Feyter P, van Urk H, Pieterman H (1993) Accurate displacement sensing device provides reproducible intravascular ultrasound images. Intravascular ultrasound. Eds. Roelandt, Gussenhoven, Bom; Kluwer Academic Press, 1993 pp 157–166.

11. Wenguang L, Gussenhoven WJ, Zhong Y, The SHK, Di Mario C, Madretsma S, van Egmond F, de Feyter P, Pieterman H, van Urk H, Rijsterborgh H, Bom N (1991) Validation of quantitative analysis of intravascular ultrasound images. Int J Card Imaging; 6: 247–253.

12. Wenguang L, Gussenhoven WJ, Bosch JG, Mastik F, Reiber JHC, Bom N (1990) A computer-aided analysis system for the quantitative assessment of intravascular ultrasound images. Proceedings of computers in cardiology. Los Alanitos, IEEE Computer Society Press: 333–336.

13. The SHK, Gussenhoven EJ, du Bois NAJJ, Pieterman H, Roelandt JRTC, Wilson RA, van Urk H (1991) Femoro-popliteal bypass grafts studied by intravascular ultrasound. Eur J Vasc Surg; 5: 523–526.

14. van Urk H, Gussenhoven WJ, The SHK, Pieterman H, Bom N (1993) Intravascular ultrasound assessment of luminal dimension: a comparison with angiography. Angiology; 44: suppl. 13–14.

15. Gerritsen GP, Gussenhoven EJ, The SHK, Pieterman H, van de Lugt A, Li W, Bom N, van Dijk LC, Du Bois MD, NAJJ, van Urk H (1993) Intravascular ultrasound before and after intervention: in vivo comparison with angiography. J Vasc Surg (in press).

16. Davidson CJ, Sheikh KH, Harrison K, Himmelstein SI, Leithe ME, Kisslo KB, Bashore TM (1990) Intravascular ultrasonography versus digital subtraction angiography: a human in vivo comparison of vessel size and morphology. J Am Coll Cardiol; 16: 633–636.

17. Tabbara M, White R, Cavaye D, Kopchok G (1991) In vivo human comparison of intravascular ultrasonography and angiography. J Vasc Surg; 14: 496–504.

18. Sheikh KH, Davidson CJ, Kisslo KB, Harrison JK, Himmelstein SI, Kisslo J, Bashore TM (1991) Comparison of intravascular ultrasound, external ultrasound and digital angiography for evaluation of peripheral artery dimensions and morphology. Am J Cardiol; 67: 817–822.

19. Deaner ANS, Caubukcu A, Scott PJ, Essop AR, Williams GJ (1992) Comparison of angiography and intravascular ultrasound in the detection of early atherosclerosis. Br Heart J; 68: 120–121.

20. van Urk H, Gussenhoven WJ, Gerritsen GP, Pieterman H, The SHK, van Egmond F, Lancée CT, Bom N (1991) Assessment of arterial disease and arterial reconstructions by intravascular ultrasound. Int J Card Imaging; 6: 157–164.

21. Cavaye DM, White RA, Tabbara MR, Kopchok GE (1992) Intravascular ultrasonography. Surg Clinics N Am; 72: 823–842.

22. Werner GS, Corovic D, Buchwald A, Sold G, Kreuzer H, Wiegand V (1990) Intravaskuläre Ultraschalldiagnostik. In-vivo-Befunde vor und nach Angioplastie bei peripherer arterielle Verschlußkrankheit. Dtsch Med Wschr; 115: 1259–1265.

23. White CJ, Ramee SR, Collins TJ, Jain A, Mesa JE (1992) Catheterization and Cardiovascular diagnosis 26: 200–203.

24. Katzen BT (1992) Radiol Clin North Am 30: 5. 895–905.

25. Tabbara MR, Mehringer M, Cavaye DM, Schwartz M, Kopchok GE, Maselly M, White RA (1992) Sequential intraluminal ultrasound evaluation of balloon angioplasty of an iliac arterty lesion. Ann Vasc Surg; 6: 179–184.

Section IV
Angioscopy

Coronary Angioscopy

K. Mizuno

Introduction

Coronary angioscopy is a new diagnostic tool that permits nonoperative imaging of intravascular structures through the use of a fiber optic system. Coronary angioscopy is playing an ever-expanding role in research and in clinical practice because it provides a precise, full-color, three-dimensional perspective of the interior surface morphology of coronary arteries whereas ordinary coronary arteriography provides only two-dimensional black and white lumenograms. Angioscopy now permits detailed examination of the macromorphology of coronary artery disease that hitherto was unavailable except during autopsy. The ability to discriminate among colors in angioscopy makes it relatively easy to distinguish between a thrombus and a plaque, even if the clot is very small [1–3]. Furthermore, angioscopy can also distinguish between types of plaque (e.g., xanthomatous versus white plaque) and types of thrombus (e.g., red versus white thrombus) [4, 5]. The three-dimensonal perspective and high resolution of angioscopic images can disclose luminal changes in minute plaque ruptures, ulceration, intimal flap, or torn tissue strands not typically appreciated by coronary angiography. Therefore, angioscopy is helpful not only in correlating anatomical and pathological features that cannot be detected in routine coronary arteriography but also in monitoring coronary interventions such as thrombolytic therapy, percutaneous transluminal coronary angioplasty (PTCA), atherectomy, laser angioplasty, and stenting. This chapter explores the development of coronary angioscopy, technical considerations, clinical results, as well as areas for future research and development.

The Angioscopic Imaging System

The angioscopic system (Fig. 1, 2), consists of angioscope, a charge-coupled device color camera, a lamp light source, a cathode ray tube, a video documentation system, and an image processor. In addition to video tape, angioscopic images can be stored on individual photographic stills, on cinematographic moving film, or on any combination of the two.

Angioscope

The coronary artery is small and tortuous. Therefore very thin, flexible, high-resolution imaging optic fibers are required to obtain high-quality angioscopic images. The utility of a fiber optic bundle depends upon its flexibility, which should be maximal, and the reliability of the transmitted image, which should be minimally distored. Minimizing the number of fibers maximizes the flexibility, but the fewer the number of fibers the more distorted is the image; conversely, maximizing the number of fibers minimizes distortion while minimizing flexibility. A compromise is achieved by using thousands of extremely small diameter fibers to make up the bundle; each fiber corresponds to one pixel of the image. Newer technology employs individual fibers less than 3 μm in diameter which are free to slide over each other throughout the body of the fiberoptic bundle; the fibers are bound together at each end. This technology allows much greater flexibility as well as miniaturization of the angioscopic probe. For percutaneous transluminal coronary angioscopy fiber optic bundles of 0.2–0.3 mm diameter containing 2000–3000 individual fibers are used. Larger diameter fiberoptic bundles containing up to 10 000 individual fibers can be used for intraoperative coronary angioscopy. A tiny lens is attached to the distal end of the bundle typically allowing a view-

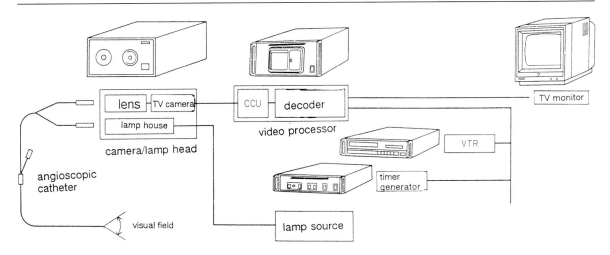

Fig. 1. Angioscopic imaging system

ing angle of 50°–90°. The energy (light signal) output of the fiberoptic bundle is far too small to be viewed directly; therefore it is converted to an electrical signal and transmitted to a television monitor. Light-transmitting fibers are required to illuminate the field of view. These are generally composed of multicomponent glass fiber or fused silica and may be set around the image-conducting fibers or packed together as a single illumination bundle. The illumination source most commonly employed is a high-intensity (300 W) xenon light. Adjustment of the light intensity is a dynamic process and depends upon the focal length, viewing angle of the distal lens, diameter of the vessel lumen, and aperture of the video camera lens. Depending on the system used, angioscopic images can be then stored either on videotape [3, 6], cine film [7], or still photographs [8, 9]. When videotape is utilized, a high-resolution 3/4-in. video tape recorder is used for storing the live angioscopic images. If still photography is utilized, ultrahigh-speed daylight type color reversal film (ASA 1600) is used.

Angiscopic Catheter

To deliver the angioscope percutaneously to the target lesion within the coronary tree accurately and without trauma we [6] first developed a 1.2-m-long angiscopic catheter with 1.55 mm outer diameter (Fig. 3). The distal end (10 cm) is tapered to an outer diameter of 1.10 mm. The catheter is made of polyvinyl chloride or polyethylene and has three or four channels. One channel (0.5 mm

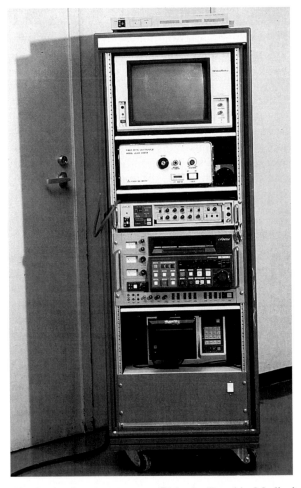

Fig. 2. Angioscopy system (Fukuda Denshi, Medical Science, Tokyo). This system includes a high-resolution color video monitor, video camera, illumination source, and video tape recorder

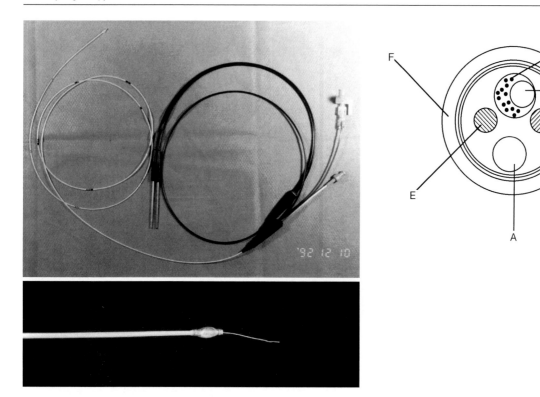

Fig. 3. Angioscopic catheter (Mitsubishi Cable, Itami Hyogo-ken). *Left above*, whole view of the angioscopic catheter. *Left below*, tip of the angioscopic catheter. *Right*, cross-section of the angioscopic catheter. *A*, Irrigation and guide wire lumen; *B*, objective lens (image guide); *C*, light guide; *D*, seal of balloon lumen; *E*, angulation lumen; *F*, balloon

in diameter) is designed for irrigation and placement of a PTCA guide wire of up to a 0.36 mm (0.014 in.). One channel is designed for balloon inflation. The remaining channels contain the image and the light guide fibers, respectively. This angioscopic catheter (Fig. 3) has an inflatable balloon at the tip of the catheter used to obstruct the blood flow and to replace it completely with a translucent medium thereby allowing for an optimum visibility. Similar systems are now commercially avaible and used by many investigators. In these angioscopic systems interventional devices such as PTCA, laser, and atherectomy catheters can be introduced independently into the coronary artery over a long guide wire. A monorail coronary angiscope [10] may be more cost effective and simpler to use. Recently a more sophisticated angioscopic catheter, employing a movable optic bundle with an outer catheter, has been introduced [11]. The angioscope (movable optic bundle) and its guide (outer catheter, 4.8 F) compose unit, and both are advanced over the guide wire. By inflation of an occlusion cuff on the outer catheter and by moving of the optic bundle, the coronary lumen can be observed in 5-cm-long segments. However, this system may need more flushing solution because there is no occlusion cuff.

Angioscopic Procedure

In our system all angioscopic catheters are tested prior to use for minimum focus, special resolution, and chromatic aberration; color balancing is controlled automatically. If a balloon is present in the catheter, air leakage from the balloon is checked by immersion in a liquid (usually physiological saline). Heparin (5000 IU) is administered intravenously immediately before the angioscopic examination. To obtain access to the coronary artery for the angioscopic catheter, a large lumen, 8-F coronary angioplasty guide catheter is positioned percutaneously into the ostium of the coronary artery. Nitroglycerin (0.1 mg) or isosorbide dinitrate (2 mg) is injected into the coronary artery to prevent coronary spasm. One arm of the

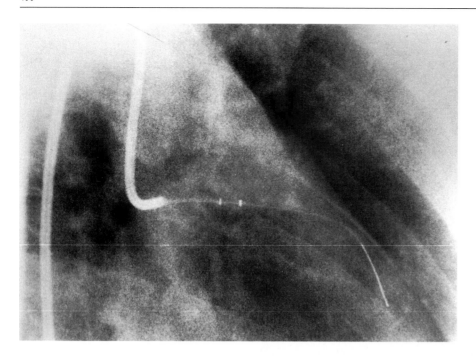

Fig. 4. The 0.36-mm angioplasty guide wire permits the angioscope to reach almost any branch of the coronary tree accurately and safely. The tip of the angioscope is accurately confirmed by the marker

angioplasty Y connector (Advanced Catheter System) is attached to the proximal end of the guide catheter and connected to a standard manifold for both pressure monitoring and injection of contrast material. The angioscopic catheter is introduced into the other arm of the Y connector and directed to the coronary artery by the guide catheter. Another Y connector is connected to the end of the irrigation channel of angioscopic catheter. The 0.36-mm angioplasty guide wire is advanced through this Y connector and passed over the target lesion. If the target lesion is a complete occlusion, the guide wire is advanced to a positon immediately before the complete occlusion. The angioscopic catheter is then advanced over the guide wire to the target lesion. The location of the tip of the angioscopic catheter is easily confirmed by te marker (Fig. 4).

After reaching the lesion to be imaged, blood must be cleared from the viewing field using 5 cc normal saline flush injection to visualize the surface of the vessel lumen. Then the balloon is inflated with carbon dioxide using a small syringe (0.2–0.5 ml, 0.5 tm). In some systems the balloon is inflated by physiological saline or contrast ma-

terial. For subsequent continuous irrigation via the guide wire channel, physiological saline with heparin (10 U/ml saline solution) or Ringer's lactate with 5 % dextrane are used. The irrigation fluid is maintained at 37 °C by a warming coil and can be used to prevent arrhythmias. After balloon inflation the system is flushed with 2.0–8.0 ml saline injected manually using a 10-ml syringe. The irrigation flow rate of our angioscopic catheter is 0.6 ml/s. An angioscope without a balloon may require a relatively large volume of irrigation fluid (15–20 ml) to flush the system and provide visibility. The irrigation volume is adjusted manually to the diameter of the lumen and severity of stenosis. The irrigation is maintained during entire viewing. Visualization is maintained for 3–5 s in one irrigation. Average visualization duration for one patient is 30 s on average the whole angioscopic procedure lasts 13 min. During observation of the inner lumen light intensity must be adjusted to prevent halation. Continuous ECG monitoring is mandatory during the entire procedure. During injection of saline solution transient (10–30 s) T wave inversions with or without ST segment depression may develop without associated symptoms. These changes usually resolve spontaneously (Fig. 5).

Achieving good coaxial alignment in the curved coronary artery lumen is always a challenge. It is sometimes necessary to withdraw the angioscopic

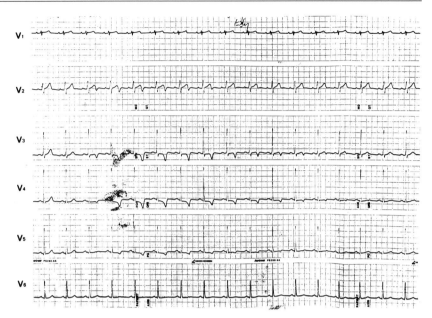

Fig. 5. Electrocardiogram during irrigation of physiological saline. Transient T wave inversion developed in most patients

catheter somewhat to obtain the coaxial alignment of the angioscope necessary for adequate visualization of the artery lumen. If the tip of the angioscope can be deflected away from the artery wall, intimal surface features can be imaged. The catching of the wall with the tip of the angioscope is a problem even in the over-the-wire system. Several techniques have been used to control the tip of the angioscope, among which are an angulation mechanism [6], in which the distal tip is angulated from the proximal side of the angioscopic catheter, and a guide wire system [3] in which tip manipulation is accomplished by manufacturing a series of bends in the distal portion of the steering guide wire. These techniques are still quite limited, and mechanisms to provide finer control of the distal tip have yet to be developed.

Indications for Coronary Angiscopy

Coronary angiscopy may be indicated for all patients with coronary artery disease and those with coronary artery bypass grafts or allografts. Angioscopy is also indicated to investigate the pathogenesis of atherosclerosis in the coronary artery. However, there are recognizable limitis; at our institute angiscopy is not attempted in patients with left main disease or pronounced distal coronary artery disease, or when affected coronary arteries are too small for insertion of the angioscope.

Complications

Coronary angioscopy is an invasive diagnostic modality and can produce transient ischemia. Several complications may occur during irrigation. The complications that have occurred during transluminal coronary angioscopy in the 394 patients studied at our institute is presented below. Transient ST elevation with or without chest pain occurred (Fig. 6) in 22 patients; these symptoms were alleviated by deflating the balloon and/or withdrawing the angioscopic catheter from the site of observation to the proximal coronary artery. Coronary spasm occurred in two patients; an intracoronary injection of nitroglycerin or isosorbide dinitrate successfully alleviated the spasm. Ventricular tachycardia occurred in one patient with variant angina pectoris; the normal rhythm was restored by direct current (DC) cardioversion. A transient complete arteriovenous block occurred in one patient; according to Bonan [12], complete arteriovenous block has also been reported by other investigators. A coronary embolism responsible for ST elevation occurred in one patient, but this dissolved after several injections of contrast material. Coronary occlusion occurred in one patient with unstable angina; subsequent angioplasty alleviated the coronary occlusion, and creatine phosphokinase was not elevated in this case. In addition, there was one instance of balloon rupture, and eight patients complained

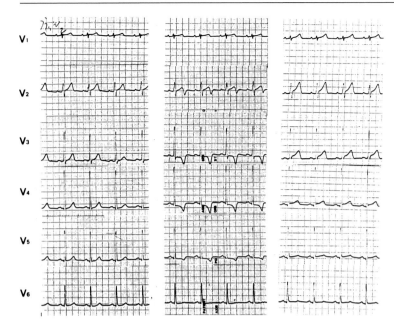

Fig. 6. Transient ST elevation during coronary angioscopy. A few seconds after of T inversion (*middle*) ST elevation occurrred in V_1–V_4 leads (*right*). ST elevation returned to baseline 30 s later upon withdrawing of the angioscopic cather

of chest pain. Thus, in our 394 patients no major complications (e.g., acute myocardial infarction or death) occurred during or as a sequalae to angioscopy. However, two cases of acute myocardial infarction have been reported by Uchida et al. [13] and a coronary artery rupture and a pseudoaneurysm formation by Wolff et al. [14].

Definition and Classification of Intraluminal Findings

There is no formally established classification system nor definition of angioscopic findings. However, the findings may be grouped into seven categories according to color, mobility, irregularity of intraluminal surface, shape or protrusion into the inner lumen: thombus, hemorrhage, dissection, intimal flap, intimal split, ulceration, and stable atheroma (Table 1). This classification system used in our institute is based upon generally recognized definitions, as follows.

Thrombus is defined as a red and/or white solid material adhering to the intima or protruding into the inner lumen despite flushing with normal saline.

Hemorrhage is defined as a nonmoving flat red color on the inner lumen that persists despite flushing with saline. It is sometimes difficult to differentiate between hemorrhage and a red mural thrombus, especially on still photographs. In

such cases serial still photos, video tapes, or cinematographic techniques demonstrating movement are needed to discriminate between the two conditions. If shaggy or nappy movement is detect in the red area a fresh mural thrombus is suggested. Similarly, a white thrombus can be distinguished from the inner wall by its mobility in serial cine frames. A thrombus that shows no movement and presents, with a highly polished surface, is considered to be an old thrombus.

Complex plaques is divided into four categories: intimal dissection, intimal flap, intimal split, and ulceration. This classification is based on morphologic appearance and cleft orientation. Intimal flap is defined as a small, thin, white, disrupted fragment floating in the lumen (Fig. 7a, b). Intimal dissection is defined as large longitudinal dissection plane encroaching on the inner lumen (Fig. 7c). Intimal split is defined as sharp cleft in the inner wall; we use this term only after PTCA (Fig. 7d). Ulceration is defined as a crater like lesion suggesting a gap in the intima (Fig. 7e). Intimal flap and intimal split are usually observed after interventions, for example, PTCA, and intimal dissection and ulceration are observed in acute coronary syndromes, such as acute myocardial infarction and unstable angina. Ramee et al. [3] describe two types of dissection: thin shaggy white, mobile fronds adhering to the arterial wall and protruding into the lumen, and large thick flaps that appear to have a longitudinal dissection plane and encroach on the lumen. In our terminol-

Table 1. Definition and classification of intraluminal findings

	Color	Mobility	Surface and shape	Protrusion to inner lumen
Thrombus	Red	Fresh thrombus present	Fresh thrombus nappy	Intraluminal thrombus present
	Red + white	Old thrombus absent	Old thrombus smooth luster	Mural thrombus absent
	White			
Hemorrhage	Red	Absent	Smooth	Absent
Intimal dissection (atheroma rupture)	Yellow	Part of cross section may move	Irregular	Present
	White		Thick cross-section	
Intimal flap	Yellow	Present	Irregular	Present
	White		Thin cross-section	
Ulceration	Yellow	Absent	Irregular	Absent
	White		Cave-in	
Intimal split	Yellow	Absent	Irregular	Absent
	White		Sharp split to outer wall	
Stable atheroma	Yellow	Absent	Smooth	Absent
	White			

ogy the former dissection is called „intimal flap" and the latter „intimal dissection."

Quantification in Angioscopy

Quantification in angioscopy, such as determining luminal area or size of the thrombus, is still far from exact. Geometric distortion of the image by the wide-angle lens makes quantification of luminal cross-sectional dimensions quite difficult [15]. The relationship between image size and lens-to-object distance is nonlinear because of divergence of angioscopic images. In addition, suitable references in angioscopic pictures are usually not available. Nevertheless, some quantification efforts have been reported. Barbeau et al. [16] have reported that divergence of images can be calculated by measuring the distance of movement of angioscopic catheter, and Johnson et al. [17] have reported that thrombus deposition in angioscopy can be quantified by digitized measurement of the percentage luminal area occluded by thrombus. At our institute we have developed a simple quantitative method using the guide wire itself as a reference marker. Luminal area (Fig. 8) is obtained by the following equation: luminal area=

$(A/B) \times C$, where A is the luminal area on the angioscopic image, B is the guide wire area on the angioscopic image, and C is the actual area of the guide wire (using a 0.36 mm diameter guide wire, C is 0.102 mm^2). A and B ware calculated by planimetry or computer digitization.

In a stenotic model using a Folly catheter, the catheter is cut proximal to the stenotic section for measurement by surface planimetry. A good correlation is obtained between the luminal area obtained by angioscopy and the actual luminal area calculated by surface planimetry. In clinical use, however, the correlation is diminished because precise alignment of the angioscopic catheter in the coronary artery is not possible, and because the coronary artery is not straight but curved. These two factors, coaxial alignment and curvature of the artery, generate erroneous estimates, of luminal area. More recently, using a transfer ring of fibero-optically transmitted laser light from the guide wire at a known distance, Spears et al. [18] were able to measure luminal dimensions with a high degree of accuracy. Although it is possible to calculate the luminal area by this method, it cannot be used to calculate the volume of a thrombus because its depth cannot be measured.

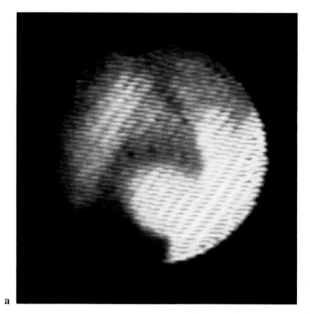

a

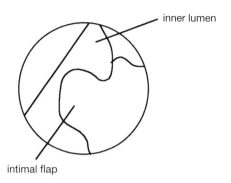

inner lumen

intimal flap

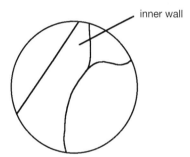

inner wall

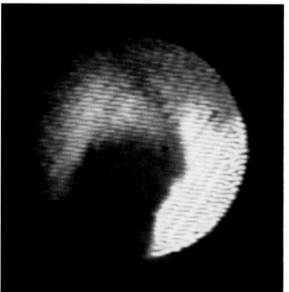

b

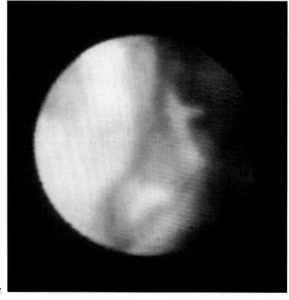

c

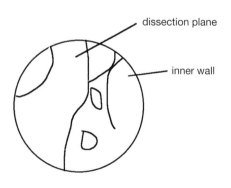

dissection plane

inner wall

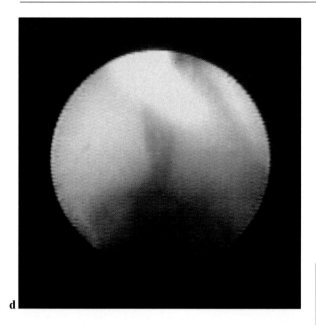

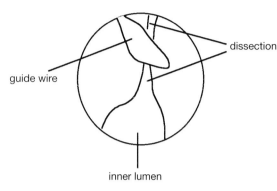

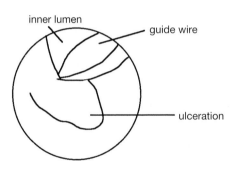

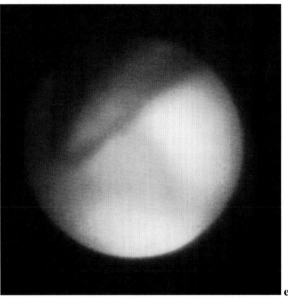

Fig. 7. a Intimal flap. A thin white fragment protrudes into the lumen. **b** Intimal flap. Flap adheres to the arterial wall. **c** Intimal dissection. Large longitudinal dissection plane is observed (*left*). **d** Intimal split. A sharp cleft in the inner wall is observed after PTCA. **e** Ulceration. A craterlike lesion suggests a gap in the intima

Effectiveness of Coronary Angioscopy in Detecting Intraluminal Changes: Comparison with Arteriography

We have investigated the feasibility of using angioscopy as a diagnostic tool for detecting intraluminal pathologic changes. Twelve patients with acute coronary syndromes (e.g., acute myocardial infarction or unstable angina) who showed no complete occlusion and 20 patients who underwent PTCA were selected for a comparison of the diagnostic accuracy of angioscopy versus arteriography in terms of detection of thrombi and complex plaques. The arteriographic morphology of the coronary stenosis at the site of angioscopy was described according to the following criteria: (a) a coronary artery thrombus as a filling defect surrounded by contrast medium at the site of stenosis, or luminal staining at the site of stenosis; (b) complex coronary stenosis morphology as a stenosis with irregularity, overhanging, dissection, or intimal flap; and (c) simple stenosis with smooth regular borders.

The thrombus, as detected in angioscopy, is defined above. The complex coronary morphology

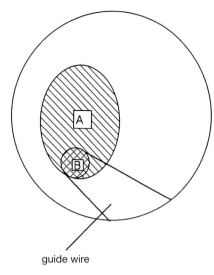

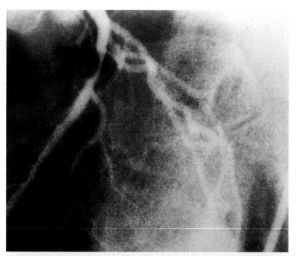

Fig. 8. The method of quantification of luminal area: $(A/B) \times C$. *A*, Luminal area on the angioscopic image; *B*, guide wire area on the angioscopic image; *C*, actual area of the guide wire

of angioscopy is defined as intima dissection, intimal split, ulceration, or intimal flap (Table 1). Thrombi and complex coronary morphologies were detected more frequently by angioscopy than by arteriography (Fig. 9) and were observed even in smooth wall lesions seen by arteriography. Sher-

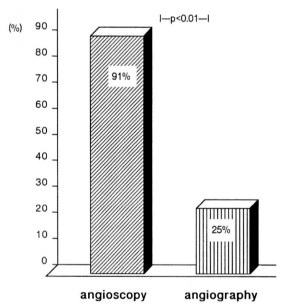

Fig. 9. Comparison of the detection of thrombi between arteriography and angioscopy. The thrombi were detected more frequently by angioscopy than by arteriography. (From [30])

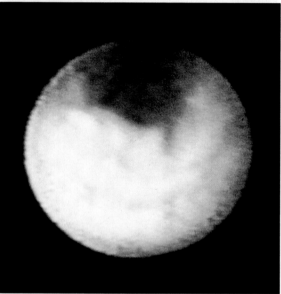

Fig. 10. Coronary arteriography (*above*) and angioscopy (*below*) of the left coronary artery in a patient with unstable angina. Irregular surface with ulceration is observed by angioscopy. (From [1])

man et al. [2] and Ramee et al. [3] have also reported that angioscopy is more sensitive than arteriography for the detection and precise morphologic definition of thrombi and complex lesions.

Clinical Implications: Pathogenesis of Coronary Artery Disease

Sherman et al. [2] demonstrated the presence of complex plaques or thrombi not detected by coronary angiography in the coronary arteries of all patients who underwent bypass surgery for un-

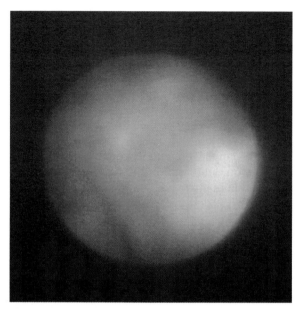

Fig. 11. Xanthomatous plaque in a patient with acute myocardial infarction. A large plaque rupture occurred at the site of yellow plaque

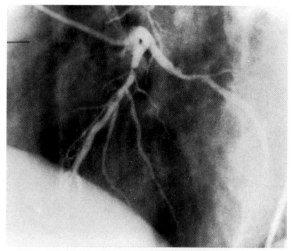

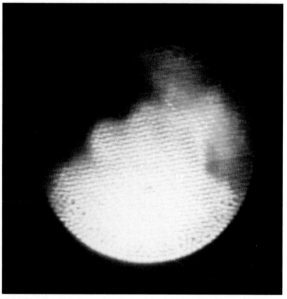

Fig. 12. Arteriography (*above*) and angioscopy (*below*) of the left coronary artery in a patient with unstable angina. White thrombi are observed by angioscopy. (From [5])

stable angina. They speculated that the ulceration of plaques may increase the frequency and severity of effort angina, and that the subsequent development of partially occlusive thrombi may cause unstable rest angina. On the basis of their study Forrester et al. [19] proposed that each coronary syndrome has a distinct intimal cause. The thrombus overlying a rupture in the lining of the plaque plays an important role in acute coronary syndromes such as acute myocardial infarction or unstable angina. We and other investigators have observed plaque rupture or ulceration (Fig. 10) in patients with acute coronary syndromes. However, the findings leave unanswered crucial pathophysiological questions. For example, what type of plaque precedes plaque rupture and formation of a coronary thrombus? In our study yellow plaque was more common in patients with acute myocardial infarction, recent myocardial infarction, and unstable angina than in patients with stable angina and old myocardial infarction. Many sites of plaque ruptures or ulcerations (Fig. 11) were observed on xanthomatous plaque. Conversely, smooth white plaques were seen in patients with stable angina and old myocardial infarction. Recently Nesto et al. [20] have confirmed our observation. Yellow plaque is likely to be lipid rich, and the fibrous cap is always thin. Routine coronary arteriography usually does not

help in predicting the location of a subsequent myocardial infarction. However, angioscopy may predict the location of a subsequent plaque rupture when xanthomatous plaque is observed.

Allograft coronary artery disease is a major cause of morbidity and mortality in cardiac transplant recipients. Coronary angioscopy is more sensitive than arteriography in detecting coronary artery disease [1–3]. Intravascular ultrasound is also a sensitive technique for detecting the allograft coronaropathy, but it does not provide information on detailed plaque surface morphology. Angioscopy typically demonstrates two types of

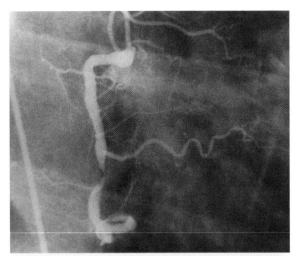

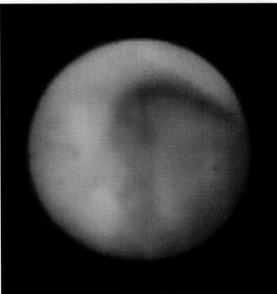

Fig. 13. Coronary arteriography (*above*) and angioscopy (*below*) of right coronary artery of a patient with acute inferior myocardial infarction. Red thrombi are observed by angioscopy. (From [1])

coronary surface morphologies, yellow and white plaques. These lesions may represent either two different types or two different stages of allograft coronary diseases in cardiac transplant recipients [21]. Similar yellow and white plaques have also been demonstrated by angioscopy in saphenous vein grafts [20]. At present a study is under way concerning the ability of angioscopy to predict complications during PTCA based on differences in plaque surface morphology.

Angioscopy is clearly more sensitive in detecting thrombus than is intravascular ultrasound or coronary angiography. A number of authors have

observed the process of thrombolysis during acute myocardial infarction. In generall, all authors report that occlusive or intraluminal thrombi ware found in the offending artery. Inoue et al. [8] reported that angioscopy can be used to identify a subset of patients with incomplete clot lysis who may be prone to reocclusion. Sherman et a. [2] and we [5] have confirmed that thrombi exit in patients with unstable angina as well as in those with acute myocardial infarction. Coronary angioscopy in our study showed that thrombi observed in unstable angina differ from those observed in acute myocardial infarction. Patients with unstable angina ware frequently observed to have white thrombi (Fig. 12), but none is seen in patients with acute myocardial infarction. In contrast, reddish thrombi (Fig. 13) are observed in any patient with acute myocardial infarction and in only a few patients with unstable angina. Differences in color probably reflect differences in the composition of the thrombus, and may be related in part on the different ages of thrombi.

Coronary Interventions

Angioplasty

If percutaneous angiscopy comes to have an important clinical role, it will be in association with coronary interventions such as angioplasty, atherectomy, or stenting. Angioscopy shows coronary surface damage that is largely undetectable by arteriography. Immediately after the procedure intimal flap, fissure, or disruption is observed in most patients [3, 23, 24] (Fig. 14). In our study the thrombi or fibrin deposit was observed in two-thirds of the patients despite the use of anticoagulants and antiplatelet agents before and during procedure [25]. A better understanding of the mechanisms of thrombus formation at the angioplasty sites may provide insights into the pathogenesis of both acute closure and restenosis following angioplasty.

Jain et al. [26] performed percutaneous coronary angioscopy in ten patients following abrupt occlusion occurring immediately after balloon angioplasty. The primary cause of the abrupt occlusion was thrombus in two patients and occlusive dissection in eight. Seven of the occlusive dissections were associated with nonocclusive mural thrombi. These findings suggest that angioscopy may allow the selection of the optimum

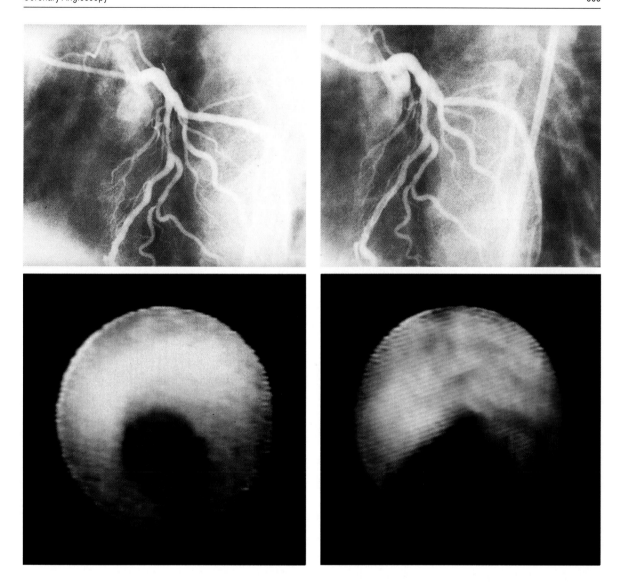

Fig. 14. Coronary arteriography (*above*) and angioscopy (below) before (*left*) and after (*right*) PTCA. After angioplasty intimal split and red mural thrombus are observed by angioscopy. (From [6])

therapy (thrombolysis, long balloon inflations, atherectomy, or stents) in patients with acute occlusion.

Atherectomy and Stent

Atherectomy or laser treatment are believed to result in smoother surfaces than angioplasty. However, Ramee et al. [27] found no qualitative difference in angioscopically viewed surface mor-

phology following directional atherectomy or balloon angioplasty. Angiosopy also reveals a high incidence of intimal flap or thrombus immediately after excimer laser angioplasty of coronary arteries [28]. Transluminal extraction catheter atherectomy in saphenous vein grafts creats deep dissection and obstructive intimal flaps [29]; coronary thrombi and flaps have been observed in the stents. The highly traumatic outcome of percutaneous revascularization interventions may contribute to the similar outcomes and complications. Thrombolysis or redilation may be carried out during angioscopy. In preliminary studies realistic decisions regarding modifications of ongoing stenting can already be made on the basis of concurrent angioscopic information [30]. Angioscopic monitoring of coronary interventions may prove useful in determing the optimum strategies and thus in improving the outcome.

Future Directions

As certain lesions or vessel characteristics may predispose vessels to restenosis or abrupt reocclusion, coronary angioscopy may improve our ability to select candidates for PTCA based on lesion morphology. In addition, it is possible that angioscopy can aid in the selection of candidates for specific coronary revascularization procedures. For example, stenting may not be indicated in patients whom thrombus is revealed by angioscopy. Angioscopy may also allow us to better predict which atheroma will progress or regress. Since coronary angioscopy can differentiate the character of thrombi in acute coronary syndromes, this new tool should help immeasurably in deciding which therapy, for example, thrombolysis or PTCA, should be chosen in dealing with acute coronary syndromes.

References

1. Mizuno K, Miyamoto A, Satomura K, et al. (1991). Angioscopic coronary macromorphology in patients with acute coronary disorders. Lancet 337: 809–812.
2. Sherman CT, Litvack F, Grundfest W, et al. (1986). Coronary angioscopy in patients with unstable angina pectoris. N Engl J Med 315: 913–919.
3. Ramee SR, White CJ, Collins TJ, Mesa JE, Murgo JP (1991). Percutaneous angioscopy during coronary angioplasty using a steerable microangioscope. J Am Coll Cardiol 17: 100–105.
5. Mizuno K, Miyamoto A, Isojima K, et al. (1992a). A serial observation of coronary thrombi in vivo by a new percutaneous transluminal coronary angioscope. Angiology 43: 91–99.
5. Mizuno K, Satomura K, Miyamoto A, et al. (1992b). Angioscopic evaluation of coronary-artery thrombi in acute coronary syndromes. N Engl J Med 326: 287–291.
6. Mizuno K, Arai T, Satomura K, et al. (1989a). New percutaneous transluminal coronary angioscope. J Am Coll Cardiol 13: 363–368.
7. Uchida Y, Tomaru T, Nakamura F, Furuse A, Fujimori Y, Hasegawa K (1987). Percutaneous coronary angioscopy in patients with ischemic heart disease. Am Heart J 114: 1216–1222.
8. Inoue K, Kuwaki K, Ochiai H, Ueda K, Takano E, Minato H (1989). Percutaneous transluminal coronary angioscopy as the guiding therapy for intracoronary thrombolysis and angioplasty. In: Vogel JHK, and King SB III (ed.) Interventional cardiol-

ogy: future directions. St. Louis, The CV Mosby Company, pp. 1–17.
9. Hombach V, Hoher M, Hopp H, et al. (1988). The clinical significance of coronary angioscopy in patients with coronary heart disease. Surg Endosc 2: 1–4.
10. Nanto S, Mishima M, Hirayama A, Koretsune Y, Lee J, Kodama K (1988). Monorail coronary angioscope with movable guide wire (abstract). Circulation 78 (suppl II): II–84.
11. Nesto RW, Sassower M, Koch JM, Manzo K, Abela GS (1992). Angioscopic features of ruptured plaques in patients with unstable coronary syndromes. Circulation 86 (suppl I): I–651.
12. Bonan R (1989). Percutaneous coronary angioscopy. In: Vogel JHK, and King SB III (ed.) Interventional cardiology: future directions. St. Louis, The C. V. Mosby Company, pp. 28–35.
13. Uchida Y, Fujimori Y, Hirose J, Oshima T (1992). Percutaneous coronary angioscopy. Jpn Heart J 33: 271–294.
14. Wolff MR, Resar JR, Stuart RS, Brinker JA (1993). Coronary artery rupture and pseudoaneurysm formation resulting from percutaneous coronary angioscopy. Catheterization and Cardiovascular Diagnosis 28: 47–50.
15. Spears JR, Spokojny AM, Marais JH (1985). Coronary angioscopy during cardiac catheterization. J Am Coll Cardiol 6: 93–97.
16. Barbeau GR, Friedl SE, Abela GS (1990). Quantitative angioscopy: a new technique for evaluation of residual lumen area. J Am Coll Cardiol 15: 105A.
17. Johnson CC, Ritchie JL, Stratton JR, Reichenbach DD (1990). Fiberoptic angioscopy: a method for quantification of intravascular thrombosis. J Am Coll Cardiol 15: 66A.
18. Spears JR, Raza SJ, Ali M, Iyer GS, Cheong WF, Crilly RJ (1993). Quantitative angioscopy: a new method for measurement of luminal dimensions by use of a „lightwire." J Am Coll Cardiol 21: 133A.
19. Forrester JS, Litvack F, Grundfest W, et al. (1987). A perspective of coronary disease seen through the arteries of living man. Circulation 75: 505–513.
20. Nesto RW, Sassower MA, Manzo KS, et al. (1993). Angioscopic differentiation of culprit lesions in unstable versus stable coronary artery disease. J Am Coll Cardiol 21: 195A.
21. Ventura HO, Jain A, Collins TJ, et al. (1993). Angioscopic surface morphology of early allograft artery disease in cardiac transplant recipients with atherosclerosis documented by intravascular ultrasound. J Am Coll Cardiol 21: 62A.
22. Komiyama N, Nakanishi S, Nishiyama S, Fuse K, Seki A (1992). Angioscopic evaluation of saphenous vein grafts longterm after coronary artery bypass grafting. J Am Coll Cardiol 19: 319A.
23. Mizuno K, Miyamoto A, Shibuya T, et al. (1988). Changes of angioscopic macromorphology following coronary angioplasty (PTCA). Circulation 78: II–289.
24. Uchida Y, Hasegawa K, Kawamura K, Shibuya I (1989). Angioscopic observation of the coronary luminal changes induced by percutaneous transluminal coronary angioplasty. Am Heart J 117: 769–776.

25. Mizuno K, Miyamoto A, Sakurada M, et al. (1989b). Evaluation of coronary thrombi after PTCA by angioscopy. Circulation 80: II–523.

26. Jain SP, White CJ, Collins TJ, Escobar A, Ramee SR (1993). Etiologies of abrupt occlusion after PTCA; angioscopic morphology. J Am Coll Cardiol 21: 484A.

27. Ramee SR, White CJ, Collins TJ, Jain SP, Escobar A (1993). A comparison of the angioscopic coronary surface morphology following directional atherectomy with balloon angioplasty. J Am Coll Cardiol 21: 78A.

28. Kvasnicka J, Nakamura F, Dupouy P, Dubois-Rande JL (1992). Angioscopic assessment of coronary arteries following excimer laser coronary angioplasty. Circulation 86 (supple I): I–654.

29. Moses JW, Lieberman SM, Knopf WD, et al. (1993). Mechanism of transluminal extraction catheter (TEC) atherectomy in degenerative saphenous vein grafts (SVG), an angioscopic observational study. J Am Coll Cardiol 21: 442A.

30. Mizuno K, Yanagida T, Shibuya T, Arakawa K, Arai T, Satomura K, Isojima K, Kurita A, Nakamura H (1992). The effectiveness of coronary angioscopy in detecting intraluminal pathologic changes. Jpn Circ J 56: 586–591

31. Teirstein PS, Schatz RA, Rocha-Singh KJ, Chiu Wong S, Strumpf R, Heuser RR (1992). Coronary stenting with angioscopic guidance. J Am Coll Cardiol 19: 223A.

Peripheral Angioscopy

C. M. Gross and G. Biamino

Introduction

In recent years new percutaneous revascularization techniques have been increasingly used in interventional angiology worldwide [1, 2, 5, 13–15, 20]. The growing application of these techniques has generated interest in the direct visualization of obliterative vascular processes, on the one hand to evaluate the efficacy of the various angioplastic procedures, and on the other hand to supplement angiographic finding. Only exact data on the nature of vascular pathology will give us a precise understanding of the pathophysiological effects of percutaneous interventions [9].

Conventional or computer-assisted angiography represents the gold standard for identification, localization, and determination of the distribution and severity of arteriosclerosis both in the peripheral and in the coronary vascular region [20]. The two-dimensional projectional imaging in angiographic techniques is a major limitation. Using angiography, it is possible to visualize protruding arteriosclerotic lesions even in small vessels. However, the definition of the lesion is only indirect, i.e., the area not opacified by contrast solutions is exposed. Although it is possible to quantify approximately the severity of the vascular obstruction, it cannot be denied that this quantification is subject to error [19], making a quantitative analysis of the nature, size, and composition of the obstructive vascular material is inadequate by means of angiography.

The above-mentioned disadvantages of angiography determine what type of data is required by the new intravascular imaging technology. Apart from the necessary data on the extent and degree of stenosis, data regarding the size, structure, and fine morphology of the occlusive vascular processes are needed. In peri-interventional settings, for example, data on the integrity of the vascular wall and potential complications such as vascular dissection or thrombosis following interventions are of the utmost interest. With such data a therapeutic interventional method could be selected to fulfil the requirements of a particular situation. For vascular surgical procedures, details of the area of the anastomoses and the integrity of the bypass graft are important factors in determining long-term results.

The requirements made by interventional angiology and vascular surgery on a modern vascular imaging system are, at least partially, fulfilled by percutaneous transluminal angioscopy. In comparison with angiography, angioscopy provides a more precise, three-dimensional color view of the vascular surface, thus enabling a direct real time examination of the vascular surface. Therefore, pathomorphological differences in the arteriosclerotic process can be distinguished.

Angioscopy was first introduced in vascular surgery using rigid vascular endoscopes [24]. At that time it became evident that angiographic examination techniques were, at least partially, surpassed; however, due to the rigidity of the optical probes, and the limited quality of the color pictures clinical utility remained limited. Technological progress with developments of glass fiber optics, miniature video cameras and effective lighting systems enabled clinical applications of percutaneous angioscopy, particularily in conjunction with vascular interventions.

Therefore, the aims of this chapter are to provide an overview of the state of the art of peripheral percutaneous angioscopy and to present data to support its increasingly prominent role in interventional angiology.

Technical Aspects of the Modular Microangioscopic System MASY

The modular microangioscopic system MASY (AD Krauth) consists of four main components: a charge-coupled device (CCD) miniature color video camera, a lighting system, highly flexible angioscopic probes, and a guiding catheter. The

CCD camera weighs about 25 g and has a diameter of 17.5 mm and a total length of 43 mm. The resolution of the camera is around 360 000 pixels. Shutter speeds of 1/60 s or 1/1000 s for fast sequences can be chosen. The minimum working light level should be 3 Lux. The camera can be focussed on an object (1 : 1.6; 7.5 mm) via a TV adapter (PAL or MTSC) while, at the same time, using the zoom function, intravascular structures can be magnified from 1 mm to infinity.

To date there have been two types of flexible probes available, with diameters of 1.4 and 0.96 mm and 10 600 and 9600 incorporated optic fibers, respectively. The large number of extremely thin (about 1 μm) light wave conductors ensures a high resolution for each angioscopic image without unduly influencing flexibility. With this device even branched vascular sections can be examined with adequate precision. At the tip of the angioscope there are various lens systems which permit the viewing of intravascular structures from angles of 50°, 65°, or 140°. Probe lengths vary from 0.5 to 1.5 m. A special manufacturing process is used to ensure that probes do not break easily. Thus bends of <40 mm radius can be tolerated without damage. Angioscopic probes with exter-

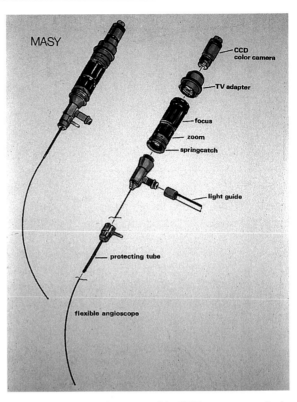

Fig. 2. MASY angioscope with CCD camera and objective lens

nal diameters of 0.7–0.5 mm are now becoming available for the coronary area.

Lighting with nearly 20 000 Lux is achieved through the use of a light source of sufficient capacity (Osram 250-W halogen lamp) via a highly flexible light conducter. The light intensity required depends on the angle of the lens system, focus, lens aperture, and vessel diameter.

Methodology and Clinical Experience with Peripheral Angioscopy

Methodologically, the procedure follows standard techniques. After application of a local anesthetic and after antegrade or retrograde puncture of the femoral artery, an F8 or F9 sheath is positioned using the Seldinger technique. With the guide wire in place, the angioscope and the guiding catheter are introduced via the sheath. Using "roadmapping" and visual control aided by the light from the system, the probe is positioned at the desired location. Digital angiography performed

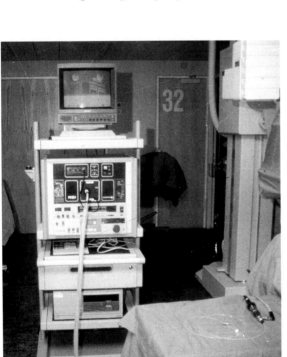

Fig. 1. Angioscopic MASY system with color monitor, camera-conducting device, and video recorder with video printer

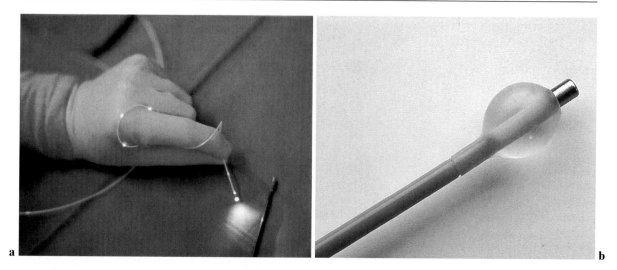

Fig. 3a, b. Angioscope with blue guiding catheter with inflatable balloon at the end

Fig. 4a–d. Angiographic and angioscopic presentation of a superficial femoral artery stenosis. Angiogram (**a**) shows a 50% stenosis in the distal segment of the vessel. In contrast, angioscopic images (**b–d**) reveal a high grade stenosis with only a minimum residual patency

previously now makes possible a global view of the local, obstructive arteriosclerosis and precise positioning of the angioscopic probe. Positioning of the angioscope is thus much easier, and the vascular structures to be investigated can now safely be found. The guiding catheter is introduced via the Y-connector frequently used with percutaneous transluminal coronary angioplasties (PTCAs).

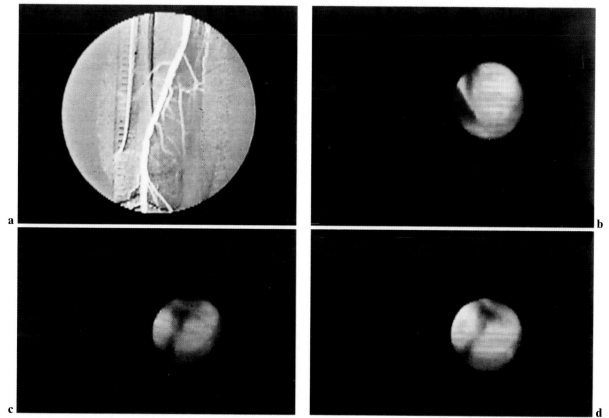

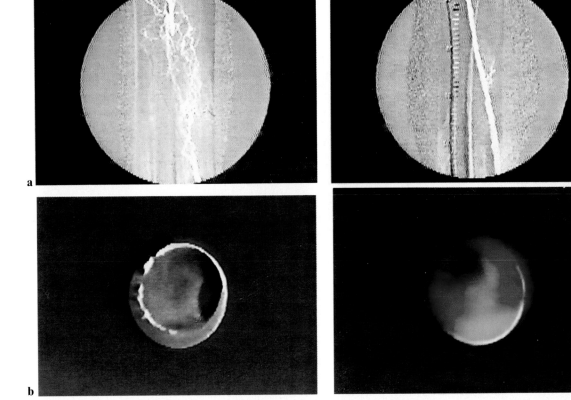

Fig. 5a–d. Angiographic (**a,c**) and angioscopic (**b,d**) presentations of a chronic closure of the superficial femoral artery before (**a,b**) and after (**c,d**) excimer laser and balloon angioplasty

Before each examination, 5000 IU heparin is administered.

In conjunction with peripheral interventional therapy such as PTA, atherectomy, and last but not least laser angioplasty, the progress and success of each procedure can be monitored and asessed. Angioscopy can, with great precision, distinguish between intervention-related complications, such as intimal flaps, and dissection or parietal thrombus, so that the therapeutic procedures can be modified or extended, with for example thrombolysis or stent implantation. By inserting the angioscope through the central channel of the laser catheter, we were able to completely document all the steps involved in the procedure of excimer laser recanalization. With this technique, early recognition of complications caused by excimer laser angioplasty was possible. For assessing intravascular morphology, the vessels must be completely or nearly free of blood.

To avoid view obstruction a guiding catheter with an inflatable balloon was developed. Through intermittent blockage of the blood flow using a balloon (10 mm long, maximum diameter, 14 mm) inflated with a mixture of physiological saline and a contrast agent, positioning the angioscope precisely at the tip of the guiding catheter and continuously rinsing with small quantities of heparinized saline solution, it is possible to view the intravascular structures directly. The angioscopic color pictures can be stored in the memory of a video recorder or they can be printed as color hard copy using a high-resolution video printer.

Rinsing the tip of the angioscope with about 10–20 ml solution allows intravascular structures to be viewed for up to about 20 s depending on collateral flow.

Fig. 6a–h. Serial angioscopic documentation of excimer ▶ laser recanalization of a mainly thrombotic closure of the superficial femoral artery. Shown are the intial vessel closure (**a**), the predominantly thrombotic and liposclerotic occluding material (**b**), the progress of the excimer laser recanalization (**c–g**) with the circular "firing" laser fibers (**f,g**) and the end-result (**g**)

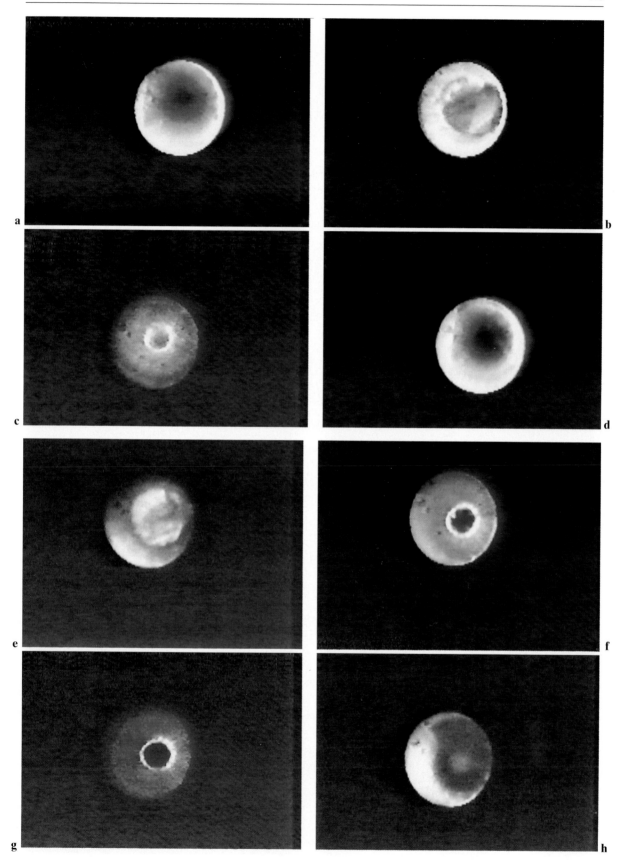

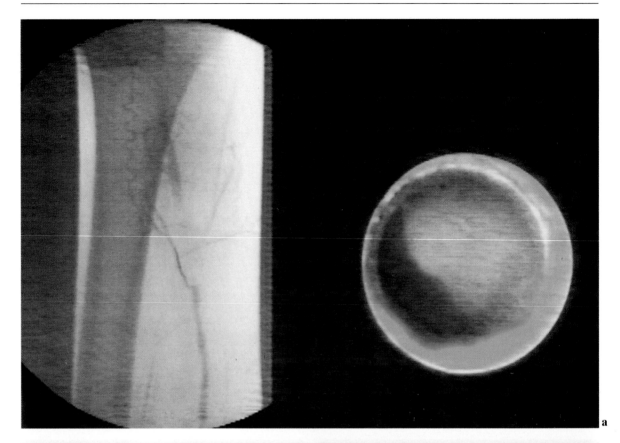

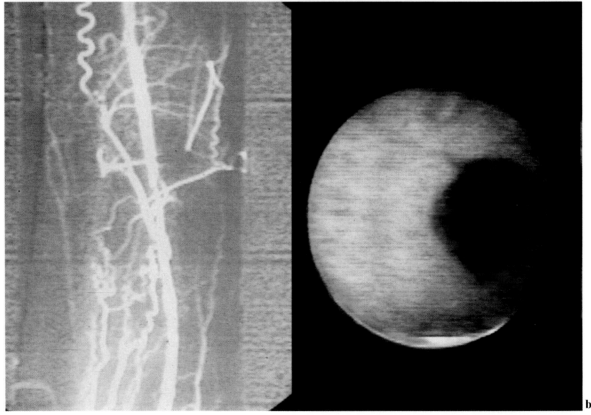

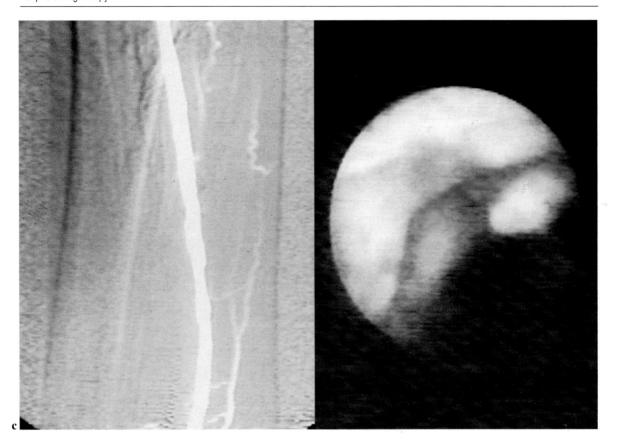

◀ **Fig. 7a–c.** Angiographic (*left panels*) and angioscopic (*right panels*) documentation of a short complete occlusion of the superficial femoral artery prior intervention (**a**), following excimer laser recanalization (**b**) and following adjunctive balloon angioplasty (**c**)

Indications for Peripheral Angioscopy

In our laboratory we have used peripheral angioscopy most frequently to diagnose peripheral arterial occlusions before using standard angiography. The femoral artery was studied most frequently with these examinations, followed by the popliteal artery. Angioscopy of the tibial arteries was performed only rarely to answer specific inquiries, such as to determine whether lysis of a thrombotic occlusion could be carried out or whether excimer laser recanalization was possible. In about half of the patients angioscopic control was performed before or during Excimer laser recanalization and again after the procedure.

Clinical Examples

The digital subtraction angiography (DSA) angiogram in Fig. 4 shows up to 50% stenosis of the superficial femoral artery in the lower third of the vessel projecting just above the patella. In comparison, the angioscopic image shows a nearly complete closure of the vessel with a very thin lumen and a collateral artery at the end. These angioscopic findings correlated better with this 60-year-old patient's inability to walk for more than 100 m.

Figure 5 shows a case of complete closure of the superficial femoral artery. For many years the patient suffered from claudication, finally limiting the walking distance to 150 m. Figure 5, above left, shows the angioscopic image before Excimer laser angioplasty. The closure is characterized very clearly, showing moderate calcification with a yellowish adhering lipomatosis with thrombotic layers and minimal residual lumen. There is also a small collateral artery at the end. The rather fibrous heterogenic structure is noticeable. This must be interpreted as a result of a closure of long

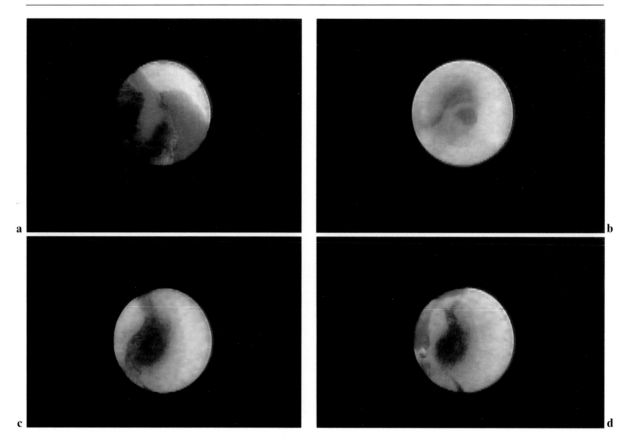

Fig. 8a–d. Angioscopic documentation of a subtotal occlusion of the femoral superficial artery with spontaneous thrombus formation (**a**) as well as obstructive lipomatosis, sclerosis and thrombosis in the vascular segment situated further distally (**b–d**)

duration, probably of many years. The lower left section of the figure shows the result after excimer laser and subsequent balloon angioplasty. The recanalization channel clearly displays thrombotic layers attached to the wall. However, flaps or intimal dissections are not present. The angiogram (on the right) shows that the vascular segment is well opacified. There are no contrast defects or deposits of it. The fact that the collateral arteries have not taken up much contrast also indicates the good result of the angioplasty.

Figure 6a–h shows excimer laser recanalization of a chronically occluded superficial femoral artery assisted by angioscopy in a 49-year-old patient. The angioscope was inserted via the central channel of the excimer laser catheter, thus enabling a continuous visual control of the entire procedure. First (images a and b), the occlusion was charac-

terized mainly as thrombosis and liposclerosis clearly seen as a yellowish crescent. Then, the progress of the excimer laser revascularization was documented (images c through g). The ring-shaped "firing" laser fibers were clearly seen during laser activation (images f,g). Approximately half-way through the 12 cm long occlusion predominantly sclerotic occlusive material indicated by the rough surface of the adjoining wall sections was encountered (image e). Finally, following the complete recanalization of the occluded segment the distal patent lumen was visualized (image h).

Figure 7a–c shows a short complete occlusion of the femoral artery occurring in the distal third of the vessel. Angioscopically the occlusion is characterized by lipomatosis and sclerotic obliteration. One can clearly see a collateral artery branching off near the occlusion. Figure 7b, c shows the state of the vessels after excimer laser recanalization and subsequent conventional PTA. The smooth recanalization channel achieved after laser ablation is noticeable (Fig. 7b). In Fig. 7c, after PTA, an obvious discrepancy between the angiographic and angioscopic vascular presentation is apparent. We observed such discrepancies

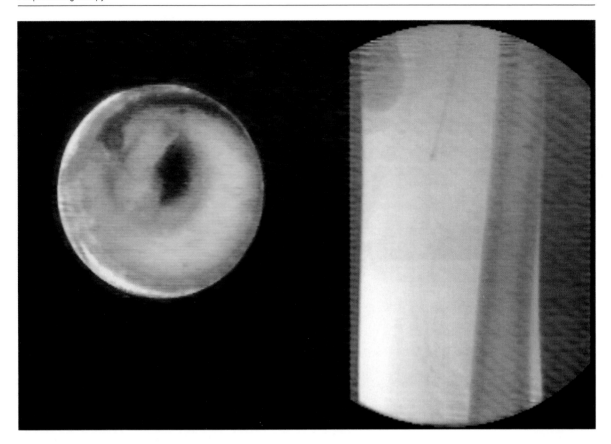

Fig. 9. Sclerotic stenosis and stenosis due to severe calcification of the femoral superficial artery in a proximal vascular segment viewed by angioscopy (*left*) and angiography

frequently. The arterial DSA, after complete recanalization, shows a smooth vascular lumen with adequate contrast solution flow, demonstrating the success of revascularization. Angiographically, however, the vascular lumen shows a diffuse border with local intimal dissections and spontaneous thrombosis on the vascular wall.

Peripheral angioscopy is a useful tool in peripheral peri-interventional settings. It is easy to use, it is safe, and it only rarely causes complications. If the angioscopic probe is positioned coaxially, the complete area of the vascular lumen can be seen at an angle of 65°. This is the case not only in diagnostic procedures but also in peri-interventional settings. With the exception of a few obliteration sites, the angioscope can be inserted and led to the lesion without difficulty. Only in some very proximal stenoses of the superficial femoral artery is the procedure limited. Localization of such stenoses prevents the movement of the angioscopic probe towards the lesion. A very intensive retrograde blood flow can also prevent clear documentation of the view. In such cases, the injection of a rinsing solution is not usually sufficient to remove the blood from the angioscopic tip. In contrast, in cases of total closure or subtotal stenosis a blockage of the balloon catheter is not necessarily required, as the catheter has already obstruction the remaining lumen. Only small amounts of rinsing solution are sufficient for precise documentation of the findings. In our experience the view of the region of interest is excellent or good in 80 % of all cases.

If angioscopy is used for evaluating the results of angioplastic procedures, the intensive orthograde blood flow can prevent a complete inspection of the vessel in spite of sufficient rinsing and the fully inflated balloon. This explains why the recanalization results can only be visualized in fragments, as the angioscopic tip cannot be kept free of blood.

It should be stressed that the angiographic findings can deviate from the angioscopic documentation of vascular obstruction. In our experience, in

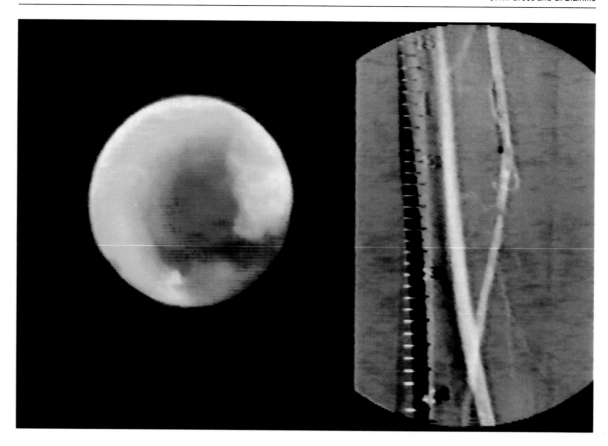

Fig. 10. Stenosis due to severe lipomatosis of the superficial femoral artery with calcificated ulcerous plaque and subtotal occluding distal thrombosis documented by angioscopy (*left*) and DSA

12 % of cases the angiographic findings show a lesser degree of stenosis than do the angioscopic findings. In addition, mural thrombosis often remains undetected in angiography (Fig. 4). Angioscopic inspection of the vascular area after angioplastic procedures, such as Excimer laser recanalization, facilitates good documentation of interventionally induced vascular lesions. Local thrombosis of the vascular wall, intimal flaps, or wall dissections can easily be detected and therapy with a particular aim can be undertaken, such as stent implantation or local lysis, or the therapeutic strategy can be modified at an early stage.

Apart from the angioscopic monitoring of the interventional therapy, angioscopy allows qualitative assessment of the vascular surface pathology. Table 1 summarizes the angioscopic vascular findings and their pathological significance in the arteriosclerotic process.

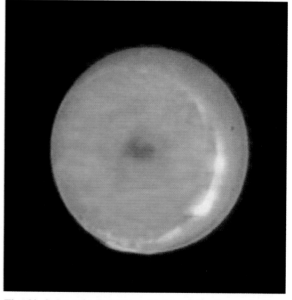

Fig. 11. Subtotal sclerotic occlusion of the femoral artery documented by angioscopy

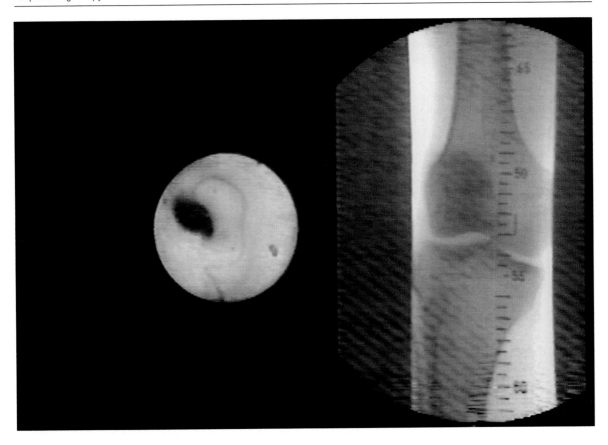

Fig. 12. Severe stenosis of the femoral artery distal to the adductor channel. Smooth border of remaining sclerotic lumen without thrombotic layers documented by angioscopy (*left*)

In the angioscopic image the intima of a healthy peripheral or coronary artery appears as a round cross-section with a pale-pink to a whitish-gray coloring. In comparison to the pathologically altered vessel, there are no or only a small amount of blood adhesions on the intima surface, which

Table 1. Angioscopic findings of peripheral arteriosclerosis

	Surface	Color	Adhesions
Normal	Smooth Reflecting	Whitish Pink	None
Lipoidosis	Smooth/rough Reflecting	Yellow White	Partially thrombotic
Sclerosis	Cleft Rough Rough	Yellow	With and without thrombotic material
Calcification	Cleft Reflecting Rough/smooth	Yellow	Usually without thrombotic material
Atheroma	Cleft Crater shaped Rough	Yellow Red	Massive thrombotic material, partially floating

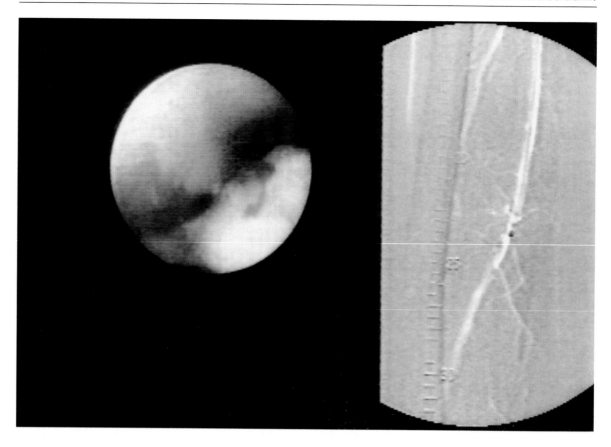

Fig. 13. Intimal dissection of the femoral artery in a distal vascular section caused by excimer laser intervention, showing a true and a false lumen documented by angioscopy (*left*) and DSA

has a smooth overall appearance. Clearly visible layers of a yellow substance with a rough or folded surface which sometimes even reaches into the lumen can be differentiated as liposclerosis. This type of pathology occurs with and without vascular obstruction and can be found especially in vascular segments taken from distal femoral arteries. Often it is found in pathological specimens and documented in angiography as so-called intramural calcifications.

Severe stenosing arteriosclerosis shows a characteristic narrowing of the lumen, of which two types can be distinguished: in one type plaque is found which nearly completely obstructs the lumen. It is yellow in color with a rough, partially cleft surface and has a moderate amount of adhesive thrombotic material. In the second type, in addition to the above-described severe stenosis, calcification is found, which is angiographically described as "native". The angioscopic picture shows athero-

matosis with an extremely rough vascular surface and layers of thrombotic, partially floating, material. The vascular lumen can, in such cases, be closed almost completely, leaving only a slit-like aperture.

We have also experienced that flat, partially floating parietal thrombi in vascular sections with light pathological changes can be found without stenosing or occlusive lesions. This observation, however, has not been duplicated in the coronary vascular system. In the peripheral vascular area such structures seem to occur relatively often.

Complete vascular occlusions can easily be examined and allow, depending on collateral flow, a sufficiently long observation time. Thus, the structure of the occlusion can be adequately evaluated. Mainly thrombotic occlusions are found which are easily recognized due to the red thrombotic material and can be differentiated from sclerotic occlusions. The latter are characterized mainly by gray to yellowish coloring and a relatively smooth occlusion surface.

The relative value and limitations of descriptive angioscopy must be mentioned here. Angioscopic observation is a method that only evaluates the

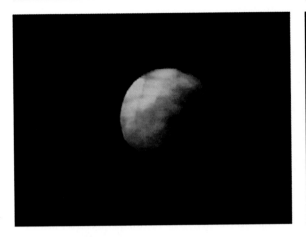 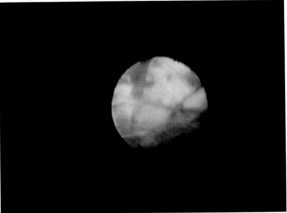

Fig. 14. Angioscopic presentation of the femoral artery after recanalization and Palmaz-Schatz stent implantation

surface of the vascular wall, thus differing from intravasal echo. Subintimal wall changes cannot be seen using angioscopy. Furthermore, it is not always possible to see the colors clearly. For example, the light reflections of vascular bends do not allow differentiation between white and yellow surfaces, thus obscuring the findings. However, it has been confirmed by a number of investigators that angioscopic findings can be interpreted to give a dependable classification of morphologic phenomena in spite of the above-described limitations. There is no doubt that intima dissections and floating structures can also be recognized and detected following interventional procedures [11, 24]. In this respect, angioscopy can surely be called a unique procedure without competition.

In agreement with other investigators, the results achieved to date only underline the diagnostic value of this procedure [6, 8, 10]. Examples of its advantages are: diagnostic classification of inflammatory, arteriosclerotic, or radiologically induced vascular pathology, angioscopically guided lysis of vascular occlusion, stent implantation, or intima biopsies [2, 4, 7, 11, 22].

To a certain extent angioscopic viewing of a vascular occlusion enables follow-up comparisons to be made. In some cases information about the age of the lesions can be obtained. Old vascular occlusions are seen to be fibrous with a greenish to brownish surface structure. Our experience showed that in this type of closure the danger of excimer laser-induced perforation is especially high due to the heterogeneity of the occlusive material.

There is still controversy in the literature as to whether or to what extent angioscopy can also provide a quantitative definition of the arteriosclerotic processes [14, 22, 25]. Limiting factors are the effects of magnification depending on the distance of the angioscopic tip to the object and in some cases incomplete viewing of the vascular wall. It should also be mentioned that through rinsing of the tip of the angioscope the distal vascular segment can be dilated, thereby altering the true dimensions of the vessel. The role of angioscopy in quantitative evaluations of vascular pathology remains to be determined.

References

1. Bauriedel G, Höfling B (1988) Adjunctive angioscopy during percutaneous artherectomy. Eur Heart J [Suppl A] 9: 132
2. Beck A, Nako N (1989) Angioscopische Kontrolle der perkutanen Gefäßendoprothese. Erfahrungsbericht über ein speziell entwickeltes transmurales Gefäßendoprothesenmodell und dessen angioskopische Kontrolle in situ. Cor Vasa 3: 119–125
3. Beck A, Blum U (1989) Die Angioskopie der percutanen transluminalen Angioplastie (PTA) von Subclaviastenosen. Cor Vasa 3: 87–93
4. Beck A, Milic St, Dinkel E, Blum U, Papacharalampous X (1989) Arterielle Gefäßendoskopie und Lysetherapie. CV World Report 2: 190–195
5. Biamino G, Kar H, Dörschel K, Skarabis P, Gross M, Stefan G, Böttcher H, Flesch U, Witt H, Müller H (1990) Laserangioplastie und andere in der Entwicklung befindliche Rekanalisationstechniken. In: Rudolph W (ed) Therapie der koronaren Herzerkrankung. Springer, Berlin, Heidelberg, New York, pp 22–136

6. Biamino G, Ragg JC, Gross M, Böttcher H, Witt H (1992) Möglichkeiten des intravaskulären Ultraschalls und der Angioskopie. Jahrbuch der Radiologie. Biermann, Zülpich, pp 103–121

7. Chaux A, Lee M, Blanche C, Kass R, Shermann T, Hickey A, Litvack F, Grundfest W, Forrester J, Metloff F (1986) Intraoperative coronary angioscopy. J Cardiovasc Surg (Torino) 92: 972–976

8. Ennker J, Gross CM, Biamino G, Hetzer R (1992) First clinical experiences with a new angioscopic system for diagnosing peripheral vascular changes. Thorac Cardiovasc Surg 40: 33–37

9. Forrester JS, Litvack F, Grundfest W, Hickey A (1987) A perspective of coronary disease seen through the arteries of living man. Circulation 75: 505–513

10. Gross M, Biamino G (1991) Transkutane Angioskopie der atherosklerotischen Gefäßerkrankungen: eine Verbesserung der Diagnostik? Z Kardiol 80: 293

11. Grundfest WS, Litvack F, Sherman F, Carrol R, Lee M, Chaux A (1983) Delineation of peripheral and coronary detail by intraoperative angioscopy. Radiology 148: 161–166

12. Grundfest W, Litvack F, Sherman T (1986) Definition of a new pathophysiologic mechanism and altered decisions: an outcome of intravascular angioscopy. J Am Coll Cardiol 7: 173A

13. Grundfest W, Forrester J, Jakubowski A, Hickey A, Litvack F (1989) Coronary and peripheral vascular angioscopy. In: Vogel J, King S (eds) Interventional cardiology: future directions. Mosby, St. Louis, pp 36–53

14. Hombach V, Höher M, Hannekum A, Hügel W, Buran B, Höpp H, Hirche H (1986) Erste klinische Erfahrungen mit der Koronarendoskopie. Dtsch Med Wochenschr 111: 1135–1140

15. Isner J, Clark R (1986) Laserangioplasty (1986) Unravelling the Gordian knot. J Am Coll Cardiol 7: 705–711

16. Kensey K, Nash J, Abrahams C, Lake K, Zarins C (1986) Recanalization of obstructed arteries using a flexible rotating tip catheter. Circulation II 74: 457

17. Lee G, Carcia JM, Corso PJ, Chan MC, Rink JL, Pichard A (1986) Correlation of coronary angioscopy to angiographic findings in coronary artery disease. Am J Cardiol 58: 238–241

18. Lesperance J, Hudon G, White GW (1989) Comparison by quantitative angiographic assessment of coronary stenoses of one view showing the severest narrowing in two orthogonal views. Am J Cardiol 64: 462–465

19. Marcus ML, Skorton DL, Johnson MR (1988) Visual estimates of percent diameter coronary stenosis: "a battered gold standard". J Am Coll Cardiol 11: 882–885

20. Sanborn T, Rygaard J, Westbrook B, Lazar H, McCormick J, Roberts A (1986) Intraoperative angioscopy of saphenous vein and coronary arteries. J Thorac Cardiovasc Surg 91: 339–343

21. Sawton T (1987) Intraoperative angioscopy of saphenous vein and coronary arteries. J Thorac Cardiovasc Surg 9: 339

22. Spears JR, Spokojny AM, Marais HJ (1985) Coronary angioscopy during cardiac catheterization. J Am Coll Cardiol 6: 93–97

23. Vallbracht C, Süss B, Awiszus H, Prignitz E, Liermann G, Vollath J, Landgraf H, Schoop W, Kaltenbach M (1988) Low speed rotational angioplasty – acute results and complications in 33 patients with chronic vessel obstruction. Eur Heart J [Suppl 1] 9: 333

24. Vollmer J, Junghans K (1969) Die Arterioskopie. Langenbecks Arch Klin Chir 325: 1201

25. Wendt Th (1990) Neue Einblicke – Angioskopie und Mikroendoskopie. C Hofmann, Frankfurt

26. White G, White R, Kopchok G (1987) Intraoperative video angioscopy compared with arteriography during peripheral vascular operations. J Vasc Surg 6: 488–495

Subject Index

– follow-up after interventional procedures 433
– ghosting 436
– iliac vessels 431
– intrapopliteal trajectory 431
– maximum intensity projection 437
– metallic clips 436
– movement artifact 435
– pedal vessels 431
– peripheral vascular disease 431
– in-plane flow saturation 434
– popliteal trajectory 431
– poststenotic signal void 437
– preoperative tumor evaluation 433
– protocols 427
– retrograde flow 435
– venography 433
phaeochromocytoma 203
phase contrast angiography (PCA), MRA 379
phase substraction technique, MRA 402
PICA (posterior inferior cerebellar artery) 228
plaque rupture 483
plethysmography 19, 25, 26
PO_2, transcutaneous 20, 28
portal veins, ultrasonography 139 ff.
– hypertension 142
portosystemic shunts, ultrasonography 140, 149
posterior fossa veins 233
pregnancy, contrast agents 204
pressure examination, segmental 20
pulmonary
– angiography 297
– embolism, CTA 451
– thromboembolism (PTE) 298
pulse
– palpation 7
– repetition interval (TR) 363

quantitative coronary angiography (QCA) 267 ff.
– calipers 267
– categories of coronary lesions 273
– computerized quantitative angiography 268
– coronary divices 281
– coronary interventions 281
– directional atherectomy 286
– excimer laser 288
– interpolated technique 281
– lesion severity 270
– percentage diameter stenosis 281
– percutaneous transluminal coronary angioplasty 281
– qualitative characteristics 272

– rotational abrasion 288
– stenting (see also there) 283, 345
– type lesions (A, B, C) 273
– videodensitometry 268
quantitative (periinterventional) coronary angiography 277 ff.
quantitative ultrasonography 129 ff.
– carotid 129
– far wall 129
– femoral arteries 129
– lumen diameter 133
– near wall 129

radiation protection 183, 184
radiofrequency excitation, MRI 355
radiographic angiography 177 ff.
– archiving 190
– calibration 187
– cardiac 186
– cine imaging 187
– collimation 182
– fluoroscopy 186
– gantry 179
– image intensifiers 183
– image processing 185
– imaging system 182
– radiation protection 183, 184
– system geometry 181
– table 180
radiographic venography 329 ff.
relaxation parameters, MRI 356
renal arteries
– in angiography 307, 308
– in CTA 457
– in ultrasonography 153–155
renal transplant 156
renal veins 154, 155
– occlusion 155
– vein compression 341
renovascular hypertension 307
Rosenthal, veins of 232
rotating frame of reference, MRI 356

S/N ratio, MRI 369
SCAs (superior cerebellar arteries) 231
Scavenger receptor 41
segmental pressure examination 20
signal void, poststenotic, peripheral MR imaging 437
spin-echo, MRI 359
spinal arteries, anterior 228
splenic arteries 152
splenic vein 140, 146, 336
– thrombosis 146
Stemmer' skin fold sign 8
stenotic arterial murmur 7

stents/stenting 283, 345, 475
– coronary 283, 475, 505
– Gianturco-Rösch stent 345
– Gianturco Z stent 345
– Palmaz-Schatz stent 283, 345
– Wallstent 283, 345
– Wiktor stent 283
subclavian
– arteries 100
– vein, compression 336, 337
superior vena cava (SVC) 331, 341

T_1 relaxation 356
T_2 relaxation 356
table, radiographic angiography 180
Takayasu's arteritis 307
TCD (transcranial Doppler sonography) 115–121
– arteriovenous malformations 119
– brain death 120
– dolichoectatic arteries 119
– fistulas 119
– functional investigations 121
– intracranial
–– collateralization of significant extracranial lesions 118
–– pressure 120
– monitoring 120
– stenosis and occlusion 116
– transcranial color Doppler flow imaging 121
– vasospasm in subarachnoid hemorrhage 118
thermometry (see also peripheral microcirculation) 26, 27
thoracic and upper extremity arteriography 295 ff.
– arterial occlusive diseases 295
– arteriovenous malformations (AVMs) 295, 298
– bronchial 299
– hemodialysis access 296
– pulmonary angiography 297
– pulmonary thromboembolism (PTE) 298
– thoracic outlet syndrom 296
– trauma 296
thoracic outlet syndrome 336
thrombolytic therapy, local 342
thrombosis 24, 171, 332, 334, 335, 337, 410
– effort (spontaneous) thrombosis 337
– MRA 410
– peripheral vascular ultrasonography 171
– portal vein 146
– splenic vein 146
– superior mesenteric vein 147
– splenic vein 336
– upper extremity 335
thrombus 483, 498, 504